Extreme Stress and Communities:
Impact and Intervention

NATO ASI Series

Advanced Science Institutes Series

A Series presenting the results of activities sponsored by the NATO Science Committee, which aims at the dissemination of advanced scientific and technological knowledge, with a view to strengthening links between scientific communities.

The Series is published by an international board of publishers in conjunction with the NATO Scientific Affairs Division

A	Life Sciences	Plenum Publishing Corporation
B	Physics	London and New York
C	Mathematical and Physical Sciences	Kluwer Academic Publishers
D	Behavioural and Social Sciences	Dordrecht, Boston and London
E	Applied Sciences	
F	Computer and Systems Sciences	Springer-Verlag
G	Ecological Sciences	Berlin, Heidelberg, New York, London,
H	Cell Biology	Paris and Tokyo
I	Global Environmental Change	

PARTNERSHIP SUB-SERIES

1.	Disarmament Technologies	Kluwer Academic Publishers
2.	Environment	Springer-Verlag / Kluwer Academic Publishers
3.	High Technology	Kluwer Academic Publishers
4.	Science and Technology Policy	Kluwer Academic Publishers
5.	Computer Networking	Kluwer Academic Publishers

The Partnership Sub-Series incorporates activities undertaken in collaboration with NATO's Cooperation Partners, the countries of the CIS and Central and Eastern Europe, in Priority Areas of concern to those countries.

NATO-PCO-DATA BASE

The electronic index to the NATO ASI Series provides full bibliographical references (with keywords and/or abstracts) to more than 50000 contributions from international scientists published in all sections of the NATO ASI Series.
Access to the NATO-PCO-DATA BASE is possible in two ways:

– via online FILE 128 (NATO-PCO-DATA BASE) hosted by ESRIN,
Via Galileo Galilei, I-00044 Frascati, Italy.

– via CD-ROM "NATO-PCO-DATA BASE" with user-friendly retrieval software in English, French and German (© WTV GmbH and DATAWARE Technologies Inc. 1989).

The CD-ROM can be ordered through any member of the Board of Publishers or through NATO-PCO, Overijse, Belgium.

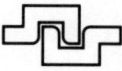

Series D: Behavioural and Social Sciences – Vol. 80

Extreme Stress and Communities: Impact and Intervention

edited by

Stevan E. Hobfoll
Applied Psychology Center,
Kent State University,
Kent, Ohio, U.S.A.

and

Marten W. de Vries
Department of Psychiatry & Neuropsychology,
Section of Social Psychiatry & Psychiatric Epidemiology,
University of Limburg
and
the International Institute for Psycho-social and Socio-ecological Research (IPSER),
Maastricht, The Netherlands

Kluwer Academic Publishers

Dordrecht / Boston / London

Published in cooperation with NATO Scientific Affairs Division

Proceedings of the NATO Advanced Research Workshop on
Stress and Communities
Château de Bonas, France
June 14–18, 1994

A C.I.P. Catalogue record for this book is available from the Library of Congress.

ISBN 0-7923-3468-X

Published by Kluwer Academic Publishers,
P.O. Box 17, 3300 AA Dordrecht, The Netherlands.

Kluwer Academic Publishers incorporates the publishing programmes of
D. Reidel, Martinus Nijhoff, Dr W. Junk and MTP Press.

Sold and distributed in the U.S.A. and Canada
by Kluwer Academic Publishers,
101 Philip Drive, Norwell, MA 02061, U.S.A.

In all other countries, sold and distributed
by Kluwer Academic Publishers Group,
P.O. Box 322, 3300 AH Dordrecht, The Netherlands.

Printed on acid-free paper

All Rights Reserved
© 1995 Kluwer Academic Publishers
No part of the material protected by this copyright notice may be reproduced or utilized in any form or by any means, electronic or mechanical, including photocopying, recording or by any information storage and retrieval system, without written permission from the copyright owner.

Printed in the Netherlands

Dedication

S. E. H. *In memory of Barry Tarshes (1953-1982) and dedicated to his parents Beverly and Jack, who were there to call on when I needed their help.*

and

M. W. deV. *To the people whose lives, triumphs, and suffering have provided the substance of this volume in the hope that it will be helpful to others.*

Table of Contents

Contributors to this volume	xi
Participants in the NATO Advanced Research Workshop	xv
Acknowledgements	xix

Preface
   Stevan E. Hobfoll and Marten W. deVries   xxi

Section I: Introduction: Focusing on the Community in the Case of Extreme Stress
   Stevan E. Hobfoll, Marten W. deVries and Rebecca P. Cameron   1

1. The Community Context of Disaster and Traumatic Stress: An Ecological Perspective from Community Psychology
   Edison J. Trickett   11

Section II: Basic Stress Concepts and Where They Lead in the Study of Community Stress
   Stevan E. Hobfoll, Rebecca P. Cameron and Marten W. deVries   27

2. Disasters, Stress and Cognition
   Donald Meichenbaum   33

3. Temperament Risk Factor: The Contribution of Temperament to the Consequences of the State of Stress
   Jan Strelau   63

4. Coping with the Loss of a Family Member: Implications for Community-Level Research and Intervention
   Camille B. Wortman, Katherine B. Carnelley, Darrin R. Lehman, Christopher G. Davis and Julie Juola Exline   83

5. Individual and Community Stress: Integration of Approaches at Different Levels
   Matthias Jerusalem, Krzysztof Kaniasty, Darrin R. Lehman, Christian Ritter and Gordon J. Turnbull   105

Section III: Resources to Offset Stress: Applications to the Community Context
Stevan E. Hobfoll, Rebecca P. Cameron and Marten W. deVries 131

6. Community Stress and Resources: Actions and Reactions
   Stevan E. Hobfoll, Sylvester Briggs and Jennifer Wells 137

7. Optimistic Self-Beliefs as a Resource Factor in Coping with Stress
   Ralf Schwarzer and Matthias Jerusalem 159

8. Stress and Social Support
   Irwin G. Sarason, Barbara R. Sarason and Gregory R. Pierce 179

Section IV: Bridges to Community Stress
Stevan E. Hobfoll, Rebecca P. Cameron and Marten W. deVries 199

9. Prevention of the Consequences of Man-Made or Natural Disaster at the (Inter)National, the Community, the Family, and the Individual Level
   Joop T.V.M. de Jong 207

10. The Pathogenic Effects of War Stress: The Israeli Experience
    Zahava Solomon 229

11. Stress and Diasaster
    Alexander C. McFarlane 247

12. Methodological Issues in Designing Research on Community-Wide Disasters with Special Reference to Chernobyl
    Evelyn J. Bromet 267

13. Research Methods and Directions: Establishing the Community Context
    Fran H. Norris, John R. Freedy, Anita DeLongis, Lucio Sibilia and Wolfgang Schönpflug 283

Section V: Long-Term Effects of Community Stress
Stevan E. Hobfoll, Rebecca P. Cameron and Marten W. deVries 301

14. Long-Term Consequences of Disasters
    Bonnie L. Green 307

15. Endurance and Living: Long-Term Effects of the Holocaust
    Jacob Lomranz 325

16. Reverberation Theory: Stress and Racism in Hierarchically Structured Communities
   James S. Jackson and Marita R. Inglehart   353

17. Culture, Community and Catastrophe: Issues in Understanding Communities under Difficult Conditions
   Marten W. deVries   375

Section VI: Prevention and Intervention
   Stevan E. Hobfoll, Rebecca P. Cameron and Marten W. deVries   395

18. Preventive Psychosocial Intervention after Disaster
   Lars Weisæth   401

19. The Treatment of Post Traumatic Stress Disorder
   Bessell A. van der Kolk, Onno van der Hart and Jennifer Burbridge   421

20. Strategies of Disaster Intervention for Children and Adolescents
   Robert S. Pynoos, Armen Goenjian and Alan M. Steinberg   445

21. Catalyzing Community Support
   Noach Milgram, Barbara R. Sarason, Ute Schönpflug, Anita Jackson and Christine Schwarzer   473

22. Prevention and Treatment of Community Stress: How to be a Mental Health Expert at the Time of Disaster
   Charles Figley, Robert Giel, Stefania Borgo, Sylvester Briggs and Mika Haritos-Fatouros   489

23. Intervention Strategies for Emergency Response Groups: A New Conceptual Framework
   Roderick J. Ørner   499

Conclusions: Addressing Communities under Extreme Stress
   Stevan E. Hobfoll, Marten W. deVries and Rebecca P. Cameron   523

Index   529

Contributors to this Volume

Stefania Borgo
  Centro di Ricerca in Psicoterapia e Scienze del Comportamento, Italy
Sylvester Briggs
  Ohio Department of Rehabilitation and Correction, OH, USA
Evelyn J. Bromet
  State University of New York at Stony Brook, NY, USA
Jennifer Burbridge
  Harvard Medical School, MA, USA
Rebecca P. Cameron
  Kent State University, OH, USA
Katherine B. Carnelley
  University of Wales, College of Cardiff, United Kingdom
Christopher G. Davis
  University of British Columbia, British Columbia, Canada
Joop T. V. M. de Jong
  International Institute for Psychosocial and Socio-Ecological Research (IPSER), University of Maastricht, and Free University of Amsterdam, the Netherlands
Anita DeLongis
  University of British Columbia, British Columbia, Canada
Marten W. deVries
  University of Limburg and the International Institute for Psychosocial and Socio-Ecological Research (IPSER), the Netherlands
Julie Juola Exline
  State University of New York at Stony Brook, NY, USA
Charles Figley
  Florida State University, FL, USA
John R. Freedy
  Medical University of South Carolina, SC, USA
Robert Giel
  Academisch Ziekenhuis Groningen, the Netherlands
Armen Goenjian
  University of California at Los Angeles, CA, USA
Bonnie L. Green
  Georgetown University, Washington, DC, USA
Mika Haritos-Fatouros
  Aristotelian University of Thessaloniki, Greece
Stevan E. Hobfoll
  Kent State University, OH, USA
Marita R. Inglehart
  University of Michigan, MI, USA

Anita Jackson
  Kent State University, OH, USA
James S. Jackson
  University of Michigan, MI, USA
Matthias Jerusalem
  Humboldt-Universität zu Berlin, Germany
Krzysztof Kaniasty
  Indiana University of Pennsylvania, PA, USA
Darrin R. Lehman
  University of British Columbia, British Columbia, Canada
Jacob Lomranz
  Tel Aviv University, Israel
Alexander C. McFarlane
  University of Adelaide and South Australia Mental Health Service, Australia
Donald Meichenbaum
  University of Waterloo, Ontario, Canada
Noach Milgram
  Tel Aviv University, Israel
Fran H. Norris
  Georgia State University, GA, USA
Roderick J. Ørner
  Lincolnshire Joint Emergency Services, United Kingdom
Gregory R. Pierce
  Hamilton College, NY, USA
Robert S. Pynoos
  University of California at Los Angeles, CA, USA
Christian Ritter
  Kent State University, OH, USA
Barbara R. Sarason
  University of Washington, WA, USA
Irwin G. Sarason
  University of Washington, WA, USA
Ute Schönpflug
  Freie Universität Berlin, Germany
Wolfgang Schönpflug
  Freie Universität Berlin, Germany
Christine Schwarzer
  Heinrich Heine Universitat, Germany
Ralf Schwarzer
  Freie Universität Berlin, Germany
Lucio Sibilia
  Universita degli Studi di Roma "La Sapienza," Italy

Zahava Solomon
  Israeli Defense Forces Medical Corps and Tel Aviv University, Israel
Alan M. Steinberg
  University of California at Los Angeles, CA, USA
Jan Strelau
  University of Warsaw, Poland
Edison J. Trickett
  National Institute of Mental Health and the University of Maryland, MD, USA
Gordon J. Turnbull
  Ticehurst House Hospital, United Kingdom
Onno van der Hart
  Harvard Medical School, MA, USA
Bessel A. van der Kolk
  Harvard Medical School, MA, USA
Lars Weisæth
  University of Oslo and The Joint Norweigian Armed Forces Medical Services Department of Psychiatry, Norway
Jennifer Wells
  Kent State University, OH, USA
Camille B. Wortman
  State University of New York at Stony Brook, NY, USA

Participants in the NATO Advanced Research Workshop

Jasem Al-Khawaj, Ph.D.
  SHAAB, P.O. Box 35642, Postcode 36057, Kuwait
Dina Birman, Ph.D.
  Refugee Mental Health Branch, Center for Mental Health Services, Substance Abuse and Mental Health Services Administration, Rockville, MD 20857, USA
Stefania Borgo, M.D.
  Centro di Ricerca in Psicoterapia e Scienze del Comportamento, P.zza O. Marucchi, 5, 00162 Roma, Italy
Sylvester Briggs, Ph.D.
  North Regional Psychological Services Administrator, Ohio Department of Rehabilitation and Correction, 1050 Freeway Drive North, Columbus, OH 43229, USA
Evelyn J. Bromet, Ph.D.
  Department of Psychiatry & Behavioral Science, State University of New York at Stony Brook, Putnam Hall--South Campus, Stony Brook, NY 11794-8790, USA
Joop de Jong, Ph.D.
  Coordinator IPSER Cross-Cultural Program, P.O. Box 214, 6200 AE Maastricht, The Netherlands
Anita DeLongis, Ph.D.
  Department of Psychology, University of British Columbia, 2136 West Mall, Vancouver, British Columbia V6T 1Y7, Canada
Marten W. deVries, M.D., Ph.D.
  IPSER, P.O. Box 214, 6200 AE Maastricht, The Netherlands
Charles Figley, Ph.D.
  Director, Marriage and Family Center, Florida State University, Tallahassee, FL 32306, USA
John Freedy, Ph.D.
  Department of Psychiatry and Behavioral Sciences, Medical University of South Carolina, Crime Victims Research and Treatment Center, 171 Ashley Avenue, Charleston, SC 29425-0742, USA
Rob Giel, Ph.D.
  Academisch Ziekenhuis Groningen, Sociale Psychiatrie, P.B. 30.001, 9700 RB Groningen, The Netherlands
Bonnie Lepper Green, Ph.D.
  Department of Psychiatry, School of Medicine, Georgetown University, 3800 Reservoir Road NW, Washington, DC 20007-2197, USA
Mika Haritos-Fatouros, Ph.D.
  Department of Psychology, Aristotelian University of Thessaloniki, Thessaloniki, 540 06, Greece

Ivonne H. Hobfoll, Ph.D.
  Hudson Psychological Associates, 5 Atterbury Boulevard, Hudson, OH 44236, USA
Stevan E. Hobfoll, Ph.D.
  Applied Psychology Center, Kent State University, Kent, OH 44242, USA
Anita Jackson, Ph.D.
  Adult, Counseling, Health, and Vocational Education, Kent State University, Kent, OH 44242, USA
James Jackson, Ph.D.
  Institute for Social Research, University of Michigan, Room 5118 ISR, Ann Arbor, MI 48106, USA
Matthias Jerusalem, Ph.D.
  Humboldt-Universität zu Berlin, Fachbereich Erziehungswissenshaften, Institut für Pädagogische Psychologie, Unter den Linden 9-12, 10099 Berlin, Germany
Krzysztof Kaniasty, Ph.D.
  Department of Psychology, Indiana University of Pennsylvania, Clark Hall, Indiana, PA 15705-1068, USA
Darrin R. Lehman, Ph.D.
  Department of Psychology, University of British Columbia, 2136 West Mall, Vancouver, British Columbia V6T 1Z4, Canada
Jackie Lomranz, Ph.D.
  The Herczeg Institute on Aging, Tel Aviv University, P.O. Box 39040, Ramat Aviv, 69978 Tel Aviv, Israel
Alexander C. McFarlane, Ph.D.
  University of Adelaide, Department of Psychiatry, South Australian Mental Health Service, P.O. Box 17, Eastwood. 5063, South Australia
Catherine McFarlane, M.D.
  Department of Psychiatry, Flinders Medical Centre, Bedford Park. 5042, South Australia
Donald Meichenbaum, Ph.D.
  Department of Psychology, University of Waterloo, Waterloo, Ontario, N2L 3G1, Canada
Vijaya L. Melnick, Ph.D.
  Director, Center for Applied Research and Urban Planning, MB4802, University of District of Columbia, 4200 Connecticut Avenue N.W., Washington, DC, 20008, USA
Noach Milgram, Ph.D.
  Department of Psychology, Tel Aviv University, Ramat Aviv 69978, Israel
Fran Norris, Ph.D.
  Department of Psychology, Georgia State University, University Plaza, Atlanta, GA 30303-3083, USA

Roderick J. Ørner, Ph.D.
  District Department of Clinical Psychology, North Lincolnshire Health Authority,
  Baverstock House, St. Anne's Road, Lincoln LN2 5RA, United Kingdom
Robert Pynoos, M.D.
  UCLA Neuropsychiatric Institute, 300 Medical Plaza, Los Angeles, CA 90024,
  USA
Christian Ritter, Ph.D.
  Department of Sociology, Kent State University, Kent, OH 44242, USA
Barbara R. Sarason, Ph.D.
  Department of Psychology, University of Washington, Seattle, WA 98195, USA
Irwin G. Sarason, Ph.D.
  Department of Psychology NI-25, University of Washington, Seattle, WA 98195,
  USA
Ute Schönpflug, Ph.D.
  Inst. f. Allg. u. Vergl. Erziehungswissenschaften, der Freien Universität Berlin,
  Fabeckstr. 13, 14195 Berlin, Germany
Wolfgang Schönpflug, Ph.D.
  Institut für Psychologie (WE 7), Freie Universität Berlin, Habelschwerdter Allee
  45, 14195 Berlin, Germany
Christine Schwarzer, Ph.D.
  Heinrich-Heine-Universität Düsseldorf, Abt. für Bildungsforschung und
  Pädagogische Beratung, Universitätsstr. 1, Geb. 23.03, 40225 Düsseldorf, Germany
Ralf Schwarzer, Ph.D.
  Institut für Psychologie (WE 7), Freie Universität Berlin, Habelschwerdter Allee
  45, 14195 Berlin, Germany
Lucio Sibilia, M.D.
  1st Terapia Medica Sist, Univ. Di Roma "la Sapienza", Via Policlinico, 00161
  Roma, Italy
Susan D. Solomon, Ph.D.
  Violence and Traumatic Stress Research Branch, Division of Applied and Services
  Research, National Institute of Mental Health, 5600 Fishers Lane, Room 18-105,
  Rockville, MD 20857, USA
Zahava Solomon, Ph.D.
  Bob Schapell School of Social Work, Tel Aviv University, 69978 Ramat Aviv,
  Israel
Charles D. Spielberger, Ph.D.
  Center for Research in Behavior Medicine and Health Psychology, University of
  South Florida, Tampa, FL 33620, USA
Jan Strelau, Ph.D.
  Wydzial Psychologii, Uniwersytet Warszawski, ul. Stawki 5/7, 00-183 Warszawa,
  Poland

Edison J. Trickett, Ph.D.
   Department of Psychology, University of Maryland, College Park, MD 20742-4411, USA
Gordon J. Turnbull, M.D.
   Ticehurst House Hospital, Wadhurst, East Sussex TN5 7HU, United Kingdom
Bessel van der Kolk, M.D.
   Massachusetts General Hospital Trauma Center, Harvard Medical School, 25 Staniford Street, Boston, MA 02114, USA
Abdul Wali Wardak, Ph.D.
   Department of Psychology, University of Hull, Hull HU6 7RX, United Kingdom
Lars Weisæth, M.D., Ph.D.
   University of Oslo, Division of Disaster Psychiatry, P.O. Box 39 Gaustad, N-0320 Oslo, Norway
Camille B. Wortman, Ph.D.
   Department of Psychology, State University of New York at Stony Brook, Stony Brook, NY 11794-2500, USA

Acknowledgements

We have many people to thank for making the NATO Advanced Research Workshop on Community Stress and this volume possible. Both the NATO International Scientific Exchange Programmes and Kent State University generously funded the projects. At Kent State, the offices of the Provost, Research and Graduate Studies, the College of Liberal Arts and Sciences, and the Department of Psychology supported our efforts financially and by providing personnel and resources. At the Institute of Psycho-Social and Socio-Ecological Research (IPSER), The University of Limburg, program directors and support staff helped with the initial tasks of writing the proposal, helping secure NATO funding, supported the writing up by authors and Kent State Staff, and rendered the work visible in the European community. The people at the Chateau de Bonas were gracious hosts for the meeting. Madame Simon and Mr. Stockman were consummate hosts and made every effort to ensure an atmosphere that was conducive to the intensive efforts we hoped to accomplish.

At Kent State Ms. Judy Jerkich and Ms. Sadhana Moneypenny helped organize the meeting and prepare the manuscript for publication. Ms. Rebecca Cameron not only helped write some of the connective pieces of the volume, but also helped organize the volume. At IPSER Yvonne Habets, Sara Legg and Marie-Jose Duchateau helped organize the flow of papers, facilitating the editing efforts of the Kent State personnel.

Finally, our wives, Dr. Ivonne Hobfoll and Dr. Nancy Nicolson were both very supportive of our efforts and also helped directly with the Bonas meeting. We are lucky to share our lives both personally and professionally with two such extraordinary women.

Preface

This volume grew out of our interest in promoting the concept of community, within the study and practice of response to large-scale traumatic events. Partially because of a media that today connects the world and partially because of changes in world politics, technology, and natural circumstances (e.g., global warming), there has been an increase in both the awareness and occurrence of extreme stress events that communities undergo. These include war, nuclear fallout, political upheaval, international terrorism, and natural and technological disasters. However, mental health professionals and social scientists have continued to focus on the individual, and not the community. Without losing sight of the individual, our primary goal was to expand the understanding of researchers and interventionists regarding the role of communities in these events.

In order to achieve a community perspective we formed an international, multidisciplinary working group consisting of many of the foremost experts in the field of extreme stress, including psychologists, psychiatrists, public health-epidemiologists, anthropologists, and sociologists. We began by sharing our past work and corresponding with one another from our various worksites around the world. Next, we disseminated a group of working papers that advanced the main themes presented in this volume. Finally we met for four days of intensive discussion and reflection on these themes at the Chateau de Bonas, France. Here we were able to immerse ourselves in advancing our thinking, sharing our ideas, and hopefully resurfacing with a more enriched perspective.

This volume is the written product of this process. We, as editors, were humbled to work with such a senior group, consisting of representatives from such varied disciplines and nations. The field of traumatology has developed in response to landmark events that shook the world. The participants in this project included researchers and interventionists who did pioneering work on many of these events, such as the Lockerbie Plane Bombing, Hurricane Andrew, the Armenian Earthquake, the Australian Bush Fires, the Lebanon Hostage Crisis, the North Sea Oil Disaster, Three-Mile Island, and the wars in Israel and the former Yugoslavia.

This process allowed us to come to a better understanding of how stressors that affect large groups are different from individually experienced traumas. We began to see patterns emerging that related to a number of factors: the presence or absence of social and instrumental resources available to the community, the differential impact of events that affect more than a certain threshold of the community, and the community response to extreme events. We examined how issues of poverty, education, and racism play a role in exacerbating or limiting the degree of trauma experienced. In some ways we rediscovered the obvious: that communities are a powerful context helping to define and influence our lives as individuals and families. In situations where we can depend on our community in times of crisis, we have a powerful resource at our disposal. In situations where communities are either not forthcoming in their support, are too devastated to act on our behalf, or are the agent of aggression, we lose an important stress resistance ally.

We became more appreciative of how communities shape people's experience even at the seemingly personal level of perception. Stories are shared, folk wisdom and traditional beliefs become expressed, and people's appraisals are molded along certain common lines. Interventions have often attempted to work through the media to shape these processes with such messages as, "we are surviving," "there is light at the end of the tunnel," and "we share the grief of the families who have lost loved ones." Yet, our knowledge about how to do this is in its most nascent stage.

This volume begins by presenting basic areas of importance to stress researchers, establishing these as building blocks for our task of understanding extreme stress. We then examine personal, social, and instrumental resources that have been found to aid adaptation to major stressful circumstances. With this basis formed, we turn to strategies for research and intervention at the community level. We address key community concepts, immediate, mid-term, and long-term responses to war and disasters, and modes of intervention. Our intervention emphasis is on intervention in the broadest sense, including prevention, education, pre and post disaster strategies, and treatment.

Overall, we hope this volume becomes an important handbook for communities and professionals interested in aiding communities in times of extreme stress. We simultaneously recognize that we have only begun to open the door to the study of how communities influence and are influenced by the individuals who comprise them. We hope that readers are aided by what we have written, and also use our work as a steppingstone for further advancing the science and practice of responding to extreme community stress.

INTRODUCTION: FOCUSING ON THE COMMUNITY IN THE CASE OF EXTREME STRESS

Stevan E. Hobfoll, Kent State University, Kent, Ohio, USA
Marten W. deVries, University of Limburg, Maastricht, the Netherlands
Rebecca P. Cameron, Kent State University, Kent, Ohio, USA

In the 1990s the enormity of both the individual and social problems related to trauma have become even more visible and apparent throughout the world. Global communication compels us to directly share the suffering and helplessness of millions of people subjected to social upheaval or disaster. Dramas ranging from incest and violence on city streets to systematic torture, war, and even genocide have become daily venue. Although not new historical developments, their sheer bulk in relation to our capacity to understand challenges the adequacy and scope of our knowledge and our ability to respond. National and international relief agencies, instead of cooperating with each other, often clash about even obsolete solutions. This volume aims to update and shape conceptual and practical knowledge of stress in communities by contributing insight into community responses under extremely stressful conditions.

Extreme stressors, such as disasters and war, are unlikely to occur at any given moment, and are the kind of event that people expect will only happen to some unidentified other in some far-away place. However, when disasters do strike, they often affect large numbers of people, and millions of people are involved at some time in their lives in such events. When discussing extreme community stress in this volume we mean circumstances that threaten the physical self, property, or security of large numbers of people who share a common living, work, or temporary setting (e.g., airplane passengers). These include such events as natural and technological disasters, war, social upheaval and resultant refugee flight, famine, and large scale epidemics. Although modern countries are somewhat buffered from the most devastating effects of disasters of human and natural origin, earthquakes, war, political upheaval, and technological catastrophes happen worldwide and affect all those involved deeply.

When extreme stressors strike, individuals', families', and communities' coping resources are put to the test. People do not know just how they, their family, their community, or their nation will respond in such extreme circumstances. We naturally base our beliefs on the data provided us by everyday life experiences. Because extreme events typically do not occur in the same place with great frequency, we have little experience judging how we will react. Even in the case of some chronic community stressor, such as ongoing war, there are few communities where enough cycles of the event have occurred to create a body of knowledge and understanding about how people will likely face these shattering events.

Some lessons learned as early as the first two world wars have largely been forgotten, but recalling them is instructive. The experience of World War II, especially, taught that most people can continue to function under highly stressful conditions. However, a very high percentage will also break down either physically or emotionally. For example, nearly one in four soldiers who landed in the Normandy invasion had to be relieved of duty owing to psychiatric difficulties (Marlowe, 1979).

Looking at different military units also reveals the importance of the community's influence. Following the failed defense of Pearl Harbor, those units involved in the defense continued to have very high levels of psychiatric breakdown throughout the war, even after significant turnover of the soldiers actually involved. This high rate of breakdown can be contrasted with the 442nd Regimental Combat Team of Nisei (second generation Japanese-American) fighters who shared a cultural background and had very high motivation to prove their loyalty to America. Despite being involved in some of the heaviest combat in the Italian campaign, they experienced little or no psychiatric breakdown in combat (Marlowe, 1979). A community can create a certain morale level that affects the stress experience. An Israeli psychiatrist was reviewing troops involved in staving off the Syrian invasion during the Yom Kippur war. In his expert and experienced evaluation these troops required immediate combat relief, having fought a sustained three days with little or no sleep and having experienced heavy casualties. Their response was to prepare their tanks for continued battle (Herzog, 1984).

Today, the best data source for extreme stress is a world-base of knowledge. In order to seek out the common elements and special circumstances that may occur following extreme stress, we need to look at as many events worldwide as possible. Inevitably this will be a daunting task, because by looking across communities, states, nations, and world regions, elements of differential history, widely varying economic situations, and variations in culture will enter the picture as important variables in the ultimate equation of understanding. Yet, this is our task, and we should come to appreciate the wealth of information that adding these larger contextual variables will bring to our emerging understanding. Even in the same country, for the same general kind of event, such as a hurricane, the response in Louisiana and Florida will be different. Indeed, different subcultures and economic classes who share the same region and disaster, may differ markedly in their responses (Norris & Thompson, in press). We must nevertheless begin to untangle this complicated web.

There is certainly an emerging base of knowledge in the study of extreme stress. Over the past 20 years, nearly 200 or more English-language articles concerning the psychological impact of natural and technological disasters have been published (Blake, Albano, & Keane, 1992). Simultaneously, there has been a marked increase in intervention into and study of war-related trauma (Milgram, 1986; Hobfoll, Lomranz, Eyal, Bridges, & Tzemach, 1989). The end of the Cold War has brought an unprecedented number of small wars, disputes, refugee flights, and situations of economic chaos. At the same time, mental health interventionists and researchers are showing increased interest in lending their expertise to aid people whose lives are disrupted by these events. Despite this level of attention, much remains to be learned concerning the linkages between extreme stress, coping, and psychological adjustment.

We know that disasters and war elicit both acute (e.g., Freedy, Kilpatrick, & Resnick, 1993) and prolonged psychological distress (e.g., see Green, Lindy, Grace, Gleser, Leonard, Korol, & Winget, 1990). However, beyond a very hazy, global view that there is a pathogenic effect of extreme stress, great ambiguity exists regarding the elements of disaster exposure responsible for adjustment difficulties. Most conceptual definitions emphasize acute factors such as injury or extreme threat. Other definitions emphasize ongoing factors including a range of adversities within the post-disaster environment (e.g., residential displacement, job disruption) (Freedy, Resnick, & Kilpatrick, 1992). By empasizing a community context, however, much more is being learned, and the future of this area of work is showing increasing promise.

A Communal-Ecological Approach to Extreme Stress

Most of what is known about reactions to extreme stress is organized around individuals' responding. Although our empirical study of community-level stress is in its infancy, there is already a trend to individualize its study and our intervention responses. Albee (1980) wrote about the danger of thinking that we can provide an individualized mental health response to the problems of our society, given the numbers in need of mental health services and the limited resources available to provide services. If communities are unable to meet their mental health needs in the face of everyday stress, how could they possibly respond using individual-based models when whole segments of communities are impacted, often including the very professionals who normally serve in mental health service roles?

Hence, this volume attempts to address extreme stress on the level of the community. As Trickett (this volume) notes in his chapter on the ecological context of community stress, we need to become aware of the ecological diversity of communities and populations who are beset by extreme stress. Given the research and attempts at intervention that have been ongoing in many countries, with diverse populations, involving circumstances and situations ranging from floods to the Holocaust, we have a wealth of material to study and understand. To emerge from this with deeper insights, however, he emphasizes that we must learn to appreciate the variability in the way such events unfold among differing populations experiencing different circumstances. We can use these community-level insights to better understand the interventions that individuals find most effective in responding to events of such major proportions across widely varying ecological niches. This work can help us challenge and advance the underlying conceptualizations of theorists whose work has derived from clinical and normative populations.

The study of community stress also differs from the study and understanding of the experience of individual victims of extreme stressors, such as rape or violence. Of course, there will be different common patterns that emerge when individuals are exposed to traumatic stress alone, versus when this occurs as a shared event with a community. However, even these differences can only be understood if we give more directed thought to the nature and circumstances of community stress.

The Current Volume

Basic Stress Concepts and Where They Lead in the Study of Community Stress

Following an introduction to the ecological perspective in Section I (Trickett, this volume), Section II addresses some of the basic principles formulated by stress experts in the course of their research. Chapters examine principles of cognitive appraisal and treatment (Meichenbaum, this volume), biological aspects of the stress response (Strelau, this volume), myths about individual responding to extreme stress (Wortman, Carnelley, Lehman, Davis, & Exline, this volume), and develop a schema for conceptualizing how the individual and community perspective compare and contrast (Jerusalem, Kaniasty, Lehman, Ritter, & Turnbull, this volume).

Extreme stress often engenders a need to create a new storyline for people's lives. The stories that were useful for guiding their understandings of the world are often shattered by traumatic events. What explained the world as it was, no longer explains the world as it has radically changed. This appraisal process is similar in many ways whether it involves individual responses to extreme personal events or community responses to extreme community events (Meichenbaum, this volume). Similarly, emerging research on the influence of temperament in the stress response calls attention to the biological involvement in the stress process when studying large scale stress.

Resources to Offset Stress: Applications to the Community Context

We have made the case that severity of exposure to extreme stress is of primary importance, but many community, social, and individual resources can affect psychological outcomes as well. Resources and conditions that facilitate or impede the employment of resources play a central role in determining how victims react to extreme stressors, and what physical and mental health consequences these reactions produce. Studies of the effects of resources and resource-facilitating circumstances help identify those victims likely to develop prolonged effects.

In Section III, authors examine general resource theories and specific resources that may be critical in adjustment to extreme stress. In particular, the role of mastery, optimistic beliefs (Schwarzer & Jerusalem, this volume), social support (Sarason, Sarason, & Pierce, this volume), and having a generally enriched reservoir of resources (Hobfoll, Briggs, & Wells, this volume) are explored. How these resources may be applied to conditions of extreme stress is delineated.

One important class of disaster resources is the community context. Community circumstances that may be important include the extent of community disruption, the centrality of the event (e.g., an airplane crash involving a group of strangers would be peripheral rather than central; see Green, 1982), the setting of the community (e.g., rural versus urban), and the nature of the community's official disaster response (e.g., adequate versus ineffective).

Community-level factors may be more important than the event itself. For example, a positive community response to the 1976 Teton Dam collapse was met by remarkably effective recovery (Golec, 1983). Despite major property loss and social disruption, recovery was facilitated by several community attributes: adequate warning (resulting in a low death/injury rate), a homogeneous (Mormon) population, maintenance of the community's social fabric, adequate financial compensation, a surplus of resources for immediate needs, and an organized regional disaster response. Section III examines many of these issues in depth and provides a sound theoretical base for future research and intervention based on resource acquisition, maintenance, and sharing.

Bridges to Community Stress

In Section IV the focus on the community elements of extreme stress is applied to specific issues relevant to extreme community stress. The cultural context is raised as a centerpoint for thinking about community stress events. Given that many disasters and wars occur in financially underdeveloped communities, but that disaster responses are often organized by Western interventionists, there is always the danger of culture clash (de Jong, this volume).

Specific issues of war and disaster are raised separately. However, bridges between the two are often made apparent. This section also develops methodological insights for evaluation of the impact of disasters and other extreme stressors. The chaos engendered by such events makes research difficult. However, a balanced approach involving no small measure of ingenuity has been successfully applied, and other researchers and interventionists may learn from these prior experiences. Solomon (this volume) explores critical findings regarding myths versus facts in the study of post-traumatic stress disorder in the aftermath of war. McFarlane (this volume) examines the influence of disasters from the viewpoint of both a clinician and a traumatic stress researcher. Bromet (this volume) and Norris, Freedy, DeLongis, Sibilia, and Schönpflug, (this volume) make recommendations for studying extreme stress on a community level.

Long-Term Effects of Community Stress

Extreme stressors cast a long shadow, apparent for decades following the initial event. Section V examines the long-term effects of stress, invoking once again the importance of culture and context. Each chapter emphasizes that an event's importance is deeply shaped by the historical and social context in which it occurs and how these interact with the unfolding story of the lives of those affected.

Green (this volume) looks at how disasters in the United States may affect people's lives over time through reports of a series of carefully conducted follow-up studies. She looks at initial severity, loss of resources, and the ongoing intactness of the community as prominent among the variables that influence disaster's long-term effects. Lomranz (this volume) applies a life-span developmental approach to achieve a better understanding of the long-term effects of the Holocaust. Now examining mostly elderly victims, he delves into the interplay between their original experience, the impact of Israeli culture upon them, and how they helped shape Israeli culture. Jackson and Inglehart (this volume) make similar points in their study of the effects of chronic racism. They develop the thesis that racism not only victimizes its target group, but that its effects reflect back in changes in the racist group and the larger society. Finally, deVries (this volume) examines how culture itself should always be considered, both for its influence on how events affect people and for its self-perpetuating tendencies during extremely stressful periods.

Prevention and Intervention

Section VI discusses how intervention has been used to reverse or modify the negative sequelae that follow in the wake of extreme stress. Traumatology has chiefly been concerned with post-traumatic stress disorder (PTSD), and intervention has mainly focused on individual, clinical intervention. This section also provides a state of the art review of individual-based clinical intervention (van der Kolk, van der Hart, & Burbridge, this volume). However, a community approach sees the individual approach as only one small component of necessary intervention. Rather, the focus is on pre- and post-disaster preventive efforts. These are aimed at reducing the numbers of people who will need individualized therapy. Further, a community approach highlights the fact that most individuals will never be treated for their maladies, further emphasizing the importance of prevention and group intervention.

Pynoos, Goenjain, and Steinberg (this volume) discuss intervention with children amidst war and disaster. They provide insightful accounts based on their work worldwide. Milgram, Sarason, Schönpflug, Jackson, and Schwarzer (this volume) discuss how community support can be catalyzed. They highlight that the community itself is taxed in the case of extreme stress and that a planful approach must both consider ways to shape people's understanding of the event and its meaning and act to limit widespread and chronic resource loss. Figley, Giel, Borgo, Briggs, and Haritos-Fatouros (this volume) offer a rich overview of intervention planning.

They present a strategic map for intervention efforts. Finally, Ørner looks at intervention with interventionists. He suggests that the overwhelmingly popular technique of critical events debriefing may not be effective and offers a more global understanding of aid to emergency service workers.

In the conclusion, we return to each of these issues and offer suggestions for future research and intervention based on the comments and criticisms found throughout the volume. We highlight the community context of the volume and emphasize the ecological perspective for guiding the work of interventionists and researchers who, rather bravely and with great difficulty, approach this critical area of work.

References

Albee, G. W. (1980). A competency model must replace the defect model. In L. A. Bond & J. C. Rosen (Eds.), Competence and coping during adulthood (pp.75-104). New Hampshire: University Press of New England. (need city of publication)

Blake, D. D., Albano, A. M., & Keane, T. M. (1992). Twenty years of trauma: Psychological Abstracts 1970 through 1989. Journal of Traumatic Stress, 5, 1-8.

Bromet, E. J. (this volume). Methodological issues in designing research on community-wide disasters with special reference to Chernobyl. In S. E. Hobfoll & M. W. deVries (Eds.), Extreme stress and communities: Impact and intervention. Dordrecht, the Netherlands: Kluwer.

de Jong, J. T. V. M. (this volume). Prevention of the consequences of man-made or natural disaster at the (inter)national, the community, the family, and the individual level. In S. E. Hobfoll & M. W. deVries (Eds.), Extreme stress and communities: Impact and intervention. Dordrecht, the Netherlands: Kluwer.

deVries, M. W. (this volume). Culture, community and catastrophe: Issues in understanding communities under difficult conditions. In S. E. Hobfoll & M. W. deVries (Eds.), Extreme stress and communities: Impact and intervention. Dordrecht, the Netherlands: Kluwer.

Figley, C., Giel, R., Borgo, S., Briggs, S., & Haritos-Fatouros, M. (this volume). Prevention and treatment of community stress: How to be a mental health expert at the time of disaster. In S. E. Hobfoll & M. W. deVries (Eds.), Extreme stress and communities: Impact and intervention. Dordrecht, the Netherlands: Kluwer.

Freedy, J. R., Resnick, H. S., & Kilpatrick, D. G. (1992). A conceptual framework for evaluating disaster impact: Implications for clinical intervention. In L. S. Austin (Ed.), Responding to disaster: A guide for mental health professionals. Washington, DC: American Psychiatric Press.

Freedy, J. R., Kilpatrick, D. G., & Resnick, H. S. (1993). The psychological impact of the Oakland Hills fire. Final report for supplement to National Institute of Mental Health grant no. 1R01 MH47508-01A1, submitted to the Violence and Traumatic Stress Research Branch.

Golec, J. A. (1983). A contextual approach to the social psychological study of disaster recovery. International Journal of Mass Emergencies and Disasters, 1(2), 255-276.

Green, B. L. (1982). Assessing levels of psychosocial impairment following disaster: Consideration of actual and methodological dimensions. The Journal of Nervous and Mental Disease, 17(9), 544-552.

Green, B. L. (this volume). Long-term consequences of disasters. In S. E. Hobfoll & M. W. deVries (Eds.), Extreme stress and communities: Impact and intervention. Dordrecht, the Netherlands: Kluwer.

Green, B., Lindy, J., Grace, M., Gleser, G., Leonard, A., Korol, M., & Winget, C. (1990). Buffalo Creek survivors in the second decade: Stability of stress symptoms. American Journal of Orthopsychiatry, 60(1), 43-54.

Herzog, C. (1984). The Arab-Israeli Wars (2nd ed.). London: Arms & Armour Press.

Hobfoll, S. E., Briggs, S., & Wells J. (this volume). Community stress and resources: Actions and reactions. In S. E. Hobfoll & M. W. deVries (Eds.), Extreme stress and communities: Impact and intervention. Dordrecht, the Netherlands: Kluwer.

Hobfoll, S. E., Lomranz, J., Eyal, N., Bridges, A., & Tzemach, M. (1989). Pulse of a nation: Depressive mood reactions of Israelis to the Israel-Lebanon War. Journal of Personality and Social Psychology, 56, 1002-1012.

Jackson, J. S., & Inglehart, M. R. (this volume). Reverberation theory: Stress and racism in hierarchically structured communities. In S. E. Hobfoll & M. W. deVries (Eds.), Extreme stress and communities: Impact and intervention. Dordrecht, the Netherlands: Kluwer.

Jerusalem, M., Kaniasty, K., Lehman, D. R., Ritter, C., & Turnbull, G. J. (this volume). Individual and community stress: Integration of approaches at different levels. In S. E. Hobfoll & M. W. deVries (Eds.), Extreme stress and communities: Impact and intervention. Dordrecht, the Netherlands: Kluwer.

Lomranz, J. (this volume). Endurance and living: Long-term effects of the Holocaust. In S. E. Hobfoll & M. W. deVries (Eds.), Extreme stress and communities: Impact and intervention. Dordrecht, the Netherlands: Kluwer.

Marlowe, D. H. (1979). Cohesion, anticipated breakdown, and endurance in battle: Considerations for severe and high intensity combat. Unpublished manuscript, Division of Neuropsychiatry, Walter Reed Army Institute of Research, Washington, DC.

McFarlane, A. C. (this volume). Stress and disaster. In S. E. Hobfoll & M. W. deVries (Eds.), Extreme stress and communities: Impact and intervention. Dordrecht, the Netherlands: Kluwer.

Meichenbaum, D. (this volume). Disasters, stress and cognition. In S. E. Hobfoll & M. W. deVries (Eds.), Extreme stress and communities: Impact and intervention. Dordrecht, the Netherlands: Kluwer.

Milgram, N. A. (1986). Stress and coping in time of war: Generalizations from the Israeli experience. New York: Brunner/Mazel.

Milgram, N., Sarason, B. R., Schönpflug, U., Jackson, A., & Schwarzer, C. (this volume). Catalyzing community support. In S. E. Hobfoll & M. W. deVries (Eds.), Extreme stress and communities: Impact and intervention. Dordrecht, the Netherlands: Kluwer.

Norris, F. H., Freedy, J. R., DeLongis, A., Sibilia, L., & Schonpflug, W. (this volume). Research methods and directions: Establishing the community context. In S. E. Hobfoll & M. W. deVries (Eds.), <u>Extreme stress and communities: Impact and intervention</u>. Dordrecht, the Netherlands: Kluwer.

Norris, F. H., & Thompson, M. P. (in press). Applying community psychology to the prevention of trauma and traumatic life events. In J. Freedy and S. E. Hobfoll (Eds.), <u>Traumatic stress: From theory to practice</u>. New York: Plenum.

Ørner, R. J. (this volume). Intervention strategies for emergency response groups: A new conceptual framework. In S. E. Hobfoll & M. W. deVries (Eds.), <u>Extreme stress and communities: Impact and intervention</u>. Dordrecht, the Netherlands: Kluwer.

Pynoos, R. S., Goenjian, A., & Steinberg, A. M. (this volume). Strategies of disaster intervention for children and adolescents. In S. E. Hobfoll & M. W. deVries (Eds.), <u>Extreme stress and communities: Impact and intervention</u>. Dordrecht, the Netherlands: Kluwer.

Sarason, I. G., Sarason, B. R., & Pierce, G. R. (this volume). Stress and social support. In S. E. Hobfoll & M. W. deVries (Eds.), <u>Extreme stress and communities: Impact and intervention</u>. Dordrecht, the Netherlands: Kluwer.

Schwarzer, R., & Jerusalem, M. (this volume). Optimistic self-beliefs as a resource factor in coping with stress. In S. E. Hobfoll & M. W. deVries (Eds.), <u>Extreme stress and communities: Impact and intervention</u>. Dordrecht, the Netherlands: Kluwer.

Solomon, Z. (this volume). The pathogenic effect of war stress: The Israeli experience. In S. E. Hobfoll & M. W. deVries (Eds.), <u>Extreme stress and communities: Impact and intervention</u>. Dordrecht, the Netherlands: Kluwer.

Strelau, J. (this volume). Temperament risk factor: The contribution of temperament to the consequences of the state of stress. In S. E. Hobfoll & M. W. deVries (Eds.), <u>Extreme stress and communities: Impact and intervention</u>. Dordrecht, the Netherlands: Kluwer.

Trickett, E. J. (this volume). The community context of disaster and traumatic stress: An ecological perspective from community psychology. In S. E. Hobfoll & M. W. deVries (Eds.), <u>Extreme stress and communities: Impact and intervention</u>. Dordrecht, the Netherlands: Kluwer.

van der Kolk, B. A., van der Hart, O., & Burbridge, J., (this volume). The treatment of post traumatic stress disorder. In S. E. Hobfoll & M. W. deVries (Eds.), <u>Extreme stress and communities: Impact and intervention</u>. Dordrecht, the Netherlands: Kluwer.

Wortman, C. B., Carnelley, K. B., Lehman, D. R., Davis, C. G., & Exline, J. J. (this volume). Coping with the loss of a family member: Implications for community-level research and intervention. In S. E. Hobfoll & M. W. deVries (Eds.), <u>Extreme stress and communities: Impact and intervention</u>. Dordrecht, the Netherlands: Kluwer.

THE COMMUNITY CONTEXT OF DISASTER AND TRAUMATIC STRESS: AN ECOLOGICAL PERSPECTIVE FROM COMMUNITY PSYCHOLOGY

Edison J. Trickett,
National Institute of Mental Health
Rockville, Maryland, U.S.
and
University of Maryland
College Park, Maryland, U.S.

The present paper integrates an ecological perspective developed in community psychology with research and intervention following disasters and traumatic stress. I approach this topic as a community psychologist who has spent a professional life developing ways of understanding the interdependence of individuals and the community contexts in which they are embedded. The perspective I have found useful is an ecological one, called the "ecological analogy" or "ecological metaphor" by its originator, James Kelly and his colleagues (Kelly, 1968, 1979, 1986, Kelly, Azelton, Burzette, & Mock, 1994; Trickett, Kelly, and Todd, 1972; Trickett, 1984; Trickett and Birman, 1989). To understand the relevance of this metaphor to the area of disaster and traumatic stress, it may be useful to sketch the origins of the field of community psychology, since the substantive areas of community psychology and disaster and traumatic stress spring from different roots.

Community psychology in the United States began during the 1960's as one of psychology's reactions to the broader U.S. society as well as to conceptual limitations related to the dominant psychological paradigms of the time, particularly in clinical psychology. The broader context was one of social turmoil, centering on the lack of participation and power of disenfranchised groups, including their access to and participation in psychology, and a focus on how social institutions and policies affected the well-being of various groups. The paradigm concerns with clinical psychology focused on (1) its tendency to ignore or minimize the contributions of history, culture, and context in the interpretation of individual behavior (see Sarason, 1981), (2) its attendant focus on problems or weaknesses of people rather than attending to their sources of strength and competency (see Bennett et al., 1966, for the seminal document of the origins of the field), and (3) a doctor-patient image of the helping relationship where power to define both the problem and the solution rested primarily if not exclusively with the professional.

The self-proclaimed task of community psychology was to develop antidotes to paradigms which decontextualized individual behavior, focused on individual pathology, and defined the role of the professional as expert rather than collaborator. The intent was to focus attention away from the individual level of analysis of behavior onto a person-in-context or person-in environment level. This in turn meant developing ways of conceptualizing the social environment. In addition, the relationship between scholar or interventionist and citizen would be based on an image of collaboration rather than viewing citizens as "subjects" for whom or on whom research and interventions would be conducted (see Rappaport, 1981, for a useful perspective on the contrasting images of working with vs. working on people). Together, these shifts were intended to illuminate the contextual contributions to individual and community life and develop mutually beneficial relations between professionals and citizens.

Further, such context-grounded understanding of behavior would help place the issue of diagnosis in a framework respectful of culture, history, and local context. Current debate of the diagnosis of antisocial personality represents an example of the larger issue. While there are many complications to this issue, one aspect relevant to this discussion involves whose frame of reference one adopts in deciding on the diagnosis. Does one view its defining nature as involving behavior that is maladaptive or disrespectful of larger dominant culture social norms, or does one look to see whether or not in the community of interest the behavior represents an adaptive response to a particular kind of environment? Does it matter how the individual living in that context assesses his or her behavior, or is it a matter for professionals to decide? (see Richters and Cichetti, 1993, for a compelling discussion of this issue. Their title, "Mark Twain meets DSM III-R", highlights one of the many differential implications for diagnosis when one adopts an acontextual or a contextual interpretation of behavior).

An Ecological Perspective on Disaster and Traumatic Stress: A Distinctive Opportunity for Theory and Intervention

While not an expert in the area of disaster and traumatic stress, I have read many papers of those contributing to other chapters in this volume. In reading these papers, I became increasingly aware of the ecological diversity of communities and populations involved in this area of scholarship and intervention. Research is ongoing in many countries, with diverse populations, involving circumstances and situations ranging from floods to the Holocaust. This variability of population and circumstance places stress researchers in a unique position to appreciate the range of adaptive options that individuals find useful in coping with life's vicissitudes across widely varying ecological niches. This work is in a unique position to challenge the values and assumptions underlying theorists whose work has derived from either clinical or normative populations who live in predominantly Western countries. The adolescent in El Salvador who is both victim and student-perpetrator of war, the Holocaust survivor coping with old age, and the unpredictable courage of ordinary citizens in helping their neighbors in times of a hurricane; all these examples provide insight into human resilience and the range of the possible not usually accounted for by theories of human development. Such diversity of culture, context, and historical circumstance provides a rich resource for an ecological perspective.

Fifteen years ago I wrote a paper with Roger Mitchell summarizing our view of social network research at that time (Mitchell and Trickett, 1979). Our conclusion specified the overarching ecological question for the social/network/social support area. "Our hope", we wrote, "was to leave the reader with an appreciation of the question: What types of social networks are most useful for which individuals in terms of what particular issues under what environmental conditions?" Translated to the disaster and traumatic events field, it becomes "What kinds of disasters and traumatic events have what consequences for whom under what environmental conditions?" This question refers to four sources of variability; (1) in the nature of the event, (2) its outcomes, (3) its participants, and (4) its context. Much research in the disaster and traumatic stress area focuses on the first three of those four aspects; the nature of the events, of outcomes, and of individual differences in response to the events. The ecological metaphor is intended to build on this body of work by elaborating on the fourth source of variability: "under what environmental conditions?".

Assumptions of an Ecological Perspective

The ecological approach addresses the question "under what environmental conditions?" by focusing on ways to describe the context surrounding the person and the person-context interaction. The term "context" can range across a variety of phenomena, but most generally refers to the world outside the individual which provides both constraints and opportunities for development, healing, and pain. Some theorists such as Roger Barker define the ecological context as independent of people's perception of it (see Barker, 1968), while others, such as Rudolf Moos, define it in terms of the shared perceptions of groups of people (see Moos, 1974, 1975, 1979).

Bronfenbrenner (1979; Bronfenbrenner and Weiss, 1983) has provided perhaps the best known conceptualization of the ecological environment or the context surrounding individual behavior. He describes the ecological environment as a nested hierarchy of systems that both directly and indirectly affect individuals. The smallest unit of analysis is the microsystem involving two or more people in a specific setting such as the family; the largest system, or macrosystem, involves the impact of culture on individuals. In between are the systems of systems which mediate the impact of the ecological environment on individuals. Thus, the mesosystem might be comprised of the relationship between the two microsystems of family and school.

This nested environmental hierarchy has both direct and indirect influences on the individual. When the relevant settings are ones in which the individual participates, the influences are direct. Thus, the relationship between the child's life in school and in the home may directly affect the success of school-based intervention to aid the adaptation of children who have seen classmates killed in a school bus accident (Pynoos, 1993). Indirect effects occur when those settings having influence over the experience are not participated in by the individual. For example, the policies governing the functioning of different community agencies may directly affect their ability to coordinate services before, during, and after a disaster, thus indirectly affecting the well-being of those needing services. Within this overarching model both direct and indirect influences are always present, though not always equally salient.

In addition to its more general heuristic value, Bronfenbrenner's perspective is important because of its insistence that variability in behavior can meaningfully be understood from multiple levels of the ecological context acting by themselves and in combination. Understanding behavior from multiple levels has implications for both understanding and the design of interventions. Not only does it force a contextual understanding on the behavior of individuals, it promotes a multi-level approach to interventions. For example, if we understand the multiple levels of influence over a particular phenomena, such as community mobilization in times of crisis, we are in a better conceptual position to develop multiple additive interventions intended to affect these multiple sources of influence. Efforts at individual change can thus be complemented by institutional or policy change at the community level (see Trickett and Birman, 1990).

One aspect of context, described in Bronfenbrenner's model as the macrosysyem, is that of culture. The term itself is perhaps as elusive as "context", having been described in over 150 different ways in the anthropological and cross-cultural psychology literature (see Lonner, 1994). I use it here to refer to a loose set of rules, understandings, and beliefs passed down over generations among a group. It is a group-level set of traditions, rituals, and bits of folk wisdom, that taken together, provide a sense of collective identity. Although there is wide variation in how members of any particular culture interpret and act in terms of these broad cultural norms, there are nonetheless identifiable group-level patterns that have substantive meaning for understanding individuals in the particular culture.

Context, Culture, and the Meaning of Events

A focus on the multiple levels of context and culture provides a mind-set for questions central to understanding disaster and traumatic stress from a community perspective. One central issue in this field involves the importance of the appraisal of events (Lazarus and Folkman, 1984) as mediators of the impact of such community stresses. An ecological perspective centering on context and culture would suggest that the appraisal of events occurs within a sociocultural matrix and specific sets of contextual conditions. According to McFarlane (1994, unpublished manuscript), however, "no attempt has been made to look at social and cultural influences affecting the perception of trauma" (p. 12).

However, the same events surely must be appraised differently in different contexts and in different cultures. For example, the popular press in the United States has reported that many Vietnamese women fleeing their homeland in boats are attacked at sea and often raped. If they know they are running this risk, if their reasons for leaving Vietnam involve other potential or real atrocities, if they are among a community of women who know these risks and may provide a community of support should these or other atrocities happen, does this not place rape in a different context of meaning than the isolated instance in a U.S. suburban parking lot, as it is inflicted on someone leading a generally predictable and contented life? Or consider the situation around discipline facing Russian Pentecostals refugees in the United States. This recently arrived group has brought with them a long-standing belief in the value of using the belt to discipline their children, a practice which has resulted in frequent clashes with the child welfare system in the U.S. (see Birman, 1994). But is the meaning of such discipline the same for these children as for the child welfare workers who call it abusive, or does its cultural and historical context provide for them a different context of meaning? And if so, does this appraisal affect the outcome of this practice for the well-being of these children? Would we expect children to have the same reaction if such discipline were done in an upper middle-class community where it was not the norm, not contextualized in tradition, and where local culture may ostracize rather than support the family?

The more general conceptual importance of context and the role of culture as part of that context are illustrated in the work of several authors in the present volume. Milgram's (1993) analysis of principles of traumatic stress prevention in Israel includes a discussion of community and cultural preventives, including varied "stress-resistant" processes of inoculation and indoctrination of the public to help them anticipate and cope with tragedy. He further discusses the cathartic role of cultural rituals, such as encouraging families to create a book memorializing a son or daughter lost through war or terrorism. Lomranz (1990), in describing the long-term adaptation of Holocaust survivors provides many examples of how "culture and history may facilitate or hinder people's ability to cope" (p. 115). He emphasizes the importance of including a "historical-cultural time-line" in the assessment of the adaptation to such long-term stressors. This time-line contextualizes the meaning and consequences of the event in a particular culture at a particular historical moment (see also Solomon, 1989). While such perspectives are indeed present in the disaster and traumatic stress literature, they seem more the exception than the rule; to borrow a Gestalt image, they seem more ground than figure.

An Ecological Metaphor

An ecological approach to disaster and traumatic stress in the community context reverses this figure-ground emphasis; context and culture are figure, not ground. In my role as Editor of the American Journal of Community Psychology I have been fascinated by a regularly occurring phenomena in the reporting of community-based research; namely, that comments about context and culture appear regularly, but most frequently in the discussion section of papers, where they are invoked as post hoc explanations for why the data did not turn out as expected. The ecological metaphor is intended to elevate such post-hoc musings to the status of theory guiding the initial conceptualization of research and intervention.

As a perspective emanating from community psychology, the ecological metaphor focuses primarily on communities and individuals in communities as the levels of analysis. Further, it is a heuristic rather than a theory, a distinction well-captured years ago by Katz and Kahn (1968) in their influential book The Social Psychology of Organizations. In that book, they introduced the notion of systems theory to the study of organizations in the following words:

> In some respects open-system theory is not a theory at all; it does not pretend to the specific sequences of cause and effect, the specific hypotheses and tests of hypotheses which are the basic elements of theory. Open-system theory is rather a framework, a metatheory, a model in the broadest sense of that over-used term. Open-system theory is an approach, a conceptual language for understanding and describing many kinds and levels of phenomena (p.452).

The origins of the ecological metaphor in community psychology come not from systems theory per se, but from field biology, a discipline expressly committed to understanding the functioning of biological communities--a community level of analysis. It revolves around four ecological processes that field biologists have found useful in understanding the functioning and evolution of plant and animal communities over time. These four principles are those of adaptation, cycling of resources, interdependence, and succession. Each provides a somewhat different emphasis on the nature of context and person-in-context.

Adaptation. In biological communities, the adaptation principle focuses attention on what is required to survive in a particular environment; what its adaptive requirements are. The adaptation principle thus draws attention to context writ large. When applied to human communities, it focuses on traditions, norms, processes, structures, and policies which, taken together, constitute the environment which both constrains and promotes certain kinds of adaptations for individuals and groups.

The adaptation principle focuses attention initially on understanding what kinds of adaptive demands different kinds of disasters and traumatic situations place on people. One way to think about this is through efforts to create a taxonomy of events. For example, Bonnie Green (1982) provides one such useful distinction with respect to disaster. She suggests the importance of the degree to which disasters are central or peripheral to a community, using the flood and the plane crash as contrasting events. The flood affects an entire community directly, while the plane crash affects any particular community to the degree that members of that community were on the plane. Lomranz provides another kind of distinction when he states that "the concentration camp experience is unlike other war experiences because it is personally directed and aims at extinction, not defeat" (1990, p. 104). Efforts to move toward such taxonomies represent one very useful way of developing a way of contrasting the wide array of circumstances involved in trauma and disaster and the kinds of coping they require.

But the adaptation principle suggests something more to attend to: that each event is itself surrounded by an ecological context which particularizes its meaning, its resources, and its outcomes. It is conceptually important to remember that the Buffalo Creek disaster took place in Buffalo Creek, the Chernobyl nuclear accident in Chernobyl. The cultures, local histories, available resources for providing help, and differences in citizen attitudes toward the government as a resource differentiate the meaning and impact of events over and above characteristics of the events themselves. For example, Soviet citizens were not initially told by the government about the accident in Chernobyl. Taxonomic approaches, while potentially useful, can do a disservice to a contextual understanding of events if they themselves are taken out of their community and cultural context.

Overall, however, the adaptation principle is intended to create a broad mindset for appreciating the ways in which community level phenomena and culture inform our understanding of people and communities coping with stress.

Cycling of Resources. In biological communities, cycling of resources refers to the manner in which energy or nutrients relevant to the survival and evolution of the community are generated and cycled through the community. Applied to human communities, it advocates for the analysis of the manifest and latent resources available for problem-solving and community development.

The concept of resources emphasized by this aspect of the ecological metaphor is becoming increasingly salient in the disaster and traumatic stress area through Hobfoll's (1988) "Conservation of resources" model for conceptualizing stress and its impact on individuals. This perspective delineates four kinds of personal resources relevant to coping with stress; objects, conditions, personal characteristics, and energies. As such, it furthers our appreciation of individuals in terms of the resources they have at their command. In addition, it draws attention to the importance of environmental resources as relevant to individual outcomes (see Hobfoll, Briggs, & Wells, this volume).

The ecological metaphor emphasizes the importance of assessing resources at the community level of analysis. Just as individuals have competencies, resilience, access to outside networks for additional resources, and specialized talents, so too do communities. They may be characterized by effective interorganizational connections, traditions for coping with adversity, and social settings that facilitate the resolution of conflict or the organizing of support in times of crisis. They may provide religious institutions that serve both the spiritual and tangible needs of those unwilling to deal with the formal service system, and celebratory or commemorative events that promote a sense of belonging or a collective reminder that adversity has been overcome before. An analysis of the community context of disaster and traumatic stress includes an assessment of the personal and social resources in the community as well as the individual resources of those affected by the event.

When thinking about individual resources, however, the ecological metaphor is reluctant to specify what is a resource and what is liability without an explicit consideration of the environmental demands required for successful adaptation. From this perspective, every asset may be a liability, every benefit a potential cost, depending on circumstance and context--there is no free lunch. Pynoos (1993) captures this complexity in his description of the match between personal qualities and coping requirements for children dealing with traumatic events: He writes: "Factors contributing to resilience may not necessarily be positive mental health attributes; similarly, factors contributing to vulnerability may not be negative ones. Lack of empathy in a conduct-disordered child may lead to less overt acute distress. Conversely, intelligence and empathy can increase distress when, for example, such a child more fully recognizes that behavior of a hostage taker is erratic and disturbed" (p.215). Solomon and Smith (1994) provide another example in their potentially paradoxical finding that women with excellent spouse relationships had worse outcomes following disaster than those with weaker spousal ties. What presumably constitutes an ongoing source of strength becomes a risk factor under certain circumstances.

Even resources often assumed to be positive, such as money, can constrain rather than create options in certain contexts. Carol Stack (1972), in her beautiful ethnography of a poor black community All Our Kin, shows how the acquisition of money within this particular community context was a liability as well as an asset. Having money incurred obligations on the individual to give back to those kin who had nurtured this person or their family in the past, and increased pressure on the individual to stay in the community rather than use money as a ticket out. Thus, the cycling of resources principle on both a community and individual level ties the definition of resources to local conditions and suggests that all resources have costs as well as benefits.

Interdependence. The interdependence principle asserts the interconnectedness of aspects of the community, be it biological or human. It assesses how the various parts of the community fit together in an interdependent whole where the function of each part is affected by how the other parts function.

At the community level, the interdependence principle focuses on such sets of relationships as how the various help-providing organizations work or do not work together, or how churches and other informal networks get along with professionals. It also focuses on the interaction among smaller systems, such as the how the relationship between work and family environment affect the stress experienced by managers (Phelan, Schwartz, Bromet, Dew, Parkinson, Schulberg, Dunn, Blaine, & Curtis, 1991), or how the traumatic reaction of a family member, perhaps diagnosed PTSD, causes ripple effects among other family members and their extended social networks (Solomon, Waysman, Levy, Fried, Mikulincer, Benbenishty, Florian, & Bleich, 1992).

A critical topic suggested by this principle involves the importance of understanding how intervention efforts are integrated into the communities in which they occur. One aspect of this involves the interdependence between the content and values of the intervention and those of the host environment. Does the intervention support local norms about what form of help-giving are acceptable to the community? Does the entrance of an outside intervention team of professionals affect the ongoing naturally occurring informal helping networks that existed before the disaster or traumatic event?

Giel (1990) provides an example of how interdependence operates in the area of social values in his description of the political issues involved in rebuilding houses after an earthquake in Peru. The tension for the interventionists involved whether or not to support a housing project based on egalitarian principles or conform to the wishes of authorities in building housing that conformed to or replicated patterns of pre-existing social stratification existing before the earthquake.

The interdependence principle is also relevant for understanding the coping behavior of individuals. This principle suggests that behavior adaptive in one setting may not be so in others and, perhaps more paradoxically, that one may choose to behave in a manner that may seem maladaptive in a particular setting because of the importance of other settings in that person's life. Consider the following example of an inner-city high school student whose coping style I discovered as part of a longitudinal study of a racially mixed, inner-city alternative high school (Trickett, 1991). The school was not strict; students would often hang out in the halls rather than attend class. Among the "regulars" was a 19 year-old black student, who drove a new expensive automobile to school, dressed in costly clothes, and always carried a large and visible roll of bills. During the school day he would hang out in the halls or outside the building talking with peers. After school was over, however, he would return for tutoring by one of his teachers.

The explanation offered by this student's teacher was that adapting to the school by going to class would conflict with his highly valued street image. However, the student also knew he needed to learn to read. His way of adapting was to flaunt his irreverence for the dominant norms of the school by showing up, but not attending class. However, he found a way to learn those school-related skills he felt necessary without compromising his street image. From the outside, his behavior may have seemed maladaptive; from the inside, it represented a balancing of the many life spheres of importance to him. The interdependence principle thus argues against assessing an individual's behavior in a single life sphere without knowing something about the individual's larger life space.

Succession. The final principle focuses on the time dimension of biological and human communities, or "how the community came to its current form of adaptation". Assessing the history of a community includes a look at such factors as cultural history, prior attempts at dealing with crisis, and how local norms about service delivery have evolved.

The importance of history as a community level characteristic is nowhere more striking than in the papers of several Israeli psychologists represented in this volume (see the Lomranz, Milgram, Sarson, Schönpflug, Jackson, Schwarzer, and Solomon chapters, this volume). Indeed, these psychologists show how the very theories of stress and coping which emerge are themselves embedded in cultural and historical experience. Thus, it is not fortuitous that the greatest emphasis on the positive rather than negative long-range adaptations of individuals to traumatic events, be they the Holocaust (Lomranz, 1990) or more recent wars (Solomon, Waysman, Neria, Ohry, & Wiener, 1994), should come from the inquiries of the Israelis; that the value of looking for strength in adversity emerges from a country and a culture for which history has provided all too many opportunities for such a quest. Neither is it fortuitous that descriptions of the role of culture, ritual, and social events as buffers and inoculators against the adverse reactions to stress should come from social scientists in a country that has been forced to maintain a systemic preparedness for attack (e.g. Milgram, 1993). This in no way denies or minimizes the importance of trauma and disaster in other countries. Rather, it is intended to draw attention to the importance of how social and cultural history informs our understanding of theory. In contrast to the emphasis in Israel, in the U.S. theory has focused on the impact of discrete natural disasters, events seen as anomalies in the ongoing lives of people.

One implication of the succession principle involves the potential longitudinal role of community and cultural supports when interpreting positive and negative consequences of disaster and traumatic stress on individuals. As McFarlane notes, "the quality of the post-disaster environment, particularly in disaster-affected communities where an individual's physical living circumstances may have been severely changed as a consequence of the event, may have important interactive effects with the traumatic exposure...Current models do not take account of the environmental, social, or cultural context within which the individual attempts to adapt to their acute post traumatic reactions" (1994, p. 22). This may suggest, for example, that the long term adaptations of Holocaust survivors may be partially explained by the ongoing supportive structures and culture of Israel in the ensuing years. Similar kinds of inquiry can be made about short and long-term outcomes in other contexts.

While appreciating the formative power of the past, the Succession Principle also reminds us of the importance of understanding the hopes and dreams we all have for the future. It draws attention to how opportunity arises from the ashes of disaster. Giel (1990) exemplifies this issue in his description of the community whose response to the aftermath of a volcanic eruption was to rebuild aspects of the town and harbor for community development. "They realized that the useful area of the harbor could be doubled, that the vast quantities of ash could provide a basis for the manufacturing of building blocks, that (the town of) Heimay could be turned into a tourist center, and that by planting grass seed they might succeed in binding the ash together and accelerate its decomposition into soil" (p. 16). The Succession Principle further reminds us that the theories we build often lack the time dimension. Lomranz (1990), for example, has found great variability in adaptation among long-term Holocaust survivors. He has noted that if one takes a life-span developmental perspective, the theoretical notion that traumatic events overwhelm individual differences in responding to them is quite temporally bound, if true at all.

The Succession Principle views traumatic events and disasters as occurring in communities with a past and an anticipated future. It draws attention to how past events, crises, and characters in a community have helped that community crystallize a sense of current collective identity and future aspirations.

Concluding Comments: Ecological Means for Appreciating Diversity

The ecological metaphor represents one paradigm for approaching the area of coping with disaster and traumatic stress. It is a perspective for dignifying the role of context and culture in such research. It adopts a community as well as person-in-context level of analysis. It is a perspective which shifts the figure-ground relationship between individuals and places found in so much psychological research and intervention. Most importantly, it represents one way to further our understanding of the great variability or diversity in peoples' responses to disaster or traumatic stress (e.g. Wortman & Silver, 1989; Lomranz, 1990). Collectively, the papers in this volume attest to the great variability people show in appraisal, in coping style, and in the short and long-term adaptations both within and between populations. This variability represents both an opportunity to appreciate diversity and resilience and provides a resource for theory about human capability not adequately explored at present. Dignifying variability requires an empathic appreciation of the diversity of adaptive behavior. It calls for an acknowledgement of cultural constraints, a from-the-inside-out look at the circumstances and realistic options facing individuals in different situations, networks of relationships, and community contexts. It requires a widening of the outcomes of interest to allow both resilience and pathology, both courage and despair, to emerge as individuals and communities cope with stress. Variability can be accounted for by a more dedicated exploration of context and culture and a broadening of definitions of successful adaptation. In this spirit I offer the following five orientations to research and theory that can illuminate ecological contributions to this diversity.

(1) <u>Investigate context and culture as a conceptual resource for theory building and theory testing</u>. Link the study of trauma to the historical and community context where it occurs. Make figure out of ground by making explicit the tacit knowledge researchers and interventionists have accumulated about community dynamics and cultural forces in the varied communities and cultures where this work has occurred.

(2) <u>Widen the methods used to generate knowledge and evaluate interventions</u> to create insider accounts as a heuristic for theory building and hypothesis testing. Quantitative work needs to be informed by local knowledge best appreciated through qualitative and ethnographic approaches. DeVries and Kaplan (1994) make a similar plea in their call for methods which aim "to return the experience of the patient in his or her natural environment to its rightful place in a psychiatry that is in danger of losing its balance by trading off for premature universals before the hard work of exhaustive classification of local variation has been locally done" (p. 1). It will take

multiple methods to dignify the validity of variability and reduce the myths associated with the stress and coping field (Wortman, 1989).

(3) <u>Reframe the interpretation of existing literature</u>, transforming what has been ground into figure. For example, the chapters in this volume report an enormous number of gender differences in the appraisal of and response to disaster and traumatic stress. Not only are men and women at risk for different kinds of traumas, but in traumas that appear similar from the outside, men and women act in dissimilar ways and may often seem to have dissimilar outcomes (see Solomon & Smith, 1994, for example). Investigating the social and cultural contexts of men and women in these circumstances represents one way of reversing the figure-ground priority. A similar perspective may be taken to investigate race or ethnic differences. It means starting from an analysis of gender, race, ethnicity, and their intersection and building theory about coping and adaptation from that contextually grounded perspective.

(4) <u>Ferret out the latent assumptions implicit in existing theory</u>. Beginning with Freud (1966), and reaching through Kuhn (1970), is the idea that not only our behavior but our theories involve implicit assumptions of which we are not fully aware but which nonetheless guide our behavior. Wortman and Silver's (1989) analysis of the myths of coping with loss highlights this issue. As they show, data do not support theory about how we assume the grief process is supposed to work, and these normative expectations limit both our understanding of variability and limit our appreciation of diversity in adaptive behavior. Where do these myths of coping come from? Where do our implicit definitions of adaptive outcomes, or what constitutes a resource, come from? I believe that such introspection will take us inside the mythology of our culture, class, race, ethnicity, or gender. Such assumptions as the importance of "working through", for example, probably reflects both a culture and class bias. And why do we think people are supposed to recover from loss? Unearthing these assumptions, these myths, is not only good psychoanalysis, but good for a science of how culture and context affects coping with stress.

(5) <u>Appreciate cultural pluralism</u> and explore the potential of indigenous psychologies for theory and research. The area of disaster and traumatic stress, like many other areas of research and intervention, is heavily influenced by the intellectual traditions and assumptions of Western culture more generally and the United States more particularly. These traditions and assumptions are embodied in the theories tested, the measures employed, and, indeed the implicit definitions of mental health contained in the choice of outcome variables. Without in any way diminishing the importance of these traditions, I end by voicing a hope for additional work focused on the indigenous psychologies of people in different cultures and contexts. Such work may complement, refine, replace, or confirm existing theories and measures evolving from Western psychological thought. But, from an ecological perspective, such a quest may have an important role in understanding the variability in human response to stress.

References

Barker, R.G. (1968). Ecological psychology. Stanford, CA.: Stanford University Press.
Bennett, C.C., Anderson, L.S., Cooper, S., Hassol, L., Klein, D.C., & Rosenblum, G. (Eds.). (1966). Community psychology: A report of the Boston Conference on the Education of Psychologists for Community Mental Health. Boston: Boston University Press.
Birman, D. (1994). Mental health needs of Soviet evangelical Christian Refugees. Rockville, MD: Refugee Mental Health Branch, Center for Mental Health Services, U.S. Department of Health and Human Services.
Bronfenbrenner, U.(1979). The ecology of human development: Experiments by nature and design. Cambridge: Harvard University Press.
Bronfenbrenner, U. & Weiss, H. (1983). Beyond policies without people: An ecological perspective on child and family policy. In E. Zigler, S.L. Kagan, & E. Klugman (Eds.), Children, families, and government: Perspectives on American social policy. Cambridge, England: Cambridge University Press.
deVries, M.W. & Kaplan, C.D. (1994). Missing links in mental health research. Paper presented at the 1993 World Congress of the World Federation for Mental Health. Makuhari, Japan.
Freud, S. (1966). Introductory lectures on psychoanalysis. New York: W.W. Norton.
Giel, R. (1990). Psychosocial processes in disasters. International Journal of Mental Health, 19(1), 7-20.
Green, B.L. (1982). Assessing levels of psychosocial impairment following disaster: Consideration of actual and methodological dimensions. The Journal of Nervous and Mental Disease, 17(9), 544-552.
Hobfoll, S. (1988). The ecology of stress. Washington, DC: Hemisphere.
Hobfoll, S. E. (1989). Conservation of resources: A new attempt at conceptualizing stress. American Psychologist, 44(3), 513-524.
Hobfoll, S. E., Briggs, S., & Wells J. (this volume). Community stress and resources: Actions and reactions. In S. E. Hobfoll & M. W. deVries (Eds.), Extreme stress and communities: Impact and intervention. Dordrecht, the Netherlands: Kluwer.
Katz, D., & Kahn, R.L. (1968). The social psychology of organizations. New York: Wiley.
Kelly, J.G. (1968). Toward an ecological conception of preventive interventions. In J.W. Carter, Jr. (Ed.). Research contributions from psychology to community mental health. New York, NY: Behavioral Publications.
Kelly, J.G. (Ed.) (1979). Adolescent boys in high school: A psychological study of coping and adaptation. New Jersy: Lawrence Erlbaum.
Kelly, J.G. (1986). Content and process: An ecological view of the interdependence of practice and research. American Journal of Community Psychology, 14, 581-589.

Kelly, J. G., Azelton, L.S., Burzette, R., & Mock, L.O. (1994). Creating social settings for diversity: An ecological thesis. In E.J. Trickett, R. Watts, & D. Birman (Eds.), Human diversity: Perspectives on people in context. San Francisco: Jossey-Bass.

Kuhn, T. H. (1970). The structure of scientific revolutions. Chicago: University of Chicago Press.

Lazarus, R.S. & Folkman, S. (1984). Stress, appraisal, and coping. New York: Springer.

Lomranz, J. (1990). Long-term adaptation to traumatic stress in light of adult development and aging perspectives. In M.A. Parris, Stevens, Crowther, S.E. Hobfoll, & D.L. Tennenbaum (Eds.), Stress and coping in later life families. Washington, D.C.: Hemisphere Publishers.

Lomranz, J. (this volume). Endurance and living: Long-term effects of the Holocaust. In S. E. Hobfoll & M. W. deVries (Eds.), Extreme stress and communities: Impact and intervention. Dordrecht, the Netherlands: Kluwer.

Lonner, W.J. (1994). Culture and human diversity. In E.J. Trickett, R. Watts, & D. Birman (Eds.), Human diversity: Perspectives on people in context. San Francisco: Jossey-Bass.

McFarlane, A.C. (1994). The severity of the trauma: Issues about its role in post traumatic stress disorder. Greenacres, South Australia, University of Adelaide Department of Psychiatry, unpublished manuscript.

Milgram, N. (1993). War-related trauma and victimization: Principles of traumatic stress prevention in Israel. In J.P. Wilson & B. Raphael (Eds.) International Handbook of Traumatic Stress. New York: Plenum Press.

Milgram, N., Sarason, B. R., Schönpflug, U., Jackson, A., & Schwarzer, C. (this volume). Catalyzing community support. In S. E. Hobfoll & M. W. deVries (Eds.), Extreme stress and communities: Impact and intervention. Dordrecht, the Netherlands: Kluwer.

Mitchell, R.E. and Trickett, E. J. (1979). Social networks as mediators of social support: An analysis of the effects and determinants of social networks. Community Mental Health Journal, 18(1), 27-44.

Moos, R.H. (1974). Evaluating treatment environments: A social ecological approach. New York: Wiley.

Moos, R.H. (1975). Evaluating correctional and community settings. New York: Wiley.

Moos, R.H. (1979). Evaluating educational environments. San Francisco: Jossey-Bass.

Phelan, J., Schwartz, J.E., Bromet, E.J., Dew, M.A., Parkinson, D.K., Schulberg, H.C., Dunn, L.O., Blaine, H., & Curtis, E.C. (1991). Work stress, family stress and depression in professional and managerial employees. Psychological Medicine, 21, 999-1012.

Pynoos, R.S. (1993). Traumatic stress and developmental psychopathology in children and adolescents. In J.M. Oldham, M.B. Riba, & A. Tasman (Eds.), <u>American Psychiatric Press Review of Psychiatry, Vol. 12</u>. Washington, D.C.: American Psychiatric Press.

Rappaport, J. (1981). In praise of paradox: A social policy of empowerment over prevention. <u>American Journal of Community Psychology, 9</u>, 1-25.

Richters, J.E. & Cicchetti, D. (1993). Mark Twain meets DSM-III R: Conduct disorder, development, and the concept of harmful dysfunction. <u>Development and Psychopathology</u>, 5, 5-29.

Sarason, S.B. (1981) <u>Psychology misdirected</u>. New York: Free Press.

Solomon, S.D. (1989). Research issues in assessing disaster's effects. In R. Gist & B. Lubin (Eds.), <u>Psychosocial aspects of disasters</u>. New York: Johm Wiley & Sons.

Solomon, Z. (this volume). The pathogenic effect of war stress: The Israeli experience. In S. E. Hobfoll & M. W. deVries (Eds.), <u>Extreme stress and communities: Impact and intervention</u>. Dordrecht, the Netherlands: Kluwer.

Solomon, S.D. & Smith, E.M. (1994). Social support and perceived control as moderators of responses to dioxin and flood exposure. In R.J. Ursano, B.G. McCaughey, & C.C. Fullerton (Eds.), <u>Individual and community responses to trauma and disaster</u>. Cambridge, England: Cambridge University Press.

Solomon, Z., Waysman, M., Levy, G., Fried, B., Mikulincer, M., Benbenishty, R., Florian, V., & Bleich, A. (1992). From front line to home front: a study of secondary traumaticization. <u>Family Process</u>, 31, 289-302.

Solomon, Z., Waysman, M.A., Neria, Y., Ohry, A., & Wiener, M. (1994). Psychological growth and dysfunction following war-captivity. Tel Aviv, Israel: Bob Shapell School of Social Work, unpublished manuscript.

Stack, C. B. (1972). <u>All our kin</u>. New York: Harper & Row.

Trickett, E. J. (1991). <u>Living an idea: Empowerment and the evolution of an inner city alternative high school</u>. Cambridge, MA: Brookline Books.

Trickett, E. J., Kelly, J. G., & Todd, D. M. (1972). The social environment of the high school: Guidelines for individual change and organizational development. In S. olann and C. Eisdorfer (Eds.). <u>Handbook of community mental health</u>. New York: Appleton Century Crofts (pp. 331-406).

Trickett, E. J. (1984). Towards a distinctive community psychology: An ecological metaphor for training and the conduct of research. <u>American Journal of Community Psychology</u>, 12, 261-277.

Trickett, E. J. & Birman, D. (1989). Takng ecology seriously: A community development approach to individually based preventive interventions. In L. A. Bond & B. E. Compas (Eds.), <u>Primary prevention and promotion in the schools</u>. Newbury Park, CA.: Sage (pp. 361-390).

Wortman, C. & Silver, R.C. (1989). The myths of coping with loss. <u>Journal of Consulting and Clinical Psychology</u>, 57(3), 349-357.

SECTION II: BASIC STRESS CONCEPTS AND WHERE THEY LEAD IN THE STUDY OF COMMUNITY STRESS (OVERVIEW)

Stevan E. Hobfoll, Kent State University, Kent, Ohio, USA
Rebecca P. Cameron, Kent State University, Kent, Ohio, USA
Marten W. deVries, University of Limburg, Maastricht, the Netherlands

The tension between individual and community approaches to extreme stress is a central theme of this book. Trickett (Chapter One) has provided an ecological framework from which to begin incorporating community perspectives into research on disasters and traumatic stress. He covers key concepts relevant to a community approach and outlines fundamental issues to be addressed by community theorists and researchers. Community approaches offer a counterpoint to the traditional individually-focused mainstream of psychology by emphasizing contextual factors, including history and culture, by focusing on people's strengths and resilience, and by viewing psychologists and the people they serve as equal partners in whatever task is being undertaken, whether it is research- or treatment-oriented. Trickett invokes the four elements of the ecological analogy as useful concepts in understanding communities: adaptation, cycling of resources, interdependence, and succession. Among his recommendations are: to pay attention to context and culture as integral components of theory-building; to use of a variety of methodologies, including those that are not mainstream; to reexamine and reinterpret the existing literature; to question the assumptions upon which existing theories are based; and to respect and seek to understand cultural diversity. Following Trickett's lead, each of the chapters in this section addresses a particular facet of the experience of community stress in such a way as to illuminate the tension between community and individual approaches and to illustrate the creative consequences of adopting an ecological-contextual stance.

In Chapter Two, Meichenbaum takes a cognitive approach to the impact of disasters. The cognitive processing of disaster could be understood as an essentially internal, individual phenomenon. Indeed, Meichenbaum begins with questions posed by mental health workers regarding how to differentiate between individuals in terms of their vulnerability and the adaptiveness of their coping responses. However, he does not limit his answer to individual differences: rather, he emphasizes the communal processes that facilitate or inhibit successful cognitive processing by individuals and groups. Meichenbaum proposes, in his constructive narrative approach, that the accounts people develop of their traumatic experiences profoundly influence their adaptation. These accounts are developed in context: they involve social comparisons, social roles, and socially sanctioned symbols and rituals. Communities, especially religious communities, provide common metaphors with which to imbue personal accounts with meaning, settings for the public sharing of stories, and commemorative activities that facilitate coping with loss. Meichenbaum differentiates between aspects of narratives that promote healing and those that prolong distress. Interestingly, he cites evidence that it is the relative quantity of positive to negative thinking that predicts positive outcomes, rather than an absolute level of either one. The sharing of personal accounts with others appears to be a critical element of the construction of healing narratives, although the willingness of community members to listen appears to fluctuate over time. These interpersonal processes, and their dynamics over time, require further research attention. In addition, the changes that personal narratives undergo over time present a challenge and opportunity to researchers. Questions of causality need to be addressed, and the links between cognitive processes, behavior, physiological changes, and the status of objective resources need to be clarified. Cultural variables, including locus of control, typical or appropriate expressions of distress, and culturally-relevant metaphors need to be considered. Meichenbaum has provided stress researchers with an intriguing approach to understanding adaptation to disaster that can be applied to individuals or groups, but which captures many of the contextual elements of timing, culture, and interpersonal interdependence emphasized by community researchers. He follows up his chapter with an instrument that can be used to assess the vulnerability of individuals and groups to post-disaster maladjustment. This instrument provides data rich with contextual and narrative information.

Strelau (Chapter Three) echoes the need to consider both the individual and her or his environment as elements in the stress-adaptation process. He provides a more biologically-based view of the individual's contribution to this process, focusing on temperamental vulnerability to stress. As does Meichenbaum with cognitive processing, Strelau begins with the highly individual concept of temperament risk factor (TRF), but then develops the concept as inevitably understandable only in terms of contextual variables. The concept of temperament risk factor that he proposes is most relevant when it encompasses behavior that provides a poor adaptive fit with certain contexts of excessive, persistent, or recurrent stress. The TRF represents relative, not absolute risk, and can be measured by the ratio of maladaptive outcomes for those with the temperamental trait(s) as compared to maladaptive outcomes for those without the trait(s), given the same stress experience. Importantly, a TRF for one set of circumstances may not be a TRF in another set of circumstances.

Strelau proposes five models that could be invoked to describe the nature of the relationship between individuals and their environments as it relates to the risk for maladaptive outcomes. These five models provide hypotheses and alternatives that can be tested empirically. The first model involves simple additive effects of temperament and environment. The second model proposes an interactive effect, in which the presence of a TRF makes the individual more susceptible to the negative effects of a predisposing environment. The third model presents a more active view. The TRF in this model serves to increase the individual's exposure to a predisposing environment, through behavioral mediators. Finally, Strelau discusses two models that represent combinations of the first three. In one, simple additive effects are combined with interactive effects. In the other, additive effects are combined with temperamental control over exposure to the predisposing environment.

After describing each model, Strelau briefly reviews evidence from the literature, including studies of children, adolescents, and adults, that illustrate the importance of temperamental traits such as arousal level and trait anxiety in predicting the effects of stress on functioning. Since temperamental factors may contribute to the occurrence of stressors, since risk factors often interact to potentiate each other, and since risk factors such as temperament are relatively stable, Strelau argues that researchers cannot afford to ignore the role that temperament plays with regard to stress and its consequences. With regard to appropriate methodology, Strelau endorses the use of causal modeling techniques to address the complexities of person-environment interactions.

Wortman, Carnelley, Lehman, Davis, and Exline (Chapter Four) provide a nice illustration of the application of Trickett's advice to question assumptions underlying existing research and theory. Their discussion of the process of coping with grief highlights the limitations of theories that are accepted without adequate empirical support because they fit our Western, and specifically U.S., cultural biases. Our embeddedness in a culture that values individualism and stoicism, and that denies death, has limited our insight and effectiveness as researchers, theorists, and service providers. Thus, our collective discomfort with grief serves as a risk factor for those who grieve, whether we are in professional or personal roles. The importance of disclosure and sharing of trauma, introduced by Meichenbaum in Chapter Two, is again cited as a helpful coping mechanism. However, Wortman et al. examine our societal reluctance to participate helpfully as listeners. Instead, we often become punitive, minimizing, or avoidant, thus reducing the potential for healing through disclosure. Mourners may choose to isolate rather than deal with others' negative reactions, although this is a less-than-optimal means of coping.

Wortman et al. challenge several popularly held beliefs about grief: that it follows an orderly stage process, that it should be resolved in a preordained amount of time, that it must be accompanied by intense distress in order to be resolved properly. Although more research is needed to test these assumptions thoroughly, it appears that grief often fails to conform to an orderly, linear progression through a set of stages, that it is never fully resolved for many people, and that it is often not accompanied by intense distress at any point. Wortman et al. call attention to the individual focus of the existing grief literature and outline barriers to effective community interventions, including the reluctance of bereaved community members to seek mental health services. They propose that the appropriate site of intervention may be with those close to the bereaved, but suggest that the discrepancy between people's cognitive understanding of how to be helpful and their actions may limit the effectiveness of educational programs. Finally, they comment on the difficulties faced by professionals attempting to assist the bereaved, including the possibility of vicarious traumatization. Wortman et al.'s chapter closes with a discussion of as-yet unanswered research questions. Already, these authors consider the problems of those grieving traumatic loss in our society to be sufficiently widespread as to constitute a legitimate target for community stress intervention. It is clear that in order to provide appropriate empirically-based interventions for traumatic bereavement in the context of large-scale disasters, much more research will need to be done. Cultural attitudes towards grief are of paramount importance in understanding lay and professional responses, and it can easily be inferred that cross-cultural efforts to intervene with those suffering traumatic loss need to be conducted with caution.

Jerusalem, Kaniasty, Lehman, Ritter, and Turnbull (Chapter Five) struggle with the issue of differentiating community from individual stress, and then propose a heuristic for placing a stressor on this continuum. They ask whether community stress processes parallel individual stress processes, or whether there are qualitative or quantitative differences in the two experiences. They reject the obvious distinctions one could make between community and individual stresses: suddenness, severity, number of victims, valence, controllability, duration, source of stress, and presence of secondary problems do not adequately differentiate the two categories. Although the distinction between objective and subjective stress is of limited value in distinguishing community and individual stress, the concept of appraisals becomes a key to their heuristic.

Jerusalem et al. propose that there are three levels of stress, that can be distinguished by the nature of appraisals, coping, and resource mobilization undertaken by the affected community. At level one (individual level stress), more than one person has experienced a stressor, but there is no common awareness of the problem, and no public effort to cope. At level two (moderate community stress), there is a detectable amount of community awareness and concern about the stressor, but public resources are not yet mobilized. This is often the case when a disenfranchised group or a small number of community members are affected, or when a group of experts has begun to identify the problem. At level three (high community stress), the larger community has identified the problem as a threat, and has mobilized public resources and begun communal coping efforts. These three stages may, but do not necessarily, reflect temporal stages of a stressor, and it is not necessary that a stressor begin at any particular level. There is room for much within-level variability in the degree of public awareness and public coping. Jerusalem et al. discuss the role of community agencies and the media in influencing the level of community appraisal and resource mobilization. Community and personal values, social comparisons, and the construction of meaning are all relevant. Particular risk may be associated with the period following initial outpourings of public resources and coping efforts, as people are left to resume individual coping efforts, but with greatly reduced resources.

In keeping with Strelau's proposed temperament risk factors that only operate within particular contexts of poor fit, Jerusalem et al. suggest that personality factors such as internal control may cause a poor fit between individuals and large-scale relief efforts and agencies. As a result of these personality factors, that appear to vary across as well as within cultures, community risk and individual risk may be increased or decreased during different phases of disaster relief as a function of the stage of public resource mobilization. Jerusalem et al. call attention to the inequities in resource allocation, even at times of high communal coping, and to the vulnerability of those left with inadequate resources and disrupted patterns of social interaction. Characteristics of a disaster, such as ambiguity and issues of blame allocation, may also interfere with communal coping efforts. These authors provide a comprehensive discussion of the reciprocal relationships between community and individual stress. Their discussion provides a rich source of research questions to be followed up, including how to facilitate successful community coping that minimizes the inevitable shortfall of resources and the inequities in distribution while capitalizing on the strengths of a community response to stress.

Essential aspects of community stress research that are emphasized throughout this section are: the need for methodological creativity, including the use of methodologies that can illustrate temporal issues such as stability and change over the course of disaster and recovery, or assess reciprocal influences of stressors, coping attempts, and consequences; the need for explicit attention to the contexts and cultures in which disasters occur; and the complexities of relationships between individuals and the groups which they comprise. Perhaps the most fundamental questions being addressed are what makes some people and certain communities more resilient than others? And what is the difference between an individual understanding and a community understanding of this question?

DISASTERS, STRESS AND COGNITION

Donald Meichenbaum
University of Waterloo
Waterloo, Ontario, Canada

I have a "story" to tell, an "account" to share about my involvement in the topic of "disasters, stress and cognition." For the last several years, I have presented two- and five-day workshops on post-traumatic stress disorders, consulted with mental health workers who conduct critical incident stress debriefing with disaster victims, and worked with clinicians who are responsible for the treatment of traumatized clients with PTSD and other clinical disorders. These activities have taken me around the world. In the course of conducting these presentations, I have developed a "condition" or "symptom" of what psychiatrists call "ideas of reference," namely, the belief that an individual can cause important events to occur. Consider the following litany of recent experiences that I have encountered. When I presented in Cape Cod, Massachusetts, Hurricane Bob arrived; in Clearwater, Florida, the largest flood of the century occurred; in Los Angeles on two occasions there were major earthquakes during the time of my consultation, and on my latest visit, there were major mudslides. When I visited Milwaukee the water supply went bad. When I visited Hong Kong the talks between China and England broke off. When I visited Israel a few years ago, the Lebanon war broke out, and when I was in Valencia, Spain, a coup occurred and a rebel general and his troops commandered the city. Moreover, while driving home from a consultation at a center for traumatic brain-injured clients in Toronto, Ontario, on two separate occasions in the exact same spot on the major highway, my car was involved in life-threatening accidents. On one occasion a passing truck dropped a metal drum through my windshield, and more recently, at the same point on the highway my brand-new car was struck by lightning.

Are these events mere "illusory correlations" between my presence and the occurrence of disastrous things happening? As my wife observed, perhaps I should switch research topics or stay home. One of the critical questions is why don't these events cause me to experience symptomatic distress, let alone PTSD? Why is it that some individuals who are exposed to such traumatic events demonstrate lingering symptoms, such as persistent intrusive memories, while others merely incorporate such events into their biographical accounts, and "move on" (ever so carefully).

This paper is designed to help answer the question of individual and group differences in response to traumatic events. Moreover, there is a need for a theoretical framework that explains such differences. It is proposed that a constructive narrative perspective that examines, in detail, how individuals and groups tell their "stories" of stress and coping provides a useful framework for understanding the different levels of adjustment. More specifically, I will examine briefly:

(a) the incidence of traumatic events;
(b) the impact of having been exposed to disasters;
(c) the factors that have been implicated in accounting for the marked variability of response to disasters;
(d) the variety of theoretical models that have been offered to explain such variability;
(e) the nature of the "stories" people tell in response to disasters; and
(f) the implications for research.

Consistent with a constructive narrative perspective, I began this paper with a "story" for several reasons. First, the research by Pennebaker (1989) indicates that not describing or confronting traumatic events can have negative psychological and physiological consequences, and that this is especially true for men who should be encouraged to confront their traumatic experiences through talking and writing (Pennebaker & Susman, 1988). Second, as we will see, this book is about the "telling of stories," and each of the chapters will highlight some specific aspect of a two part story of "the impact of disasters and how people cope with them." The authors will use a variety of explanatory schemes and metaphors to discuss the impact of disasters (e.g., biological changes, diagnostic categories, conditioning models, conservation of resources, "shattered" assumptions, social supports, and the like). I will focus on the characteristics of the "stories" or "accounts" that the victims of disaster relate.

My account begins with a consideration of what constitutes disasters? Disasters are traumatic events that are so extreme or severe, so powerful, harmful or threatening that they demand extraordinary coping efforts. They may take the form of an unusual event, or a series of continuous events, that subject people to extreme, intensive, overwhelming bombardment of perceived threats to themselves, or to significant others. Such traumatic events may overwhelm a person's or a community's sense of safety and security. These events may be brief and powerful, often lasting no more than a few minutes or hours, or they may last for a prolonged, if not an indefinite period, as in the case of nuclear or toxic accidents. These disastrous events may leave behind long-term secondary stressors (Bolin, 1988; Green, 1990, this volume; Kleber et al., 1992; Lomranz, this volume). Disasters present salient, powerful, highly emotionally threatening, critical events that are not easily accounted for or assimilated by the victims/survivors.

Just how widespread are such disastrous events? Consider the illustrative epidemiological facts enumerated in Table 1. In addition to the impact of major disasters, Freedy and his colleagues (1994) have reported on the negative impact of cumulative low magnitude events and the cumulative impact of such traumatic events that can occur over a lifetime. A major finding that emerges from the research on the impact of both low and high magnitude disasters is that it is not just the objective features (e.g., severity, degree, frequency) of the disaster, but the subjective features or meanings attached to the disaster that are critical in accounting for individual differences and influencing PTSD and accompanying sequelae (Solomon & Smith, 1993).

Table 1

How Widespread are Disastrous Traumatic Events?
Some Illustrative Data

1. Over the past two decades, natural disasters and other calamities have killed about 3 million people worldwide and adversely affected the lives of at least 800 million more people (Weisaeth, 1992).

2. In the U.S., approximately 2 million households experience injuries and physical damage each year from fire, floods, hurricanes, tornadoes, severe tropical storms or windstorms, and earthquakes (Solomon & Green, 1992).

3. Between 1974 and 1980, there were 37 major catastrophes in the U.S. alone (Freedy et al., 1993).

4. At present, there are 48 countries in the world who are at war or where there is violent internal strife (Vogel & Vernberg, 1994).

What is the impact of being exposed to such disasters? Both the immediate and long-term impact of natural and technological disasters have been studied extensively. For example, Solomon and Green (1992) have concluded that the effects of natural disasters may persist for many years, but for most individuals symptoms abate within 18 months. It has been estimated that the prevalence of psychiatric disorders in a disaster-affected community will increase approximately 20% (McFarlane, 1989). It is worth noting that the initial response to traumatic events (anxiety, dissociative response, sadness) are often predictive of future adjustment (Cardena & Spiegel, 1993; Lonigan et. al., 1994). Both adult and children's responses to disasters may cover a wide range of symptoms including fears, anxiety, depression, sadness, grief reactions, guilt, anger, physical symptoms, interpersonal problems, as well as PTSD symptoms (Wilson & Raphael, 1993). PTSD symptoms are more likely to occur in disasters with sudden onset and high life threat, while anxiety and depression, alienation and mistrust are more likely to occur after technological disasters (Vogel & Vernberg, 1993). For example, stressful events like the Three Mile Island incident can cause symptomatology that did not reach the level of diagnosable illness, but can be clinically important (Baum et al., 1993). The exposure to such continual stressors can contribute to apathy, resigned coping methods, and a lowered ability to deal with additional stressors, potentially furthering the illness process (Dew et al., 1987). Such forms of distress have been found to persist for years (e.g., 17 years in the Buffalo Creek disaster, 6 years in the Three Mile Island incident, and 8 years for an oil rig disaster -- see respectively, Green et al., 1994; Baum, 1990; and Holen, 1991).

But such a distressing picture is only part of the story. In studies of some 52 disasters, Rubonis and Bickman (1991) have reported that there was only a 17% increase in the prevalence of psychopathology, as compared to control groups, or as compared to pre-disaster levels of psychopathology. Freedy et al. (1994) have noted the remarkable resilience of human beings when faced with traumatic experiences. The vast majority of individuals do not require extended mental health services following natural disasters and the majority of adults do not experience irreversible losses due to natural disasters, especially in industrialized nations.

The critical questions that have been posed to me by the various mental health workers with whom I consult are: (i) Which individuals are most vulnerable or at most "high risk" for developing PTSD and other signs of maladjustment in response to traumatic events? and (ii) What distinguishes those who cope versus those who do not cope with such traumatic events? In answering these questions, researchers have implicated characteristics of the disaster, characteristics of the community response or recovery environment, and characteristics of the individual or group. Based on my reading of this literature (e.g., Baum et al., 1993; Bromet, 1989; Giel, 1990; Gleser et al., 1978; Goenjian, 1993; Green, 1982; Green et al., 1990; Kleber et al., 1992; Lindy et al., 1981; Lonigan et al., 1994; McFarlane, 1989; Raphael, 1986; Smith et al., 1990; Vogel & Vernberg, 1993; Wilson & Raphael, 1993; and others), I have put together a compendium of factors that have been implicated in the adjustment process (see Appendix A). The items and accompanying questions in Appendix A cover both objective and subjective features of disasters; pre-disaster characteristics; reactions during and after the disaster for the individual, family, and community.
Accompanying each factor is a question designed to tap that variable. These specific questions have not been validated as a formal scale; thus, Appendix A should be viewed as an "educated hunch" of what makes an individual, family, or group, more vulnerable to the negative effects of having lived through a disaster. The questions are designed to assess the individual's and group's appraisal of the disaster, its context, and perceived meaning.

It is one thing to enumerate some 50 variables (as noted in Appendix A) that have been implicated in disaster research; it is another to consider how these multiple variables can be integrated into a theoretical framework to explain individual differences. Investigators have not shied away from this task. One can find in the literature on disasters many diverse theoretical models that have been offered to explain the occurrence of PTSD and related disorders. Given the complexity of people's reactions to disasters, it is not surprising that theorists with very diverse orientations would emphasize different features of the stress response. Some theorists have emphasized the biological features of how people react to traumatic events (e.g., van der Kolk, 1987), while others have proposed a behavioral conditioning framework to explain such stress reactions (e.g., Keane et al., 1992). Yet, others adopt a psychodynamic perspective (Horowitz, 1986; Marmar & Horowitz, 1988), an information and emotional processing model (Foa et al., 1989; Rachman, 1980; Thrasher et al., 1994), a schema-based model (Janoff-Bulman, 1990; McCann & Pearlman, 1990) and a constructivist perspective (Harvey et al., 1990, 1992; Meichenbaum & Fitzpatrick, 1993; Meichenbaum & Fong. 1993). Others have explored the social dimension of people's responses to traumatic events in terms of the loss of resources (Freedy et al., 1993, 1994; Hobfoll, 1991; Hobfoll & Lilly, 1993). Space does not permit a comparison of each of these explanatory models, and the interested reader should see Goodman et al. (1993) for a more detailed discussion, and especially, Silver and Wortman's (1980) critique of stage models of emotional reactions to traumatic events.

Of these various models the three that highlight the role of cognition will be examined. Before considering (1) the information processing, (2) schema-based, and (3) constructivist perspectives, it is important to keep in mind that the term "cognition" reflects a variety of diverse processes. These include (i) cognitive events or conscious readily retrievable automatic thoughts, images, and "internal dialogue"; (ii) cognitive processes or the manner in which individuals selectively attend, retrieve, access mental heuristics, and integrate information; and (iii) cognitive structures that reflect the implicit beliefs, schemas, frames of reference, and readiness sets, that provide the "if...then" rules by which people function. These cognitive structures or tacit assumptive worlds guide and influence both cognitive events and cognitive affective processes. Each of the respective cognitive perspectives of stress responses emphasize different aspects of cognition and employ different metaphors to describe the individual's response to traumatic events.

1. The <u>information processing perspective</u> highlights that the stress response to traumatic events, especially diagnosable PTSD when it occurs, should be viewed as an anxiety disorder. Individuals who have been exposed to traumatic events (e.g., rape, combat, and disasters), and who are also high on PTSD symptomatology, exhibit perceptual biases for trauma-related material and are hypersensitive to false alarm responses (Foa et al., 1989; Jones & Barlow, 1990; Thrasher et al., 1994). It has been proposed that those individuals who do not recover and who evidence maladjustment in response to traumatic stressors have specific fear structures in long-term memory

that are readily triggered and exhibit deficits in emotional processing (Rachman, 1980). Distressed individuals remain "fixated" on the trauma as evident in their performance on information processing tasks such as the Stroop, and in their persistent intrusive ideation.

The information processing perspective emphasizes such features as encoding, accessing mental heuristics, emotional processing, integrating, or reframing information (all from a computer-based metaphor) to explain individual differences in responses to traumatic events.

2. The <u>schema-based perspective</u> of traumatic stress regard the rapid loss of resources as causing changes that "threaten," "challenge," "violate," "invalidate," "shatter," "attack" people's basic values and world views (Hobfoll, 1991; Janoff-Bulman & Frieze, 1983; McCann & Pearlman, 1990). Traumatic events are viewed as challenging people's basic beliefs about themselves, others, and the world. This invalidation of core beliefs lead to a compensatory search for meaning. When such a search persists over a prolonged period of time and is not "completed," then psychological and physical distress are often evident (e.g., Silver et al., 1983). As Janoff-Bulman and Frieze (1983) observe, the impact of traumatic events "shatters" the very basic assumptions and beliefs that victims hold about the operation of the world and that give structure and purpose to their lives. The primary metaphors used to describe the schema-based approach are those derived from Piaget's model, namely, assimilation and accommodation.

3. A <u>constructive narrative perspective</u> focuses on the "accounts" or "stories" that individuals offer themselves and others about the important events in their lives. Harvey et al. (1990) define "account-making" as people's story-like constructions of events that include descriptions of behavioral and affective reactions, explanations, and predictions. Individuals routinely develop accounts or stories of significant life events that entail changes and losses in their lives in an effort to infuse these occurrences with some coherence and meaning (Harvey et al., 1990, 1992; Sarbin, 1986). As Mair (1990) observed, "we live in and through stories." There are several aspects of account-making and story-telling that are worth considering as possible sources of explanation for how people respond to traumatic events.

When bad things happen to people they are prone to engage in an internal dialogue or construct a narrative account that focuses on trying to answer questions (especially, "why" questions) that provide explanations. It is proposed that some individuals get "stuck" in the following narrative.

> "What happened to me, to us?", "This can't be happening to me.", "Why me?", "Only if I(we) would have...", "I should have...", "Why did I live and why did they die?", "How did I survive?", "Why did it have to happen?", "Just when...", "Had I(we) only...", "What more could I have done?", "Am I going crazy?", "Why won't it end?", "Why do these things happen?", "Why has God forsaken us?"

The formulation of these questions preclude or reduce the likelihood of the individual accepting, resolving, or finding meaning in the "loss." There are few satisfactory answers to "why" questions. The importance of finding meaning and moving beyond the traumatic events is highlighted by many theorists in the field who propose that victims of disasters must "assimilate the traumatic experience," "resolve issues of meaning," "digest the aftermath," "confront and accept the reality of permanent losses," "rearrange or reorganize their life stories," "come to terms with the meaning of the traumatic event," "find a mission or personal meaning," "rebuild assumptive worlds," "restore positive memories," and "synthesize events." These theorists tend to view PTSD more as a "disorder of meaning," than as a "disorder of anxiety," *per se*.

When operationalized, what do these various mandates for coping have in common? They each are calling for the victims of disasters and other traumatic events to tell their "stories" differently. The "accounts" that victims offer become the "final common pathways" to change. What else does the research literature on coping with traumatic stress tell us about the "stories" that victims tell?

In order for people to "integrate" traumatic experiences into their meaning systems so they do not live in the past, so that traumatic events only become one chapter in their autobiographical memories (and as Herman, 1992, observes, not the most interesting chapter), the victims must employ various cognitive mechanisms as part of their story-telling. Taylor (1990) and Taylor et al. (1983) have identified five such cognitive mechanisms that people report using to cope with distressing situations. These include: (i) comparing oneself with those who are less fortunate; (ii) selectively focusing on positive attributes of oneself in order to feel advantaged; (iii) imagining a potentially worse situation; (iv) construing benefits that might derive from the victimizing experience; and (v) manufacturing normative standards that make one's adjustment seem "normal."

Meichenbaum and Fitzpatrick (1993) have noted that as individuals begin to script and rescript their reactions to traumatic events they recast their roles. Like good story tellers, survivors redefine, embellish, alter their accounts, as they reconstrue what they expect or want from a given situation. The narrator may adopt a stance of resigned acceptance in the form of a fatalistic outlook or impose a culturally shared religious belief or societal ritual as a way to remember in a more benign and accepting fashion.

Prayer, religion, rituals, culturally prescribed commemorative acts, and ceremonies, each help individuals remember in a more adaptive fashion. For instance, in an insightful article, Jay (1994) analyzes how Judaism provides survivors with an organizing metaphor of the "wall of wailing" to tell their stories differently, to see their emotional pain as part of a whole people's suffering. Annual ceremonies and religious holidays enforce the idea that survivors are obligated to remember -- "'Thou shalt remember!" Traumatic memories are to be "contained" and 'sanctified," and not avoided, obliterated, or denied, for such efforts are likely to fail. (Keep in mind research indicating that subjects who attempted to "suppress" specific thoughts are twice as likely to have such thoughts at a later time than those who do not attempt to suppress such ideation; Wegner, 1992). Religious rituals provide meaningful ways to restory an experience. The Vietnam memorial, the Holocaust museum, the visit by a soldier to the parents of a buddy who accidentally he had killed in "friendly fire," the telling of the story of the visit to the childhood site of one's "imprisonment" (e.g., see Breznitz, 1993), and so forth, each become powerful metaphors of the "restorying" process. The following case study illustrates this process in the instance of a natural disaster.

The small Southern town in Piedmont, Alabama is used to storms and destruction, but on Palm Sunday of March, 1994, no one was ready for the tornado that tore through the Goshen Methodist Church, which was filled with parishioners. The storm killed 20, including the minister's four year old daughter. As reported in the New York Times (April 3, 1994), the surviving parishioners used their faith and religious rituals to cope; these acted like "anchors in a turbulent sea." The survivors struggled with such questions as, "But why? Why a church? Why those little children? Why? Why? Why?"

As reported, this incident hurt them in a place usually safe from hurt, it was like a "bruise on the soul." The minister noted that while their "faith is shaken it is not the same as losing it." Events like this only strengthen one's faith as one church-goer commented, "those who die inside any church will find the gates of heaven open wide." Another resident noted, "As long as we have our faith, we are strong. Because no matter how dark it is, if I have faith, I have a song in the night. Our beliefs trembled, but did not break." In response to the persistent questions of "why," the Reverend noted: "There is no reason. Our faith is not determined by reason. Our faith is undergirded by belief, where there is no reason."

For many, if not most, when disaster strikes, when stressors that meet criterion A of DSM-III R are experienced, it is religion and ritual, it is a coherent belief system that represents the central means of coping. Religion and ritual provide powerful culturally accepted metaphors and a framework to construct a new adaptive narrative. Religion provides an acceptable ritual to cognitively reframe events and a means to provide guidance for healing.

As Vernberg and Vogel (1993) observe, rituals serve several important psychological functions including:

1) "opportunities for public expressions of shared grief and mutual support;
2) reassurance that disaster victims are remembered;
3) recapitulation and interpretation of disaster experiences; and
4) provides a degree of closure on a painful period" (p. 496).

Rituals can play an important role in the recovery process (e.g., grieving, talking through the stress, restoring positive memories, finding meaning by taking actions such as bearing witness, publishing memories, engaging in educational missions,

Table 2
Illustrative Metaphors Offered by Traumatized "Victims"
to Describe Their Experience

I. <u>Describe their affective state</u> (hypersensitivity)
   1. Time bomb ticking.
   2. I'm at my breaking point.
   3. I walk a thin red line, walk on egg shells.
   4. I am an emotional yo-yo.
   5. Emotional jack-in-the-box.

II. <u>Describe feelings of being blocked and trapped</u> (psychic numbing)
   1. I am a spectator to life.
   2. I run on auto-pilot, no feelings.
   3. My emotions have been castrated, neutered.
   4. I am a time machine.
   5. I live in partial anesthesia, a robot with no feelings.

III. <u>Describe intrusive thoughts</u>
   1. My mind has run amok. A constant time slide.
   2. My thoughts visit me.
   3. My thoughts have a life of their own.
   4. Indelible, engraved, memories.
   5. A nightmare that cannot stop. My memories are not digestible.

IV. <u>Describe a sense of loss</u>
   1. Hole in me, not complete.
   2. Part of me died.
   3. Wear different lenses. Tunnel vision.
   4. Robbed me of my...social dignity, personhood, innocence, trust, intimacy, ability to relate to others.
   5. Live in no man's land.

V. <u>Describe past traumatizing events</u>
   1. This disaster opened a can of worms.
   2. Skeletons in my closet.
   3. Blackhole (vacuum) in my history.
   4. Baggage I carry with me.
   5. Opened Pandora's Box.

VI <u>Describe characteristics of self</u>
   1. Prisoner of the past.
   2. Damaged goods, crippled.
   3. Deadened, no guideposts.
   4. Counterfeit world.
   5. Stuck in trauma, in a rut, a dead end.

commemorative ceremonies, and taking political action). Another occasion for finding meaning are anniversaries of the event.

An anniversary of the traumatic event can provide an opportunity to look back, "take stock" of how far the individuals, group, or community have come since the disaster. Such ceremonial efforts provide opportunities for bonding, solidarity, and constructing a new narrative. Rituals and ceremonies are each forms of account-making.

Lakoff and Johnson (1980) have highlighted the powerful role that metaphors play in people's story telling. They observe that "we define our reality in terms of metaphors and then proceed to act on the basis of the metaphors. We draw inferences, set goals, make commitments, and execute plans, all on the basis of how we in part structure our experience, consciously or unconsciously, by means of metaphors" (p. 158). When one speaks to individuals who have been traumatized they have very interesting ways to describe their experiences. Words often prove inadequate to describe their distress so in their own way, victims become "poets" (of sorts), as they resort to the use of metaphors to tell their stories. They have specific ways of describing their experience that interestingly coincide with the various clusters of DSM-III-R symptoms of PTSD and related disorders. I have spent quite a bit of time listening to the stories of individuals who have survived traumatic events, both natural and those of intentional human design. Table 2 provides an abbreviated list of the metaphors individuals employ as part of their narratives. Imagine the impact of individuals telling themselves and others their stories using such metaphors. If we go back to my opening account of the various "near death" experiences and mishaps I have encountered, we can now begin to co-construct the nature of what I would have had to say to myself (and to others) in order to develop PTSD and related distress. You, the reader, could now begin to predict what must be present and absent from my account if I am to evidence maladaptive versus adaptive behavior.

Before scripting a too harsh narrative, it is worth noting that Meichenbaum and Fitzpatrick (1993) have reported that it is not merely the presence of stress engendering "negative thoughts" that distinguishes those who cope versus those who do not cope with stressful events. Individuals who adjust more effectively on some occasions, or early on in response to disasters, may also employ stress-engendering metaphors. It is not the absence of "negative thinking" *per se*, but rather it is the ratio of "positive" to "negative" thinking (2 to 1, respectively) that correlates with adaptive coping. Thus, those individuals who experience traumatic events often include positive metaphors in their story telling (see Table 3). As Baumeister (1989) has proposed, one's narrative should reflect the "optimal margin of illusion. It may be most adaptive to hold a view of self that is a little better than the truth -- neither too inflated nor too accurate" (p. 189). Baumeister is calling for a specific style of narrative to facilitate coping.

Another critical feature of story telling is the need to share one's story with others. Pennebaker's (1989) program of studies indicated that having individuals such as Holocaust survivors, adults who have been terminated from their job, and first year college students who are adjusting to a new setting, as well as victims of an earthquake, write or talk about the upsetting events, resulted in improved psychological and physical well-being (e.g., improved long-term immune functioning, lowered autonomic nervous system activity, reduced visits to physicians, and improved self-reports of adjustment). The findings about the earthquake victims are particularly relevant to this volume. During the initial two or three weeks after the earthquake the victims were preoccupied with thoughts about the upheaval. At the same time, their social contacts increased and people were able to openly express their anxieties, thoughts, and feelings to others. During this initial time, <u>negligible changes</u> in health problems, nightmares, and social conflicts occurred. Between 3 and 6 weeks after the earthquake there was a significant decrease in the opportunity to talk about the upheaval, but many individuals continued to have thoughts about the earthquake and its aftermath. It was during this "inhibition phase" that social conflicts, disturbing dreams, and health problems surfaced. It was also during this "inhibition phase" when many significant others did <u>not</u> want to hear other people talk about the earthquake, although many survivors wished to talk about it. This "inhibitory" atmosphere was epitomized by the sale of T-shirts that read, "Thank you for <u>not</u> sharing your earthquake experience." After 6 weeks for most individuals the psychological upheaval was over and signs of distress receded (Pennebaker & Harber, 1994).

Table 3
Illustrative Metaphors Offered by Traumatized "Victims"
to Convey Their Hope for Change

I want to write a new chapter.
I want to join the world, join life.
Bear witness.
Be reborn again.
Get back in the driver's seat.
make peace with the past.
Take charge of my life.
I want to be a gardener, not just the florist.
Recharge my batteries.
I want to be the person before all this happened.
In the same way I don't trust everything I read in the newspapers, I want to learn not to trust everything I say to myself.
I want to believe in order and purpose again. As Einstein said, "God doesn't play dice with the world."
I want this trauma to lose its gripping quality.

What is it about the writing or the speaking about a traumatic upheaval that is healing? What is it about constructing a narrative that proves helpful? While we do not know the exact answers to these questions we can, nevertheless, begin to speculate. As noted earlier, traumatic events can provoke an increased number of intrusive, fragmented, and disorganized thoughts about the upheaval and its aftermath. In fact, Baum et al. (1993) have reported that the more the individual has intrusive memories of the traumatic event, the more symptoms of somatic chronic distress he/she will experience (as evident by increased urinary cortisol and norepinephrine levels, heightened systolic blood pressure, as well as poorer attentional performance). Intrusive memories appear to be less diagnostically significant early in post-accident situations, but they become more and more diagnostically significant as time passes. Nolen-Hoeksma (1990) also report that the level of rumination is highly correlated with measures of anxiety, depression, and sleep disturbance. Such intrusive ideation reflects a particular form of constructive narrative.

Writing and talking about distressing events can help change this pattern by:

a) facilitating the expression and labeling of feelings;
b) making one's thoughts and feelings about the events more organized (i.e., since language is both structured and social, talking and writing forces one's thoughts to be implicitly more integrated, less fragmented, leading to a more coherent explanation, and to an increased likelihood of accepting the unchangeable aspects of the situation);
c) influencing the accessibility of the thoughts and feelings (i.e., not being as preoccupied as a result of putting their stories into words), and also soliciting feedback from others;
d) fostering a new perspective, reframing of the stressful situation, and increasing the likelihood of reaching some degree of acceptance and closure; and
e) fostering a sense of control and nurturing hope.

As Pennebaker and Francis (in press) conclude, "Failure to translate upsetting experiences into language [or some other form of expression] can result in psychological conflict and stress-related health problems" (p. 21). In short, there is increasing evidence from a variety of sources to indicate that how individuals construct narratives and how they tell their stories about traumatic events play a critical role in their adjustment process. This is clearly a critical tenet of those who have conducted Critical Incident Stress Debriefing (e.g., see Mitchell and Everly, 1994).

The research challenge for those who propose such a constructive narrative perspective is to develop reliable coding systems of survivors' "accounts," and to relate them to concurrent and predictive levels of adjustment. A challenging question will be to determine if the changes in survivors' accounts, over time, relate to changes in various PTSD symptomatology (e.g., intrusive ideation avoidance/numbing and increased arousal), as well as, to various measures of information processing (e.g., Stroop performance), and to measures of altered belief systems? Are the changes in the survivors' accounts a mere "epiphenomenon" that reflects changes in adjustment, or are the "stories" that victims offer critical causative factors that influence adjustment? Are the physiological changes that accompany intrusive ideation (a la Baum, Pennebaker) also evident when the unit to be analyzed is the survivor's "account" (e.g., metaphors, presence of cognitive mechanisms a la Taylor, as well as behavioral indicators, such as engaging in healing activities)? Moreover, how do such narrative accounts relate to various indicators of resource losses (a la Hobfoll, Freedy), and to the other factors enumerated in Appendix A?

If one adopts a biopsychosocial perspective of response to traumatic events a research agenda can be established that begins to examine the complex interdependencies across various levels of response to disasters. We can begin to study how, when, with whom, and with what effect, do "victims" tell their stories to others (as well as share stories with themselves as in the form of personal diaries). Moreover, how do these stories change over time, with or without social supports, with and without psychological interventions?

Finally, it would be an oversight to adopt a parochial, Westernized perspective on the relationships between disasters, stress, and cognition. There is a need to adopt and maintain a cross-cultural perspective and not allow a Western mentality to impose an ethnocentric prism on our search for answers. Since non-Western countries constitute more than two thirds of the world population, any consideration of the role that stress and cognition play in response to disasters need to take a cross-cultural perspective into consideration. For instance, in non-Westernized societies the human suffering that accompany both natural and man-made disasters are more likely to be viewed as an expression of external forces, and are more likely to be expressed in the form of somatizing behaviors. As Nikelly (1992) observes, "the cognitive dimension of sufferers from non-Westernized countries is much less marked, and bodily organs are cited metaphorically to convey 'pain' and 'conflict' (e.g., 'My heart aches', 'My liver is eating at me.'). Non-westerners often attribute their emotional condition to forces outside themselves" (p. 18). Such culturally-different explanatory styles must be taken into consideration in any description of the relationships between disasters, stress, and coping.

Finally, I am pleased and relieved to report that nothing untoward happened during the course of the NATO conference. This is just the type of disconfirming data, if repeated, that will cause me to give up my "ideas of reference."

References

Baum, A (1990). Stress, intrusive imagery, and chronic distress. Health Psychology, 9, 653-675.
Baum, A., Cohen, L., & Hall, M. (1993). Control and intrusive memories as possible determinants of chronic stress. Psychosomatic Medicine, 55, 274-286.
Baumeister, R.F. (1993). Meanings of life. New York: Guilford Press.
Bolin, R. (1988). Response to natural disasters. In M.L. Lystad (Ed.), Health response to mass emergencies: Theories and practice. New York: Brunner/Mazel.
Breznitz, S. (1993). Memory fields. New York: Alfred Knopf.
Bromet, E.J. (1989). The nature and effects of technological failures. In R.Gist & B. Lubin (Eds.), Psychosocial aspects of disaster. New York: Wiley.
Cardena, E., & Spiegel, D. (1993). Dissociative reactions to the San Francisco bay area earthquake of 1989. American Journal of Psychiatry, 150, 474-478.
Dew, M.A., Bromet, E., & Schulberg, H.C. (1987). A comparative analysis of two community stressors' long-term mental health effects. American Journal of Community Psychology, 15, 167-184.
Foa, E.B., Steketee, G., & Olasov-Rothbaum, B. (1989). Behavioral/cognitive conceptualizations of post-traumatic stress disorder. Behavior Therapy, 20, 155-176.
Freedy, J.R., Kilpatrick, D.G., & Resnick, H.S. (1993). Natural disasters and mental health. Journal of Social Behavior and Personality, 8, 49-103.
Freedy, J.R., Saladin, M.E., Kilpatrick, D.G., Resnick, H.S., & Saunders, B.E. (1994). Understanding acute psychological distress following natural disaster. Journal of Traumatic Stress, 7, 257-274.
Giel, R. (1990). Psychosocial processes in disasters. International Journal of Mental Health, 19, 7-20.
Gleser, G.C., Green, B.L., & Winget, C.N. (1978). Quantifying interview data in psychic impairment of disaster survivors. Journal of Nervous and Mental Disease, 166, 209-216.
Goenjian, A. (1993). A mental health relief programme in Armenia after the 1988 earthquake: Implementation and clinical observations. British Journal of Psychiatry, 163, 230-239.
Goodman, L., Koss, M., & Russo, N.F. (1993). Conceptualizations of posttraumatic stress. Applied and Preventive Psychology, 2, 123-130.
Green, B.L. (1982). Assessing levels of psychological impairment following disaster: Consideration of actual and methodological dimensions. Journal of Nervous and Mental Disease, 170, 544-550.
Green, B. L. (this volume). Long-term consequences of disasters. In S. E. Hobfoll & M. W. deVries (Eds.), Extreme stress and communities: Impact and intervention. Dordrecht, the Netherlands: Kluwer.

Green, B.L., Grace, M.C., Vary, M.G., Kramer, T.L., Gleser, G.C., & Leonard, A.C. (1994). Children of disaster in the second decade: A 17-year follow-up of Buffalo Creek survivors. Journal of American Academy Child and Adolescent Psychiatry, 33, 71-79.

Green, B.L., Lindy, J.D., et al. (1990). Buffalo Creek survivors in the second decade: Stability of stress symptoms. American Journal of Orthopsychiatry, 60, 43-54.

Harvey, J.H., Orbuch, T.L., Weber, A.L., Merbach, N., & Alt, R. (1992). House of pain and hope: Accounts of loss. Death Studies, 16, 99-124.

Harvey, J.H., Weber, A.L., & Orbuch, T.L. (1990). Interpersonal accounts: A social psychological perspective. Oxford, England: Basil Blackwell.

Herman, J.L. (1992). Trauma and recovery. New York: Basic Books.

Hobfoll, S.E. & Lilly, R.S. (1993). Resource conservation as a strategy for community psychology. Journal of Community Psychology, 21, 128-148.

Hobfoll, S.E. (1991). Traumatic stress: A theory based on rapid loss of resources. Anxiety Research, 4, 187-197.

Holen, A. (1991). A longitudinal study of the occurrence and persistence of post-traumatic health problems in disaster survivors, Stress Medicine, 7, 11-17.

Horowitz, M.J. (1986). Stress-response syndromes (2nd ed.). Northvale, NJ: Aronson.

Janoff-Bulman, R. (1992). Shattered assumptions: Towards a new psychology of trauma. New York: Free Press.

Janoff-Bulman, R., & Frieze, I.H. (1983). A theoretical perspective for understanding reactions to victimizations. Journal of Social Issues, 39, 1-17.

Jay, J. (1994). Walls for wailing. Common Boundary, May/June, 30-35.

Jones, J.C., & Barlow, D.H. (1990). The etiology of posttraumatic stress disorder. Clinical Psychology Review, 10, 299-328.

Keane, T.M., Gerardi, R.J., Quinn, S.J., & Litz, B.T. (1992). Behavioral treatment of posttraumatic stress disorder. In S.M. Turner, K.S. Calhoun and H.E. Adams (Eds.), Handbook of Clinical behavior therapy. Second Edition. New York: Wiley.

Kleber, R.J., Brom, D., & Defares, P.B. (1992). Coping with trauma: Theory, prevention and treatment. Amsterdam: Swets & Zectlinger.

Lakoff, G., & Johnson, M. (1980). Metaphors we live by. Chicago: University of Chicago Press.

Lindy, F.D., Grace, M. C., & Green, B.L. (1981). Survivors: Outreach to a relevant population. American Journal of Orthopsychiatry, 31, 468-478.

Lomranz, J. (this volume). Endurance and living: Long-term effects of the Holocaust. In S. E. Hobfoll & M. W. deVries (Eds.), Extreme stress and communities: Impact and intervention. Dordrecht, the Netherlands: Kluwer.

Lonigan, C.J., Mitsuko, S.P., Taylor, C.M., Finch, A.J., & Sallee, F.R. (1994). Children exposed to disaster: II. Risk factors for the development of post-traumatic symptomatology. Journal of American Academy of Child and Adolescent Psychiatry, 33, 94-105.

Mair, M. (1990). Telling psychological tales. International Journal of Personal Construct Psychology, 3, 121-135.

Marmar, C., & Horowitz, M.J. (1988). Diagnosis and phase-oriented treatment of post-traumatic stress disorder. In J. Wilson, Z. Harel, & B. Kahana (Eds.). Human adaptation to extreme stress: From the holocaust to Vietnam. New York: Plenum Press.

McCann, I.L., & Pearlman, L.A. (1990b). Psychological trauma and the adult survivor: Theory, therapy and transformation. New York: Brunner/Mazel.

McFarlane, A.C. (1989). The etiology of post traumatic morbidity: Predisposing precipitating and perpetuating factors. British Journal of Psychiatry, 154. 221-228.

Meichenbaum, D., & Fitzpatrick, D. (1993) A constructivist narrative perspective on stress and coping. Stress inoculation applications. In.L. Goldberger and S. Breznitz (Eds.) Handbook of stress: Theoretical and clinical aspects. (Second Edition). New York: Free Press.

Meichenbaum, D., & Fong, G. (1993). How individuals control their own minds: A constructive narrative perspective. In D. M. Wegner & J. W. Pennebaker (Eds.). Handbook of Mental control. New York: Prentice Hall.

Mitchell, J.T., & Everly, G.S. (1994). Preventing work related post-traumatic stress: The Critical Incident Stress Debriefing (CISD). In G.S. Everly & J.M. Lating (Eds), Psychotraumatology. New York: Plenum Press.

Nikelly, A.G. (1992). Can DSM-III-R be used in the diagnosis of non-Western patients? International Journal of Mental Health, 21, 3-22.

Nolen-Hoeksma, S. (1990). Sex differences in depression. Stanford, CA: Stanford University Press.

Pennebaker, J.W. (1989). Confession, inhibition, and disease. In L. Berkowitz (Ed.), Advances in experimental social psychology, Vol. 22. Orlando, FL: Academic Press.

Pennebaker, J.W., & Francis, M.E. (1994). Cognitive, emotional, and language processes in writing. Unpublished manuscript, Southern Methodist University, Dallas, TX.

Pennebaker, J.W., & Harber, K.D. (1993). A social stage model of collective coping: The Loma Prieta earthquake and the Persian Gulf war. Journal of Social Issues, 49,. 125-146.

Pennebaker, J.W., & Susman, J. (1988). Disclosure of traumas and psychosomatic processes. Social Science and Medicine, 26, 327-332.

Rachman, S. (1980). Emotional processing. Behavior Research and Therapy, 18, 15-60.

Raphael, B. (1986). When disaster strikes. London: Hutchinson.

Rubonis, A.V., & Bickman, L. (1991). Psychological impairment in the wake of disaster: The disaster -psychopathology relationship. Psychological Bulletin, 109, 384-399.

Sarbin, T.R. (1986). The narrative as a root metaphor for psychology. In T.R. Sarbin, Narrative psychology. New York: Praegar.

Silver, R.L., & Wortman, C.B. (1980). Coping with undesirable life events. In J. Garber & M.E.P. Seligman (Eds.), Human helplessness: Theory and applications (pp.279-340). New York: Academic Press.

Silver, R.L., Boon, C., & Stones, M.H. (1983). Searching for meaning in misfortune: Making sense of incest. Journal of Social Issues, 39, 81-102.

Smith, E.M., North, C.S., McCool, R.E., & Shea, J.M. (1990). Acute postdisaster psychiatric disorders: Identification of persons at risk. American Journal of Psychiatry, 147, 202-206.

Solomon, S.D. & Green, B.L. (1992). Mental health effects of natural and human made disasters. PTSD Research Quarterly, 3, 1-8.

Solomon, S.D., & Smith, E.M. (1993). Social support and perceived control as moderators of responses to dioxin and flood exposure. In R. Ursano, B. McCaughey, & C. Fullerton (Eds.). Individual and community responses to trauma. New York: Guilford.

Taylor, S.E. (1990). Positive illusions. New York: Basic Books.

Taylor, S., Wood, J., & Lichtman, R. (1983). It could be worse: Selective evaluation as a response to victimization. Journal of Social Issues, 39, 719-740.

Thrasher, S.M., Dalgesh, T., & Yule, W. (1994). Information processing in posttraumatic stress disorder. Behaviour Research and Therapy, 32, 247-253.

van der Kolk, B.A. (1987). Psychological trauma. Washington, D.C.: American Psychiatric Press.

Vernberg, E.M., & Vogel, J.M. (1993). Interventions with children after disasters. Journal of Clinical Child Psychology, 22, 485-498.

Vogel, J.M., & Vernberg, E.M. (1993). Children's psychological responses to disasters. Journal of Clinical Child Psychology, 22, 464-484.

Wegner, D.M. (1989). White bears and other unwanted thoughts. New York: Viking Press.

Weisaeth, L. (1992). Prepare and repair: Some principles in prevention of psychiatric consequences of traumatic stress. Psychiatria Fennica, 23, 11-18.

Wilson, J.P. & Raphael, B. (Eds.) (1993). International handbook of traumatic stress syndromes. New York: Plenum Press.

Appendix A

Possible Vulnerability Factors:
Who is at "High Risk" for Developing PTSD and Other Forms of Maladjustment?

The vulnerability factors and accompanying questions are divided into three categories:

(i) Characteristics of the disaster (essentially within disaster characteristics)
   a) Objective (factors that can be independently corroborated)
   b) Subjective (based primarily on individual's or group's perceptions)

(ii) Characteristics of the post-disaster response and environmental recovery factors
   a) Reactions of the individual and group
   b) Reactions involving others

(iii) Characteristics of the individual and group (pre-disaster characteristics)

First the factor is highlighted and then it is framed in the form of a "yes", "no" questions that can be directed to the "victim(s)". The more "yes" answers, the greater the proposed risk for developing PTSD and related forms of distress.

I. Characteristics of the Disaster

<u>Objective factors directly affecting the "victim" and "significant others"</u>

1.	Proximity to disaster and duration of the stressor	Was the individual close or "relatively" close to the site of the disaster? Did the individual experience a "narrow escape?" (The greater the proximity, intensity and duration, the poorer the level of adjustment).
2.	Degree of physical harm or injury	Was the individual physically injured?

3.	Intentionality of injury or harm along a "continuum of deliberateness"	Was the individual injured "on purpose"?
4.	Witness violence	Did the individual witness physical violence?
5.	Witness violent or sudden death of others -- like one's loved one or of a child or a friend	Did the individual witness the death of a "significant other"? Was there violent or sudden death to loved ones? Has the parent lost a child? Did the individual helplessly witness such deaths?
6.	Exposure to grotesque or mutilating deaths of others -- exposure to mass deaths or human remains	Was the individual exposed to grotesque sights, sounds and smells (e.g., mutilated and severed bodies)? Was the individual exposed to scenes of death and destruction? If there was injury or death, was there disfigurement, mutilation and other grotesque sights? Was the individual exposed to mutilated or burned bodies? Was the individual exposed to mass deaths or mass dying? Was the individual exposed to traumatic events that were vivid and emotionally powerful? Were children among the injured and dead? Does the individual identify with the victims?
7.	Degree of property damage to "victim" and others ($5,000+)	Did the individual experience a substantial degree of property damage to the point where his/her home is uninhabitable? Is the individual living in make-shift quarters? Was there sudden and severe property loss to others, as well? Will the property damage take a long time to repair? Is the landscape devastated?

8. Learning of one's exposure to further potential threats — Is the individual or group at continued "high risk" for future stressors?

9. Irreversibility of resource losses (prolonged environmental disruption) — Is the individual, family, group <u>unable</u> to reverse losses (i.e., failure to recover lost possessions, property, job, income, and other personal losses)? Is there continual displacement? Is there loss of both home <u>and</u> job or livelihood?

10. Escape blocked or experience impossible choices — Was escape blocked for the individual? Was the individual faced with impossible choices such as help others at great risk to one's own survival?

11. Constant reminders -- remain in or near epicenter — Are there constant reminders of the accident or traumatic event? Is the individual(s) chronically exposed to reminders of the traumatic events? Is there an absence of a "safety signal?"

12. Signs of injury — Is the impact of the traumatic event evident to the individual, but "invisible" or not readily noticeable to others?

13. Involve noxious agents — Was the individual or loved ones exposed to noxious agents or experienced continuing threat from potential toxicity or radiation? Are there continuing concerns and uncertainty about possible long-term health consequences?

14. Degree of physical injury and death to others and loved ones — Was there violent, sudden or severe injury or death to a "loved one," or friend or neighbor (e.g., number of friends killed)? Did the individual have to wait a prolonged period to hear about the fate of loved ones?

15.	How information of death was conveyed	If there was death that was not witnessed was the news of the death conveyed in a non-supportive fashion? Not told why he/she cannot view body of significant other?
16.	Description of social supports -- both immediate and long-term	(i) Was the individual separated from family members during or immediately after the disaster? (ii) Was there significant disruption of social supports and kin networks with accompanying loss of proximity to friends and relatives?

"Subjective" factors related to the "victim" and "significant others"

17.	Perception of the disaster	(i) Was the disaster viewed as unexpected, unpredictable, sudden, as compared to a predictable disaster (e.g., seasonal flooding)? (ii) Was the threat <u>not</u> known to exist?
18.	Perception of the "intensity" of threat to life or bodily integrity to self or family	Did the disaster cause "threat" to life survival or to physical integrity? Is the traumatic event perceived as being continually threatening to one's life or well-being or to his/her loved ones?
19.	Perception of "psychological" and "physical" demands	Did the disaster cause excessive demands and entail extended exposure?
20.	Perception of cause of the disaster	Did the individual(s) perceive the disaster as being due to callousness ... irresponsibility ... greed ... stupidity? Does the individual(s) feel the disaster was preventable and controllable? Is there someone to blame?

21.	Perception of preparation	Did the individual(s) feel unprepared for the disaster? Was there lack of training for such disasters? Was there an opportunity to warn potential victims ahead of time, so they could take precautions, but the warning was not given? Were the potential victims unable to take precautions after the warning? Did the individual fail to respond to anticipatory warnings? Could the event have been prevented or the injury/destruction reduced?
22.	Perception of lack of personal control	Does the individual feel a loss of control over social processes that are generally perceived as being in control? ... Does the disaster represent a breakdown in a "system" that is not supposed to falter? Does the individual experience a loss of personal control?
23.	Perception of assistance offered	Did the individual offer assistance to others that proved to be unhelpful ... futile ... or even made things worse (e.g., further property loss)?
24.	Perception of personal responsibility -- blame self	Does the individual see himself/herself as being in a role that resulted in injury or death to others because of what he/she did or failed to do?
25.	Perception of social supports	Does the individual(s) feel he/she has no, or few, family members, friends, neighbors to turn to for help? Did the disaster interfere with peer support?

II. Characteristics of the Post-disaster Response

Reactions of the Individual

26. Intense initial emotional reactions to disaster. For example, symptomatic response/ panic/anxiety/dissociation/ sadness/depression

    In the immediate aftermath of the traumatic event did the individual develop high levels of anxiety and/or evidence dissociative reactions? In children did they evidence being sad, grieving over potential and realized losses, feel alone during and immediately after the traumatic event? Does the individual experience the "pressure" of PTSD symptoms?

27. Feelings of helplessness

    Did the individual experience terror and feel helpless and powerless during and after the event?

28. Symptomatic responses/sleep disturbance/insomnia/agitation

    In subsequent weeks following the disaster, did the individual evidence insomnia or agitation?

29. Presence of continual intrusive ideation

    a) Does the individual have persistent intrusive thoughts, images, dreams, nightmares of the traumatic experience?
    b) Does the individual continue to repetitively "relive" and reexperience the event and its aftermath? (Note, 3 months following the event is usually taken as a guidepost when such intrusive symptoms should become less frequent and less disruptive)

30. Degree of bereavement

    Is the individual acquainted with the victims? Is the individual grieving the loss of significant others?

31.	Presence of evidence to "work through" and "resolve" trauma	Is the individual having difficulty "integrating" or constructing "a new world view," or having difficulty "moving beyond" this event (i.e., a constructive resolution)? Does the individual, family or group lack a coherent framework (e.g., religious or philosophical outlook) that would help make sense of what has happened? Is the individual continuing to "search for meaning" by pursuing the answer to "why" questions, for which there are no acceptable answers?
32.	Self-disclosure opportunities	Is the individual unable or unwilling to talk with others about the trauma and his/her reactions?

Reactions involving significant others -- environment recovery factors

33.	Opportunity for self-disclosure, working through and resolution	Does the individual think about the upheaval a good deal, but have limited access or opportunity to share his/her feelings and thoughts with others?
34.	Lack of social support	Are kin or neighbors/friends available to provide material and social support? Has the family failed to share their different experiences about the disaster?
35.	Extent of dislocation or displacement (move often and move furthest away against one's will - involuntary relocation)	Was (Is) the individual and his/her family placed in an unfamiliar environment due to the disaster (dislocated)? Is the nuclear family still apart? Does the relocation plan fail to take into consideration family or neighborhood patterns and wishes? Was relocation done arbitrarily? (What is the length of time in so-called "temporary housing?")

36.	Disruption social support	Was there significant disruption of social support and kin networks with accompanying loss of proximity to friends and relatives?
37.	Impact of disaster on social support providers	Are the kinfolk or neighbors/friends who are providing support also "victims" of the disaster or "victims" of its aftermath?
38.	Stress of receiving social support	Has the evacuee individual or family "worn out his/her welcome" with the host family (e.g., stayed longer than 1 month)?
39.	Resumption of normal routines -- exposure to continued adversities such as financial strain, lack of transportation, residential displacement, jobless	Has the individual and his/her family and community been unable to reestablish "normal" routines (e.g., sleeping arrangements, communication, transportation arrangements, work and school schedules)? Is there still dislocation and unemployment? Has the individual or group failed to engage in any proactive actions (e.g., attempts to change things)?
40.	Stress reactions of significant others	Did the parent(s) evidence exaggerated emotional response at the time of the disaster or at the reunion? Do "significant others" (e.g., parents) evidence continual distress? Is the individual exposed to a social network of negative rumors that acts like a stress contagion or what has been called a "pressure cooker effect"? Are parents intolerant of their child's proclivity to engage in regressive behavior?

41. Community efforts at rebuilding and social support -- evidence of community solidarity, group cohesion and a common purpose and programs

Has the community failed to organize efforts to rebuild or cope in some <u>acceptable</u> fashion? Does the community evidence little concern and lack a supportive response? Is there absence of any temporary community near the disaster site for victim families? Has the group or community <u>failed to</u> engage in any group bereavement or memorial service (i.e., did <u>not</u> provide ritual healing ceremonies)? Is there disruption in community life and routines? Is there a shortage of food and petrol and health care services? Is there a lack of counseling?

42. Nature of information

Is the information following the disaster seen as confusing, inconsistent or contradictory? Is there an absence of an ascribed individual or designated group who gathers and disseminates information to combat negative rumors?

43. Nature of designated leadership

Are the authorities in charge seen as being untrustworthy, secretive, and inconsistent, and as a result suffering from a loss of credibility, leading to general mistrust?

44. Mitigating factors to recovery

Is the recovery process being hampered by extensive media coverage, litigation hearings, difficulty over insurance claims, unavailability of contractor or unscrupulous behaviors by contractors/repairmen/storekeepers, dispute with authorities about recovery procedures such as decontamination, lack of information about permanent housing, long term loans, and the like?

45.	How community views victim(s) -- stigmatization	Does the community (society) view the individual ("victim") who has gone through the traumatic events in a "negative" fashion? Is there a "stigma" attached to asking for help?
46.	Secondary victimization	Did the individual experience "secondary victimization" (e.g., from agencies such as police, doctors, courts, insurance companies)? Has the individual experienced a loss in the market value of his/her home as a result of the disaster?

III. Characteristics of the Individual and Group

47.	High risk factors -- Is the individual a member of a group who lives on the "margin" of society or is likely to be "overlooked" or "forgotten" (e.g., geographically isolated, frail and elderly, homeless, physically or mentally ill, lack financial or social resources.	Is the individual at particular risk because he/she is a single parent, middle aged with responsibility to both children and parents, frailed elderly, or from a lower SES level, or a child separated from his/her family as an immediate aftermath of the disaster? Is the individual or parent unemployed or work for low wages? Is the individual single, widowed, divorced? Is the child of a single, divorced or separated parent? Does the child not reside with family members?
48.	Prior history of adjustment problems to stressors and other traumatic events	Did the individual and family members adjust poorly to prior major losses or stressors?
49.	Prior history of mental illness (e.g., anxiety, depression, substance abuse)	Does the individual have a history of mental illness? For example, is there a personal or family history of anxiety disorders? In children is there evidence of high trait anxiety prior to the disaster?

50. Presence of comorbidity — Is the individual evidencing anxiety, phobias, depression, addictive behaviors and somatization?

51. Prior exposure, to traumatic events, anniversary effects, reactive unresolved conflicts (e.g., prior violent crime victimization) — Were there prior stressors that influenced the present reactions to the disaster (e.g., anniversary effects), or exposure to prior stressful events? Did the events reactivate prior unresolved conflicts and reactions from prior victimization?

52. Premorbid evidence marital and familial distress — Was there marital or familial discord prior to the disaster?

53. Family vulnerability — Is the family "vulnerable" as evident in the "pile-up" of family life changes and demands? Does the family have a history of irritability with each other, depression, despair and family instability?

54. Family style of communicating — Do the family members engage in what are called "hot reactions," tending to blow-up small events into larger crises, use language that is blaming, critical, inflames reactions, and other similar "high expressed emotional" behaviors (e.g., being overprotective unwittingly reinforcing overdependent behaviors)?

55. Exposure to sustained anticipatory alerts — Was the individual or group exposed to a sustained anticipatory alerts?

56. Degree of preparedness — Does the individual/group/community lack experience and/or training in dealing with such traumatic events (disasters)? Has the individual been assigned (as compared to volunteering) for this recovery work or involuntarily assigned to live in this residential area? Is the individual or group unable to use rescue skills that he/she was trained for?

57. Exposure to low magnitude pre-existing non-traumatic, stressful life events in the last year

Was the individual (family, group) exposed to a series of low magnitude stressful events in the last year?

58. Exposure to traumatic events over the course of a lifetime.

Was the individual (family, group) exposed to a series of traumatic events over the course of a lifetime?

TEMPERAMENT RISK FACTOR: THE CONTRIBUTION OF TEMPERAMENT
TO THE CONSEQUENCES OF THE STATE OF STRESS

Jan Strelau
University of Warsaw, Faculty of Psychology
Warsaw, Poland

An individual differences approach may be applied to the phenomena of: stressors, the state of stress, coping with stress, and consequences of stress as expressed in psychophysiological and psychological costs. There exists an enormous number of factors that, in interaction with each other, determine the individual-specific components of stress. A list of some of them has been presented elsewhere (Strelau, 1989a). Among the many determinants of individual differences, considerable attention has been devoted to personality characteristics. The latter have been mostly considered as moderators of stress. Considerable research has been devoted to such more or less stable characteristics as: hardiness (e.g., Kobasa, 1979; Kobasa & Puccetti, 1983), repression-sensitization (e.g., Krohne, 1986), self-esteem (e.g., Chan, 1977; Ormel & Schaufeli, 1991), locus of control (e.g., Ormel & Schaufeli, 1991; Parkes, 1984), self-confidence (e.g., Holohan & Moos, 1986), and sense of coherence (Antonovsky, 1987). Among personality attributes a special place in research on stress should be given to temperament to which this chapter refers.

The Main Constructs Under Consideration

Before entering the subject of this chapter it is necessary to define the main constructs under discussion. This avoids misunderstandings and confusion.

Temperament as a Moderator of Stress

For the purpose of this chapter temperament is defined as referring to basic, relatively stable personality traits that are present from early childhood on, and occur in man and animals. Being primarily determined by biological factors, temperament undergoes slow changes caused by maturation and individual-specific genotype-environment interactions.

In several temperament theories the assumption that temperament plays an important role in moderating stress is incorporated as one of the most important postulates. For example, Kagan (1983) considered the two types of temperament distinguished by him--inhibited and uninhibited temperaments--as representing differential vulnerability to experience stress under situations of unexpected or unpredictable events. According to Nebylitsyn (1972) and Strelau (1983) the functional significance of temperament is evident when individuals are confronted with extreme situations or demands.

In arousal-oriented theories of temperament, which refer to the concepts of optimal level of arousal or stimulation, temperamental characteristics are regarded as moderators in experiencing the state of stress under extreme levels of stimulation, as exemplified in the domain of extraversion (Eysenck, 1970; Eysenck & Eysenck, 1985), stimulus screening (Mehrabian, 1977), reactivity (Strelau, 1983, 1988), sensation seeking (Zuckerman, 1979, 1994), or approach-withdrawal tendencies (McGuire & Turkewitz, 1979).

The question arises, why temperamental traits should be considered as important variables, moderating stress phenomena. Being more or less nonspecific characteristics, they penetrate all kinds of behavior, whatever the content or direction of this behavior. In so doing they contribute to a variety of stress phenomena. Connected mainly with energetic and temporal characteristics of behavior they take part as moderators in all stress phenomena that may be characterized by means of energy and time. Many temperament characteristics are related to emotions, as expressed in a tendency to generate emotional processes. As commonly accepted (see e.g., Lazarus, 1991, 1993), emotions are one of the core constructs for understanding stress.

The statements drawn above may be illustrated by referring to temperament with respect to the four following stress-related events: (1) the impact of temperament in determining the intensity of stressors; (2) the role of temperament as a co-determinant of the state of stress; (3) the moderating effect of temperament in coping with stress; and (4) the contribution of temperamental traits to the psychophysiological and psychological costs of the state of stress.

The Understanding of Stress Phenomena

There is no agreement regarding the understanding of stress and related phenomena, thus, before entering the main object of this paper some explanations are needed regarding my own position among the different conceptualizations in the domain of stress.

Stressors and psychological stress. I refer to the understanding of psychological stress as a state that is characterized by strong negative emotions, such as fear, anxiety, anger, hostility, or other emotional states evoking distress, accompanied by physiological and biochemical changes that evidently exceed the baseline level of arousal. Neuroendocrine changes are inherent attributes of emotions, thus, they cannot be ignored as components of psychological stress. This statement is based on strong empirical evidence, of which, the most representative are the studies conducted by Frankenhaeuser (1979, 1986) with respect to adrenal-medullary and adrenal-cortical changes as a reaction to stressors. This view differs from from that of Lazarus (1993). In his definition of stress he does not recognize the place of arousal as a component of stress. In fact he reduces the state of stress to emotions.

Most researchers on stress differ regarding the causes determining the state of stress. According to my own view (Strelau, 1988), the state of stress is caused by the lack of equilibrium (occurrence of discrepancy) between demands and the individual's capability (capacity) to cope with them. Such a conceptualization of stress can be also found in the literature (see Laux & Vossell, 1982; McGrath, 1970; Schulz & Schonpflug, 1982). The magnitude of the state of stress is a function of the size of discrepancy between the demands and capacities, assuming, the individual is motivated to cope with the demands with which he or she is confronted.

The demands are regarded as stressors or stress-inducing situations. The following factors may be considered as demands: unpredictable and uncontrollable life events, hassles, significant life changes, situations of extreme high or extreme low stimulative value, internalized values and standards of behavior. Demands exist in two forms: objective and subjective, the latter as a result of individual-specific appraisal.

Demands that exist objectively, act as such independently of the individual's perception. This refers to traumatic or extreme life changes, such as death, bereavement, disaster and war. However, objectively existing stressors may be modified by the process of appraisal that results in elevating or reducing the effect of objective stressors. As shown by Holmes and Rahe (1967) there is a very high degree of consensus between groups and among individuals about the significance of life events. The fact that there exist correlations about .9 across age, sex, marital status and education in the intensity and time necessary to accommodate to specific life events speaks in favor of the existence of objective, universal stressors (see Aldwin, Levenson, Spiro III & Bosse, 1989; Freedy, Kilpatrick & Resnick, 1993; Pellegrini, 1990).

The individual's capability to cope with demands depends on the following characteristics: intelligence, special abilities, skills, knowledge, personality and temperamental traits, features of the physical make-up, experience with stress-inducing situations, coping strategies and the actual (physical and psychic) state of the individual.

Depending on the specificity of the demands different individual characteristics influence individuals' capability. Capabilities, too, may occur in two forms. They exist objectively, and as such they may be subject to measurement. But they also may be subjectively experienced, the latter being a result of individual-specific appraisal. In both forms (objective and subjective) the imbalance between them may be considered as a source of psychological stress. What is underlined here is the fact that the state of stress is a result of interaction between real or perceived demands and individuals' response capability as it exists in reality or as it is perceived by them.

The interactional approach to the causes of the state of stress is present in different conceptualizations, however with views differing in specific aspects of the interactional processes (see e.g., McGrath, 1970; Lazarus, 1991; Lazarus & Folkman, 1984).

Also if we define stress in terms of resources, which has become more recently a popular view (see Hobfoll, 1989; Schonpflug, 1993; Schonpflug & Battman, 1993), potential or actual loss of valued resources regarded here as the causes of the state of stress can be understood only if we take into account the interaction between invested and gained resources. Important in conceptualizations defining stress in terms of resources is the fact that not only perceived but also actual (objectively existing) loss or lack of gain is regarded as a source of stress. This is especially evident in the theory of conservation of resources developed by Hobfoll (1989). The extension of causes of stress to objectively existing factors, a position I do share, does not violate the interactional approach to stress in which the individual plays an important role in regulating the balance between demands and capacities, or, regarding stress from another perspective, in regulating the balance between resources allocated and resources gained.

Coping with stress. The state of stress is inseparable from coping. Coping with stress is understood in this chapter as a regulatory function that consists of maintaining the adequate balance between demands and capacities or of reducing the discrepancy between demands and capacities. Efficient coping, which results in match or goodness of fit between demands and capacities, reduces the state of stress whereas inefficient coping leads to the increase of the state of stress (see Vitaliano, DeWolfe, Maiuro, Russo & Katon, 1990). As underlined by Lazarus (1993; Lazarus & Folkman, 1984) in respect to subjectively experienced stressors, coping is a process that consists of managing specific demands appraised as overwhelming or taxing. "Coping is highly contextual, since to be effective it must change over time and across different stressful conditions" (Lazarus, 1993, p. 8).

Coping, that leads to resolving the state of stress, may be also considered from the point of view of a resource management process in terms of gains and loss (Schonpflug & Battmann, 1993). The benefits of coping consists of gains in or savings of resources, whereas the costs of coping incorporate allocation, loss and consumption of resources. The individual copes with stress by means of replacement, substitution, or investment of resources (Hobfoll, 1989). The intensity, extent, and persistence with which coping attempts are applied refer to effort expenditure, a construct broadly discussed by Schonpflug (1993) with taking into account the individual differences approach.

Consequences of stress. Maladaptive functioning and behavior disorders, including pathology resulting from excessive or chronic stress are regarded in this chapter as consequences or costs of stress. Excessive stress consists of extremely strong negative affects accompanied by unusually high elevation of the level of arousal. Chronic stress is regarded as a state of stress not necessarily excessive but experienced permanently or frequently. As a consequence of both excessive and chronic stress, changes in the organism occur which may result in problems in psychological functioning, such as increased level of anxiety and depression, or in physiological or biochemical disturbances expressed in psychosomatic diseases or other health problems. Not all excessive or chronic states of stress lead to the negative consequences described above. Stress should be regarded as one of the many risk factors (external and internal) contributing to maladaptive functioning and disorders. When the state of stress is in interaction with other factors that decrease or dampen the consequences of stress, maladjustment or behavioral disturbances may not occur.

Temperament as a Moderator of Consequences of Stress: The Temperament Risk Factor (TRF)

Having now defined the major constructs I will concentrate on the relationship between temperament and stress limiting this chapter to the relationship between temperament characteristics and consequences of stress. The considerations presented herein should be regarded not as arguments based on conclusive evidence, but rather as a starting point for formulating hypotheses regarding some aspects of the "temperament-stress" relationship.

As already mentioned it is excessive or chronic stress that leads to behavior disorders, maladaptive functioning, and pathology. Thomas and Chess (1977; Thomas, Chess & Birch, 1968) should be regarded as pioneers who have shown that behavior disorders in children cannot be explained by the unfavorable environmental factors (stressors) only, and that an essential part of the variance in behavior disorders refers to a given configuration of temperamental traits called by them "difficult temperament". The pattern of difficult temperament comprises such categories as irregularity (in biological functions), slow adaptability to changes in the environment, intense negative mood, and withdrawal responses to new situations or strange persons. The number and quality of temperamental traits (categories) that constitute the pattern of a difficult temperament has changed from study to study and from author to author. Essential for most of the conceptualizations in respect to the difficult temperament is that a given configuration of temperamental characteristics (difficult temperament) does not by itself lead to development of behavior disorders. Only if the difficult temperament is in interaction with an inappropriate environment (e.g., family conflicts, divorce, parent-child dissonance), which is experienced by the child as a chronic or excessive state of stress, then there is a risk that behavior disorders or maladaptive functioning may develop.

In spite of Thomas and Chess' intention to give the concepts of "difficult temperament", meaning only when considered in interaction with the environment, these concepts have been criticized, among other things, for their personological and evaluative context (e.g., Bates, 1980; Plomin, 1982; Strelau & Eliasz, 1994). The term "difficult" suggests that it is the individual's temperament that causes difficulties and it also implies a negative meaning attributed to the individual.

To underline the fact that disturbances of behavior and pathology in children occur only when temperament characteristics predisposing a child to poor fit interact with an unfavorable environment, Carey (1989) introduced the concept of temperament risk factor (TRF). However, he limited this concept to excessive interactional stress experienced by children. To give the TRF a more universal meaning that allows us to extend this concept to the whole human population, the definition of TRF has been modified (Strelau 1989b). By temperament risk factor I mean any temperamental trait or configuration of traits that in interaction with other factors acting excessively, persistently or recurrently (e.g., physical and social environment, educational treatment, situations, the individual's characteristics) increases the risk of developing behavior disorders or pathology, or that favors the molding of a maladjusted personality.

Assessing temperamental traits as being risky or not risky is meaningful only under conditions that given temperamental traits or configurations of traits are considered within the context of other variables with which they interact. Among other things, this means that a particular configuration of temperamental traits considered as a TRF in one situation or for a given environment may not be at all a TRF in other situations or for other environments. Using the concepts of absolute and relative risk behaviors as understood by Jeffery (1989), one may say that TRF belongs to the category of relative risk. TRF may be assessed by the ratio of the chance of behavior disorders as consequences of exposure to stressors in individuals with given temperamental traits, compared to the risk of behavior disorders in response to the same stressors in individuals who do not have these temperamental traits.

Hypothesized Relationships between TRF and Behavior Disturbances

By studying the contribution of temperament to unfavorable consequences of the state of stress it is important to consider that there exist many risk factors contributing to behavior disorders and psychopathology.

The epidemiological aspects of these disorders and pathology, with taking into account temperament as one of the many risk factors, have been broadly discussed from a theoretical and methodological perspective by Carey and McDevitt (1989, 1994), Chess and Thomas (1984), Garrison and Earls (1987), Maziade (1988), Pellegrini (1990), and Rutter (1991). Kyrios and Prior (1990) postulated a theoretical model for the development of early childhood behavioral disturbances, in which, among such risk factors as childhood stress, child health problems, parental adjustment, developmental influences, child-rearing practices, and language abilities, the place of temperament in co-determining behavioral disorders has been shown.

Maziade (1988) postulated that children with an adverse temperament, an equivalent to difficult temperament, when in interaction with adverse environmental factors, present special vulnerability (liability) to clinical disorders. Developing an additive and synergistic model of adverse temperament-adverse environment interaction, Maziade referred to Kendler and Eaves' (1986) models for the joint effect of genotype and environment on liability to psychiatric illness. The authors postulated that etiology of psychiatric disorders consists of the interactional effect between genes and environment. The joint effect of genes and environment on liability to psychiatric disorders may be comprised by three basic models: (1) additive effects of genotype and environment, (2) genetic control of sensitivity to the environment, and (3) genetic control of exposure to the environment.

Taking the three basic models as introduced by Kendler and Eaves (1986), and Maziade (1988) as a starting point, I adapted these models to the construct of temperament risk factor. Instead of limiting the consequences of stress to liability to illness, they have been extended also to behavior disorders that can be found in a normal population when exposed to stress-inducing environments. Genotype has been replaced in the models by temperament. As postulated by many temperament researchers (see Buss & Plomin, 1984; Eysenck, 1970; Strelau, 1994; Zuckerman, 1994) the genetic endowment plays an essential role in determining the variance of temperamental traits. Also Kendler and Eaves (1986), when exemplifying the contribution of genes to liability to psychiatric disorders, referred to such temperament traits as impassivity and emotional instability as being influenced by genes, thus contributing, in interaction with a predisposing environment, to illness.

Without specifying the temperamental traits or composition of traits that constitute the TRF, and which can be different for different environments, a distinction should be made between present and absent temperament risk factors. TRF present means that, given the presence of temperamental traits or configuration of traits vulnerability to behavior disorders will be evidenced. Temperament risk factor absent implies that temperamental traits are different from those typical for TRF present, and that they do not constitute a risk factor for behavior disorders.

Regarding environment, the distinction has been made, according to Kendler and Eaves (1986), between protective and predisposing environments. Protective environment means in this context a lack of excessive or chronic stressors, which diminishes the probability of behavior disorders and pathology. In turn, predisposing environment which can be characterized in terms of chronic or excessive stress-inducing environments, increases the probability of behavior disorders and pathology. Further, when using the term behavior disorders, pathology is also meant as a possible consequence, although this would imply extreme poorness of fit between temperament and environmental demands.

In line with Kendler and Eaves' (1986) considerations, five models for joint temperament and environment effect on vulnerability to behavior disorders or pathology are presented below in order to show the different ways in which temperament and environment may interact with each other in producing the risk of behavior disorders.

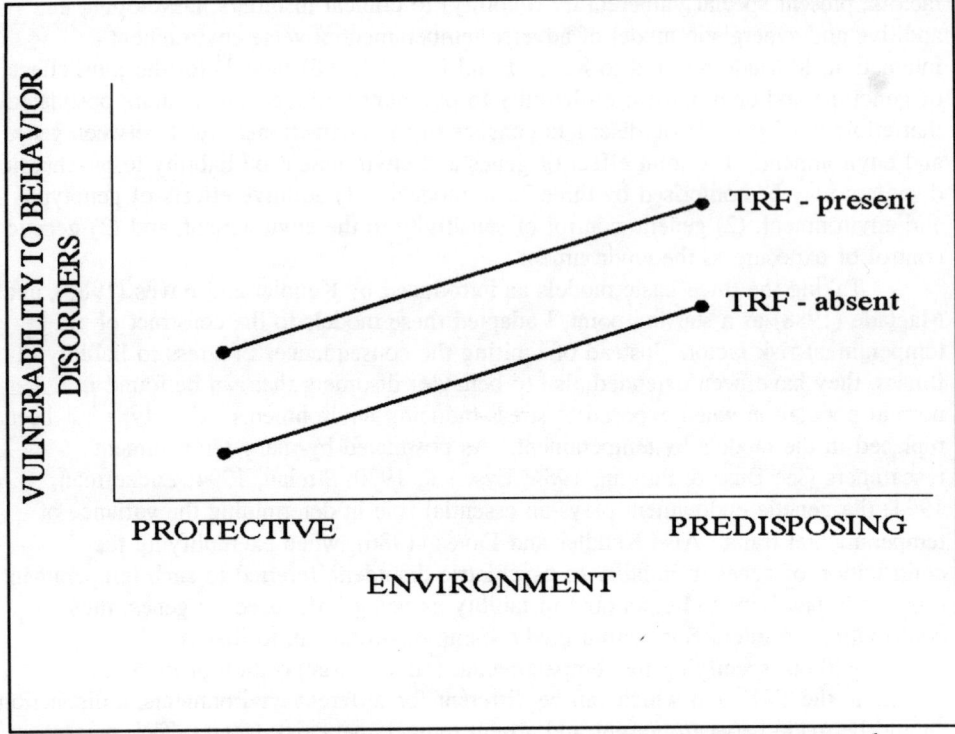

Figure 1. Vulnerability to behavior disorders as a function of temperament and environment with additive effects of both.

(1) <u>Temperamental and environmental control of behavior disorders</u>. This model, depicted in Figure 1, postulates that vulnerability to behavior disorders is a function of temperament and environment with additive effects of both temperament and environment. Individuals in whom the TRF is present, show in comparison with individuals in whom the TRF is absent, higher vulnerability to behavior disorders and pathology. This tendency occurs independently of the kind of environment, whether protective or predisposing to vulnerability. In turn, the effect of exposure to protective or predisposing environment is the same regardless of the individual's temperament characteristics. This model underlines the significance of temperament itself as predisposing the individual to poor fit, thus, as a predisposition for developing behavioral disorders. As may be exemplified by Eysenck's (1992) understanding of psychoticism, this temperamental trait is directly related to pathology and behavior disorders.

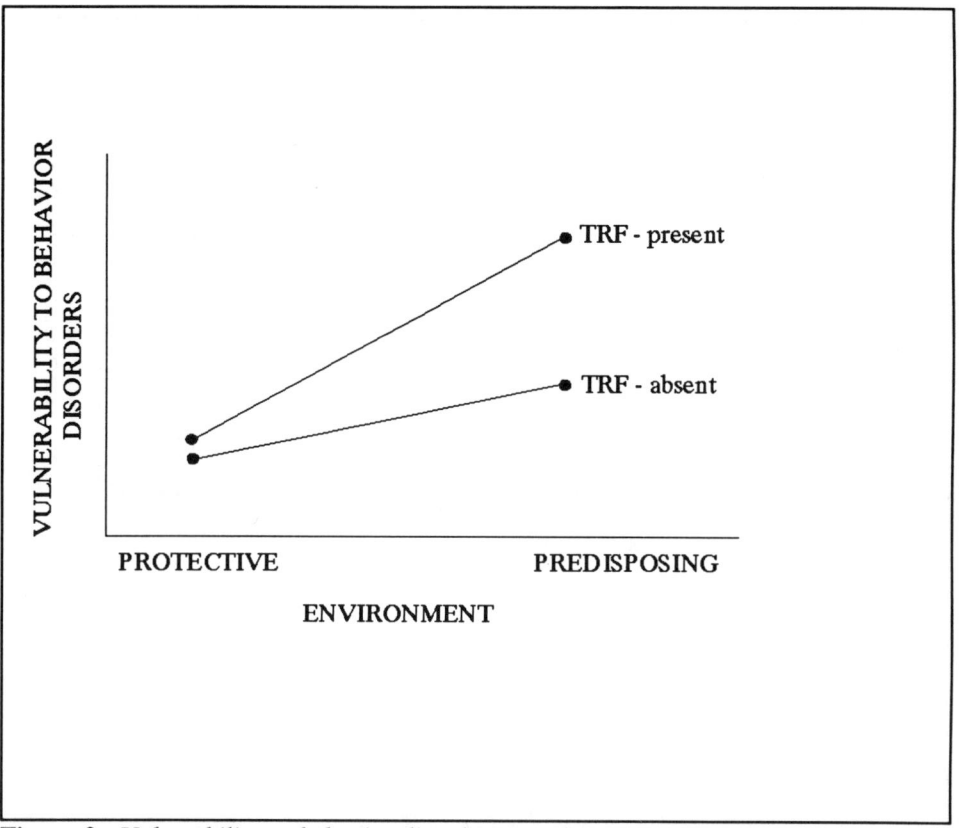

Figure 2. Vulnerability to behavior disorders as a function of temperament and environment with temperament control of sensitivity to the environment.

(2) <u>Temperamental control of sensitivity to the environment</u>. It is hypothesized by this model (see Figure 2) that vulnerability to behavior disorders is a function of temperament and environment with temperament influencing sensitivity to the environment. Given temperament traits or configurations of traits, regarded here as TRF, moderate the intensity of stressors by elevating sensitivity to stress-inducing situations. As a consequence of increased sensitivity to the predisposing environment, vulnerability to behavior disorders is higher in individuals in whom the TRF is present. Such temperamental traits as high anxiety, neuroticism, and emotionality heighten the tendency to experience negative affects in terms of their frequency and intensity.

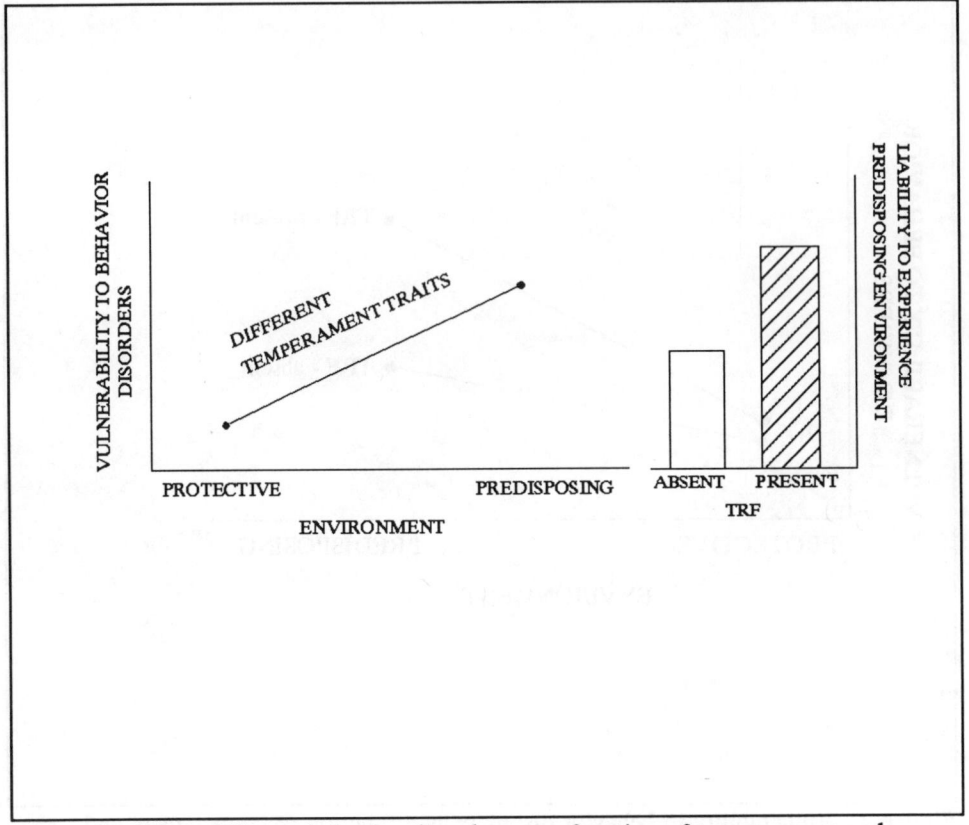

Figure 3. Vulnerability to behavior disorders as a function of temperament and environment with temperamental control of exposure to the environment.

(3) <u>Temperamental control of exposure to the environment</u>. Temperament may influence the vulnerability to behavior disorders by means of the individual's behavior which consists of selecting, creating or approaching such environments that are predisposing or protective with respect to vulnerability of behavior disorders (see Figure 3). TRF is composed of such temperamental traits that expose the individual to excessive or chronic stressors predisposing to behavior disorders. Sensation seeking, characterized by undertaking risky activities and approaching risky environments (Stacy, Newcomb & Bentler, 1993; Zuckerman, 1979), exemplifies the temperamentally determined exposure to predisposing environments.

The two remaining models are secondary to the three described above. Probably they are closer to real life situations in which the interactions between temperament and environment are more complex in producing the risk of behavior disorders or pathology as a consequence of chronic or excessive stress.

(4) <u>Temperamental control of behavior disorders and sensitivity to the environment</u>. This model consists of the combination of model (1) and model (2). As depicted in Figure 4, it postulates a synergistic effect of temperament with environment. TRF makes the individual more vulnerable to behavior disorders in a predisposing environment, whereas the absence of TRF protects the individual from negative consequences of the predisposing environment. In other words, TRF increases the risk of behavior disorders when in interaction with predisposing environment.

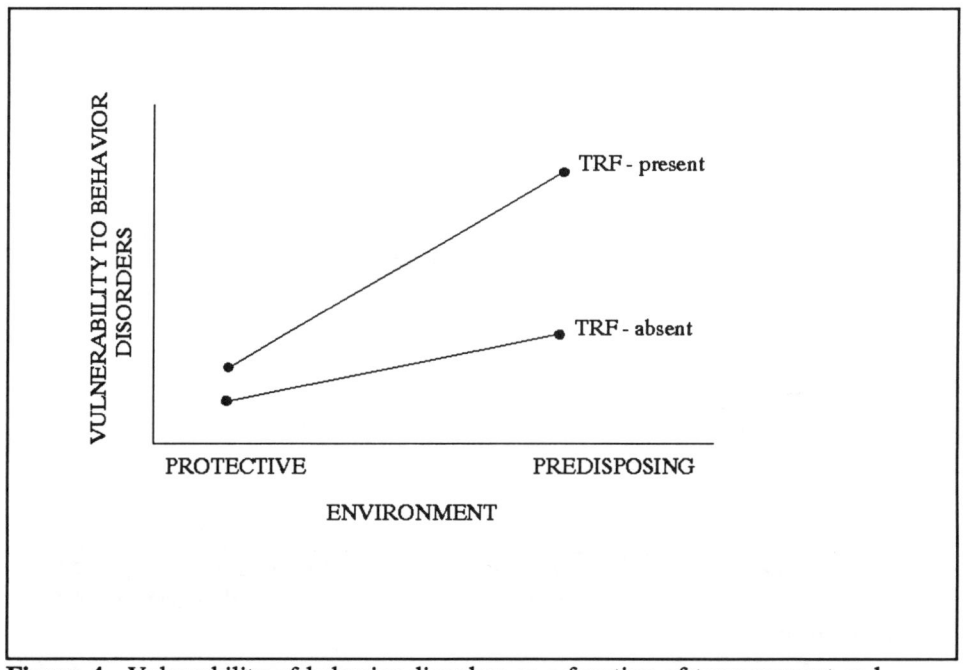

Figure 4. Vulnerability of behavior disorders as a function of temperament and environment with temperamental control of vulnerability to behavior disorders and sensitivity to the environment.

(5) <u>Temperamental control of behavior disorders and exposure to the environment</u>. This model, depicted in Figure 5, consists of a combination between models (1) and (3). On the one hand, temperament by itself predisposes people to

vulnerability to behavior disorders. On the other hand, temperament controls the exposure to a predisposing environment. Thus, there exists a cumulative effect of the temperament risk factor on vulnerability to behavior disorders. First, the effect results from temperamental traits that contribute to the risk of behavior disorders. Second, due to these temperamental traits the risk of exposure to predisposing environment increases, thus elevating the vulnerability to behavior disorders and pathology.

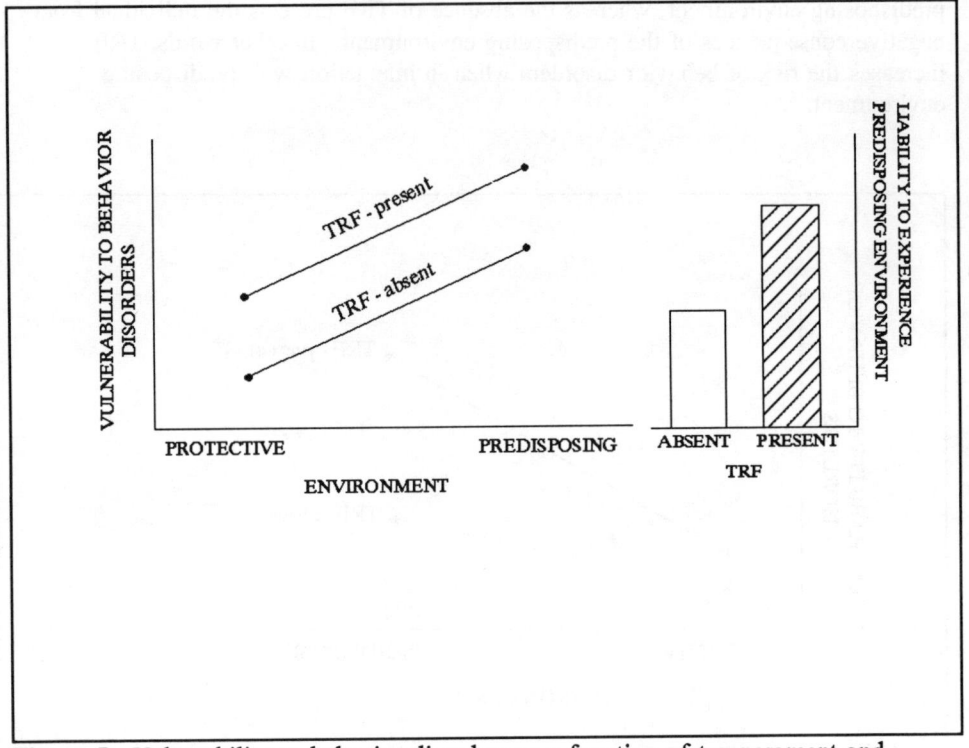

Figure 5. Vulnerability to behavior disorders as a function of temperament and environment with temperamental control of vulnerability to disorders and exposure to the environment.

The models presented above reflect the ways studies have been conducted or can be conducted in order to show the significance of temperament in producing the consequences of stress. They may also serve as a starting point for putting forward hypotheses regarding the role temperament plays as a moderator of behavior- and health- consequences of chronic or excessive state of stress.

Selected Findings

Several books (e.g., Chess & Thomas, 1984, 1986; Garrison & Earls, 1987; Thomas et al., 1968) and many papers have been published in order to show the role temperamental traits play in interaction with adverse environments in producing maladjusted personality, behavior disorders and pathology. Many of the studies have been conducted in children, mainly under the influence of the two senior child temperament researchers--Thomas and Chess. Studies on adults stem mostly from different theories of temperament, not necessarily related to these two New York psychiatrists. A very selective review limited to studies on adolescents and adults, and on causal modeling which reflects most evidently the complex interactions between risk factors of behavior disorders is given below.

Evidence from studies on adolescents and adults. Windle (1989) has shown that among five temperament factors (extraversion, emotional stability, activity, adaptability and task orientation) in late adolescents and early adults, it was mainly emotional instability and introversion that were the strongest predictors of mental health as composed of such factors as anxiety, depression, loss of control, and emotional ties. Kohn, Lafreniere and Gurevich (1991) demonstrated the moderating effect of temperament on stress and the consequences of stress in undergraduate students. Hassles and trait anxiety both contributed to perceived stress, hassles and temperament reactivity both had significant impact on minor ailments, and hassles and trait anxiety had a significant effect on psychiatric symptomatology. Another study conducted by Mehrabian and Ross (1977), also on university students, has shown that high arousability (the opposite pole of stimulus screening), when in interaction with long-lasting arousal states caused by life changes, may be regarded as a TRF for incidence of illness as judged by means of subjective ratings. Type A behavior pattern in adolescents expressed in activity of high stimulative value, when in interaction with high reactivity regarded in this study as a TRF, increased, in comparison with low reactivity, the probability of developing a high level of anxiety (Strelau & Eliasz, 1994).

Complex studies focused on the TRF. In some of the studies listed above multivariate analysis was applied to show some causal relationships between the variables under control. Causal modeling has become the most fruitful approach to studying the contribution of temperament, in interaction with other risk factors, to behavior disorders and pathology. A few more detailed examples are given below in order to show not only the diversity, but also the complexity of approaches to the issue of temperament risk factor.

A longitudinal study conducted by Kyrios and Prior (1990) on 3-4 year old children, and based on a "stress resilience" model of temperament, has shown the moderating role of high reactivity-low manageability and low self-regulation in behavioral adjustment under family stressors. These two temperamental characteristics influenced behavioral disturbances directly, as well as indirectly, by moderating the parental maladjustment, a family stressor, which was causally related to children's behavioral disturbances. This study exemplifies to a large extent Model 5. Using a broad statistical approach which was comprised of factor analysis, correlational procedures, multiple regression and path analysis of the obtained data, the authors arrived at the conclusion that temperamental characteristics are the most predictive variables of child behavioral adjustment. Low self-regulation, and high reactivity-low manageability, regarded in the Kyrios-Prior study as TRFs, contributed most to the variance of behavioral disturbances at the age of 3-4 years, and high reactivity-low manageability was the strongest predictor of behavioral maladjustment at the age of 4-5 years.

Studies conducted by Maziade and co-workers (Maziade, Cote, Bernier, Boutin & Thivierge, 1989; Maziade et al., 1990) in the domain of psychiatric disorders have shown that extreme temperaments, in terms of easy and difficult temperament, when taken alone, are bad predictors of clinical outcome. However, when these temperament constellations are considered in interaction with stressors, consisting in these studies of family dysfunctional behavior control, they became essential predictors of psychiatric disorders. This finding was replicated in several longitudinal studies at different ages.

The data reported by Maziade et al. (1990) showed that there was no statistically significant difference between extreme temperament at age 7 and the presence of definite psychiatric diagnosis at age 16. However, a statistically significant relationship occurred between temperament and internalized and externalized symptoms. Children with difficult temperament had significantly more reported symptoms. The results analyzed by means of stepwise logistic regression have shown that all children with extremely difficult temperament who lived in dysfunctional families, an environment which might be considered as a chronically acting stressor (predisposing environment), were diagnosed as having psychiatric disorders. In turn, for children in families with superior behavior control functioning (an example of a protective environment), there was no difference in psychiatric outcome between easy and difficult temperament. This study exemplifies the powerful role of interaction between temperament and environment in determining consequences of experienced stress.

A study which shows the role of one temperamental trait, emotionality, in moderating the effect of stressors on the vulnerability to behavior disorders has been conducted on over one thousand adult men by Aldwin and co-workers (1989). This study showed that individuals characterized by high emotionality report more stressors as compared with low-emotional persons. Most important, however, is that a high position on this temperament dimension predicted mental health symptoms. Thus, high emotionality, under the conditions studied by Aldwin et al. (1989), may be regarded as TRF. Using multivariate analysis of data the authors have shown that emotionality had a stronger effect on mental health than hassles and life events, but that together, emotionality, life events, and hassles accounted for almost 40% of the variance in mental health symptoms.

Final Remarks

The aim of this chapter was to show the place of temperament in studies on consequences of stress. My intention was to demonstrate that temperament is one of the many personal variables that cannot be ignored for a proper understanding of human functioning under stress, including community stress, especially when analyzing behavior disturbances resulting from excessive or chronic states of stress.

A special position has to be given to the temperament risk factor because of the far-reaching consequences individuals experiences as a result of excessive and chronic stress to which temperament may contribute in different ways. Among the many risk factors regarded as causes of behavior disorders and pathology, temperament plays to a given extent a specific role because of its low susceptibility to modification. Whereas some risk factors acting as stressors can be avoided or diminished by the individual him/herself (e.g., noise, crowd, job overload, parent-child conflict, etc.), others are not easily modified or cannot be avoided at all. As Pelligrini (1990, pp. 206-207) emphasized, "some risk factors are more likely to be preventable or modifiable once they occur (e.g., marital discord), others simply are not (e.g., gender) or are less likely to be so (e.g., difficult temperament)."

One of the senior researchers of child temperament, Rutter (1979), who studied protective factors in children's responses to stress, has shown the powerful influence of increasing numbers of risk factors for the epidemiology of behavior disorders. The probability of behavior disorders increases with the number of risk factors taken into account. The rate of behavior disorders was in practice the same for an individual with only one risk factor as compared with an individual being free from this risk factor. But when the number of risk factors acting jointly extended to four or more, the rate of behavior disorders increased to 20 percent. This finding is a strong argument for taking into account temperament as one of the many possible risk factors contributing to psychological, psychophysiological and pathological consequences of stress.

Author's note

I thank Stevan E. Hobfoll for his help in preparing this manuscript. Part of this research was supported by Grant 1108-9102 for the Committee for Scientific Research.

References

Aldwin, C. M., Levenson, M. R., Spiro III, A., & Bosse, R. (1989). Does emotionality predict stress? Findings from the normative aging study. Journal of Personality and Social Psychology, 56, 618-624.

Antonovsky, A. (1987). Unraveling the mystery of health: How people manage stress and stay well. San Francisco: Jossey-Bass.

Bates, J. E. (1980). The concept of difficult temperament. Merrill-Palmer Quarterly, 29, 89-97.

Buss, A. H., & Plomin, R. (1984). Temperament: Early developing personality traits. Hillsdale, NJ: Erlbaum.

Carey, W. B. (1989). Introduction: Basic issues. In W. B. Carey & S. C. McDevitt (Eds.), Clinical and educational applications of temperament research (pp. 11-20). Lisse: Swets & Zeitlinger.

Carey, W. B., & McDevitt, S. C. (Eds.). (1989). Clinical and educational applications of temperament research. Lisse: Swets & Zeitlinger.

Carey, W. B., & McDevitt, S. C. (Eds.). (1994). Prevention and early intervention: Individual differences as risk factors for the mental health of children. New York: Brunner/Mazel.

Chan, K. B. (1977). Individual differences in reactions to stress and their personality and situational determinents: Some implications for community mental health. Social Science and Medicine, 11, 89-103.

Chess, S., & Thomas, A. (1984). Origins and evolution of behavior disorders: From infancy to early adult life. New York: Brunner/Mazel.

Chess, S., & Thomas, A. (1986). Temperament in clinical practice. New York: The Guilford Press.

Eysenck, H. J. (1970). The structure of human personality (3rd ed.). London: Methuen.

Eysenck, H. J. (1992). The definition and measurement of psychoticism. Personality and Individual Differences, 13, 757-785.

Eysenck, H. J., & Eysenck, M. W. (1985). Personality and individual differences: A natural science approach. New York: Plenum Press.

Frankenhaeuser, M. (1979). Psychoneuroendocrine approaches to the study of emotion as related to stress and coping. In H. E. Howe, & R. A. Dienstbier (Eds.), Nebraska Symposiom on Motivation, 1978 (pp. 123-161). Lincoln: University of Nebraska Press.

Frankenhaeuser, M. (1986). A psychobiological framework for research on human stress and coping. In M. H. Appley & R. Trumbull (Eds.), Dynamics of stress: Physiological, psychological, and social perspectives (pp. 101-116). New York: Plenum Press.

Freedy, J. R., Kilpatrick, D. G., & Resnick, H. S. (1993).Natural disasters and mental health: Theory, assessment, and intervention. Journal of Social Behavior and Personality, 8, 49-103.
Garrison, W. T., & Earls, F. J. (1987). Temperament and child psychopathology. Newbury Park, CA: Sage Publications.
Hobfoll, S. E. (1988). The ecology of stress. Washington, DC:Hemisphere.
Hobfoll, S. E. (1989). Conservation of resources: A new attempt at conceptualizing stress. American Psychologist, 44, 513-524.
Holmes, T. H. & Rahe, R. H. (1967). The Social Readjustment Rating Scale. Journal of Psychosomatic Research, 11, 213-218.
Holohan, C. J., & Moos, R. H. (1986). Personality, coping, and family resources in stress resistance: A longitudinal analysis. Journal of Personality and Social Psychology, 51, 389-395.
Jeffery, R. W. (1989). Risk behaviors and health: Contrasting individual and population perspectives. American Psychologist, 44, 1194-1202.
Kagan, J. (1983). Stress and coping in early development. In N. Garmezy, & M. Rutter (Eds.), Stress, coping and development in children (pp. 191-216). New York: McGraw-Hill.
Kendler, K. S., & Eaves, L. J. (1986). Model for the joint effect of genotype and environment on liability ot psychiatric illness. The American Journal of Psychiatry, 143, 279-289.
Kobasa, S. C. (1979). Stressful life events, personality and health: An inquiry into hardiness. Journal of Personality and Social Psychology, 37, 1-11.
Kobasa, S. C., & Puccetti, M. C. (1983). Personality and social resources in stress resistance. Journal of Personality and Social Psychology, 45, 839-850.
Kohn, P. M., Lafreniere, K., & Gurevich, M. (1991). Hassles, health, and personality. Journal of Personality and Social Psychology, 61, 478-482.
Krohne, H. W. (1986). Coping with stress: Dispositions, strategies, and the problem of measurement. In M. H. Appley, & R. Trumbull (Eds.), Dynamics of stress: Physiological, psychological, and social perspectives (pp. 209-234). New York: Plenum Press.
Kyrios. M., & Prior, M. (1990). Temperament, stress and family factors in behavioural adjustment of 3-5-year-old children. International Journal of Behavioral Development, 13, 67-93.
Laux, L., & Vossell, G. (1982). Theoretical and methodological issues in achievement-related stress and anxiety research. In H. W. Krohne, & L. Laux (Eds.), Achievement, stress, and anxiety (pp. 3-18). New York: Hemisphere & McGraw-Hill.
Lazarus, R. S. (1991). Emotion and adaptation. New York: Oxford University Press.
Lazarus, R. S. (1993). From psychological stress to the emotions: A history of changing outlooks. Annual Review of Psychology, 44, 1-21.
Lazarus, R. S., & Folkman, S. (1984). Stress, appraisal, and coping. New York: Springer.

Maziade, M. (1988). Child temperament as a developmental or an epidemiological concept: A methodological point of view. Psychiatric Developments, 3, 195-211.

Maziade, M., Caron, C., Cote, R., Merette, C., Bernier, H., Laplante, B., Boutin. P., & Thivierge, J. (1990). Psychiatric status of adolescents who had extreme temperaments at age 7. American Journal of Psychiatry, 147, 1531-1536.

Maziade, M., Cote, R., Bernier, H., Boutin, P, & Thivierge, J. (1989). Singificance of extreme temperament in infancy for clinical status in pre-school years. 1: Value of extreme temperament at 4-8 months for predicting diagnosis at 4.7 years. British Journal of Psychiatry, 154, 535-543.

McGrath, J. E. (Ed.). (1970). Social and psychological factors in stress. New York: Holt, Rinehart and Winston.

McGuire, I., & Turkewitz, G. (1979). Approach-withrawal theory and the study of infant development. In M. Bortner (Ed.), Cognitive growth and development: Essays in memory of Herbert G. Birch (pp. 57-84). New York: Brunner/Mazel.

Mehrabian, A. (1977). Individual differences in stimulus screening and arousability. Journal of Personality, 45, 237-250.

Mehrabian, A., & Ross, M. (1977). Quality of life change and individual differences in stimulus screening in relation to incidence of illness. Psychological Reports, 41, 267-278.

Nebylitsyn, V. D. (1972). Fundamental properties of the human nervous system. New York: Plenum Press.

Ormel, J., & Schaufeli, W. B. (1991). Stability and change in psychological distress and their relationship with self-esteem and locus of control: A dynamic equilibrium model. Personality and Social Psychology, 60, 288-299.

Parkes, K. R. (1984). Locus of control, cognitive appraisal, and coping in stressful episodes. Journal of Personality and Social Psychology, 46, 655-668.

Pellegrini, D. S. (1990). Psychosocial risk and protective factors in childhood. Journal of Developmental and Behavioral Pediatrics, 11, 201-209.

Plomin, R. (1982). The difficult concept of temperament: A response to Thomas, Chess, and Korn. Merril-Palmer Quarterly, 28, 25-33.

Rutter, M. (1979). Protective factors in children's responses to stress and disadvantage. In M. W. Kent, & J. E. Rolf (Eds.), Primary prevention of psychopathology (Vol. 3, pp. 49-74). Hannover, NH: University Press of New England.

Rutter, M. (1991). Nature, nurture, and pschopathology: A new look at an old topic. Development and Psychopathology, 3, 125-136.

Schonpflug, W. (in press). Effort regulation and individual differences in effort expenditure. In G. R. J. Hockery, A. W. K. Galillard, & M. G. H. Coles (Eds.), Energetics and human information processing. Dordrecht: Nijhoff.

Schonpflug, W., & Battmann, W. (1993). Two pieces in resource management. In Spielberger, C.D., Kulscar, S., & G. van Heck (Eds.), Stress and emotion. Washington: Hemisphere.

Schulz, P., & Schonpflug, W. (1982). Regulatory activity during states of stress. In H. W. Krohne, & L. Laux (Eds.), Achievement, stress, and anxiety (pp. 51-73). New York: Hemisphere & McGraw-Hill.

Stacy, A. W., Newcomb, M. D., & Bentler, P. M. (1993). Cognitive motivations and sensation seeking as long-term predictors of drinking problems. Journal of Social and Clinical Psychology, 12, 1-24.

Strelau, J. (1983). Temperament, personality, activity. London: Acedemic Press.

Strelau, J. (1988). Temperamental dimensions as co-determinants of resistance tostress. In M. P. Janisse (Ed.), Individual differences, stress, and health psychology (pp. 146-169). New York: Springer.

Strelau, J. (1989a). Individual differences in tolerance to stress: The role of reactivity. In C. D. Spielberger, I. G. Sarason, & J. Strelau (Eds.), Stress and anxiety (Vol. 12, pp. 155-166). Washington, DC: Hemisphere.

Strelau, J. (1989b). Temperament risk factors in children and adolescents as studied in Eastern Europe. In W. B. Carey & S. C. McDevitt (Eds.), Clinical and educational applications of temperament research (pp. 65-77). Lisse: Swets & Zeitlinger.

Strelau, J. (1994). The concepts of arousal and arousability as used in temperament studies. In J. E. Bates, & T. D. Wachs (Eds.), Temperament: Individual differences at the interface of biology and behavior (pp. 117-141). Washington DC: APA Books.

Strelau, J., & Eliasz, A. (1994). Temperament risk factors for Type A behavior patterns in adolescents. In W. B. Carey, & S. C. McDevitt (Eds.), Prevention and early intervention: Individual differences as risk factors for the mental health of children (pp. 42-49). New York: Brunner/Mazel.

Thomas, A., & Chess, S. (1977). Temperament and development. New York: Brunner/Mazel.

Thomas, A., Chess, S., & Birch, H. G. (1968). Temperament and behavior disorders in children. New York: New York University Press.

Vitaliano, P. P., DeWolfe, D. J., Maiuro, R. D., Russo, J., & Katon, W. (1990). Appraised changeability of a stressor as a modifier of the relationship between coping and depression: A test of the hypothesis of fit. Journal of Personality and Social Psychology, 59, 582-592.

Windle, M. (1989). Predicting temperament-mental health relationships: A covariance structure latent variable analysis. Journal of Research in Personality, 23, 118-144.

Zuckerman, M. (1979). Sensation seeking: Beyond the optimal level of arousal. Hillsdale, NJ: Erlbaum.

Zuckerman, M. (1994). Behavioral expressions and biosocial bases of sensation seeking. New York: Cambridge University Press.

COPING WITH THE LOSS OF A FAMILY MEMBER: IMPLICATIONS FOR COMMUNITY-LEVEL RESEARCH AND INTERVENTION

Camille B. Wortman, State University of New York at Stony Brook, USA
Katherine B. Carnelley, University of Wales, College of Cardiff, Great Brittain
Darrin R. Lehman, University of British Columbia, Canada
Christopher G. Davis, University of British Columbia, Canada
Julie Juola Exline, State University of New York at Stony Brook, USA

In this chapter, we focus on how people react to the loss of an immediate family member, with special emphasis on reactions to sudden, traumatic loss. Although a few studies have examined loss as a result of community-level events such as floods or fires (see, e.g., Erikson, 1994; Green et al., 1990; Lindy, Green, Grace, & Titchener, 1983), the vast majority of published work on grief is centered around individual losses, principally the loss of one's spouse or child. In our judgment, the literature on coping with an individual loss raises a myriad of challenging issues that have considerable relevance for those planning community-level interventions. In this chapter, we explore how such losses are perceived and reacted to by those who have endured the loss, and also by those in their social environment. We maintain that even when they experience troubling symptoms that may be caused by the trauma, people who lose a family member are unlikely to seek help from community mental health services. Ways of resolving this dilemma, and enhancing the likelihood that those suffering traumatic loss will receive the care they need, are considered.

In exploring reactions to those who have encountered traumatic loss, we draw from previous work to focus on three themes. First, we describe what we have called "myths of coping" with loss (Wortman & Silver, 1989). As a society, we hold strong beliefs about the appropriate ways to cope with loss. These beliefs are so powerful and so pervasive that they have exerted a strong influence on research and intervention in the area. As we detail below, however, these beliefs have caused a variety of problems for those who have endured a major loss. We begin this section of the paper by providing a brief description of these cultural beliefs. Next, we explore the research evidence bearing on these assumptions, drawing from our own research program as well as studies completed by others. Finally we discuss the implications of these beliefs for how the bereaved are treated.

A major theme that emerges from the work on myths of coping with loss concerns a belief about the value of expressing one's emotions following loss. Whether the bereaved person is showing little grief following a loved one's death or whether he or she shows distress longer than those in the social network expect, emotional expression of one's painful feelings is believed to be beneficial. Such beliefs are held both by lay people and professionals. Putting one's feelings to words is believed to assist the bereaved in resolving the loss and finding meaning in it, and to minimize the likelihood that the suppressed feelings of grief will hasten a decline in physical health. However, this emphasis on expression of negative emotions ignores one important factor: the almost uniformly negative social response that the bereaved person is likely to elicit from others if negative feelings are conveyed. Drawing from our own and others' work, we discuss why others are often threatened and upset by the bereaved person's discussions of negative affect. We also discuss why others deal with their negative feelings in ways that are hurtful to the bereaved, such as avoiding the bereaved person or minimizing his or her problems.

Because the social environment is so intolerant of expressions of distress, some investigators have argued that in many cases, the bereaved would benefit from professional help. We attempt to show, however, that many of the factors that make it difficult for laypersons to tolerate the bereaved person's distress also hold true for professionals as well. We elaborate the situations under which professional helpers are made uncomfortable by the bereaved person's expressions of distress, and we illustrate how the feelings evoked by their bereaved clients can sometimes lead professionals to relate to the bereaved in ways that are unhelpful.

This analysis is followed by a discussion of research questions which emerge from the material we have presented. Perhaps the most central question to emerge concerns what it means when a person fails to become intensely distressed following a major loss. Is this reaction more appropriately conceptualized as denial or resilience? We describe ongoing research designed to shed light on this important issue.

We conclude with a brief discussion of the implications of our analysis for intervention efforts. We maintain that in virtually all communities, there is a substantial population of individuals who have experienced the sudden, traumatic loss of a loved one, who are having difficulties as a result, and who have not sought help from any mental health professional. Moreover, these people are unlikely to be receptive to mental health services. As our analysis suggests, they are also unlikely to be receiving adequate support from those in their social network. We maintain that the absence of intervention strategies for this group represents a critical gap in knowledge which must be filled.

Cultural Assumptions about Coping with Loss

An examination of available literature leaves little doubt that people hold strong assumptions about how individuals should cope with the loss of a loved one (Wortman & Silver, 1989). These assumptions are derived from a variety of sources, including theories of loss offered by prominent writers in the area, clinical lore about coping with loss, and our cultural understanding of the experience.

The most prominent theories in the area of loss are the so-called stage theories. One of the most important stage models was developed by Bowlby (1961), who maintained that individuals go through a series of four stages following the loss of a loved one: numbness or shock; yearning or searching for the lost person, which is accompanied by feelings of anger; giving up the attempt to find the lost loved one, which is associated with feelings of depression; and reorganization or recovery, which involves resumption of normal role activities. A highly influential stage theory has also been advanced by Kubler-Ross (1969) regarding how people react to their own impending death. According to Kubler-Ross, individuals go through the stages of denial, anger, bargaining, depression, and acceptance. Because stage models like these have been taught in thousands of medical, nursing, and social work schools for the past several years, they have become firmly entrenched among health care professionals. However, the application of stage models may not always have positive effects. Pattison (1977) reports that, as a result of the widely held belief in Kubler-Ross'(1969) stages of dying, "dying persons who did not follow these stages were labeled 'deviant,' 'neurotic,' or 'pathological' dyers. Clinical personnel became angry at patients who did not move from one stage to the next... I began to observe professional personnel demand that the dying person 'die in the right way' [p. 304]." Similarly, in our own prior work with cancer patients, we observed many situations in which patients' feelings were discounted or dismissed as "just a stage" (Wortman & Dunkel-Schetter, 1979). For example, one man with prostate cancer was accidentally given the wrong medication, and he became quite angry. He overheard one nurse say to another, "Don't worry about Mr. X. He's just going through the anger stage." In light of the widespread acceptance of these models, Silver and Wortman (1980) began a systematic examination of all empirical studies purporting to test them. To their surprise, there was virtually no evidence to support the stage models. Some evidence-- for example, the finding that among those coping with bereavement, feelings of depression often precede feelings of anger-- was inconsistent with the models (Silver & Wortman, 1980). As evidence has failed to accumulate, researchers have become more skeptical about the validity of the stage approach. For example, in an Institute of Medicine report on research on bereavement (Osterwies, Solomon & Green, 1984), it was recommended that the word "stages" not be used, because it implies a more orderly progression through the grieving process than typically occurs.

Assumptions about the Necessity of Distress

Description. Although most people no longer see bereavement as a set of discrete stages, they do see it as a process. Because assumptions about the nature of this process are likely to have a pervasive impact on how reactions to loss are evaluated, it is important to examine such assumptions carefully. One assumption that is widely held in our culture is that when a person suffers an important loss, he or she will experience intense distress. For example, the aforementioned Institute of Medicine report claimed that there is a "near-universal occurrence of intense emotional distress following bereavement, with features similar in nature and intensity to those of clinical depression" (Osterweis et al., 1984, p. 18).

A related assumption is that those who fail to react to loss with intense distress are reacting abnormally (see Wortman & Silver, 1987, for a review). This view is so firmly entrenched that negative attributions are typically made about those who do not show such distress. A bereaved person who fails to exhibit distress is often judged as a shallow, superficial person who is incapable of real attachment (cf. Raphael, 1977). Alternatively, the bereaved person may be labeled as denying the loss. It is also widely believed that the failure to grieve will result in subsequent health problems or physical symptoms (Osterweis et al., 1984).

<u>Evidence</u>. This insistence on distress following loss has been labeled the "requirement of mourning" (Dembo, Leviton, & Wright, 1956; Wright, 1983). According to this notion, outsiders "insist that the person they consider unfortunate is suffering (even when the person seems not to be suffering) or devalue the unfortunate person because he or she ought to suffer" (Dembo et al., 1956, p. 21). But in fact, the available research evidence suggests that there is considerable variability in how people react to a major loss, with a substantial percentage of respondents not showing initial distress. In a review of five longitudinal studies on how people cope with the loss of a spouse or child, respondents were classified according to their pattern of grieving (Wortman & Silver, 1990). Respondents who showed high initial depression, but low depression at a later point in time (typically two years later) were classified as showing a normal pattern of grieving. Those who exhibited little depression at either time point were classified as evidencing absent grief. Those respondents who showed high distress at both time points were classified as suffering from chronic grief. Finally, those who evidenced low initial distress, but who showed high distress at a later time point, were classified as exhibiting delayed grief.

While a detailed discussion of these data is beyond the scope of this chapter (see Wortman & Silver, 1990), we wish to highlight those findings that bear on the issues raised above. First, by examining the percentage of respondents showing a normal pattern of grief, it is clear that this is not a universal reaction: it ranged across studies from 9.4 % to 41%. Second, the number of respondents showing a delayed grief reaction ranged from 0 to 5.1%, and was typically around 1 or 2 percent, suggesting that this is not a common response to loss. Third, there was a substantial percentage of respondents, ranging from 26.2% to 77.8%, who did not show evidence of intense distress at either of the two time points. In virtually all of these studies, those respondents who did not show distress in the initial weeks or months following the loss are those who appeared to be coping most successfully several months later.

Taken together, these data raise serious questions about the universality of distress following a major loss. They also raise questions about whether the failure to show a grief response is maladaptive. These data suggest that, in fact, it is typical not to show distress in the first weeks and months following the death, and that failure to show such distress does not necessarily portend subsequent difficulties.

Implications. These findings have straightforward implications for people suffering loss. First, the expectation that people must go through a period of distress may lead them to push the bereaved into such a reaction. One guidebook stated that "it is often necessary to confront the patient gently but firmly with the reality of his situation and to force him into a period of depression while he works out his acceptance of his loss" (Nemiah, 1957, p. 146). The assumption of distress also has implications for laypersons, who may become judgmental if the bereaved person is not showing sufficient distress. For example, one of the parents in our study of loss of a child to Sudden Infant Death Syndrome, or SIDS, (Downey, Silver, & Wortman, 1990) arranged a birthday party for a sibling a few months after the loss. She was extremely hurt by the comment of the neighbor that if she really loved the baby, how could she be enjoying herself at a party such a short time after the death?

These findings also have relevance for how victims of trauma are judged in legal situations. In one well-publicized legal case, John Henry Knapp was convicted of the murder of his two young daughters, who died in a fire that destroyed their one-bedroom trailer. The principal evidence against Mr. Knapp was that immediately after the fire, he was outwardly calm, and showed no visible grief reaction (Brill, 1983; Ferrell, 1990). Similarly, Calhoun and his colleagues (Calhoun, Cann, Shelby, & Magee, 1981) found that rape victims who exhibited more emotional distress were more likely to be believed in a mock courtroom setting than rape victims who appeared to be "calm" or "numb."

Expectations about how the bereaved should react may also influence how they are treated by physicians. There is evidence that those in the medical profession practice a kind of "pharmacological Calvinism" in treating the bereaved -- that is, they are extremely reluctant to prescribe medication. Although the available evidence suggests that antidepressants and antianxiety medications often benefit the bereaved (Rando, 1993; see Jacobs, 1993, for a review), these are often not prescribed because it is believed that the person needs to experience the pain associated with the loss in order to recover (Brown & Stoudemire, 1983). There seems to be general agreement among clinicians that resolution of grief cannot proceed and reach completion without suffering on the part of the bereaved.

Assumptions about Resolution and Recovery

Description. While it is believed that bereaved persons must go through a period of distress, such a phase is not expected to last indefinitely. In fact, it is expected that over time, people should be able to resolve the loss and recover, returning to a normal state of well-being and functioning (See Lehman, Wortman & Williams, 1987, for a more detailed discussion). Clinical lore suggests that six months to a year is sufficient to recover from the loss of a spouse, and that it may take somewhat longer to recover from the loss of a child (one to two years total). Evidence of a norm that grief will usually be completed within this time frame comes from a variety of sources, including articles written by clinicians for fellow practitioners (e.g., Bellitsky &

Jacobs, 1986); self-help books written for the bereaved (e.g., DiGuilio, 1989); and numerous articles about grief that have appeared in magazines and newspapers (e.g., Horowitz, 1989). As grief expert Phyllis Silverman has emphasized, outward displays of grief are tolerated for an even shorter period of time: "there's still a tendency in this country to expect people to get over the grief and sorrow of a loved one's death almost immediately. People see grief as something that is appropriate around the time of the death and the funeral and for some brief period afterwards" (1983, p. 65).

One of the most important concepts in the literature on grief and loss concerns the notion of resolving the loss. It is widely believed that in order to recover from the loss, individuals must first be able to achieve a state of resolution regarding the death. This state has also been referred to as accommodation, closure, or completion. In describing resolution, some investigators have focused on the importance of tasks that are primarily cognitive, such as accepting the loss intellectually. For example, Parkes and Weiss (1983) have argued that people must come up with a rationale for the loss; they must be able to understand what has happened and make sense of the loss. Similarly, Craig (1977) has suggested that an essential part of coming to grips with the loss of a child involves resolving the meaninglessness of the death. Another type of resolution that has been discussed in the literature involves accepting the loss emotionally. Emotional acceptance is thought to be reached when the dead person can be recalled, and reminders confronted, without intense distress (cf. Rachman, 1980; Rubin, 1985; Volkan, 1985; Weiss, 1988). If a person fails to work through the loss successfully, it is believed that he or she will experience a variety of symptoms, including intrusive thoughts, nightmares, obsessions (Rachman, 1980), emotional constriction (Van der Kolk & Van der Hart, 1991) as well as other symptoms of Post Traumatic Stress Disorder or PTSD (Rothbaum & Foa, 1992).

Despite emphasis on the resolution process, it should be noted that those writing on the topic have been somewhat vague about how resolution is accomplished (see Tait & Silver, 1989, for a review). Most investigators regard resolution as an active process. For example, it has been suggested that for resolution to occur, the griever must examine every aspect of what happened, and sift through thoughts and memories of the deceased person again and again (see, e.g., Brown & Stoudemire, 1983; Parkes & Weiss, 1983). As is discussed below, several investigators have suggested that the process is facilitated when feelings or images associated with the trauma are turned into language (Clark, 1993; Pennebaker, 1989; Van der Kolk & Van der Hart, 1991).

Evidence. The evidence suggests that the processes of resolution and recovery may work somewhat differently than previous investigators anticipated. It is clear, for example, that a large number of people never reach a stage of resolution. In a study of people who lost a spouse or child in a motor vehicle accident, Lehman, et al., 1987 found that as long as 4 - 7 years after the loss, most of the bereaved continued to experience painful thoughts about their loved one, and could not make sense of, or find any meaning in, the loss. There is also evidence from this study indicating that people may not recover as quickly and completely as expected following the loss of a spouse or child. In this study, individuals who lost a spouse or child in a motor vehicle crash 4-7 years earlier were compared to a matched control group of respondents on various indicators of adjustment and functioning. There were significant differences between bereaved and control respondents on several measures, including depression, mortality, and (for respondents who lost a child) divorce. Other studies have supported the notion that a one or two year recovery period is unrealistic, especially if the loss is sudden and traumatic (see Parkes & Weiss, 1983; see Tait & Silver, 1989, or Wortman & Silver, 1987, for reviews). Taken together, the empirical data suggest that many people struggle with the emotional ravages of loss for the rest of their lives.

Implications. Assumptions about resolution and recovery from loss may lead others to respond judgmentally when the bereaved do not complete their grief work according to the expected timetable. In one article, a woman who lost her husband to cancer told her son that she did not want to go to a party to celebrate a friend's 25th wedding anniversary. Her son was so alarmed that he phoned their family doctor and reported that his mother was "severely disturbed and in need of psychiatric help" (Jacoby, 1984). "'After all,' the young man said, 'it's been six months since Dad died. It's time for Mom to get on with her life.'" In fact, the bereaved may apply cultural norms to their own behavior, and wonder if they are experiencing more distress than they should. Others' feedback that they should be over the loss, combined with their own assessment that they are more distressed than the norm, have led many bereaved to doubt their own sanity (Osterweis et al., 1984).

Dilemmas Surrounding Emotional Expression Following Loss

There is consistent evidence in the literature that people who have suffered a major loss value opportunities to discuss the loss (Lehman, Ellard, & Wortman, 1986). In studies involving a variety of different stressful experiences, over 85% of all respondents expressed a desire to share their feelings with others (see Pennebaker, 1993, for a review). This wish to discuss what has happened is thought to be related to a need for validation-- that is, confirmation that one's responses are normal and appropriate under the circumstances (Tait & Silver, 1989).

It is also clear that people are often encouraged to talk about what they have been through both by laypersons and by mental health professionals who believe it is harmful to keep negative feelings "bottled up" inside. In a handbook for mental health professionals dealing with trauma, for example, it was emphasized that the professional should gradually encourage clients to talk about what happened in detail, including what he or she felt or thought at the time and what they feel now (McCann & Pearlman, 1990).

There is some evidence from the work of Pennebaker and his associates that inhibition of expression about traumatic events can lead to long-term health problems (see Francis & Pennebaker, 1991). This work has shown that those who express their feelings about a trauma in writing for 3-4 sessions make fewer visits to health clinics than those who do not write about their trauma (Pennebaker & Beall, 1986; see also

Greenberg & Stone, 1992). Moreover, recent work has linked emotional disclosure to improved immune function (Pennebaker, Kiecolt-Glaser, & Glaser, 1988).

Clark (1993) has also focused attention on the benefits of talking about one's feelings among those who have experienced trauma. She has maintained that when a traumatized person enters into a conversation, a number of things happen which have beneficial consequences. According to Clark (1993), the attempt to communicate what has happened can produce important insights and a broadening of perspectives that can enhance problem solving and coping.

Unfortunately, evidence from our own and others' work suggests that any benefits from expressing one's feelings in a social context may be outweighed by the costs. There is evidence that when people try to talk about their feelings regarding a major loss, others often react negatively and respond in ways that are not comforting. Those in the bereaved person's social network frequently employ strategies to get the bereaved to inhibit displays of distress (Lehman, et al., 1986; Wortman & Lehman, 1985). These include discouraging expression of feelings (e.g., "tears won't bring him back"); minimizing the loss (e.g., "You had many good years together"), encouraging the bereaved person to recover more quickly (e.g., "You should get out and do more"); portraying their own past experiences as being similar to what the bereaved has experienced (e.g., "I know how you feel. I lost my second cousin."); and offering advice (e.g., "You should consider getting a dog. They're wonderful companions."). In many cases, such lines of conversation are likely to have the effect of closing off communication with the bereaved person.

The evidence is clear that the bereaved do not find any of these types of responses -- discouraging feelings, minimizing the loss, mentioning "similar" experiences, or offering advice -- to be helpful (Davidowitz & Myrick, 1984; Lehman et al., 1986). What they do find helpful is contact with people who have had similar experiences, or talking with others who are nonjudgmental and will allow them to express their feelings if and when they want to (Lehman et al., 1986).

Why do the bereaved consistently report that those in their social environment respond in ways that are unhelpful? There are several possible explanations. First, most people in the bereaved person's social network probably believe the myths of coping detailed above. They believe that feelings of intense sadness are experienced for a much shorter duration than may often be the case, and they expect the bereaved to recover much more quickly than they usually do. Second, in our judgement, others often see the bereaved person's continuing distress as a character weakness rather than as a legitimate response to the loss (Coyne, Wortman, & Lehman, 1988). Outsiders often believe that if bereaved people wanted to, they could control their displays of distress and resume normal functioning. Unfortunately, displays of distress are often attributed to a lack of will power; the bereaved are said to be "wallowing in their grief."

A third reason why the bereaved may generally perceive others as unhelpful has to do with the kinds of feelings that are elicited when interacting with the bereaved. We believe that interactions with a person who is suffering elicit two kinds of negative feelings in the potential helper: helplessness and vulnerability (see Wortman & Lehman, 1985, for a more detailed analysis). One of the most frustrating aspects of dealing with a bereaved person who is suffering is that there is so little one can do or say to effect any real improvement in the situation. The more distressed the individual, the more helpless outsiders are likely to feel. Regarding feelings of vulnerability, there are several theories in social psychology which suggest that the evaluations that people make about others who are less fortunate than they are determined in large part by their own needs for security and self-esteem (e.g., Lerner's, 1980 "Just World Theory"; see Coates, Wortman, & Abbey, 1979, for a review). Such feelings lead others to avoid, derogate, and blame the bereaved for their fate. By so doing, people can maintain the belief that they don't deserve to suffer and that nothing bad will happen to them. Several investigators have commented that widows often report that married friends are uncomfortable in their presence, perhaps because they serve as a reminder that death and widowhood are a real possibility (Walker, MacBride & Vachon, 1977). Reports of derogation and blame are also common. As Rando (1993) has expressed it, blaming the victim allows an individual "to achieve distance from the frightening notion that such capricious victimization can take place". In a book written for the bereaved, Lord (1988) quotes one woman whose son had been killed by a drunk driver: "Several people said,' If he had had a seat belt on, he probably would have lived.' That may be true, but it broke my heart to hear them say it" (p. 91). Another woman whose husband was killed while riding a motorcycle noted that, "My husband was killed shortly after we moved to Chicago. Several people blamed me for moving the family to that area." (p. 91).

It should be emphasized that the mere presence of a bereaved person who is distressed may be enough to evoke feelings of helplessness and vulnerability, and a consequent display of behaviors that are difficult for the bereaved person. One woman whose child was murdered confided to us that people avoided her at the supermarket, presumably because they were uncomfortable in her presence and did not know what to say. This was so painful to her that she drove to the next town to do her grocery shopping.

Intuitively, one might expect unhelpful or insensitive remarks or behaviors to be more prevalent among strangers or casual acquaintances than among the bereaved person's relatives or close friends. However, this does not appear to be the case. In one study, the results indicated that slightly more than half of all unhelpful comments were made by relatives or friends (Lehman et al., 1986). Because those closest to the bereaved person may have the greatest stake in his or her recovery, it is perhaps not surprising that they have little tolerance for the bereaved person's displays of distress. As Wortman and Lehman (1985) have suggested, family members and friends may be concerned about whether they will be able to cope effectively with such intense negative feelings on a regular basis.

Whether interacting with acquaintances or with family or friends, it is ironic that the very processes that would facilitate resolution of the loss may be very difficult for the bereaved to carry out. One element of the resolution process judged to be especially important is verbal repetition of the trauma (McCann & Pearlman, 1990). Supposedly, by repeating what has occurred a number of times, an individual will be aided in clarifying what happened to him or her. Yet repetition may be difficult for the potential helper to tolerate. As one of our clients who lost her son in a motor vehicle accident expressed it, "I needed to talk about the accident, but when I started talking to my closest friend about it for the second time, she became visibly annoyed. 'You told me about that already,' she said." Similarly, the aspects of the trauma or loss that are causing the bereaved the most distress may be the most difficult to discuss with others, even when the relationship is a close one. People who have suffered a major loss have often confided to us that aspects of the loss that were most painful for them, such as claiming a mutilated body at the morgue, could not really be discussed with anyone.

As a result of these processes, many bereaved people withdraw from others and give up on the possibility of meaningful social exchanges (see Pennebaker, 1993, for a more detailed discussion). Although it has not received much systematic study, many bereaved appear to prefer no social interaction to interaction with others who seem incapable of understanding what they are going through. Such interactions may only serve to make people feel more alienated, isolated, and alone (Coates, et al., 1979). Another reason for keeping their distress to themselves is that the bereaved may not want to upset their family and friends. Regardless of what causes their withdrawal, however, it may have negative consequences. In recent years, there has been increasing speculation that those who are unable to discuss their trauma with anyone may show an increase in ruminations about the loss and a greater number of health problems (Pennebaker, 1993, Tait & Silver, 1989). Moreover, if the bereaved fail to exhibit their distress and instead hide it from others , this will contribute further to false societal norms that displays of intense distress are atypical, or indicative of maladjustment.

Obtaining Professional Help

We have maintained that the bereaved have strong needs for close, confiding relationships in which they can express their pain and receive validation and support. For the reasons detailed above, however, such interactions are unlikely to occur spontaneously. Hence, it is worth considering whether those who have experienced traumatic loss would be helped by professional intervention. Is this an option for the bereaved that is likely to facilitate the resolution process?

One problem with looking to professional relationships as a solution for the bereaved person's problems is that only a small percentage of bereaved seek professional help (in most studies, from 1 - 5%; see Jacobs, 1993, for a review). Reluctance to enter a helping relationship may stem from a number of factors. One factor is the attitudes held by the bereaved about professional help. McCann and Pearlman (1990) have discussed several fears that lead individuals to resist therapy, or to resist disclosing their true feelings in therapy. These include the fear that they will not be believed; the fear that the therapist will be repulsed and disgusted by their feelings; fear of their own reactions to the material discussed, including intense rage and/or lack of control over their emotions; and the fear that talking about the deceased will not help, and perhaps will make things worse. As one of their clients expressed it, "I'm afraid I might fall apart if I talk about it in detail. I try to push away some of the images because if I don't, I might begin crying and never stop. I don't think I can stand the pain" (McCann & Pearlman, 1990, p. 214). Those who have suffered a loss may also resist therapy because they believe that people should be able to handle their problems on their own. Many see therapy of any sort as a crutch for weak-willed, dependent people, and they refuse to seek therapy for that reason. Because of these attitudes, Everstein and Everstein (1993) have recommended that "psychological services for traumatized people not be labelled as 'mental health services' because trauma victims will not use them" (p. 61).

Although few controlled studies are available, the available evidence suggests that therapy is usually beneficial in dealing with bereavement (see, e.g., Gerber, Wiener, Battin, et al., 1975; Marmar, Horowitz, Weiss, et al., 1988; Raphael, 1977; see Jacobs, 1993, for a review). However, therapists are likely to be vulnerable to many of the same biases discussed above, and even they may sometimes react to the bereaved in ways that are unhelpful. Many therapists have discussed how extremely difficult it is to work with people who are grieving. Administering such treatment is hard not only because of the trauma surrounding the death, but because of the depth of the client's pain. As Rando (1993) has suggested, such therapy can raise intense emotional reactions, which can lead the therapist to deny, blame, or punish the victim. McCann and Pearlman (1990) have called this process "vicarious traumatization." They suggest that people who work with the bereaved can experience profoundly disruptive and painful psychological effects that can last for months and years, if not indefinitely. Rando (1993) has noted that such reactions are particularly likely if the death was sudden and traumatic. She indicates that such deaths generate feelings of high anxiety and increased vulnerability on the part of the therapist because they repeatedly confront the therapist with the fact that victimization happens to innocent people. According to Rando, close observance of another person's world being shattered viciously and without warning can be terrifying to the therapist "and can prompt a search for meaning and existential sustenance that may be difficult to find" (Rando, 1993, P. 659). Taken together, this information suggests that contact with bereaved clients may evoke feelings that interfere with forging a successful therapeutic alliance, and with providing effective treatment.

Over time, the pressures of such work may lead therapists and other health care providers to become cynical and hardened (Rando, 1993). Consequently, they may sometimes make comments to the bereaved that add considerably to their distress. For example, a client seen by one of us (CBW) had experienced two miscarriages and two neonatal deaths. She was informed by her obstetrician that "we have a name for women like you. We call them baby wasters."

Administering treatment to a bereaved person who is suffering is not only likely to require intense commitment on the therapist's part. It is also likely to require consummate skill. Perhaps the best discussion of what is required is summarized in Rando (1993). In a book written for therapists, she includes a long list of common therapeutic errors (e.g.; failure to incorporate the use of medication when warranted; pushing the mourner too fast), as well as a list of guidelines for effective therapy (see also Worden, 1982). This material suggests that it may be difficult to establish a treatment program which relies solely on lay helpers. In fact, it implies that it may be difficult for a person to find a therapist who is experienced and comfortable working with clients who have endured loss.

Future Research Questions

In this chapter, we have challenged current views regarding how people cope with loss. In so doing, however, we have raised many more questions about the grief process than we have answered. In this section of the paper, we delineate what we believe are a number of exciting questions for subsequent research that emerge from this approach. We also include a brief description of our own current research.

Perhaps the most perplexing question to emerge from our analysis is what it means when a person fails to become intensely distressed following a major loss. We have indicated that such a reaction is far more common than previously believed, and that it is not necessarily followed with a delayed grief reaction. However, much more empirical work is necessary to clarify the meaning of such a response. Delayed grief is a difficult construct to measure, and we cannot rule out such a grief response just because respondents have evidenced no serious depression at a subsequent time interval in the study. Perhaps the measurement points did not coincide with a subsequent grief reaction for a significant percentage of respondents. For example, a respondent may have shown an inappropriately intense reaction to a minor loss that occurred between measurement periods in the study.

It is also believed that those who fail to express their grief will develop physical health problems. However, the vast majority of studies on the impact of loss have failed to include health outcome measures other than self-report. Thus, there is virtually no information available to test this provocative notion. Longitudinal studies which combine assessments of grieving and physical health measures would add immeasurably to our knowledge of these processes.

Current research suggests that for some types of loss, there is information available to suggest what kinds of reactions are "normal" following the loss. In general, the research reviewed in this paper suggests that it is normal to show distress following a sudden loss for longer than the 1-2 year period thought to be necessary for recovery. One intriguing question is whether it is helpful, shortly after a loss has been experienced, to provide the bereaved with information regarding what is known about the norms for recovery. One of us (CBW) met a woman at a conference who confided that she had lost a child 6 months ago in a sudden and traumatic incident.

She said that she was not in good shape now, but expected to be pretty much recovered by Spring. Somehow, it seemed inappropriate to say, "Actually, research has shown that your symptoms are likely to continue for a number of years."

We have suggested that because the majority of bereaved individuals learn that others do not want to hear about their difficulties. Consequently, they become less likely to convey their distress to others. Much more needs to be learned about this suppression of distress. Does it cause other problems, such as an increase in ruminations? Does suppression place more physical strain on the body, and therefore result in subsequent health problems? If research demonstrates suppression to have negative health consequences, is it better to convey one's distress and incur the social disapproval of others, or to suppress one's distress regardless of the response of one's support network?

Given that expressions of distress are believed to have positive mental and physical health consequences, but negative interpersonal consequences, are there alternative ways of expressing one's pain that are beneficial, such as artistic expression (e.g. music, poetry, painting) or keeping a diary? These modes of expression sometimes include elements thought to be therapeutic, such as achieving cognitive clarification. As noted earlier, Pennebaker and his associates (see Pennebaker, 1993, for a review) have found that individuals who write about their past trauma just a few times make fewer health center visits than respondents who do not. Writing has the advantage of permitting expression in a setting where negative social reactions from others are generally precluded.

A related series of questions concerns whether the bereaved can or should receive instruction in how to manage their distress so as to minimize its potential negative impact on others. Are people in distress less likely to alienate others if they describe their feelings verbally than if they convey negative emotions? Are some negative emotions, such as bitterness or rage, more difficult to tolerate than other negative emotions, such as anxiety, and hence especially likely to result in avoidance or derogation? Are there gender differences in the ability to tolerate others' distress, and do males or females react differently to males in pain than to females in pain? Is there anything else that those experiencing intense distress can do to minimize the likelihood of negative reactions from others? In one study (Silver, Wortman, & Crofton, 1990), we found that cancer patients who were coping poorly with their illness were judged far more negatively, across a wide range of outcome variables, than cancer patients who had the same prognosis but were attempting to do something about their fate. Thus, the bereaved may be able to minimize the likelihood that others will respond negatively if they mention any positive steps they are taking to cope with their loss. Of course, it could be argued that ethically, it is inappropriate to even suggest that people who have suffered the loss of a loved one should be made responsible for influencing the reactions of others. In our judgment, the problems described here are perpetuated by powerful sociocultural beliefs, not by the misbehavior of the bereaved themselves.

As we have maintained elsewhere (Coyne, Wortman, & Lehman, 1988), we believe that any study of interactions between the bereaved and those in their social network will be much more fruitful if it includes both parties. Because of everything they have been through, bereaved persons may be hypersensitive to criticism from others, and may perceive it where it does not exist. This possibility can only be evaluated by studying the bereaved in the context of their social network, and obtaining the perspective of the bereaved, their potential supporters, and also detached observers of the social situation.

The research reviewed above suggests that particularly in the case of sudden, unexpected losses, it may take more time to recover than is commonly believed. In subsequent research, it will be important to identify those processes through which wounds from the loss are kept open. One idea we feel is in need of further research is that people may process information differently following a major loss. For example, consider a person who has lost a child in a drunk driving crash a few years previously. That person may become upset if he or she is subsequently a guest at a cocktail party where some guests have had too much to drink. Such a person may also become distressed upon learning of another drunk driving fatality, or of reading about legislation designed to crack down on drunk drivers which is defeated in the legislature. Even ads for alcohol may elicit some emotional pain. In short, those who have been victimized may have a heightened sensitivity for certain types of information. Processing this information may contribute further to their belief that the world is a capricious, unfair place.

Until this point, we have focused our attention on interventions for the bereaved. However, it is worth considering whether the bereaved would benefit indirectly by interventions directed at those in their social network. If network members are educated about the enormous variability in response to loss and the usual timetable for the type of loss that has occurred, as well as the strategies most likely to help the bereaved, would they be more likely to behave toward the bereaved in a supportive manner? Unfortunately, there are two separate studies suggesting that this may not be the case. In the previously mentioned study by Lehman et al. (1986), most non-bereaved control respondents guessed that it would take as long, or longer, to get over the loss of a loved one than bereaved respondents did. When asked what they would say or do to be helpful, control respondents were able to generate responses that are in fact perceived as helpful, such as providing an opportunity for the bereaved person to express feelings. Similarly, in a study by Caserta and Lund (1992), nonbereaved respondents rated the coping ability of respondents who lost a spouse as significantly lower than the bereaved rated their own coping ability. In this study, nonbereaved respondents also rated the stressfulness of losing a spouse as higher than the bereaved respondents did. These findings suggest that those in the social network are not minimizing the severity of the problem, and are not overestimating the bereaved person's ability to deal with the problem. Hence, merely educating people about the experience of loss and the coping strategies that are most helpful may be insufficient to solve the problem.

We have been very intrigued by the questions raised by prior research, and have attempted to develop a comprehensive research program that would provide answers to some of these questions. Our most pressing questions center around individuals who appear to go through a major loss without experiencing major distress. Should this group be understood as evidencing pathology or resilience? To help clarify this question, we have designed an implemented two prospective studies on widowhood that begin before the spouse dies and continue after his or her death.

Both of these prospective studies are part of a large-scale project begun at the University of Michigan in collaboration with Ron Kessler and James House. The first study is part of a large scale multidisciplinary investigation of health, stress and productive activities across the lifespan. This is called the Americans' Changing Lives project. In 1986, interviews were conducted with a nationally representative sample of 3,617 adults. In 1989, 2,867 were reinterviewed. Approximately 80 respondents lost a spouse between waves of data collection. The second prospective study is the CLOC (Changing Lives of Older Couples) project. Baseline data were obtained in 1988 from 1,532 members of older couples in the Detroit area. Death records were monitored, and subjects who lose a spouse were interviewed at several intervals following the loss, including 6 months, 18 months, and 5 years later. Matched control respondents were interviewed at comparable time periods. In addition, the study includes a biomedical component which provides a comprehensive assessment of physical health.

These studies will provide the opportunity to address a variety of fascinating questions (see Wortman, Silver & Kessler, 1993, for a more detailed discussion). To clarify our understanding of individuals who fail to become distressed following a major loss, we will determine whether those who fail to show distress show other indications of mourning (e.g., preoccupation with thoughts of avoidance of reminders of the loved one). Such data should be useful in clarifying whether such a reaction is indicative of denial or repression of distress, or whether it reflects resilience.

Because health outcomes will be monitored in the CLOC study, we will be able to determine whether initial failure to experience distress results in subsequent health problems. We will also be able to determine whether there is any relationship between initial distress and long-term positive changes as a result of the loss. Are people who show little initial distress following a major loss less likely to experience personal growth than those who have experienced intense distress?

There are a variety of additional questions that can be addressed with prospective data of this sort. One question of major theoretical significance concerns the impact of prior life events on a person's ability to cope with a major loss. Some individuals have suggested that prior life events may holster a person's ability to deal with loss (Wortman & Silver, 1990). According to this view, individuals often develop new coping strategies as a response to stress that then become available for use in future crises. However, others have maintained that the impact of previous events is often negative, particularly if the prior crisis has not been satisfactorily resolved. In fact, some investigators (e.g., Haan, 1977) have suggested that a crisis may trigger "ominous meaning" or associations for people who have past unresolved conflicts.

Summary

For over a decade, we have been involved in a program of research designed to clarify how people come to terms with major losses in their lives. We have summarized evidence suggesting that people's reactions to loss are based on powerful cultural assumptions that are often not acknowledged.

It is widely assumed that people become extremely distressed following a major loss, that failure to show distress is indicative of pathology, and that within a relatively short time (1-2 years), people resolve what has happened and recover their former level of functioning. However, available evidence provides little support for these firmly entrenched views.

Much of the chapter focuses on the interpersonal consequences of these myths about coping with loss. There is considerable evidence that people who are going through a crisis benefit from social support (see Wortman & Silver, 1990, for a review). Unfortunately, those who have suffered the loss of a loved one rarely receive effective support from others. We have attempted to demonstrate how beliefs in the myths of coping undermines support by leading others to respond judgmentally to the bereaved. Moreover, there is evidence to suggest that contact with the bereaved can evoke feelings of vulnerability and helplessness. These feelings can result in behaviors toward the bereaved that are unhelpful, such as avoidance, offering advice, or minimizing the bereaved's problems. We maintain that these difficulties in relating effectively to the bereaved are experienced not only by acquaintances, friends and family members of the bereaved, but also by health care professions. We suggest that particularly when the loss is sudden and traumatic, professionals may experience a kind of "vicarious traumatization" that makes it difficult to establish an effective therapeutic alliance.

It is clear from the literature that sudden, traumatic death is the leading cause of death of people under 50 (Lehman et al., 1987). We also know that the vast majority of people who suffer such losses do not seek psychotherapy. If the analysis presented here is accurate, such people may also have great difficulty eliciting effective support from their family and friends.

Despite the prevalence of traumatic loss, there are only a handful of controlled studies (see Jacobs, 1993 for a review) evaluating specific treatments. This suggests that in virtually all communities, there are pressing unmet needs for this highly vulnerable group.

Above, we have delineated a variety of research questions that would help clarify how victims of traumatic loss could best be supported through their loss. We hope that as a result of this discussion, greater research attention will be directed toward this group. Much more needs to be understood about whether those who have endured traumatic loss can profit from peer support. Mechanisms for encouraging those who have suffered such losses to seek professional help should also be studied. Finally, it would be extremely useful to know what steps, if any, victims of traumatic loss could take to strengthen their own support networks. Hopefully, studies focusing on topics such as these will contribute to a knowledge base on treatment of traumatic loss over time. This will help ensure that those suffering from traumatic loss will have access to the kinds of help they so badly need.

References

Belitsky, R., & Jacobs, S. (1986). Bereavement, attachment theory, and mental disorders. Psychiatric Annals, 16(5), 276-280.

Bowlby, J. (1961). Process of mourning. The International Journal of Psychoanalysis, 42, 317-340.

Brill, S. (1983, December). An innocent man on death row. The American Lawyer, pp.1, 84-91.

Brown, J. T., & Stoudemire, G. A. (1983). Normal and pathological grief. JAMA, 250(3), 378-382.

Calhoun, L. G., Cann, A., Selby, J. W., & Magee, D. L. (1981). Victim emotional response: Effects on social reaction to victims of rape. British Journal of Social Psychology, 20, 17-21.

Caserta, M. S., & Lund, D. A. (1992). Bereavement stress and coping among older adults: Expectations versus the actual experience. OMEGA, 25(1), 33-45.

Clark, L. F. (1993). Stress and the cognitive-conversational benefits of social interaction. Journal of Social and Clinical Psychology, 12, 25-55.

Coates, D., Wortman, C. B., & Abbey, A. (1979). Reactions to victims. In I. H. Frieze, D. Bar-Tal & J. S. Carroll (Eds.), New approaches to social problems (pp. 21-52). San Francisco: Jossey-Bass.

Coyne, J. C., Wortman, C. B., & Lehman, D. R. (1988). The other side of support: Emotional overinvolvement and miscarried helping. In B. H. Gottlieb (Ed.), Marshaling social support: Formats, processes and effects (pp. 305-330). Newbury Park: Sage.

Craig, Y. (1977). The bereavement of parents and their search for meaning. British Journal of Social Work, 7, 41-54.

Davidowitz, M. & Myrick, R. D. (1984). Responding to the bereaved: An analysis of "helping" statements. Research Record, 1, 35-42.

Dembo, T., Leviton, G. L., & Wright, B. A. (1956). Adjustment to misfortune: A problem of social-psychological rehabilitation. Artificial Limbs, 3, 4-62.

DiGiulio, R. C. (1989). Beyond widowhood: From bereavement to emergence and hope. New York: The Free Press.

Downey, G., Silver, R. C., & Wortman, C. B. (1990). Reconsidering the attribution-adjustment relation following a major negative event: Coping with the loss of a child. Journal of Personality and Social Psychology, 59, 925-940.

Erikson, K. T. (1994). A new species of trouble: Explorations in disaster, trauma, and community. New York: Norton.

Everstine, D. S., & Everstine, L. (1993). The trauma response: Treatment for emotional injury. New York: Norton.

Ferrell, D. (1990, November 13). New clues in a trial by fire. Los Angeles Times.

Francis, M. E. & Pennebaker, J. W. (1992). Putting stress into words: The impact of writing on physiological, absentee, and self reported emotional well-being measures. American Journal of Health Promotion, 6, 280-287.

Gerber, I., Wiener, A., Battin, D., et al. (1975). Brief therapy to the aged bereaved, in Bereavement: Its Psychological Aspects. Edited by Shoenberg, B., Gerber,I.,Wiener, A., et al (pp. 310-333). New York: Columbia University Press.

Green, B. L., Lindy, J. D., Grace, M. C., Gleser, G. C., Leonard, A. C., Korol, M., & Winget, C. (1990). Buffalo Creek survivors in the second decade: Stability of stress symptoms. American Journal of Orthopsychiatry, 60, 43-54.

Greenberg, M. A. & Stone, A. A. (1992). Emotional disclosure about traumas and its relation to health: Effects of previous disclosure and trauma severity. Journal of Personality and Social Psychology, 63, 75-84.

Haan, N. (1977). Coping and defending: Processes of self-environment organization. New York: Academic Press.

Horowitz, S. (1989). How to say the right thing. Reader's Digest, 134, 161-164.

Jacobs, S. (1993). Pathological grief: Maladaption to loss. Washington, DC and London: American Psychiatric Press, Inc.

Jacoby, S. (1984). "You'll be your old self again soon". McCall's, 111, 38-43.

Kubler-Ross, E. (1969). On death and dying. New York: Macmillan.

Lehman, D. R., Ellard, J. H., & Wortman, C. B. (1986). Social support for the bereaved: Recipients' and providers' perspectives on what is helpful. Journal of Consulting and Clinical Psychology, 54, 438-446.

Lehman, D. R., Wortman, C. B., & Williams, A. F. (1987). Long-term effects of losing a spouse or child in a motor vehicle crash. Journal of Personality and Social Psychology, 52, 218-231.

Lerner, M. J. (1980). The belief in a just world: A fundamental delusion. New York: Plenum.

Lindy, J. D., Green, B. L., Grace, M., & Titchener, J. (1983). Psychotherapy with survivors of the Beverly Hills Supper Club fire. American Journal of Psychotherapy, 37, 593-610.

Lord, J. H. (1988). Beyond sympathy: What to say and do for someone suffering an injury, illness or loss. Ventura, CA: Pathfinder Publishing.

Marmar, C. R., Horowitz, M. J., Weiss, D. S., et al. (1988). A controlled trial of brief psychotherapy and mutual help group treatment of conjugal bereavement. American Journal of Psychiatry,145, 203-209.

McCann, I. L., & Pearlman, L. A. (1990). Psychological trauma and the adult survivor: Theory, therapy, and transformation. New York: Brunner/Mazel.

Nemiah, J. C. (1957). The psychiatrist and rehabilitation. Archives of Physical Medicine and Rehabilitation, 38, 143-147.

Osterweis, M., Solomon, F., & Green, M. (1984). Bereavement: Reactions, consequences and care. Washington, DC: National Academy Press.

Parkes, C. M., & Weiss, R. S. (1983). Recovery from bereavement. New York: Basic Books.

Pattison, E. M. (1977). The experience of dying. Englewood Cliffs, NJ: Prentice-Hall.

Pennebaker, J. W. & Beall S. (1986). Confronting a traumatic event: Toward an understanding of inhibition and disease. Journal of Abnormal Psychology, 95, 274-281.

Pennebaker, J. W., Kiecolt-Glaser, J. K., Glaser, R. (1988). Disclosure of Traumas and Immune Function: Health implications for psychotherapy. Journal of Consulting and Clinical Psychology, 56(2), 1-7.

Pennebaker, J. W. (1989). Confession, inhibition, and disease. In L. Berkowitz (Ed.), Advances in experimental social psychology. Vol. 22. New York: Academic Press.

Pennebaker, J. W. (1993). Social mechanisms of constraint. In D. M. Wegner, & J. W. Pennebaker (Eds.), Handbook of mental control (pp. 200-219). Englewood Cliffs, NJ: Prentice Hall.

Rachman, S. (1980). Emotional processing. Behaviour Research and Therapy, 18, 51-60.

Rando, T. A. (1993). Treatment of complicated mourning. Champaign, IL: Research Press.

Raphael, B. (1977). Prevention intervention with the recently bereaved. Archives of General Psychiatry, 34, 1450-1454.

Rothbaum, B. O. & Foa, E. B. (1992). Cognitive-behavioral treatment of posttraumatic stress disorder. In P. Saigh (Ed.), Posttraumatic stress disorder: A behavioral approach to assessment and treatment (pp. 85-110). Boston: Allyn and Bacon.

Rubin, S. (1985). The resolution of bereavement: A clinical focus on the relationship to the deceased. Psychotherapy, 22, 231-235.

Silver, R. L. & Wortman, C. B. (1980). Coping with undesirable life events. In J. Garber & M. E. P. Seligman (Eds.), Human helplessness: Theory and applications (pp. 279-340). New York: Academic Press.

Silver, R. C., Wortman, C. B., & Crofton, C. (1990). The role of coping in support provision: The self-presentational dilemma of victims of life crises. In B. R. Sarason, I. G. Sarason & G. R. Pierce (Eds.), Social support: An interactional view (pp. 397-426). New York: Wiley.

Silverman, P. (1983). Coping with grief - it can't be rushed. U. S. News & World Report, Inc., 65-68.

Tait, R., & Silver, R. C. (1989). Coming to terms with major negative life events. In J. S. Uleman and J. A. Bargh (Eds.), Unintended thought (pp. 351-382). New York: Guilford Press.

Van der Kolk, B. A., & Van der Hart, O. (1991). The intrusive past: the flexibility of memory and the engraving of trauma. American Imago, 48(4), 425-454.

Volkan, V. (1985). Psychotherapy of complicated mourning. In V. Volkan (Ed.), Depressive states and their treatment. Northvale, NJ: Jason Aronson.

Walker, K. N., MacBride, A., & Vachon, M. L. S. (1977). Social support networks and the crisis of bereavement. Social Science and Medicine, 11, 35-41.

Weiss, R. S. (1988). Loss and recovery. Journal of Social Issues, 44, 37-52.

Worden, J. W. (1982). Grief counseling and grief therapy: A handbook for the mental health practitioner. New York: Springer.

Wortman, C. B., & Dunkel-Schetter, C. (1979). Interpersonal relationships and cancer: A theoretical analysis. Journal of Social Issues, 35, 120-155.

Wortman, C. B., & Lehman, D. R. (1985). Reactions to victims of life crises: Support attempts that fail. In I. G. Sarason & B. R. Sarason (Eds.), Social support: Theory, research and applications (pp. 463-489). Dordrecht, The Netherlands: Martinus Nijoff.

Wortman, C. B., & Silver, R. C. (1987). Coping with irrevocable loss. In G. R. VandenBos & B. K. Bryant (Eds.), Cataclysms, crises, and catastrophes: Psychology in action (Master Lecture Series), 6, 189-235. Washington, DC: American Psychological Association.

Wortman, C. B., & Silver, R. C. (1989). The myths of coping with loss. Journal of Consulting and Clinical Psychology, 57, 349-357.

Wortman, C. B., & Silver, R. C. (1990). Successful mastery of bereavement and widowhood: A life course perspective. In P. B. Baltes & M. M. Baltes (Eds.), Successful aging: Perspectives from the behavioral sciences (pp. 225-264). New York: Cambridge University Press.

Wortman, C. B., Silver, R. C. & Kessler, R. C. (1993). The meaning of loss and adjustment to bereavement. In M. S. Stroebe, W. Stroebe & R. O. Hansson (Eds.), Bereavement: A sourcebook of research and interventions (pp. 349-366). London: Cambridge University Press.

Wright, B. A. (1983). Physical disability - A psychosocial approach (2nd ed.). New York: Harper & Row.

Authors' Notes

Preparation of this chapter was supported by the National Institute on Aging Program project grant A605561 to Dr. Camille Wortman, Principal Investigator. The authors thank Charles Figley, Donald Meichenbaum and Zahava Solomon for feedback on the ideas presented here. Inquires or requests for reprints should be directed to Dr. Camille B. Wortman, Director, Social/Health Graduate Training Program, Department of Psychology, SUNY-Stony Brook, NY 11794.

INDIVIDUAL AND COMMUNITY STRESS: INTEGRATION OF APPROACHES AT DIFFERENT LEVELS[1]

Matthias Jerusalem, Humboldt-Universität zu Berlin, Berlin, Germany
Krzysztof Kaniasty, Indiana University of Pennsylvania, Indiana, PA, USA
Darrin R. Lehman, University of British Columbia, Vancouver B.C., Canada
Christian Ritter, Kent State University, Kent, OH, USA
Gordon J. Turnbull, Ticehurst House Hospital, Wadhurst, UK

Introduction: Many Facets of Stress

The last two decades have witnessed a dramatic increase of theoretical and empirical efforts aimed at understanding the nature of the human stress process. The contemporary literature includes many theoretical propositions, integrative models, and research findings that have advanced our ability to predict and explain people's responses to stressful life circumstances (e.g., Ensel & Lin, 1991; Goldberger & Breznitz, 1993; Hobfoll, 1988; Jerusalem, 1993; Jerusalem & Schwarzer, 1989; Lazarus, 1991; Lazarus & Folkman, 1984; Moos, 1986; Pearlin, 1989). However, the vast majority of this literature has focused on the analysis of the stress process at the level of the individual. We know a great deal about how a single person in the context of his or her own personal resources, stress appraisals, coping efforts and environmental constraints confronts a variety of stressful circumstances. In contrast, community stress processes, that pertain to the issue of what happens when an entire community is affected by a common stressor, have been examined less frequently. Are there parallels between the essentials of individual stress processes and the dynamics of stress at the community level? Is it possible to conceptually differentiate between both stress processes and to integrate them into a common theoretical framework? Certainly, there are no readily available answers to these challenging questions.

The existing literature on stressful encounters at the community level has examined a variety of rather heterogeneous stressors. Among them are natural disasters, nuclear and toxic hazards, industrial accidents, wars, political oppression and

---

[1] The authors would also like to acknowledge the members of the working group whose contributions were incorporated into this chapter: Jan Strelau, Charles D. Spielberger, Abdul Wali Wardak, and Camille Wortman.

violence, terrorist acts, transportation accidents, epidemics, crime, immigration, social discrimination, unemployment, and many more. What is the common denominator of these diverging events that allows them to be labeled as community stressors? Some of these upheavals are large-scale events that could simultaneously impact the majority of a community, be it at the regional or nationwide levels (e.g., natural disasters, wars). Others could be restricted to certain subgroups of the population or area (e.g., immigration, unemployment). Moreover, individual level stressors such as illness, traffic accidents, crime, or job stress, to name a few, may shift to a community level event as soon as the number of people involved substantially increases and the local community begins to regard these events as threatening. Hence, simple typologies of events have a rather limited utility as a platform for distinguishing between individual and community level stress.

Different stressors are often indexed along characteristics or features such as suddenness, severity, valence, controllability, or duration. Can these criteria help in distinguishing individual and community stress? Events such as wars or earthquakes usually occur suddenly and cause a severe impact on human beings. But the same is true for the individual level fates such as cancer, rape, or traffic accidents. On the other hand, wars and traffic accidents could also be grouped together because they tend to be more controllable than earthquakes and rape. Furthermore, earthquakes, rapes, and traffic accidents may appear similar when considering their duration -- they all are less lasting than wars, cancer, or other illnesses. However, all stressful events can spur an array of secondary stressors (see Pearlin, 1989). Thus whereas the duration of the onset may differ, all of them have the potential of evolving into lasting conditions. Similar problems surface when we try to compare other individual and community events. Undoubtedly, all kinds of stressors differ along severity, valence, controllability, or duration dimensions which determinate their significance for the individuals and communities they impact. Consequently, for our purposes, the discriminating power of these distinctions is low.

Stressors also differ in the sources from which they originate. Many stressful upheavals have a multitude of causes that generally stem from natural, human-made, political, cultural, or economic conditions. Can community and individual stressors be traced back to unique sources? Earthquakes or hurricanes have natural origins, toxic spills or industrial accidents are human-made, large-scale lay-offs are a reflection of economic conditions, wars or terrorist acts primarily are motivated by political and economic circumstances. Likewise, similar sources can be linked to individual stressors. Severe illness and traffic accidents may be a combination of natural and human-made influences; divorce can be traced back to economic problems or to differences that are cultural or political in nature. It is evident that classifying sources of stressors is of little use for our purposes because the origins of stressful events cut across individual and community events and most of these stressors are associated with a variety of causes.

Our search for differential characteristics of individual and community stress finally led us to the issue of individual differences. The experience of stress may not simply be an objective feature determined by the nature of a measurable stressor (see Lazarus & Folkman, 1984). The stress literature documents that individuals' subjective perceptions and interpretations may be most decisive in determining whether or not people experience stress (e.g., Jerusalem, 1993; Jerusalem & Schwarzer, 1992; Lazarus, 1991). From this theoretical perspective, a subjective appraisal is the key concept that may explain why some individuals suffer more from what happens to them whereas others suffer less. Possibly, the role of subjective appraisals is most evident in the case of individual level stressors, especially those whose severity may not be easily defined in objective terms. At the community level the variability of subjective appraisals may be reduced or proven less consequential because of a common experience of a larger group of people undergoing a clearly defined, and most often unambiguously stressful circumstance (see Hobfoll, 1988; Hobfoll, Briggs, & Wells, this volume for a discussion). Evidence pertaining to these considerations is at best equivocal. The literature on traumatic events such as brush-fires, hurricanes, or floods provides strong evidence that these events affect adversely the well-being of large segments of victimized populations. At the same time, however, researchers are quick to note that not everybody and not every community develop clinically significant psychological problems. Usually, only a small subset of the affected persons require mental health services, develop PTSD symptoms, or other psychopathologies (e.g., Freedy, Saladin, Kilpatrick, Resnick, & Saunders, 1994; Green, this volume; McFarlane, this volume; Norris, 1992; Rubonis & Bickman, 1991). Thus, as with individual level stressors, community level events are subject to individual differences in stress appraisals, coping behavior, and outcomes. Despite a common stressor, subjective reactions differ considerably. Consequently, objective and subjective appraisals of the stressful encounters turn out to be insufficient to provide a framework capable of distinguishing between individual and community level stress.

Our brief analysis indicates that individual and community stress are heterogenous phenomena and cannot easily be differentiated. At least attempts to differentiate them along various qualitative and quantitative features proved unsuccessful. It appears that individual and community stressors do not represent separable or distinct sociopsychological entities. They are multi-faceted and overlapping stress phenomena. However, in spite of these difficulties, we will propose a parsimonious heuristic that could serve as a first step toward differentiation between individual and community level stressors. Our proposal is based on reciprocal transactions between the two key elements of the stress experience: the number of people involved or affected by the stressful event and the amount of public concern and response associated with that event.

Transitions from Individual to Community Stress:
Three Levels of Changes in Appraisal, Coping, and Resource Mobilization

Research investigating individual level stress uses as the unit of observation the person with his or her idiosyncratic reactions. Even if data are aggregated across many individuals, the analyzed processes regarding resources, appraisals, coping efforts, and outcomes are documented and discussed at the individual level. Even if communal resources in coping with stress are taken into account (e.g., formal and informal social support systems), their influences are usually assessed from the perspective of the individual. At what point in the process of coping with stress does the community come into play? When does a stressor become a communal concern?

Before we attempt to address these questions, let us first define what we consider to be a community. Quite broadly, a community may be an intimate couple, an informal network such as a family, relatives or friends, a political organization, cultural association, city or a larger geographical region, an ethnically homogenous group, or a group of foreigners in a state. The basic formal characteristic of a community is that it consists of two or more persons linked to each other through blood or personal ties, common interests, geographical proximity, cultural solidarity, national identity, and, most importantly for our purposes, through an experience of a common stressor.

Consequently, in our view, the obvious prerequisite of a community level stress is that more than one person experiences it. Beginning with this criterion, transitions from individual to community level stress can be described along three levels or stages generally characterized by different degrees of public responses to a stressor. The following sections will examine the stages of individual stress (Level 1), moderate community stress (Level 2), and high community stress (Level 3).

Level 1: Individual Level Stress

The criterion of the prevalence rate as greater than one individual affected is necessary but not sufficient for the occurrence of community stress. Imagine, a small nuclear outfall that is kept secret or a city in an ecologically damaged region. In both cases, a certain number of people (which could be large) will exhibit negative physical and psychological reactions. As long as the victims are not aware of each other's common problems, the resulting stress remains restricted to the individual level. Level 1 is a stage of individual stress because there is no common awareness of the problem, and thus no reason for public action.

Level 2: Moderate Community Stress

Theoretically speaking, the individual level of stress is surpassed when a detectable amount of communal awareness and concern for the problem emerges. At this point, victims become a kind of stressor-related psychological community because they realize that others share the same fate. Either through mere numbers or through organized vocalization of the problem, the general public may accept the stressor as threatening, and as having relevance for the community. In other words, one can identify a transition from individual stress to community stress when the awareness and individual appraisals become a public entity. This is Level 2 of the proposed transition model. At this stage, individuals experience a stressor and the public is aware of it, but the communal stress perceptions and appraisals are not yet strong enough to motivate public action and communal coping. The resulting community stress may be either low or moderate. If the public does not judge the stressor as dangerous for communal well-being, the community stress is merely acknowledged but not acted upon. Unfortunately, it is possible that not many community members will initially be ready to act if a group of homeless elderly people gets ill due to poor sanitary conditions in inner-city dwellings, or if a minority group of foreigners is terrorized by violence of right wing political youth gangs. However, if public opinion shifts and evaluates the stressor as a source of danger to larger (or more prominent) segments of the community the amount of shared stressful experience would increase significantly. For example, if poor sanitary conditions were to affect business- and service-people working downtown, or if the violent acts of youngsters were perceived as harmful to the community's image, then, undoubtedly these stressors would become a common concern of the larger community.

Level 3: High Community Stress

Communal appraisals of distress tend to bring with them communal coping efforts. The point at which commonly judged relevance of the stressful condition leads to actual coping efforts at the community level marks the transition from moderate to high community stress. Thus Level 3 is characterized both by the community's perception of the stressor as being of high relevance to all and by the introduction of communal coping. If many people are concerned, and if the stressor endangers the functioning of the whole community, the public and authorities are challenged to act to protect against further damage. For example, if the risk of spreading disease is high, the health care system must be mobilized. If people are afraid to leave their homes at night, or businesses move away because of violent crimes, public officials are pressured to re-establish law and order.

In sum, we propose to examine the dynamics of stress processes moving across three stages. In Level 1 (individual level stress), although more than one person can be affected by the stressor, neither public awareness nor public coping are observed. In other words, community response is absent. In Level 2 (moderate level of community stress), more than one person is affected and the public awareness is emerging, although public coping is not yet observed. And in Level 3 (high level of community stress), many people are affected, public awareness is present, and coping efforts at the public level begin to emerge.

The three levels of stress are not only associated with changes in individual and public appraisals. The coping dimension, and with it the process of resource mobilization, are also important. At Levels 1 and 2, the individual primarily has to rely on his or her own coping resources. Affected individuals may have very limited access to communal resources of social or physical welfare systems (e.g., hospitalization, counselling, unemployment benefits). In fact, access to these communal resources could be determined solely by the individual's characteristics such as socio-economic status, employment, education, or psychological sense of mastery. Due to the rising public awareness of the stressor at Level 2, a detectable increase in the availability of communal resources will take place that could be relied on by those victimized. For example, one of the ways in which collective recognition augments access to resources is through a formation of mutual help groups. At Level 3, where the community as a whole, more often than not, must cope with the stressor, a great increase in availability of public resources is expected. At this stage, as compared to the individual level, the available public resources will most likely become the primary source of assistance in coping efforts.

Three Stress Levels: Discrete Classifications and Developmental Sequences

The proposed model of transitions from individual to community stress is flexible because it allows classification of both discrete stressful events (e.g., disasters) as well as those which unfold over time (e.g., AIDS epidemic). The model is not meant to be a simple enumeration of distinct stages that are independent of each other. Thus, first of all, any stressful event may originate at any particular level. For instance, severe events that threaten the lives of most members of a community (e.g., disasters, wars) can be classified instantly as Level 3 stress -- the state of emergency demands public coping. On the other hand, stressors affecting certain groups (e.g. homeless, homosexuals, foreigners) are more likely to be classified as Level 2 stress -- public awareness is present but communal coping is not yet mobilized because of the relatively minor relevance of the problem to the majority of community members.

One complicating issue is that the extent of public awareness and public coping may vary over considerable ranges, not only across levels but also within levels. For example, public awareness of a disease and its risk for the community might be present in a group of experts but absent among laypersons (Level 2 event). Some progressive groups may try to fight against hostility toward foreigners (i.e., public coping has begun) but broad masses of the society may remain indifferent to that problem (Level 3 event). Therefore, the model allows for a variety of continua of increasing degrees of communal awareness and coping.

The model also allows for developmental transitions such that an event may move across levels over time. For example, it might be that a new and unknown infectious disease will originate with a few individuals (Level 1). As the number of affected people increases, the more likely the public will become aware of it (Level 2). Further, the greater the danger for all members of a community, the higher the probability that the public will eventually try to find ways of coping with the threat, help the victims, and mobilize efforts to prevent others from the same fate (Level 3). In some instances this process could be rapid, provided that the communication between affected individuals and the public is unimpeded. Unfortunately, factors such as stigma or collective denial may also play a role and delay the breakthrough to the level of awareness at the community level. Such social forces hinder mobilization of necessary resources needed to aid the victims as well as to marshal public efforts to protect the community as a whole. One has only to briefly reflect upon the history of public awareness concerning the dangers of HIV infection to realize that stigma and denial are potent forces obstructing efforts to aid victims, understand risks, and act upon the threat.

It is not assumed, however, that every unfolding stressful event must pass through levels 1 through 3. Events may move in the opposite direction as well. Natural disasters or wars are community stressors that start at Level 3, where public coping is instantaneously mobilized to aid victims. However, over time the public interest may slowly but steadily decrease as the community moves away from the crisis phase and begins to recover. Other needs and concerns will surface and compete for resources. Consequently, some of the victims, especially those whose recovery is not complete, may be left alone and find themselves thrown back to the level of individual stress (Level 1).

In the remainder of this chapter we will attempt to illustrate some of the dynamics of community level stress. Particularly, we are interested in examining how key elements of the individual stress process -- resources, appraisals, coping, and social support -- translate to the community stress context.

Resources and Community Stress

The extent of public awareness and public coping efforts accelerates as the number of affected individuals increases and the danger to the community's well-being becomes apparent. Thus the stressor becomes a communal entity as it surpasses the individual levels of losses and begins to threaten or actually destroys communal resources as well (see Hobfoll, 1988; Hobfoll et al., this volume). Therefore, in the case of community stress both individual resources (e.g., partner support, job, self-esteem, optimism, health, etc.) and community resources (e.g., emergency equipment, transportation and communications systems, availability of employment, sense of community, social cohesion, etc.) must be considered.

The literature on disasters and other traumatic events clearly demonstrates the potential of these events to strain basic economic, social, and psychological resources valued by both individuals and their communities. Regardless of the level of its impact, it is important to remember that the stress experience always begins with the individual. When losses incurred due to a stressor surpass the individual level and cause losses for the community as well, the resulting depletion of community resources reduces the ability of the community to help its members. The individual loss cycles are accelerated (see Hobfoll & Lilly, 1993). On one hand, when the stressor damages basic public resources like water, food or fuel reserves, traffic control systems, emergency services, or communication channels, the community itself is in need of coping assistance. For many directly affected individuals these may be secondary losses but they undoubtedly reduce their ability to cope with their own fate. On the other hand, the losses at the community level extend to all residents in the community, even to those who were spared the destructive powers of the stressor and did not sustain primary losses. These residents of the affected community are also victims because the quality of their lives is dependent on the services provided by a well-functioning communal infrastructure. The irony of the community-wide resource depletion is that these "secondary victims" may now be less likely to aid the coping of those who experienced most severely the impact of the stressor. In any case, depleting community resources aggravates the crisis as the number of victims increases and the availability of both personal and community resources decreases. Thus resource loss at the communal level augments loss at the individual level.

A differential vulnerability to stress may be as much of an issue for whole communities as it is for individuals. For example, communities with a high proportion of children, elderly, or economically disadvantaged may be characterized by low levels of preevent resources. A rather rapid exhaustion of available communal resources would be especially devastating to these individuals because of their general dependence on such services as public health care, low cost housing, or social welfare systems (see deVries, this volume). Other communities may be in a better position to cope with community stress because of their greater initial levels both of individual and community resources. Communities that are better endowed with communal resources are more capable of mobilizing their efforts to block the spirals of losses experienced by their affected members. Thus the differential vulnerability at the community level is a function of resource reserves reflected in the postevent ratio of <u>depleted resources</u> to <u>resources still available</u>.

Appraisals and Community Stress

The role of subjective appraisals is continuously debated in the stress literature. Many researchers (e.g., Lazarus & Folkman, 1984) claim that subjective appraisals are key determinants of stress experiences. Others (e.g., Hobfoll, 1988) suggest that objective loss of valued resources is of greater importance. Both positions are supported by empirical evidence. Possibly, one important determinant of the role of subjective appraisals in the experience of stress, both for individuals and communities, is the level of ambiguity of the stressing agent. Natural disasters and other extreme events (e.g., airplane crashes), for example, have immediate, pervasive, and often catastrophic impacts because they directly threaten people's lives and destroy basic resources needed for survival. The extent of physical and psychological devastation cannot be denied. Immediately after such extreme events the role of the obvious and unambiguous resource loss is of dominant significance to the affected individuals. Nevertheless, the importance of subjective appraisals might increase over time as the victims begin to process the psychological meaning of the event and its consequences for their futures. On the other hand, many events may invoke more subjective appraisals more quickly because the extent of the objective losses is unclear. Nuclear accidents, toxic waste spills, or chemical contamination of natural resources might induce higher levels of subjective appraisals immediately simply because the losses and their consequences are uncertain. This ambiguity concerning the objective impact of the stressor allows for a greater range of the threat, loss, or challenge interpretations (see Lazarus & Folkman, 1984). If at some later time, consequences of such events become clear (e.g., increased morbidity in the area), the event may be reevaluated in terms of the objective losses it brought about. Thus the level of a stressor's ambiguity, in terms of losses it begets, may determine the relative importance of subjective appraisals.

However, even in cases where the extent of actual losses is not disputed, there is plenty of variability in observable distress reactions indicating that subjective evaluations are always of additional significance. It may be that subjective appraisals are particularly pervasive with respect to the evaluation of what valued resources are still remaining. Stressful encounters could be seen as transactions between different appraisal perspectives, some of which may retrospectively focus on irreversible losses while others may be prospectively oriented towards the future. Therefore, even situations of extreme stress with high and unambiguous loss may be appraised as a challenging task to regain a sense of control, to maintain an optimistic outlook, or a sense of mastery (e.g., Lazarus & Folkman, 1984; Ritter, Benson & Snyder, 1990). Evaluations of objective losses are always associated with threat or challenge appraisals because the experienced loss brings along negative implications for the future that can be faced with a more optimistic or more pessimistic approach.

Our discussion of the three levels of stress process suggests that a prerequisite of community stress is that a community must appraise an event as relevant to the collective. Is the community level appraisal a simple aggregation of individual appraisals? Probably not because collective appraisals are a function of many active forces in the community. Official declarations and interpretations of the event by political, civic, or religious leaders, information campaigns in the media, public risk assessments, all give a large number of public interpretations. The congruence or fit among these appraisals may be most important in the case of community stress. Severe events, due to their clear losses, are usually characterized by a high congruence of appraisals at different levels. Because of the dominance of the objective features of resource loss there is little or no doubt that the community is faced with danger. In other cases, however, the fit between individual appraisals must be achieved in order to reach some level of consensus needed for a public or community to respond. Local authorities, religious and political organizations, and media can play the role of "appraisal makers." For example, officials often make risk predictions and threat appraisals for the public and advocate or even mandate that precautionary steps at the communal level be undertaken (e.g., erection of dikes and dams to better protect against a flood). However, more often than not, achieving a full consensus with respect to appraisals is not simple because pervasive differences in personal values make such agreements difficult to achieve (e.g., heated debate about current abortion laws).

The fit of appraisals is not only affected by individual philosophies and belief systems but also by community values. Cultural values and political or religious worldviews bring with them different appraisals of what is at stake, what is being threatened or lost. In Western cultures, for example, the process of socialization encourages autonomy, individualism, and personal control whereas other cultures value to a greater extent group conformity, group cohesion, and collective responsibility. Thus perhaps in Western cultures the increasing rates of mortality caused by the abuse of firearms might be judged as relatively less threatening because any actions to control it would result in the endangerment of individual freedoms. On the other hand, in cultures that emphasize the importance of collectivism, individual freedoms may be easily sacrificed in the name of the collective good. In such context, for example, the oppression of dissenting factions of the population would not constitute a community threat or loss.

A few points about the role of social comparisons in the appraisal process deserve comment. The presence of other victims helps to validate one's own evaluations and judgments. In fact, through such comparisons the process of reaching an agreement on appraisals at the community level may be expedited. If most people in the affected area perceive the stressor as a loss or harm event there is little doubt that others will follow suit. On the other hand, the mere presence of other victims will affect individual appraisals as well. The fact that so many other people are experiencing the stressor may render it somewhat less threatening and severe (e.g., Jemmott, Ditto, & Croyle, 1986). Consequently, one may feel less like a victim if many other people are similarly victimized. Primary appraisals of the stressor may tend to focus on objective losses (see Hobfoll, 1988), and these appraisals may be unaffected by the social setting. However, secondary appraisals may tend to focus on more subjective circumstances surrounding the event; the fact that large numbers of people are similarly afflicted may somehow make the stressor appear less adversive. Social comparisons are also made across communities. They open up opportunities for the assessment of communal well-being either by selecting less fortunate comparison targets or by selectively focusing on positive aspects of one's circumstances (see Taylor & Lobel, 1989; Wills, 1981). For example, a community with high atmospheric pollution or crime rate may compare itself with other communities that are even worse off in that respect. On the other hand, public opinion may focus on the communal benefits of high industrialization or economic welfare and appraise problems with pollution or crime as minor nuisances. In either case, the community may appraise the situation as irrelevant or, at most, as challenging.

Coping and Community Stress

People faced with individual stressors often go through an initial period of time where they feel unable to do much in the way of active (problem-focused) coping. In short, having difficulty getting going, they may require some time before feeling up to tackling their problems. Victims of community stressors, in contrast, may often find themselves simply flung into immediate action. One reason for this is that community stressors tend to be sudden and catastrophic. (Obviously, sudden and acute personal traumas would also tend to elicit such immediate coping efforts.) But there are additional reasons why the community stressor context makes people more likely to feel compelled to "burst into action." For one thing, there is a sense that "everyone is out there doing things, so I should as well." Moreover, the community stressor context provides an important feature not often present in individual-based stressor contexts: lots of people, frequently immediately visible, who are worse off than oneself. Thus, the requirement to help others, even during one's own time of crisis, can propel individuals into extremely high activity levels almost instantly. As a character in a recent, popular movie, so eloquently put it: "We're all a little broken, but the ones who are less broken have to help those who are more broken."

There are some significant, potential benefits from this "forced," initial coping. At the most basic level, these activities often serve as useful distractors. Moreover, people coping in this way tend to focus their attention on "making things better" rather than on more dysfunctional cognitions such as "isn't this terrible." The opportunity to help, then, can be therapeutic; it can provide people with an immediate mission or purpose. Rather than focusing on the trauma of the flood, for example, victims may attend to the goals of sandbagging the river, rebuilding the bridge, or protecting a neighbor's home. On balance, it is less likely that this immediate sense of purpose will be developed within the context of individual-based stressors. One reason that these "missions" or "goals" can be so powerful is that, they, very early on, can impart to people a sense of meaning in the trauma. They can help individuals come to terms with what has happened to them.

It is also necessary to consider the potential downsides of the community stressor context, in terms of its effect on the way people cope. As with many of the other constructs to be described in this section, one hindrance to coping concerns the point at which beneficial aspects from the community stressor context are removed or simply naturally evolve and end. That is, there often comes a time when the "missions" or "goals" of a community are put behind and the next phase begins. It may be at precisely this critical juncture that a significant percentage of community members begin to have difficulties, emotionally or cognitively. For example, the salient and active phase of heroic resource mobilization that the public deploys in the aftermath of large-scale disasters inevitably has to cease. Professional helpers, voluntary aid organizations, and the media, will eventually move to other crisis sites and leave the victims alone to cope with the consequences of a stressor that really just began (see Kaniasty & Norris, in press).

Although we have suggested that initial coping activity may impart meaning to victims, the process is undoubtedly more complicated. For example, perhaps because of the high level of activity at the onset of the stressor, victims are less likely to work on resolving their own personal problems. The potentially therapeutic effects of being "forced" to cope, then, may be overshadowed by a lack of personal resolution. Empirical examinations of these conflicting processes would likely prove valuable.

Just as the community stressor context encourages people to get going quickly, it also may provide for community members their initial "positive changes" or benefits (see Lehman et al., 1993; Taylor, Kemeny, Reed, & Aspinwall, 1991). We often hear not only community officials (such as city mayors) but also ordinary citizens proclaiming, almost instantaneously following a disaster, how wonderful it is that the community is pulling together, how the disaster has brought the community closer. One's willingness to look for, and ability to see, the silver lining in disaster may be increased if one does not feel singled out as a victim. Although we know of no empirical work on this issue, it may be that once people are able to point to one positive aspect from a stressor they are more likely to arrive at additional benefits.

The literature on positive changes, or "growth" is still at the point where we need to learn more about what victims' claims of positive changes really mean (see Lehman et al., 1993, for a discussion). For example, within the context of a large-scale stressor such as an earthquake, should we consider a victim's claim about increased community cohesiveness to be a positive gain, or would it be more accurate to characterize this claim as a coping mechanism? And, is this distinction even important?

Some influential research over the past decade has focused on people's everyday assumptions about the world, and in particular, on how victimizing experiences tend to shatter these assumptions (see Janoff-Bulman, 1992, for a review). What was once assumed to be a benign world, where bad things happen only to "bad" people, is now viewed, following victimization, as one in which innocent and good people can be besieged with horrendous misfortune and consequent despair. Not surprisingly, victims often report feeling that their traumatic experience was unfair and that they were cheated (e.g., Lehman, Wortman, & Williams, 1987). In short, they seem to be psychologically caught up with understandable concerns about justice and fairness, and with their newly modified, and much more malevolent, model of the world. Community stressors, which are by definition events where lots of people are similarly afflicted, may provide a context that is less conducive to triggering concerns about justice. Thus on the one hand, because many others in their community have been victimized, and some more so than they, people may be less likely to feel that their fundamental assumptions about world have been shattered. On the other hand, some community stressors seem particularly likely to yield concerns about justice. For example, human-made disasters, such as the Chernobyl or Three Mile Island nuclear accidents, or the Exxon Valdez oil spill, tend to brutally violate people's beliefs about justice and fairness. We need to learn more about how people process such community events with respect to justice issues.

Since Wills' (1981) initial statement about the use of downward social comparison in coping, a large body of research (e.g., Hemphill & Lehman, 1991; Wood, Taylor, & Lichtman, 1985) has confirmed the importance of comparison processes in the coping context. Obviously, the community stressor context is likely to heighten such comparison processes because of the salient availability of similarly afflicted community members: downward, but also upward, social comparison targets are readily available. Whereas people tend to take a relatively active role in making social comparisons within individual-based stressor contexts, comparisons are ubiquitous when community stressors hit. Thus, community residents passively experience a great many such comparisons.

One of the recent advances in this literature is Taylor and colleagues' notion that both downward and upward comparisons have the capability of making people feel either good or bad. Whereas downward comparisons can make one feel lucky and grateful, they can also increase one's fears and anxieties about getting worse in the future. Similarly, upward comparisons can lead a person to feel frustrated and depressed because one is more unfortunate than others, but they can also have a comforting and inspirational effect by highlighting the possibility of improvement (see Taylor & Lobel, 1989, for a discussion). The community stressor context clearly provides people with opportunities for all sorts of social comparisons. To the extent that victims focus on upward contacts (for information about possible improvement) and downward evaluation targets (for affect regulation), the literature suggests they will be better off psychologically.

Another issue that seems highly relevant for coping with a community stress pertains to the responsibility or blame allocation for the event. Brickman et al.'s (1982) models of helping and coping can serve as a useful organizing framework. These authors separated attributions of responsibility for problems and solutions, and developed a 4-cell model where people view themselves (or others) as either (1) responsible for causing the problem and for solving it (moral model); (2) responsible for causing the problem but not for solving it (enlightenment model); (3) not responsible for causing the problem, but responsible for solving it (compensatory model); or (4) not responsible for either causing the problem or for solving it (medical model).

Community stressors are rarely caused by the very individuals who are forced to cope with them. Thus, Brickman et al.'s moral and enlightenment models become less relevant. The critical issue it seems, and one that dovetails nicely with more traditional work on psychological control, is whether or not people view themselves to be (at all) responsible for (or in control over) the solutions to their and their community's problems. Thus, respectively, compensatory and medical models could be operant in the context of community events. From a situationist perspective, the fact that communities, in times of crisis, are in the business of mobilizing support (e.g., preventing wide-spread damage, sending out information, administering aid), could be thought of as an environmental mechanism by which individuals lose feelings of psychological control. On the other hand, community residents themselves often tend to be the very individuals who are performing these activities. Nonetheless, community members, perhaps especially those high on internal control (Rotter, 1966), may feel a clash between their own need to be the "captains of their ship" and their perceptions that community leaders and agencies are interfering with their ability to cope themselves with their problems. Meichenbaum (this volume) has suggested that authorities and relief agencies can at times act as a "surrogate frontal lobe" for communities in crisis, thereby stripping community members of their ability to respond themselves to the call to arms.

It makes sense to assume that people high on "powerful other control" (Levenson, 1972), who feel comfortable (and perhaps even prefer) seeking guidance from knowledgeable others, will fare best, psychologically, within the community stressor context. This is because the presence of "powerful other" sources (e.g., community service agencies, disaster relief teams) is ubiquitous during these times. In terms of models of helping and coping (Brickman et al., 1982), these individuals would likely view themselves in the medical model. Conversely, people high on internal control, who have a difficult time succumbing to outside powers, are more likely to view themselves in the compensatory model.

An additional factor that differentiates individual-based stressors from community stressors is the greater involvement of the media in the latter. Although people coping with individual stressors may be affected by presentations in the media (e.g., cancer patients reading a newspaper article about cancer super-copers such as Betty Ford or Pat Nixon; see Wood, Taylor, & Lichtman, 1985), those coping with community stressors are much more likely to be exposed to such media portrayals. The disaster literature, and more generally the literature on stress and coping, could gain from an examination of the possible effects of the media on the ways people perceive and cope with stressful life experiences. How do journalists go about covering community stressors? In addition to supplying valuable information, are there certain biases that various media bring to their reporting of such events? Might these biases, moreover, create certain fears amongst community members that might not otherwise be present? A clear link exists between media coverage of community stressors and social comparison processes. For individual level stress, it is rather rare to have many potential comparison targets available, especially in the initial phases of coping with one's trauma. However, in cases of community events, television, radio, and newspapers bombard us with endless stories about successful and unsuccessful coping efforts. Whether or not people gain comfort from such "overexposure" is not clear. For example, Pennebaker and Harber (1993) reported that two to three weeks following community-wide stressful events people seemed to became tired of hearing about other people's experiences with the stressor. Similarly, Kaniasty and Norris (1991) found that some respondents in a community sample became quite "weary" of constant exposure to news about the Persian Gulf War. Furthermore, the community stressor context also has the effect of making individual residents' coping more visible, and hence more open to public scrutiny, as everyone is "looking around." So, whereas people may feel less isolated, confused, and alone, they may also be apprehensive about the public aspect of the coping process.

Social Support and Community Stress

The role of social support as a coping resource has been studied within the context of many stressful life events ranging from individual level stressors (e.g., bereavement, pregnancy, divorce, illness) to community wide events (e.g., crowding, unemployment, disaster, war). Reviews of literature (e.g., Cohen & Wills, 1985; Kessler & McLeod, 1985; Sarason, Sarason, & Pierce, this volume; Schwarzer & Leppin, 1991), while recognizing limitations of supportive relationships in times of stress, have generally concluded that social support is beneficial to psychological well-being and physical health. The vast majority of studies that provided evidence for such conclusions were conceptually based on theoretical formulations (support as a buffer stress model and the main effects model) assuming that the stressor and social support are unrelated to each other. In fact, the link between the stressor and social support, though often observed, has been largely ignored or considered as a conceptual or methodological inconvenience (see Barrera, 1986). However, both lay and empirical observations provide numerous examples of stressful life events changing the availability and quality of social ties (e.g., Coyne, Wortman, & Lehman, 1988; Eckenrode & Wethington, 1991). Although individual level events such as death of a spouse, divorce, or serious illness all potentially augment or diminish available support, we believe that linkage between the stressor and social support is particularly important when discussing the protective role of interpersonal relationships in coping with community-wide stressors. By definition, community-wide stressors such as massive lay-offs, migrations, disasters, or wars, affect great numbers of people simultaneously, many of whom are members of each other's support networks, and are mutually dependent on each other's coping efforts. Undoubtedly, these characteristics of the stressor dramatically impact the social support available to victims. This explicit realization that stressful life events alter social support is crucial in this context because it unveils other pathways through which social support may operate to foster or hinder adaptation (see Barrera, 1986). On one hand, stressors may mobilize high levels of support, on the other hand, they can also result in a deterioration of social support. We will consider the mobilization and deterioration of social support following community-wide stressors relying primarily on literature investigating coping with disasters. We recognize that some aspects of these processes may not generalize to other community events. Nevertheless, exploring the role of social support in disasters represents a useful starting point for greater elaboration of interpersonal dynamics within the context of stress at the community level.

"Altruistic Communities"

Stressors often mobilize a support network to aid victims. In essence, this is exactly what people expect from their social relationships: when help is needed, supporters provide it. Researchers studying public responses to natural disasters such as hurricanes, floods, or earthquakes, often describe high levels of mutual helping engrossing whole communities. This phase immediately following a clearly devastating, visible, and unambiguous event has been referred to as the "altruistic or therapeutic community," "postdisaster utopia or heroism," and is characterized by increased internal solidarity, disappearance of common community conflicts, utopian mood, and a general sense of altruism (see Barton, 1969; Bolin, 1993; Giel, 1990). It has been hypothesized that such heightened communal concern for each other may mitigate adverse psychological consequences of disasters (Quarantelli, 1985). Norris and Kaniasty (1994) showed, for example, that higher levels of received support following Hurricanes Hugo and Andrew protected some victims from a postdisaster decline in perceptions of social support availability, an important coping resource most directly related to psychological well-being (see the discussion below). The question remains, however: are all victims favored equally by these "therapeutic communities?"

Postdisaster helping communities give priority to those victims who experience most exposure to the disaster's destructive powers (e.g., Barton, 1969; Bolin & Bolton, 1986; Kaniasty & Norris, 1994), and thus generally distribute assistance according to the rule of relative needs. At times, a special pattern of concern may also surface. A study of victims of Hurricane Hugo (Kaniasty & Norris, 1994) found that the oldest respondents (over 70 years old), when faced with threats to their lives and health, received relatively more help than similarly affected victims from younger age groups. Unfortunately, this pattern of concern did not emerge in response to property loss. In fact, other studies (Kaniasty, Norris, & Murrell, 1990; Kilijanek & Drabek, 1978) that operationalized severity of stressor in terms of tangible losses and damages reported that older victims experienced a pattern of neglect and received considerably less help from all sources than younger people. Whereas older victims may experience both concern and neglect, depending on the nature of the stressor, the poor and minorities most often experience a pattern of neglect and have the greatest difficulties securing adequate assistance and recovering from disaster (Bolin & Bolton, 1986; Kaniasty & Norris, 1994). Thus postevent help is not distributed equally or randomly. Some victims may be excluded from, or overlooked by, helping communities and recovery programs, whereas others may have a clear advantage in securing postdisaster relief. The often talked about altruism and fellowship that the public marshals in times of crisis should not obscure the fact that not all the victims are fully participating in these emergent helping communities. Because of potentially great numbers of victims, the need usually exceeds the level of helping resources at hand, leaving some victims with their needs unfulfilled (Kaniasty & Norris, in press).

Two important points must be made about emerging "altruistic communities" following disasters. First, they do not evolve in every disaster context, and second, they are short lived. Research indicates that victims of technological disasters are not afforded the emergence of altruistic communities. Contrary to the findings of studies of natural disasters, studies that investigated technological catastrophes, such as nuclear power plant accidents or toxic chemical spills, quite frequently report increases of interpersonal conflicts and erosion of social cohesiveness in the affected communities (see Bolin, 1993; Bromet, 1989). Cuthbertson and Nigg (1987) noted that because of the ambiguity of such events, lack of visible impact, and lack of clearly identifiable low point ("worst is over") (see Baum, Fleming, & Davidson, 1983), postdisaster therapeutic communities are unlikely to develop in such contexts. Residents, local authorities, and the perpetrators (those responsible for the hazard) often dispute the severity of the actual threat and question who are the "true victims?" It is often left to those who feel victimized to gather evidence and document that harm was done. For example, Bromet (this volume) reported that her research team's involvement in the study of Chernobyl's catastrophe was to some extent instigated by a local women's organization concerned about the mental health of their children. Residents of affected areas often divide into antagonistic factions and those who consider themselves victims may be rejected, stigmatized, and discriminated against by others in the community. Even technological disasters of clearly visible impact (e.g., explosions, dam breaks) are usually followed by lasting disputes and litigations concerning the allocation of blame for the event. Such antagonisms separate and politicize whole communities (Bolin, 1993). Not surprisingly then, victims of technological disasters are found to experience greater levels of anger, alienation, suspicion and mistrust of others, loneliness, and isolation (see Bromet, 1989; Cuthbertson & Nigg, 1987; Green, Lindy, & Grace, 1994). The overall postdisaster reality of persons affected by technological catastrophes is that of deterioration of social support and erosion of sense of community.

Natural disasters may also spur social confrontations. Distribution patterns of institutionalized relief and temporary housing can potentially become a political issue and vividly expose and augment preexisting social inequalities along the lines of ethnicity, race, or socioeconomic status. Bolin and Stanford (1990) observed such developments following the Loma Prieta earthquake where in some areas shelter and housing allocation resulted in charges of racism, political and cultural discrimination, and further marginalization of minorities, elderly, and the poor. This, in turn, led to organized demands for reformation of the political process in those communities, thus creating a momentum for social change. Such movements are often resisted by a political "status quo" and can result in conflicts (Bolin & Stanford, 1990; see also, Rochford & Blocker, 1991). Jackson and Inglehart (this volume) described a process in which community stress escalates racism and confrontation for both dominant and subordinate groups in the affected populations. On one hand, postevent social dynamics may create an opportunity for empowerment of disadvantaged and social change, on the other, community stress can divide and antagonize the affected communities and neighborhoods even further.

Social Support Deterioration Process

It appears that any gains in coping resources, in the form of temporarily elevated communal cohesion and mobilization of received social support that follow disasters and other community level events, are overwhelmed by an accelerating cycle of losses. According to Hobfoll's (1988; Hobfoll et al., this volume; Hobfoll & Lilly, 1993) conservation of resources theory, resource loss is hard to prevent, more powerful, and more potent, than resource gain. Although disasters often occur suddenly, the stress they inflict is not simply acute. Disasters create an array of secondary stressors that continuously deplete available coping resources at a faster rate than the progress of recovery. Thus the initial mobilization of social support resources may not be capable of blocking the inadvertent and longer lasting deterioration in quality of social ties. Notwithstanding the macro level conflicts and political confrontations, each victim may individually experience these declines in the privacy of their homes, neighborhoods, and communities. Disasters can diminish the sense of support (see Sarason, Sarason, & Pierce, this volume) because they disrupt various vital functions of social networks. Most tragically, disasters remove significant supporters from victims' networks through death, injury, or relocation. Most often, the entire community is victimized. The likelihood is high that potential support providers are victims themselves, and as a consequence, the need for support across all those affected frequently exceeds its availability. Destruction of the physical environment alters usual patterns of social interaction by disrupting daily activities such as visiting, shopping, or recreation. Physical fatigue, emotional irritability and scarcity of resources augment the potential for interpersonal conflict and social withdrawal. The salient heroic phase, with its healing features of increased consensus and fellowship, is inevitably replaced by a harsh reality of grief, destruction, and loss. Soon after all helpful outsiders (e.g., the media, governmental emergency services, volunteer relief agencies) leave, the indigenous residents of affected communities discover that the increased sense of communality was short-lived. As a "rise and fall of utopia" (see Giel, 1990), disasters are powerful illustrations of how stress transforms community resources from initial abundance to long-term depletion (Kaniasty & Norris, in press).

Whereas the instant mobilization of helping behavior is a clear manifestation of received social support (actual receipt of help), the deterioration processes following the impact of stress are more directly related to perceived social support (the belief that help would be available if needed) and social embeddedness (quantity and type of relationships with others). Kaniasty and Norris (Kaniasty & Norris, 1993; Kaniasty et al., 1990) examined changes in perceived social support and social embeddedness following a severe and wide-spread flooding in Kentucky. Using a prospective design that controlled for preevent levels of social support their analyses clearly showed that perceptions of social support declined from preflood levels. A similar erosion in perceived social support was reported following different disasters such as hurricanes, floods, dioxin exposure (Ironson et al., 1993; Norris & Kaniasty, 1994; Solomon, Bravo, Rubio-Stipec, & Canino, 1993), and other community stressors such as unemployment or residential crowding (Atkinson, Liem, & Liem, 1986; Lepore, Evans, & Schneider, 1991). Simply, the need for support in these victimized communities may have exceeded its availability. Most importantly, a deterioration of social support can extend to all residents of an affected community, even to those who did not sustain any direct personal losses due to the stressor. For example, Kaniasty and Norris (1993) found that "secondary victims" of flooding also reported postevent decreases in perceived availability of support and sense of embeddedness. These findings were interpreted as indicating declines in the companionship domain of social support that was experienced by all in the community. According to Rook (1985), companionship entails sharing with others the moments of leisure, exchanging ideas, and participating in social activities. It appears that victimized communities may be denied for a long time this particular aspect of social relationships. Residents of disaster-stricken communities often report decreased participation in social activities with relatives, friends, neighbors, or community organizations (see Solomon, 1986). Pennebaker and Harber (1994) observed that at some time following the Loma Prieta earthquake residents in the affected areas greatly reduced their interest in hearing other victims' stories about the disaster and, in fact, possibly were "erecting barriers to prohibit others from bringing up the topic" (p. 133). Ironically, this inhibition of talking about the disaster experience did not protect them from thinking (or ruminating) about it which inadvertently may have resulted in poorer physical and mental health (see also Meichenbaum, this volume).

Altogether, an erosion of perceived support and sense of embeddedness is one path through which community stressors may exert their adverse effects on psychological well-being. Kaniasty and Norris (1993) found that primary and secondary flood victims experienced the impact of the disaster both directly, through immediate loss and exposure to trauma, and indirectly, through deterioration of perceived support and sense of embeddedness. The loss of social support has also mediated psychological consequences of Hurricanes Hugo and Andrew (Ironson et al., 1993; Kaniasty & Norris, in press). In sum, deterioration of social support is a useful way of describing possible pathways of how community stress may operate to affect psychological health (see Atkinson et al., 1986; Barrera, 1986; Ensel & Lin, 1991; Lepore et al., 1991). It also illustrates the value of conceptualizing the stress process in terms of resource loss (Hobfoll, 1988).

Conclusion

Our goal in writing this chapter was to compare and contrast stress processes at the individual and community levels, and to focus on the later. We began by speculating about the stages of dynamic transitions between the two phenomena, and a simple, 3-level heuristic was proposed. We suggested that the impact of a stressor on an individual transposes onto the community level when it reaches the collective consciousness and is no longer just a concern of individual victims. However, we pointed out that even during stressful community events people ultimately cope at the individual level. What seems significant are the reciprocal relations between collective and individual experiences of trauma, stress, coping, and recovery. We attempted, with our discussion of resources, appraisals, coping, and social support, to highlight some of these dynamics and to expose how the community context can aid or hinder the individual's process of adapting to collective upheavals. Our analysis emphasized the ecological perspective (see Trickett, this volume), demonstrating how overarching contextual factors play important roles in individual and collective processing of stressful events. The task of integrating the field's knowledge base concerning the individual and communal experience of stress has merely begun.

References

Atkinson, T., Liem, R., & Liem, J. H. (1986). The social costs of unemployment: Implications for social support. Journal of Health and Social Psychology, 27, 317-331.

Barrera, M. (1986). Distinctions between social support concepts, measures, and models. American Journal of Community Psychology, 14, 413-445.

Barton, A. M. (1969). Communities in disaster. Garden City, NJ: Doubleday.

Baum, A., Fleming, R., & Davidson, L. (1983). Natural disaster and technological catastrophe. Environment and Behavior, 15, 333-354.

Bolin, R. (1993). Natural and technological disasters: Evidence of psychopathology. In A-M. Ghadirian, & H. E. Lehmann (Eds.), Environment and Psychopathology (pp. 121-140). Springer: New York.

Bolin, R., & Bolton, P. (1986). Race, religion, and ethnicity in disaster recovery. Boulder, CO: University of Colorado.

Bolin, R., & Stanford, L. (1990). Shelter and housing issues in Santa Cruz County. In R. Bolin (Ed.), The Loma Prieta Earthquake: Studies of short-term impacts (pp. 99-108). University of Colorado: Boulder, CO.

Brickman, P., Rabinowitz, V., Karuza, J., Coates, D., Cohn, E., & Kidder, L. (1982). Models of helping and coping. American Psychologist, 37, 368-384.

Bromet, E. J. (1989). The nature and effects of technological failures. In R. Gist & B. Lubin (Eds.), Psychological aspects of disaster (pp.120-139). New York: Wiley.

Bromet, E. J. (this volume). Methodological issues in designing research on community-wide disasters with special reference to Chernobyl. In S. E. Hobfoll & M. W. deVries (Eds.), Extreme stress and communities: Impact and intervention. Dordrecht, the Netherlands: Kluwer.

Cohen, S., & Wills, T. A. (1985). Stress, social support, and the buffering hypothesis. Psychological Bulletin, 98, 310-357.

Coyne, J. C., Wortman, C. B., & Lehman, D. R. (1988). The other side of support: Emotional overinvolvement and miscarried helping. In B. H. Gottlieb (Ed.), Social support: Formats, processes, and effects (pp. 305-330). Newbury Park, CA: Sage.

Cuthbertson, B., & Nigg, J. (1987). Technological disaster and the nontherapeutic community: A question of true victimization. Environment and Behavior, 19, 462-483.

deVries, M. W. (this volume). Culture, community and catastrophe: Issues in understanding communities under difficult conditions. In S. E. Hobfoll & M. W. deVries (Eds.), Extreme stress and communities: Impact and intervention. Dordrecht, the Netherlands: Kluwer.

Eckenrode, J., & Wethington, E. (1990). The process and outcome of mobilizing social support. In S. Duck (ed. with R. C. Silver), Personal relationships and social support (pp. 83-103). London: Sage.

Ensel, W., & Lin, N. (1991). The life stress paradigm and psychological distress. Journal of Health and Social Behavior, 32, 321-341.
Freedy, J. R., Saladin, M. E., Kilpatrick, D. G., Resnick, H. S., & Saunders, B. E. (1994). Understanding acute psychological distress following natural disaster. Journal of Traumatic Stress, 7, 257-274.
Giel, R. (1990). Psychosocial process in disasters. International Journal of Mental Health, 19, 7-20.
Goldberger, L., & Breznitz, S. (Eds.) (1993). Handbook of stress. New York: The Free Press.
Green, B. L. (this volume). Long-term consequences of disasters. In S. E. Hobfoll & M. W. deVries (Eds.), Extreme stress and communities: Impact and intervention. Dordrecht, the Netherlands: Kluwer.
Green, B. L., Lindy, J., & Grace, M. (1994). Psychological effects of toxic contamination. In R. Ursano, B. McCaughey, & C. Fullerton (Eds.), Individual and community responses to trauma and disaster: The structure of human chaos (pp. 154-176). Cambridge, U.K.: Cambridge University Press.
Hemphill, K. J., & Lehman, D. R. (1991). Social comparisons and their affective consequences: The importance of comparison dimension and individual difference variables. Journal of Social and Clinical Psychology, 10, 372-394.
Hobfoll, S. E. (1988). The ecology of stress. New York: Hemisphere.
Hobfoll, S. E., Briggs, S., & Wells J. (this volume). Community stress and resources: Actions and reactions. In S. E. Hobfoll & M. W. deVries (Eds.), Extreme stress and communities: Impact and intervention. Dordrecht, the Netherlands: Kluwer.
Hobfoll, S. E., & Lilly, R. (1993). Resource conservation as a strategy for community psychology. Journal of Community Psychology, 21, 128-148.
Ironson, G., Greenwood, D., Wynings, C., Baum, A., Rodriquez, M., Carver, C., Benight, C., Evans, J., Antoni, M., LaPerriere, A., Kumar, M., Fletcher, M., & Schneiderman, N. (1993, August). Social support, neuroendocrine, and immune functioning during Hurricane Andrew. Paper presented at the 101th Annual Convention of American Psychological Association, Toronto, Canada.
Jackson, J. S., & Inglehart, M. R. (this volume). Effects of racism on dominant and subordinate groups: A reverberation model of community stress. In S. E. Hobfoll & M. W. deVries (Eds.), Extreme stress and communities: Impact and intervention. Dordrecht, the Netherlands: Kluwer.
Janoff-Bulman, R. (1992). Shattered assumptions: Towards a new psychology of trauma. New York: Free Press.
Jemmott, J. B. III, Ditto, P. H., & Croyle, R. T. (1986). Judging health status: Effects of perceived prevalence and personal relevance. Journal of Personality and Social Psychology, 50, 899-905.
Jerusalem, M. (1993). Personal resources, environmental constraints, and adaptational processes: The predictive power of a theoretical stress model. Personality and Individual Differences, 14, 15-24.

Jerusalem, M., & Schwarzer, R. (1989). Anxiety and self-concept as antecedents of stress and coping: A longitudinal study with German and Turkish adolescents. Personality and Individual Differences, 10, 785-792.

Jerusalem, M., & Schwarzer, R. (1992). Self-efficacy as a resource factor in stress appraisal processes. In R. Schwarzer (Ed.), Self-efficacy: Thought control of action (pp. 195-213). Washington DC: Hemisphere.

Kaniasty, K., & Norris, F. (1993). A test of the support deterioration model in the context of natural disaster. Journal of Personality and Social Psychology, 64, 395-408.

Kaniasty, K., & Norris, F. (1994). In search of altruistic community: Patterns of social support mobilization following Hurricane Hugo. Manuscript submitted for publication.

Kaniasty, K., & Norris, F. (in press). Mobilization and deterioration of social support following natural disasters. Current Directions in Psychological Science.

Kaniasty, K., & Norris, F. (1991). Some psychological consequences of the Persian Gulf War on the American people: An empirical study. Contemporary Social Psychology, 15, 121-126.

Kaniasty, K., Norris, F., & Murrell, S. A. (1990). Received and perceived social support following natural disaster. Journal of Applied Social Psychology, 20, 85-114.

Kessler, R. C., & McLeod, J. D. (1985). Social support and psychological distress in community surveys. In S. Cohen & S. L. Syme (Eds.), Social support and health (pp. 19-40). New York: Academic Press.

Kilijanek, T., & Drabek, T. E. (1979). Assessing long-term impacts of a natural disaster: A focus on the elderly. The Gerontologist, 19, 555-566.

Lazarus, R. (1991). Emotion and adaptation. London: Oxford University Press.

Lazarus, R., & Folkman, S. (1984). Stress, appraisal, and coping. New York: Springer.

Lehman, D. R., Davis, C. G., DeLongis, A., Wortman, C. B., Bluck, S., Mandel, D. R., & Ellard, J. H. (1993). Positive and negative life changes following bereavement and their relations to adjustment. Journal of Social and Clinical Psychology, 12, 90-112.

Lehman, D. R., Wortman, C. B., & Williams, A. F. (1987). Long-term effects of losing a spouse or child in a motor vehicle crash. Journal of Personality and Social Psychology, 52, 218-231.

Lepore, S. J., Evans, G. W., & Schneider, M. L. (1991). Dynamic role of social support in the link between chronic stress and psychological distress. Journal of Personality and Social Psychology, 61, 899-909.

Levenson, H. (1972). Distinctions within the concept of internal-external control: Development of a new scale. Proceedings of the 80th Annual APA Convention, 7, 259-260 (summary).

McFarlane, A. C. (this volume). Stress and disaster. In S. E. Hobfoll & M. W. deVries (Eds.), Extreme stress and communities: Impact and intervention. Dordrecht, the Netherlands: Kluwer.

Meichenbaum, D. (this volume). Disasters, stress and cognition. In S. E. Hobfoll & M. W. deVries (Eds.), Extreme stress and communities: Impact and intervention. Dordrecht, the Netherlands: Kluwer.

Moos, R. (Ed.) (1986). Coping with life crises. New York: Plenum.

Norris, F. (1992). Epidemiology of trauma: Frequency and impact of different potentially traumatic events on different demographic groups. Journal of Consulting and Clinical Psychology, 60, 409-418.

Norris, F., & Kaniasty, K. (1994). Receipt of help and perceived social support in times of stress: A test of the social support deterioration deterrence model. Manuscript submitted for publication.

Quarantelli, E. (1985). Conflicting views on mental health: The consequences of traumatic events. In C. Figley (Ed.), Trauma and its wake (pp. 173-218). New York: Brunner-Mazel.

Pearlin, L. (1989). The sociological study of stress. Journal of Health and Social Behavior, 33, 241-256.

Pennebaker, J., & Harber, K. (1993). A social stage model of collective coping: The Loma Prieta Earthquake and the Persian Gulf War. Journal of Social Issues, 49, 125-145.

Ritter, C., Benson, D., & Snyder, C. (1990). Belief in a just world and depression. Sociological perspective, 33, 235-252.

Rochford, B., & Blocker, T. (1991). Coping with "natural" hazards as stressors. Environment and Behavior, 23, pp. 171-194.

Rook, K. S. (1985). Functions of social bonds: Perspectives from research on social support, loneliness and social isolation. In I. G. Sarason & B. R. Sarason (Eds.), Social support: Theory, research and application. The Hague: Martinus Nijhof.

Rotter, J. B. (1966). Generalized expectancies for internal versus external control of reinforcement. Psychological Monographs, 80, (1, Whole No. 609).

Rubonis, A. V., & Bickman, L. (1991). Psychological impairment in the wake of disaster: The disaster-psychopathology relationship. Psychological Bulletin, 109, 384-399.

Sarason, I. G., Sarason, B. R., & Pierce, G. R. (this volume). Stress and social support. In S. E. Hobfoll & M. W. deVries (Eds.), Extreme stress and communities: Impact and intervention. Dordrecht, the Netherlands: Kluwer.

Schwarzer, R., & Leppin, A. (1991). Social support and health: A theoretical and empirical overview. Journal of Social and Personal Relationships, 8, 99-127.

Smith, C. A., & Lazarus, R. (1990). Emotion and adaptation. In L.A. Pervin (Ed.), Handbook of personality: Theory and research (pp. 609-637). New York: The Guilford Press.

Solomon, S. D. (1986). Mobilizing social support networks in times of disaster. In C. R. Figley (Ed.), Trauma and its wake: Vol. 2. Traumatic stress theory, research, and intervention (pp.232-263). New York: Brunner/Mazel.

Solomon, S. D., Bravo, M., Rubio-Stipec, M., & Canino, G. (1993). Effect of family role on response to disaster. Journal of Traumatic Stress, 6, 255-269.

Taylor, S. E., Kemeny, M. E., Reed, G. M., & Aspinwall, L. G. (1991). Assault on the self: Positive illusions and adjustment to threatening events. In J. Strauss & G. R. Goethals (Eds.), The self: Interdisciplinary approaches (pp. 239-254). New York: Springer-Verlag.

Taylor, S. E., & Lobel, M. (1989). Social comparison activity under threat: Downward evaluation and upward contacts. Psychological Review, 96, 569-575.

Trickett, E. J. (this volume). The community context of disaster and traumatic stress: An ecological perspective from community psychology. In S. E. Hobfoll & M. W. deVries (Eds.), Extreme stress and communities: Impact and intervention. Dordrecht, the Netherlands: Kluwer.

Wills, T. A. (1981). Downward comparison principles in social psychology. Psychological Bulletin, 106, 231-248.

Wood, J. V., Taylor S. E., & Lichtman, R. R. (1985). Social comparison in adjustment to breast cancer. Journal of Personality and Social Psychology, 49, 1169-1183.

SECTION III: RESOURCES TO OFFSET STRESS: APPLICATIONS TO THE COMMUNITY CONTEXT (OVERVIEW)

Stevan E. Hobfoll, Kent State University, Kent, Ohio, USA
Rebecca P. Cameron, Kent State University, Kent, Ohio, USA
Marten W. deVries, University of Limburg, Maastricht, the Netherlands

Section Three begins to provide answers to some of the questions raised in Section Two, regarding how to incorporate multiple perspectives into research on extreme stress. Hobfoll, Briggs, and Wells (Chapter Six) provide a theoretical approach that allows a great deal of flexibility in the way researchers attempt to understand community stress. As a general resource theory, Conservation of Resources (COR) can accommodate relatively universal resources (e.g., food, adequate roads, good health, social skills, communal pride) as well as culturally-specific resources (e.g., particular valued community identities, unique religious or secular rituals). Temporal characteristics of disaster stress and recovery can be approached in terms of loss and gain cycles. In addition, the principles of COR theory apply to both individuals and communities, allowing for a broad conceptual base that capitalizes on the commonalities between those two units of analysis. Schwarzer and Jerusalem (Chapter Seven) and Sarason, Sarason, and Pierce (Chapter Eight) provide compelling discussions of two particular resources, optimism and social support, that relate to individual and community functioning, especially during periods of stress. Schwarzer and Jerusalem make theoretical distinctions between different levels of optimism that have importance for how researchers operationalize this concept. They illustrate the application of their theoretical ideas to research through their own sophisticated work on adaptation to migration from East to West Germany. Sarason et al. provide an integrative theoretical perspective on social support that incorporates the situational and interpersonal context as well as individual-level intrapersonal factors. This perspective offers clarity as well as breadth of focus, and as such has the potential to contribute a great deal to research on the complex topic of social support.

In Chapter Six, Hobfoll et al. present the basic tenets of COR theory, and illustrate them through examples from the stress literature. A central assumption of this theory is that individuals and communities act to maximize their resources. It follows that stress is the result of being threatened with the loss of resources, actually losing resources, or investing resources without adequate return on the investment. COR theory further posits that losses of resources are more salient and influential than gains of resources, that resources are invested to achieve gains or prevent losses, and that initial losses or gains can snowball into loss cycles or gain cycles, in which the initial change in resource status results in a positive feedback loop resulting in further loss or gain. Because losses are thought to be more powerful than gains, loss cycles are more destructive than gain cycles are constructive. In addition, loss cycles have relatively more momentum than gain cycles, making them more difficult to interrupt.

As Hobfoll et al. outline, this theory provides a framework for understanding a community's historical experiences and for predicting its likely future development, given current stressors and resources. Thus, it has compelling implications for the study of and for intervention into community stress. A number of these implications are discussed. First, COR theory suggests that it is of paramount importance to interrupt or contain loss cycles that are in progress. Second, COR theory focuses attention on identifying key resources that are critical to preventing or limiting loss, and suggests the strategy of countering or preventing loss with gain cycles. Third, COR theory emphasizes the importance of prompt and intensive management of loss cycles. Fourth, it advises us to anticipate secondary losses occurring as a result of initial losses, and the consequent reduction in individual or community functioning. Fifth, it proposes that we should expect losses to spread from one category of resources to others, since resources are intertwined with each other. Sixth, it explains poor coping as often representing a last-ditch effort when appropriate means of coping are no longer available. And, seventh, COR theory suggests that even communities that are initially coping well with a stressor may lose resources and thus experience reduced resilience over time if their resources are not replenished. All of these correlates of COR theory offer insight into the strategic application of community assistance following disaster. In addition, they can serve as useful hypotheses to guide research.

Drawing on COR theory and a particular event of extreme community stress, the Lucasville prison uprising, Hobfoll et al. outline several potential roadblocks to effective community intervention. One obstacle is the presence of unidentified subcommunities within the affected community. Each subcommunity may have its own priorities, based on its particular stake in a set of resources. This can lead to competing agendas and result in less advantaged subcommunities becoming further marginalized. Thus, community interventionists must identify subcommunities, emphasize their common goals and provide equitable, rather than political, solutions to resource distribution. Other potential obstacles that are discussed in Chapter Six are the process of stress contagion (the pressure cooker effect), the operation of political agendas, and the focus on short-term needs to the detriment of long-term functioning. Hobfoll et al. suggest several approaches to counteracting and overcoming these obstacles during community stress events. These include careful emergency planning prior to the event, centralized information and communication during the event, and assistance to leaders to optimize their decision-making under stress.

One of the basic assumptions of COR theory is that objective resources are of primary importance, especially in situations of relatively high stress (e.g., impoverished or disrupted communities). Hobfoll et al. suggest that the emphasis on appraisals or perceptions found in the literature on stress and coping reflects the relatively advantaged situation of the average research participant. In the context of the surfeit of resources experienced by middle class, educated Americans, appraisals are fairly influential in determining relative well-being. In contrast, those with barely enough resources to manage daily life are more likely to be affected and differentiated by objective conditions. In addition, perceptions of resources generally do not stray far from objective reality without becoming a liability themselves. For these reasons, COR theory places emphasis on objective rather than subjective resources. However, not all theorists and researchers agree on this choice of emphasis. Issues of the role of objective versus subjective stressors and resources recur throughout this volume and the larger stress and coping literature. The next chapter, by Schwarzer and Jerusalem, takes a different perspective of the importance of subjective appraisals.

Schwarzer and Jerusalem (Chapter Seven) propose that appraisals form a mediating link between objective conditions and coping. They conceptualize objective resources as only having <u>potential</u> benefits until they are perceived and utilized. The tendency to appraise resources as available and effective has been characterized as a personality disposition called optimism. Optimism itself is a resource, as it facilitates the effective use of other resources. Schwarzer and Jerusalem review three levels of optimistic self-beliefs: explanatory style, generalized outcome expectancies, and perceived self-efficacy. All of these are helpful, but perceived self-efficacy is the level of optimism with the most potential to counteract stressful circumstances.

An optimistic explanatory style refers to the tendency to make self-serving attributions (positive events are attributed to global, stable, and internal causes and negative events are attributed to specific, situational, and external causes). A construct that relates more directly to current and future behavior, in part by explicitly referring to expectancies, is called dispositional optimism, and is characterized by positive generalized outcome expectancies. This construct encompasses a higher level of motivation and investment in planful, effective coping. It can include both action-outcome and situation-outcome expectancies, with situation-outcome expectancies reflecting a more passive optimistic stance than action-outcome expectancies. According to Schwarzer and Jerusalem, the strongest form of optimism is perceived self-efficacy, which represents a sense of capability, agency, and control over one's circumstances. Although all of the three levels of optimism are associated with better psychological and physical functioning, perceived self-efficacy is related to a more realistic assessment of situations, choosing more challenging tasks, performing better at them, and sticking with them longer, and is more closely related to mastery than to a belief in the benign nature of the universe. Rather than being limited to a generally positive view of the future, it includes the ability to size up a situation and make the most of it.

Following this review of the status of various theoretical approaches to optimism, Schwarzer and Jerusalem report data from a community stress research program that illustrate their concept of self-efficacy as a personal resource. Their research participants were East Germans migrating to West Germany during the period of German reunification. Schwarzer and Jerusalem obtained data regarding self-efficacy, partner status, and employment status at three time points during migration and resettlement. The process of migration is extremely disruptive and can easily precipitate loss cycles, as resources are lost and invested while the replenishing of resources may be delayed for years. Self-efficacy should theoretically offset the effects of migration-related stress on personal well-being. One particular risk for communities of Western refugees is that posed by long-term unemployment, with its economic and also psychological significance. Lack of employment following migration is often not the result of personal factors but is due to circumstances beyond the individual's control. In addition, the presence of an intimate partner is a particularly important antidote to the slow process of rebuilding a social network from scratch.

As hypothesized, Schwarzer and Jerusalem found that self-efficacy was an important resource for stress resistance, predicting less depressive symptomatology and fewer health complaints. In line with COR theory, objective environmental conditions also had an impact on well-being: having a job and an intimate partner were factors contributing to better well-being. Thus, a combination of personality variables and objective resources appear to be important in adjusting well to a major community-level stressor. This has implications for appropriate intervention in situations of community stress, in that reestablishing employment opportunities, providing support to couples, and establishing means for social networking may be helpful. Screening for self-efficacy and targeting interventions to those who may benefit from enhanced self-efficacy may also be a strategy for interventionists. And, since the personality characteristic of self-efficacy arises from a set of interactions with the family and the world, prevention researchers and workers may be well-advised to focus attention on enhancing and promoting self-efficacy through family and school interventions prior to the onset of extreme circumstances.

Sarason et al. (Chapter Eight) provide a thorough, yet concise review of social support as it relates to coping with stress. Social support is another variable, like self-efficacy, that partially reflects individual differences, but that also reflects a set of contextual circumstances and their influence on developmental history and current resources. Unlike self-efficacy, social support is an explicitly interpersonal construct. There is a great deal of literature that indicates that social support is a resource useful for combatting the effects of stress on psychological and physical health.

Sarason et al. first review the concept of social support, then present their interactional-cognitive view of social support, which integrates the three elements of context relevant to social support: the event, the person, and the social environment. More specifically, this model includes: situational elements of support, including the stressor being experienced and its secondary consequences; intrapersonal factors such as support perceptions and attachment style; and the interpersonal contexts of social transactions, including qualitative and quantitative aspects of particular relationships and the broader social network.

Next, Sarason et al. link social support to coping, advocating that investigators attend to a time frame that extends prior to the occurrence of a stressor, in order to clarify the reasons a stressor occurred to a particular individual or group (with obvious implications for thinking about prevention). They connect perceived social support to a self-efficacious and interpersonally effective style. Again emphasizing the temporal context of support, they indicate the role of familial experiences in forming a particularly effective or ineffective orientation toward social support. Sarason et al. discuss issues related to the effective provision of social support, such as conflict and timing, and then turn to the role of social support in the community stress context. In particular, Sarason et al. focus on two of the beneficial functions that social support can fulfill during periods of extreme community stress: anxiety reduction and facilitation of attention and coping. They call for demonstration projects on social support as a component of community stress intervention, and encourage the use of outreach and information dissemination programs within interventions. Researchers are beginning to formulate a more sophisticated understanding of social support, incorporating questions about who, under what circumstances, can provide what form of social support, to whom, so that it will be perceived as supportive, and have positive effects. The process of seeking answers to these questions will surely continue to be a complex, yet exciting undertaking.

The chapters in this section continue to demonstrate and explore the interwoven nature of communities, individuals, stressful experiences, and beneficial resources. Temporal issues again are raised, and reciprocal causality is cited: individuals are influenced by their circumstances, and then in turn, influence their circumstances; communities' attempts at coping can become the source of further stress. Meanwhile, resources beget other resources: self-efficacy leads to continuing mastery experiences, and receiving social support encourages one to access social support as needed, which in turn strengthens one's ties. The authors of the following chapters help to point the way to further productive inquiry on these issues by providing multiple perspectives on resources that can guide the formulation of research questions and intervention strategies.

COMMUNITY STRESS AND RESOURCES: ACTIONS AND REACTIONS

Stevan E. Hobfoll, Kent State University
Sylvester Briggs, Ohio Department of Rehabilitation and Correction
Jennifer Wells, Kent State University

We are concerned here with the family of stressful events and circumstances that occur to large groups of people. These include natural and man-made disasters, major epidemics, famine, war, mass violence, and severe human economic and political upheaval. The study of such traumatic events is not new, but it has concentrated on the individual level, focusing on how individuals are affected. Little attention has been paid as to how community stressors impact the group, organization, community, or society. Nor has appreciable research addressed how individuals' reactions are mediated by the way their community is impacted by community stressors. Some investigators have speculated on the community level and some have provided insightful descriptions, but usually in a piecemeal fashion, without reference to a general theoretical framework.

It is not surprising that community stress has been approached on the individual level. In part, this has been due to the fact that psychology and psychiatry are professions concerned primarily with individuals. In addition, it has been difficult to evaluate differences between community stressors, because each event is different from every other event in some critical way (McFarlane, 1994; Quarantelli, 1985). The individualistic perspective also is promoted because it is consistent with Western Eurocentric worldview, which emphasizes the role of the individual in society as the unit of interest, rather than the community. This "pull yourself up by your bootstraps," "rugged individualism" perspective dominates Western thought and dictates the very questions that we ask and the solutions we seek (Guisinger & Blatt, 1994; Riger, 1993; Triandis & Brislin, 1984). The psychosocial study of community stress must go beyond these constraints and look to communal theories to understand the consequences of major, community stressors and to arrive at working solutions to these problems.

We present Conservation of Resources (COR) theory (Hobfoll, 1988; 1989; Hobfoll & Jackson, 1991) and apply it to community stress. COR theory provides a general theoretical framework for understanding the influence community stress has on communities and how these, in turn, reverberate down to the individual level. We will use examples from research on traumatic stress and from a single community event, the disturbance at the maximum security southern Ohio correction facility in Lucasville in 1993 by a group of 409 inmates. Owing to the paucity of empirical research that addresses the community level, we will often speculate about possible outcomes in hopes of encouraging future investigation of these phenomena.

Conservation of Resources Theory

COR theory is based on the tenet that <u>individuals strive to obtain, retain, and protect those things they value</u>. The critical things that they value, or that serve as a means of helping them obtain what they value, we call resources. We proffer that communities, being made up of individuals, likewise strive to obtain, retain, and protect their resources. According to COR theory this basic tenet leads to the prediction that psychological stress occurs in one of three instances. These are:

(1) when resources are threatened with loss;
(2) when resources are actually lost; and
(3) when resources are invested without consequent gain, hence producing a net loss.

COR theory divides resources into four categories, although some resources may be depicted in more than one category. The four categories are objects, conditions, personal characteristics, and energies. Objects include material things such as home, transportation, and clothing. On a community level objects extend to the presence of roads, communal shelter, and emergency equipment (e.g., specialized equipment). Conditions are the social structures and circumstances that apply to an individual, group, or community. On an individual level these include secure work, good health, and a good marriage. On a community level they include the availability of employment, the level of emergency services, and the quality of ties between community organizations. Personal characteristics are attributes of individuals that are either esteemed in their own right or that facilitate the creation or protection of other resources. They include both personal traits, such as self-esteem and sense of mastery, and skills, such as social aplomb and having a skilled occupation. On a community level we need to translate personal characteristics to group attributes such as communal pride, psychological sense of community (Sarason, 1974), and community competence (Iscoe, 1974). The last resource category is energies, and these include money, food, knowledge, and credit. They are useful only in that they may be exchanged or used to obtain or protect other resources. On a community level they include government financing, knowledge of how to act in a crisis, and heating and transportation fuel reserves.

By emphasizing resources, COR theory highlights the objective attributes of events and circumstances, rather than their perception. Stress research has focused on individual perception of stress (Lazarus & Folkman, 1984), even defining stress as the perception of being overtaxed. Certainly, individuals' perceptions play a role in the stress process, but to say that perception in the sine qua non of stress suggests that any event is stressful to the extent that it is perceived as such. This places stress research into the realm of neurosis and leads to confounding of the study of individual differences with stress outcomes, such that we cannot say whether the individual has an anxious personality or whether they are made anxious by an event (Dohrenwend, Dohrenwend, Dodson, & Shrout, 1984; Stanton, Danoff-Burg, Cameron, & Ellis, 1994).

COR theory posits that the objective impact on resources underlies the process of stress, and that people's perceptions of these resources further influences their reactions. Moreover, these perceptions are not idiographic, but generally are reasonable interpretations of actual events. For minor hassles, interpretation may predominate, but for major, community stressors it is the objective quality of the events that are paramount. Indeed, Lazarus and Folkman (1984) stated that they are not interested in major stressors, precisely because perceptions play a lessor role in such instances. In their own words, "extreme environmental conditions result in stress for nearly everyone . . . extreme conditions are not uncommon, but their use as a model produces inadequate theory and applications" (p. 19).

For communal stressors we must address the loss and gain of resources experienced by the community. When a community is beset with a disaster, what is the extent of loss and damage? How critical are the resources that have been lost or threatened? What are the remaining reserves? Finally, what are the perceptions of these losses, threats, and gains, and what are people's expectations about future reverberations stemming from the event?

Even appraisals are based in large part on reality. Giel (1990), for example, addressed the influence of the reality-based perceptions of the role of local and state government among the affected population following the 1989 Armenian earthquake. He writes "The role of the Communist Party is limited since it has no deep roots in society [and] . . . people have little respect for their leaders," (p. 388). He further states that these events are perceived as part of a history of misfortune for the Armenian people. These current and historical perceptions, Giel suggests, lead to a feeling of helplessness that is difficult to overcome. Our point is that these perceptions are realistic given objective historic circumstances. The community or the individual are merely the catalog or camera that we ask to encapsulate the record of events. Their perception does come through a lens that may alter or distort the image, but the picture is nevertheless primarily an outgrowth of the actual world. As Iscoe (1974) pointed out in his major paper on the competent community, the perception of communal competence is an outgrowth of actual attributes of their communal history.

Principles of COR Theory

A number of principles stem from COR theory and these aid in prediction, understanding, and intervention concerning the sequelae that follow stressful circumstances.

Principle 1: The primacy of loss. The first principle that follows from COR theory is that loss of resources is more potent than resource gain. The gradient of loss is steeper than the gradient for gain. On a community level this means that when a community experiences some communal loss it is more negative than the equivalent gain would be positive. On the individual level we found that resource loss was strongly related to psychological distress (Hobfoll & Lilly, 1993). In contrast, resource gain had little direct influence on psychological distress. Indeed, gain was only important in the context of loss, such that individuals who received greater loss were more positively affected by gain than were those who had not experienced significant loss. Early work on stressful events suggested that gain would also be stressful because it was accompanied by change, but more careful research has found that if anything gain has a salutary effect (Kaniasty & Norris, 1993; Thoits, 1983).

Communities, like individuals, can experience either loss or gains. For example, in the normal course of events new monies may come to a community for bridges and roads. Because loss is more salient than gain, the positive effect of such additions will not match the opposite effect that destruction of roads and bridges would have following an earthquake. As in the individual case, we suggest that gain will also be more meaningful in the context of loss. Hence, replacement of the lost infrastructure will have greater impact than would the same gain had there not been a loss. Green, Lindy, Grace, Gleser, Leonard, Korol, and Winget (1990) have studied the long-term impact of communal losses and found that if particularly devastated, those involved in the earthquake will experience negative sequelae for decades thereafter. There is no comparable evidence that some community fortune has anything like this kind of lasting effect.

In most cases, losses also occur much more precipitously than do gains, which tend to take long periods to accumulate. Wardak (1992) has discussed the loss of cultural and religious resources in Afghanistan in the wake of the recent Civil War. He reports that this has left young people to be raised out of traditional social values. This loss occurred in a matter of a few years, but may take generations to reverse, or may never be fully reversed and may represent a death to some aspects of traditional culture.

A number of authors have discussed major losses that occur following extreme stress. Van der Kolk (1987) speaks of the loss of trust that occurs to the individual and Figley (1978) has extended this to the generation of Vietnam veterans who lost trust in government and the services that they expected to support them upon their return home. Hobfoll, Lomranz, Eyal, Bridges, and Tzemach (1989) suggested that communal stress may threaten central, defining values of a society. Studying the 1982 Israel-Lebanon war, they found that threat to defining values (e.g., seeing one's nation as moral even in war), may be more stressful even than threat of loss of life. Similarly, Jerusalem and Schwarzer (1989) found that for refugees, their flight may result on a personal level in loss of their status in the community and loss of fit of their skills with demands of their new home. Communities can absorb a certain number of such individuals, but when their number climbs there are outgrowths in the community that extend beyond the individual's or family's difficulties. When generalized to millions of people this may, in turn, give rise to nationalistic and fascistic public reaction when translated onto the larger social scale.

McFarlane (1989, 1990, 1993) has studied losses following the 1983 Australian Bush Fires. These fires killed scores of people and great number of livestock and caused enormous property and natural resource damage. He found that greater exposure to the most disturbing aspects of the fire (e.g., threat to life, witnessing loss of life, witnessing the grisly aftermath of the fire) resulted in greater likelihood of experiencing intrusive thoughts and avoidance reactions. However, those whose personal losses were greatest posed the highest risk for post traumatic stress disorder (PTSD).

Freedy, Shaw, Jarrell, and Masters (1992) examined the impact of losses related to Hurricane Hugo, which devastated Charleston, South Carolina in 1989. They hypothesized that resource loss would be a critical element in defining the impact of the hurricane. They further predicted that resource loss would have a larger impact than coping behavior and personal characteristics (e.g., gender, income, economic level). Finally, they expected that loss would not only predict greater malaise, but would constitute a risk factor for clinical levels of distress. Resource loss had an effect size that was appreciably greater than any of the other variables. Only emotion-focused coping even approached the impact of loss and since the assessments were made cross-sectionally it is likely that emotion-focused coping and emotional outcomes were confounded (Dohrenwend et al., 1984; Stanton et al., 1994). In a replication study that examined the effects of the 1991 Sierra Madre earthquake in California among an ethnically diverse sample, similar findings were noted (Freedy, Saladin, Kilpatrick, Resnick, & Saunders, 1994). Once again, resource loss was a principle ingredient in psychological distress.

Losses associated with exposure to major community stress also have long-term impact. A study of the effects of a supper club fire in northern Kentucky in 1977 examined the effect of resource losses and threat of loss, including loss of loved ones, exposure to life threat and lost lives, and prolonged waiting to hear the fate of loved ones (Gleser, Green, & Winget, 1981). Demographic factors, social support, and coping were also assessed. Resource loss accounted for most of the variance in affective outcomes two years after the event. Looking at long-term effects of a dam collapse in West Virginia in 1972, fourteen years later, prolonged exposure to threats to loss associated with the disaster still predicted PTSD diagnosis (Green et al., 1990).

Principle 2: Resource investment. Following the insightful work of Schönpflug (1985), we came to understand that people must invest resources to gain other resources, to protect resources, and to prevent rapid resource loss once initial losses occur. On an individual level, for example, self-esteem is invested to prevent the further loss of self-esteem or social support can be invested to bolster lagging self-esteem at a time of crisis (Pearlin, Menaghan, Lieberman, & Mullan, 1981). On a community level, monies that have been reserved for other matters may be required for emergency services and the community may need to call on support from neighboring communities in the form of housing, emergency personnel, and equipment.

The investment of resources to preserve other resources emphasizes two further insights provided by COR theory. First, it becomes apparent that those communities who have more resources will be better able to counteract the demands of community stress. They will have deeper reservoirs from which to call forth resources. Relatedly, they will be more likely to have the resources that fit demands, assuming that they have a breadth of resources, and not just a depth of resources. Second, because coping demands investment of resources, community coping will result in resource depletion, which is itself a loss. Hence, resources reserves become increasingly depleted, even for resource rich communities. In the case of extreme or chronic stressors, this means that even communities that are well-endowed with resources may find that demands overwhelm their resource reserves. Still, this will come later and less severely than for communities that begin with limited resources.

People employ varied resources to cope with community stress. McIntosh, Silver, and Wortman (1993) found that the importance of religion in people's lives and religious participation were helpful resistance resources illustrating how communal and personal aspects of religion aids stress resistance. Wardak (1992) suggested that religious and cultural affiliation may have similarly helped people cope with the ongoing stress of the Afghan civil war. In his own observations, Giel (1990) suggested that the Armenian Orthodox Church was not a resource for the Armenians affected by natural disaster because it did not have ties to people's daily lives. Similarly, work by Dew, Bromet, and Schulberg (1987) suggested that availability of employment in a region moderated the effects of large scale layoffs. Studying a sample of children relatively well-endowed with social resources, Oner and Tosun (1990/1991) found that they were relatively immune to the upheaval of immigration.

Resources are not limitless, however. The need to call on community resources may make aircraft disasters a special problem, illustrating how resources can be quickly depleted from a resource-poor community situation. In such cases, the survivors may have no community to call upon because following the accident they are dispersed to varied communities that have no common commitment to the disaster (Williams, Solomon, & Bartone, 1988). This may be compared to the rare case where a plane crash occurs at the site of the very community from which most survivors live, as occurred in a case reported by Hobfoll, Morgan, and Lehrman (1980) in a remote Eskimo village on an island in the Bering Sea. In this case, the community mobilized to save victims, tend their wounds, assist in burials and mourning, and help in rehabilitation. The community was deeply harmed by the event, but survivors received economic assistance, succorance, and support as did families who lost loved ones in an ongoing manner.

The case of depletion of even rich community resources is exemplified by the settlement of refugees from former East Germany into former West Germany. Enormous resources have been invested in this process, but resources available for refugees compete with needs for funds for other aspects of unification. At the same time, Germany has had to cope with settlement of refugees from other countries based on long-term liberal policies regarding refugees that are now being challenged. This community coping process of subsidized resettlement taps a common resource reservoir that is finite and has become a significant burden on the German economy and a tinderbox in German politics over the very issue of where resources should be invested. The fact that this social challenge occurred at the time of a world recession and therefore declining resources only strained the resource pool further.

Stress appraisals have been assumed to be a major mediator of stress reactions (Lazarus & Folkman, 1984). However, Jerusalem (1993) found that for recent refugees personal resources, housing resources, and employment were closely linked with appraisals of threat and loss. This suggests that appraisals may actually be aggregate self assessments of resource conditions. When individuals have objectively adequate resources to invest they maintain positive appraisals and they will do well; when they lack resources to maintain a positive summative evaluation of their conditions they will do poorly. Such appraisals do not appear to be as idiographic as Lazarus and Folkman's (1984) model assumes. Rather, they seem to be reflections of actual resource conditions. When one adds to this model that personal resources that themselves relate to appraisal (e.g., optimism, self-esteem) stem developmentally from social resources (e.g., family support, economic prosperity, availability of good schools and employment) (Allen & Britt, 1983), a more objective picture of appraisals begins to emerge. Clearly individual interpretation plays a role here as well, but we believe that this role has been greatly overestimated because so many of the middle class populations that social and behavioral scientists have studied are heavily endowed with resources. Hence, it is true enough that for them idiographic differences in perceptions would become more salient. Quite simply, poor communities do worse than wealthier communities and these differences are far more powerful than the role of individual perceptions (Weisbeth, 1991).

Principle 3: Loss and Gain Cycles. By integrating Principles 1 and 2 we arrive at Principle 3. Specifically, if stress involves loss of resources, and if people invest resources to offset loss, then following initial loss people will be more vulnerable to subsequent losses. Initial losses deplete resources and there are fewer resources available to meet subsequent demands. Each iteration of this process attacks an increasingly weakened system. This creates loss cycles that gain in momentum (i.e., speed) and strength. Translated to the community level, resources may be depleted quickly in the case of some extreme stressors or resource depletion may be ongoing in the case of chronic stressors.

Communities act to limit the onslaught of continued threat and loss and to limit the secondary consequences of such circumstances. We should pay special attention here to ecological principles, because community stressors often vie for resources that were reserved for community development and progress (Trickett, 1984). This suggests that by drawing away these resources, additional losses will occur because the community will also have difficulty meeting its normal obligations and developmental goals.

Borrowing from Meichenbaum's notions (Meichenbaum & Fong, 1992; Meichenbaum & Fitzpatrick, 1992), the ecological interplay of resource loss might, in turn, influence healthy communal narratives that facilitate community success and progress. If Meichenbaum is correct, then exposure to community stressors are milestone events for "meaning taking." Loss cycles and the devastation they leave in their path could leave a trail of meanings indicating doom, helplessness, and social alienation, or at least they have the potential to do so. COR theory suggests that actual resource loss and how resources are used to limit loss cycles will tell the tale as to what kinds of meanings are constructed, survivorship and communal cohesion or victim role and social isolation. Even in the face of chronic community stress, sustaining a sense of mastery and a belief in a just world, may aid people's stress resistance (Ritter, Benson, & Snyder, 1990). We need to know much more about the communal level of meaning and Meichenbaum's notions provide valuable insights for such work.

Prior research suggests that exposure to stress may make individuals more vulnerable to future exposure (Coleman, Burcher, & Carson, 1980) or inoculate them against the negative impact of future stress exposure (Epstein, 1983). According to Z. Solomon (1990) and Block and Zautra (1981) whether prior stress exacerbates sensitivity or inoculates people depends on the success of their stress experience. COR theory suggests a means for judging this prior experience. Specifically, those who are able to limit losses and whose resources allow them to continue a reasonable life course within perhaps a few months following their stress exposure, should experience a stress inoculation effect. It should be underscored, however, that even if their ultimate experience is one of a survivor who triumphs over adversity, if they originally experienced severe losses they should remain sensitive to future stressors. In such cases, the survivor role may include both increased stress sensitivity and a heightened sense of mastery and even leadership surrounding such events, as in the case of many women active in the organization Mothers Against Drunk Driving (MADD), many of whom have lost a child in an alcohol-related traffic accident.

On a community level, it would be interesting to examine how communities become inoculated or stress sensitized to disaster, war, and other community stressors. Work by Lomranz and his colleagues (Lomranz, Hobfoll, Johnson, Eyal, & Zemach, 1994; Hobfoll et al., 1989) examined Israelis' response to war by studying changes in depression among a series of national samples. They found that even among this population who have been frequently subjected to war, there were marked increases in depression among the population in the face of new war threat and losses. However, they also noted rather rapid recovery to normal levels of distress and it would be interesting to examine whether this quick recovery occurs for other populations less experienced about war. Following Milgram and Hobfoll's (1986) supposition, the response of Americans to Vietnam and of Israelis to the Yom Kippur war may have led to increased sensitivity because the respective communities felt they experienced greater losses--not just of life, but of meaning--in the wake of these events. Loss of valued community narratives or meaning may increase vulnerability.

S. Solomon (1986) suggested that when communities are confronted with major stress events their support systems can become overtaxed. The loss of support may itself lead to psychological stress due perhaps to feelings of isolation, loneliness, and despair (Solomon, Mikulincer, & Hobfoll, 1987). Moreover, loss of support leaves the community more vulnerable to future stressful events. Kaniasty and Norris (1993) carefully examined this hypothesis, basing their thinking on COR theory. They wrote,

> Because of the multifaceted nature of disaster impact, all kinds of provisions [of resources] may be essential to match victims' coping demands. Unfortunately, natural disasters have the capacity to deplete social support. Although disasters tend to mobilize support immediately after the impact, it also appears that need soon exceeds the availability of those supports. (p. 396)

Looking at older adults exposed to a flood, Kaniasty and Norris (1993) found that personal loss and degree of community destruction led to a reduction in perceived and actual support. This loss of support mediated negative psychological outcomes. In particular, flood related losses led to deterioration of kin and non-kin support and social embeddedness. Loss of non-kin support and social embeddedness, in turn, led to increased depression. This is an exciting, creative research approach and provides a model for both application of theory and adaption of careful methodological and analytical approaches.

Gain spirals may also occur, but COR theory suggests that they will be weaker and slower developing than loss cycles. Hobfoll, London, & Orr (1988) investigated the effects of war-related stress on Israeli soldiers following their return to civilian life. There was some indication that those who had supportive, intimate ties actually did better if they were more seriously threatened by war-related stress or experienced greater war-related losses. Gains may occur for individuals in the existential sphere, whereby survivors find greater meaning in life and in their families (Frankl, 1963; Solomon, Waysman, Neria, Ohry, & Wiener, 1994), however, the negative psychological impact is more pervasive than are the consummate effects of these gains.

Intervention Based on Resource Investment and Conservation

Many authors have discussed the importance of a resource-based approach to intervention and prevention of community stress. S. Solomon (1986) has discussed mobilization of social support resources. Weisbeth (1991, 1992) has pointed to the need to create temporary communities near the disaster site for victims' families so that they can provide mutual support, be given necessary information, and treated for grief and shock by professional staff. Ørner and Thompson (1993) have developed important principles of debriefing for emergency staff that aims at keeping their sense of mastery and esteem high. COR theory provides insights that might facilitate an understanding of how these different resource investment strategies will operate and the likely obstacles that will prevent these strategies from being implemented. Community interventionists must be aware of these principles and obstacles if they are to avert the diversion of resources to other than the most important needs or the dilution of resources, such that none of the areas of need receives a critical mass of resources.

Intervention in the Community

Hobfoll and Lilly (1993) have suggested intervention correlates of COR theory that follow from the concepts we have raised thus far. These corollaries are as follows:

1. Because loss of resources is the critical determinant of psychological and health outcomes, intervention must first concentrate on halting or limiting resource loss cycles. Mental health interventionists may even need to keep a step back at early junctures and allow emergency on other tactical interventionists to act to limit the devastation of the disaster or emergency. When psychosocial intervention is appropriate mental health professionals should consider how best to limit further losses so there is ultimately less to repair, replace, and reintegrate.

2. Although resource gain is secondary to resource loss, initiation of gain cycles can help counteract loss cycles. Enhancing victims' or a community's sense of mastery, for example, may aid them in preventing further psychosocial loss from occurring. Nevertheless, loss cycles have to be sufficiently limited if we are to (1) receive the community's or target individuals' attention, and (2) expect positive consequences of this aspect of intervention. Gain cycles may be most appropriately launched as prevention efforts prior to any disaster or community upheaval, enriching community resources for a future time when disaster or emergency will make heavy resource demands.

3. Loss cycles are more rapid in momentum and more intense in magnitude than gain cycles. This means that intervention aimed at halting loss cycles should proceed early and intensively. This is especially true when working with resource-poor communities as their natural resources are vulnerable to rapid depletion.

4. Expect secondary losses as spin-offs from the primary losses attributable to the disaster or emergency. Because resources are required for coping, resource loss will result in increased inability to master everyday stressors. Thus, the new losses lead to failures in normal life domains when individuals or systems are stripped of resources.

5. Because resources are intertwined, resource loss in one domain will reverberate to other domains. Loss of community mastery, for example, would be likely to deplete social connections in the community, and vice versa.

6. Communities that lack resources will react in odd and unexpected manners because they are basing their coping strategies on resources that have increasingly poor fit with demands. To use a metaphor, having only a square peg, they will strenuously attempt to force it into a round hole. If they had a round peg (i.e., more appropriate resources), they would use that. For example, police or army units may need to aid firefighters, despite their lack of training. Further, communities may sense the immediacy of their need to act and may use resources inappropriately in order to act quickly. Socially, this may include acts of selfishness that are ultimately self-defeating, as when residents isolate themselves from help.

7. Because even successful coping demands resources, communities that are coping well may begin to falter as their resources are depleted. It may be a better strategy therefore to aid a community with a modicum of resources before this stage occurs, rather than pouring resources into a community or situation that is already deeply in a loss spiral.

Obstacles to Intervention

Building on COR theory and the experience of the 11-day Lucasville, Ohio prison disturbance we can also see that certain common obstacles to community intervention are likely to develop. In particular, we wish to draw attention to four common obstacles:

1. Identification of communities within communities
2. Pressure cooker effects
3. Political processes and agendas
4. Avoidance of long-term needs

Identification of communities within communities. A first obstacle to intervention is that there are subcommunities within the ecology of the community (Trickett, 1984; this volume). Underestimating the diversity of the ecology of these communities can impede the ability to intervene at the various necessary levels.

From a resource perspective subcommunities will vie for protection of their community and act to limit their community's losses and halt or minimize loss cycles. At the Lucasville prison takeover one might assume that the prison was one community. Instead, those involved quickly learned that separate communities included the prisoners, the correction officers, the local prison administration, the central office prison administration, the local surrounding community, Ohioans in general, and the different protective agencies (e.g., State Police, federal troops, FBI). These communities did not stand to lose or gain the same resources to the same extent, yet understanding what each stood to gain and lose allows one to determine what their position is on any given reaction by authorities toward intervention.

Local subcommunities had both real and imagined fears of the consequences of a prison breakout. They had little empathy with the prison inmates and great empathy with the prison correction officers, many of whom were family members, church members, customers, and friends. Their call for intervention was to go in with guns blazing and to act with a great show of force. Correction officers who were not taken hostage may have harbored similar feelings, but were torn between these feelings and their deep concern for fellow guards and for themselves were they to be taken hostage on a future occasion. Prison inmates in a fortified section tried to survive the ordeal and were aware of the need to threaten, on one hand, but not cross a perceived line in the sand, on the other hand, that may have led to swift or irrevocable retribution.

This tendency for subcommunities to protect against their resource loss applies to refugee, disaster, and war situations. The poor are usually most negatively affected by disaster (Weisbeth, 1991) due to their lack of resources. They also may lack spokespersons to make their case in the clamor for resources provided by intervention. Giel (1990) has suggested that sometimes a sense of equity results in the richer community sharing resources, but it would seem that greed and a natural tendency to empathize with one's own would also be powerful motivators. Given ethnic diversity, racism may also play a role in unfair distribution of resources to the different subcommunities involved. In the Lucasville prison ordeal, prisoners were disproportionately African American (57%), whereas the prison employees (90%) and local community were mainly white. Had the local community been mainly African American, this may have caused a different kind of responding and alignment of loyalties. The poor will be less well-insured, may have less of a voice of government, and may have fewer spokespersons in the media. This can lead to their further disenfranchisement during disaster. One might think that churchleaders would provide a voice for equity and reason in their leadership in voluntary efforts or as spokespersons for the poor, but the church is the most segregated place in America, as it is in many countries where communities divide according to racial, ethnic, and economic lines on their day of holiness. As we see in the former Yugoslavia and in Israel, religious authorities are not necessarily champions of all men and women, but tend like others to align to protect their community's resources.

Successful intervention must find common goals of different subcommunities, bring them together during times of crisis, avoid making political gain out of community differences, and ensure equitable distribution of intervention resources. Identifying and working with the formal and informal leadership in communities is important in order to know what losses have occurred, what resources are necessary, and the best avenues for appropriating resources and shoring up resource loss and resource leakage (see also Kelly, 1988). Since loss increases efforts to limit further loss and to counteract those losses, interventionists can expect that the normal ecology of resource exchange will be accelerated toward efforts to retain, obtain, and protect resources by each of the subcommunities involved.

Defusing the pressure cooker effect. Stress researchers have discussed the process of stress contagion (Kessler, McLeod, & Wethington, 1985; Riley & Eckenrode, 1986), whereby people's stress is shared when they interact. Rather than decreasing the negative impact of stress, such social interaction may actually exacerbate negative stress sequelae. Hobfoll and London (1986) discussed the special case of stress contagion during shared or community stress events. Investigating Israelis' reactions to the 1982 Israel-Lebanon War, they noted that those who had more social support were more, rather than less, distressed. On debriefing study participants, they found that social interactions often focused on sharing rumors about the war, and these rumors were almost uniformly negative. They termed this the pressure cooker effect.

The pressure cooker effect emerged as a major influence in the Lucasville prison disturbance. Both among prison inmates and among the prison authorities, stress resulted in rumors whose source could never quite be tracked. Among the command center authorities there were attempts at rumor control, but the strength of the rumors generated more force than did the attempts to quell them. As found by Hobfoll and London (1986), the rumors were typically negative and extreme: "guards were being killed or tortured," "a certain maniacal prisoner has control of the situation, etc." COR theory proposes that loss is much more salient than gain and that people concentrate more on loss than on gain. It follows that rumors that indicate gains will quickly lose momentum, whereas negative rumors will reverberate on the reactions of those hearing them and be perpetuated with fear and excitement. Media looking for breaking stories add another dimension to this problem, because by reporting rumors the rumor gains a new authority. Secondary sources will even cite reported events as if they occurred by stating that an "authoritative newspaper reported that . . . ," when there was no basis for the originally reported event.

Psychosocial intervention must pay special attention to the pressure cooker process. A single authoritative source should be assigned the role of information gatherer and disseminator. They must be reasonably free and honest in sharing information, because otherwise they either lose credibility or lose their status as disseminator of information. This requires coordination of emergency and other service authorities, such that they must freely share information and not garner information to gain authority and status. This will not extinguish the pressure cooker effect, but should serve an offsetting function.

Survivors and their families must also be given special access to information. By bringing together families of plane crash victims or industrial disaster the authoritative source can work closely with them to ensure that they are updated and kept apprised of the facts to the extent that they are known. When a disaster involves an entire community information should be shared by regularly scheduled reports of updated knowledge. As rumors emerge they should be investigated and the details reported to the extent they can be verified or discredited.

Political processes and agendas. Disasters and other major community stressors are political events. As such, political processes and their own chase for resources emerge and play a major role. Leaders, including politicians and agency and department administrators, will act to limit resource loss to them and their constituencies and may even attempt to make gains from the pain and suffering of others.

In the Lucasville prison takeover, as in other community stress events, one of the first processes is that of avoiding culpability. No one wishes for the blame to be laid at their doorstep. In the case of natural disasters one can cite the hand of God or fate, but when people have created the situation there are both immediate and continued attempts to avoid responsibility. In both human made and natural disasters this process continues such that leaders try to take credit for any successes and avoid being associated with any negative fallout. This pressure can also motivate leaders to act, so as not to be faulted for complacency, but they are pressured to lose sight of the community needs that they are entrusted to serve. Those closest to the situation may also be motivated to limit their actual feelings of guilt about loss of life and human suffering, whether or not they are in fact responsible. In the Lucasville situation, the quick response of the senior prison authorities and the governor kept a problem-based focus, rather than a blame-reduction focus. Nevertheless, even as positive overall steps are being taken, it is inevitable that subplots transpire that drain energy from needed resource investment.

This social-political process is counterproductive because it is likely to engender a climate whereby action is not taken so that one does not make an error. Actions are considered for their potential negative side-effects rather than their positive impact, even if the positive impact far outweighs the negative consequences. At Lucasville, local prison authorities, statewide prison authorities, and multiple government agency leaders were quickly caught between an honest motivation to protect life and quell the disturbance and the knowledge that they were being judged in the press and by each other. Given an unclear chain of command and multiple emergency, law enforcement, and political authorities these political processes present obstacles for attention to the need to address the grave problem at hand. It is critical for senior leaders to express the need to avoid political squabbling. This often requires for senior leaders to themselves take a hands on approach.

Knowledge about how to handle emergencies is helpful in such situations, in part, because it provides a blueprint for authorities to follow. This may open the way for them to make difficult decisions and allow accumulated wisdom to defend their position. For example, despite some hot tempers, a relatively cool hand was maintained in the gruelling process of an 11 day wait for the culmination of the Lucasville prison takeover. The experience provided by other similar situations guided the policy as to how to negotiate with prison inmates, the need to wait and not overreact, and the need to be prepared to move quickly if conditions changed dramatically.

Mental health professionals can aid authorities by helping them deal with their own distress, a desire to act precipitously to end the difficult state of tension, and such problems as may be caused by their lack of sleep, attacks by the media, and fear for their own political or employment futures. In this regard, leaders are likely to feel isolated and under attack and this may lead to an us against them, siege mentality. We clearly need more research on how leaders act in community stress situations and on how to improve the decision-making process.

Addressing long-term needs. Motivation to act and invest resources to limit loss and interrupt loss cycles are critical at the time of the event. To the extent that loss cycles are halted early, they will produce less ultimate damage (Hobfoll & Jackson, 1991). However, it is also important to continue to address long-term, chronic losses associated with the event. Communities and authorities are increasingly motivated to move on to other pressing agendas. Also, resources are drained over time, and so fewer resources may be available to address long-term needs. Given that long-term problems clearly continue (Green et al., 1990), this competition for resources becomes an important tertiary problem.

We have learned that both personal and social resources may ebb as chronic community stress takes its toll (Pearlin et al., 1981; Kaniasty & Norris, 1993). Now, we must establish how to meet this ongoing process of resource loss. Freedy and Hobfoll (1994) have found that group intervention can aid in building resources for professional groups who are experiencing ongoing organizational stress and who are otherwise at risk for burnout and a group approach may lend itself to other community stress.

Examining the long-term effects of the Lucasville disturbance we can see that prison inmates, correction officers, and administrators who were involved in the crisis first hand have ongoing experience of continuing stress and distress. Long after the prison takeover was set to rest, the fears evoked by the event remain acute and the continued possibility of further unrest lays a shadow of anxiety. Correction officers fear that prison inmates may have been emboldened by the empowerment they felt and prisoners fear retribution by correction officers. Daily work at the prison serves as a constant reminder of the original traumatic experience (van der Kolk, 1987). Methods of coping are not necessarily the most adaptive, because many of those involved have no experience of this kind on which to rely and may take drastic steps to limit future loss.

Even acute community stressors can create long-term demands that strip resource reserves (Greene et al., 1990). This may especially occur when the original event caused such severe loss as to render individuals or communities handicapped in dealing with normal life events. Economic loss, familial loss, material loss to critical infrastructure (housing, factories, businesses) may make otherwise normal stressors beyond coping capacity. Where aspects of the stressor itself continue, such as in the case of living in a contaminated region or a region saddled with ongoing armed conflict, or where exposure to a contaminant or war may produce health problems that might only emerge years later, the draining of resources is even more salient (Baum, 1987). Long-term demands compete with new demands for the same diminishing set of resources. It may be difficult for communities or individuals to adopt a survivor role when they continue to be assaulted by such ongoing demands.

COR theory suggests that when resources fall below a necessary threshold that is required for ongoing coping that more severe forms of dysfunction will occur. On a community level this may translate to alienation, breakdown of social codes, and an assault on the very cultural fabric that ties communities together (Wallace, 1990; Wardak, 1992). Wallace, Fullilove, and Wallace (1992) suggest that ongoing community stressors break down personal, community, and domestic social networks that underlie a community's well-being. They show that rates of disease, violence, and behavioral pathologies (e.g., substance abuse) consequently arise in such situations.

Conclusion: No Silk Purses Out of Sow's Ears

Work on individual stress has tended to emphasize perception as the sine qua non of stress (Lazarus & Folkman, 1984). This, in turn, has led to an emphasis on reappraisal as an avenue for intervention (Meichenbaum & Fitzpatrick, 1992; Meichenbaum, this volume). COR theory, and we believe the literature on community stress in particular, argues that the objective nature of events, not just their perception, plays the major role in stress reactions. When authors have discussed increasingly social support as a means of intervention, they have not meant to merely change the perception of support (S. Solomon, 1986). When Ozer and Bandura (1990) have sought to increase formerly raped women's self-efficacy to face possible sexual assault, they did not have women just reframe the threat; they taught them aggressive martial arts. Clearly, perceptions play a role in such instances, but they follow from actual resources and the circumstances that people face. Indeed, when attempts have been made to merely have people reframe their threats, the results were clearly negative and greater distress resulted (Wiebe, 1991).

On the community level, we suggest that it is similarly the actual presence of resources and challenges to those resources that will determine a community's success in addressing major stress events. Over time, resources will become depleted, even if initial resource levels are strong. Just as individuals might benefit from social support at such times, communities may require outside help to shore resource losses and create some initial small wins that will increase community sense of mastery. Psychosocial assistance to survivors is one resource for communities that are confronted with significant stressors. In addition, social and behavioral scientists and clinicians can also help limit the impact of community stress by conducting more research on decision making, supportive communication, and potential organizational breakdowns or other obstacles that stress engenders that will otherwise impede successful adjustment. More informed consultation can then be provided in order to assist community prevention and intervention efforts aimed at limiting loss in the face of major community stress circumstances. A community's meaning taking (Meichenbaum, this volume) cannot stray far from its actual resource reservoirs without creating false hopes that may actually increase communal vulnerability.

References

Allen, L., & Britt, D.W. (1983). Social class, mental health, and mental illness: The impact of resources and feedback. In R.D. Felner, L.A. Jason, J.N. Moritsugu, & S.S. Farber (Eds.), Preventive Psychology: Theory, Research, and Practice, (pp. 149-161). New York: Pergamon.

Baum, A. (1987). Toxins, technology, and natural disasters. In G.R. Vanderbos, and B.K. Bryant (Eds.), Cataclysms, crises, and catastrophes: Psychology in action. Washington, D.C.: American Psychological Association.

Block, M., & Zautia, A. (1981). Satisfaction and distress in a community: A test of the effects of life events. American Journal of Community Psychology, 9, 165-180.

Coleman, J.C., Burcher, J.N., & Carson, R.C. (1980). Abnormal psychology and modern life (6th ed.). Glenview, IL: Scott/Foresman.

Dew, M.A., Bromet, E.J., & Schulbert, H.C. (1987). A comparative analysis of two community stressors long term mental health effects. American Journal of Community Psychology, 15, 167-184.

Dohrenwend, B.S., Dohrenwend, B.P., Dodson, M., & Shrout, P.E. (1984). Symptoms, hassles, social support, and life events: Problem of confounded measures. Journal of Abnormal Psychology, 93, 222-230.

Epstein, S. (1983). Concluding comments to section I. In D. Meichenbaum & M.E. Varenko (Eds.). Stress reduction and prevention (pp. 101-106). New York: Plenum Press.

Figley, C.R. (1978). Stress disorders among Vietnam veterans: Theory, research, and treatment. New York: Brunner/Mazel.

Frankl, V.E. (1963). Man's search for meaning. Boston: Beacon.

Freedy, J.R., & Hobfoll, S.E. (1994). Stress inoculation for reduction of burnout: A conservation of resources approach. Anxiety, Stress, and Coping, 6, 311-325.

Freedy, J.R., Saladin, M.E., Kilpatrick, D.G., Resnick, H.S., & Saunders, B.E.(1994). Understanding acute psychological distress following natural disaster. Journal of Traumatic Stress, 7, 257-273.

Freedy, J.R., Shaw, D.L., Jarrel, M.P., & Masters, C.R. (1992). Toward an understanding of the psychological impact of disasters. Journal of Traumatic Stress, 5, 441-454.

Giel, R. (1990). The psychosocial aftermath of two major disasters in the Soviet Union. Journal of Traumatic Stress, 4, 381-392.

Gleser, G.C., Green, B.L., & Winget, C. (1981). Prolonged psychosocial effects of disaster: A study of Buffalo Creek. New York: Academic Press.

Green, B.L., Lindy, J.D., Grace, M.C., Gleser, G.C., Leonard, A.C., Korse, M., & Winget, C. (1990). Buffalo Creek survivors in the second decade: Stability of stress symptoms. American Journal of Orthopsychiatry, 60, 43-54.

Guisinger, S., & Blatt, S.J. (1994). Individuality and relatedness: Evolution of a fundamental dialectic. American Psychologist, 49, 104-111.
Hobfoll, S.E. (1988). The Ecology of Stress. Washington, D. C.: Hemisphere.
Hobfoll, S.E. (1989). Conservation of resources: A new attempt at conceptualizing stress. American Psychologist, 44, 513-524.
Hobfoll, S.E., & Jackson, A.P. (1991). Conservation of resources in community intervention. American Journal of Community Psychology, 19, 111-121.
Hobfoll, S.E., & Lilly, R.S. (1993). Resource conservation as a strategy for community psychology. Journal of Community Psychology, 21, 128-148.
Hobfoll, S.E., Lomranz, J., Eyal, N., Bridges, A., & Tzemach, M. (1989). Pulse of a nation: Depressive mood reactions of Israel is to Israel-Lebanon War. Journal of Personality and Social Psychology, 56, 1002-1012.
Hobfoll, S.E., & London, P. (1986). The relationship of self-concept and social support to emotional distress among women during war. Journal of Social and Clinical Psychology, 12, 87-100.
Hobfoll, S.E., London, P., & Orr, E. (1988). Mastery, intimacy, and stress resistance during war. Journal of Community Psychology, 16, 317-331.
Hobfoll, S.E., Morgan, R., & Lehrman, R. (1980). Development of a training center in an Eskimo village. Journal of Community Psychology, 8, 80-87.
Iscoe, I. (1974). Community psychology and the competent community. American Psychologist, 29, 607-613.
Jerusalem, M. (1993). Personal resources, environmental constraints,and adaptational processes: The predictive power of a theoretical stress model. Journal of Personality and Individual Differences, 14, 15-24.
Jerusalem, M., & Schwarzer, R. (1989). Anxiety and self-concept as antecedents of stress and coping: A longitudinal study with German and Turkish adolescents. Personality and Individual Differences, 10, 785-792.
Kaniasty, K., & Norris, F.H. (1993). A test of social support deterioration models in the context of natural disaster. Journal of Personality and Social Psychology, 64, 395-408.
Kelly, J.G. (1988). A guide to conducting prevention research in the community: First steps. New York: Haworth Press.
Kessler, R.C., McLeod, J.D., & Wethington, E. (1985). The costs of caring: A perspective on the relationship between sex and psychological distress. In I.G. Sarason and B.R. Sarason (Eds.), Social support: Theory, research, and applications (pp. 491-506). The Netherlands: Martinus Nijhoff, The Hague.
Lazarus, R.S., & Folkman, S. (1984). Stress, appraisal, and coping. New York: Springer.
Lomranz, J., Hobfoll, S.E., Johnson, R., Eyal, N., & Zemach, M. (1994). A nation's response to attack: Israelis' depressive reactions to the Gulf War. Journal of Traumatic Stress, 7, 55-69.

McFarlane, A.C. (1989). The prevention and management of the psychiatric morbidity of natural disasters: An Australian experience. Stress Medicine, 5, 29-36.

McFarlane, A.C. (1990). An Australian disaster: The 1993 bushfires. International Journal of Mental Health, 19, 36-47.

McFarlane, A.C. (1993). PTSD: Synthesis of research and clinical studies: The Australian Bush fire disaster. In J.P. Wilson and B. Raphael (Eds.), International Handbook of Traumatic Stress Syndromes, (421-429). New York: Plenum Press.

McFarlane, A.C. (1994). The severity of the trauma: Issues about its role in post traumatic stress disorder. Unpublished manuscript.

McIntosh, D.N., Silver, R.C., & Wortman, C.B. (1993). Religion's role in adjustment to a negative life event: Coping with the loss of a child. Journal of Personality and Social Psychology, 65, 812-821.

Meichenbaum, D. (this volume). Disasters, stress, and cognition. In S. E. Hobfoll & M. W. deVries (Eds.), Extreme stress and communities: Impact and intervention. Dordrecht, the Netherlands: Kluwer.

Meichenbaum, D., & Fitzpatrick, D. (1992). A constructivist narrative perspective of stress and coping: Stress inoculation applications. In L. Goldberger and S. Breznitz (Eds.), Handbook of stress. New York: Wiley.

Meichenbaum, D., & Fong, G.T. (1993). How individuals control their own minds: A constructive narrative perspective. In D.M. Wegner and J.W. Pennebaker (Eds.), Handbook of mental control (pp. 473-490). Englewood Cliffs, NJ: Prentice Hall.

Milgram, N.A., & Hobfoll, S.E. (1986). Generalizations from the theory and practice in war-related stress. In N.A. Milgram (Ed.), Stress and coping in time of war: Generalizations from the Israeli experience (pp. 316-352). New York: Brunner/Mazel.

Oner, N., & Tosun, U. (1990/1991). Adjustment of the children of immigrant workers in Turkey: A comparison of immigrant and nonimmigrant Turkish adolescents. In N. Bleichrodt and P.J.D. Drenth (Eds.), Contemporary issues in cross cultural psychology: Selected papers from a regional conference of the International Association for Cross-cultural Psychology, (pp. 72-83). Amsterdam/Lisse: Swets & Zeitlinger, Inc.

Ørner, R.J. & Thompson, M. (1993). Current provision for traumatic stress reactions in N.H.S. Personnel: A survey of critical incident stress management services (CISMS) in England, Scotland and Wales. Unpublished manuscript.

Ozer, E.M., & Bandura, A. (1990). Mechanism governing empowerment effects: A self-efficacy analysis. Journal of Personality and Social Psychology, 58, 472-486.

Pearlin, C.I., Menaghan, E.G., Lieberman, M.A., & Mullan, J.T. (1981). The stress process. Journal of Health and Social Behavior, 22, 337-356.

Quarentelli, E.L. (1985). An assessment of conflicting views on mental health: The consequences of traumatic events. In C.R. Figley (Ed.), <u>Trauma and its wake: From victim to survivor: Social responsibility in the wake of catastrophe</u> (pp. 398-415). New York: Brunner/Mazel.

Riger, S. (1993). What's wrong with empowerment. <u>American Journal of Community Psychology, 31,</u> 279-292.

Riley, D., & Eckenrode, J. (1986). Social ties: Subgroup differences in costs and benefits. <u>Journal of Personality and Social Psychology, 51,</u> 770-778.

Ritter, C., Benson, D.E., Snyder, C. (1990). Belief in a just world and depression. <u>Sociological perspective, 33,</u> 235-252.

Sarason, S.B. (1974). <u>The psychological sense of community: Prospects for a community psychology.</u> Washington, D.C.: Jossey-Bass.

Schönpflug, W. (1985). Goal-directed behavior as a source of stress: Psychological origins and the consequences of inefficiency. In M. Frese and J. Sabini (Eds.), <u>The concept of action in psychology,</u> (pp. 172-188). Hunsdale, New Jersey: Laurence Erlbaum.

Soloman, S.D. (1986). Mobilizing social support networks in times of disaster. In C.R. Figley (Ed.), <u>Trauma and its wake, volume II: Traumatic stress, theory, research, and intervention.</u> (pp. 232-263). New York: Brunner/Mazel.

Solomon, Z. (1990). Does the war end when the shooting stops? The Psychological toll of war. <u>Journal of Applied Social Psychology, 20-21,</u> 1733-1745.

Solomon, Z., Mikulincer, M., & Hobfoll, S.E. (1987). Objective versus subjective measurement of stress and social support: The case of combat related reactions. <u>Journal of Clinical and Consulting Psychology, 55,</u> 577-583.

Solomon, Z., Waysman, M.A., Neria, Y., Ohry, A., & Wiener, M. (1994). <u>Psychological growth and dysfunction following war captivity.</u> Unpublished manuscript.

Stanton, A.L., Danoff-Burg, S., Cameron, C.L., & Ellis, A.P. (1994). Coping through emotional approach: Problems of conceptualization and confounding. <u>Journal of Personality and Social Psychology, 66,</u> 350-362.

Thoits, P.A. (1983). Dimensions of life events that influence psychological distress: An evaluation and synthesis of the literature. In H.B. Kaplan (Ed.), <u>Psychological Stress: Trends in Theory and Research.</u> (pp. 33-103). New York: Academic.

Triandis, H.C., & Brislin, R.W. (1984). Crosscultural psychology. <u>American Psychologist, 39,</u> 1006-1016.

Trickett, E.J. (1984). Toward a distinctive community psychology: An ecological metaphor for the conduct of community research and the nature of training. <u>American Journal of Community Psychology, 12,</u> 261-279.

Trickett, E.J. (this volume). The community context of disaster and traumatic stress: An ecological perspective from community psychology. In S. E. Hobfoll & M. W. deVries (Eds.), <u>Extreme stress and communities: Impact and intervention.</u> Dordrecht, the Netherlands: Kluwer.

van der Kolk, B.A. (1987). Psychological Trauma. Washington, D.C.: American Psychiatric Press, Inc.

Wallace, R. (1990). Urban desertification, public health, and public order: Planned shrinkage, violent death, substance abuse and AIDS in the Bronx. Social Science, 31, 801-813.

Wallace, R., Fullilove, M.T., & Wallace, D. (1992). Family systems and deurbanization: Implications for substance abuse. In J.H. Lowninson, P. Rueiz, and R. Millman (Eds.), Substance abuse: A comprehensive textbook (2nd ed.) (pp. 944-955). Baltimore: Williams and Wilkins.

Wardak, A.W.H. (1992). The psychiatric effects of war stress on Afghanistan society. In J.P. Wilson and B. Raphael (Eds.), International Handbook of Traumatic Stress Syndromes, (349-364), New York: Plenum Press.

Weisbeth, L. (1991). The information and support center: Preventing the after-effects of disaster trauma. In T. Sørensen, P. Abrahamsen, and S. Torgersen (Eds.), Psychiatric disorders in the social domain. (pp. 50-58). Oslo: Norwegian University Press.

Weisbeth, L. (1992). Prepare and repair: Some principles in prevention of psychiatric consequences of traumatic stress. Psychiatria Fennica, 23, 11-18.

Wiebe, D.J. (1991). Hardiness and stress moderation: A test of proposed mechanisms. Journal of Personality and Social Psychology, 60, 89-99.

Williams, C.L., Solomon, S.D., & Bartone, P. (1988). Primary prevention in aircraft disasters: Integrating research and practice. American Psychologist, 43, 730-739.

OPTIMISTIC SELF-BELIEFS AS A RESOURCE FACTOR IN COPING WITH STRESS

Ralf Schwarzer, Freie Universität Berlin
Matthias Jerusalem, Humboldt-Universität zu Berlin

Optimistic Self-Beliefs as a Resource Factor in Coping With Stress

When people face adversity they can appraise the encounter as being challenging, threatening, or harmful before turning to coping strategies to alleviate the stress (Hobfoll, 1988, 1989; Jerusalem & Schwarzer, 1992; Lazarus, 1991). Cognitive appraisal and coping represent two critical stages in the stress process. One's resources come into play at both stages. Resources can be material, social, health or personal assets that may be of use in the confrontation of difficult problems. But these resources represent only a potential. To be of service they have to be perceived by the individual. One has to identify the appropriate resources and to make use of them. For example, it is not enough to have a close social network one also has to mobilize it to receive actual social support in times of need. Believing in one's resources makes a difference initially when it comes to appraising the stressful encounter and it does so again later on when one copes with adversity. In the present chapter, we deal exclusively with a personality disposition that can buffer stress appraisal, coping, and stress experience. We focus on optimistic self-beliefs as an important personal resource factor. For this purpose, we will first discuss the theoretical status of three kinds of optimistic self-beliefs: explanatory style, generalized outcome expectancies, and perceived self-efficacy. We believe that the last one represents the most promising construct because of its theoretical foundation and overwhelming empirical evidence. In the subsequent section, we will present data from a longitudinal study on stressful life transitions experienced by East Germans who left their country in the wake of the breakdown of the communist system in order to support our theoretical treatise.

Functional Optimism Pertaining to Personal Resources

Individuals who have a positive outlook on life are likely to be less vulnerable to adversity as long as this optimism does not become too unrealistic. Naive or defensive optimism reflects a perception bias that distorts reality and may lead to risk behaviors (Schwarzer, 1994). On the other hand, functional optimism pertains to the belief that the future will be positive because one can control it more or less. Effort investment would then probably result in favorable outcomes. Among the manifold optimism concepts there are three major ones that we are going to explain in some detail, starting with the least functional and ending with the most functional: (a) optimistic explanatory style, (b) dispositional optimism, and (c) perceived self-efficacy.

Optimistic Explanatory Style

When Martin Seligman (1991) published his book on "learned optimism" 16 years after his landmark book on "learned helplessness", this could be understood as a portent of a historical trend. Today, positive emotions and cognitions receive most of the attention, and optimism has become a "magic bullet" in the prediction of well-being, coping behavior, and stress outcomes. Learned optimism stands for the construct of "optimistic explanatory style" that is simply the reverse of the well-known "depressive attributional style." When the Seligman group completely revised the original helplessness theory three years after its initial publication (Abramson, Seligman, & Teasdale, 1978), its key feature was the application of attribution theory to depression. Later on, individual differences in attributions became the focus of attention (Alloy & Abramson, 1988; Peterson & Seligman, 1984). It was found that people develop depression if they acquire a depressive attributional response style. This style was composed of three dimensions: locus of control (internal versus external), stability (stable versus unstable), and globality (global versus specific). Habitual responses to negative events in terms of internal, stable and global attributions ("I am a loser and always will be") were coded as depressive. A meta-analysis has demonstrated the impressive body of research that corroborates the pervasiveness of this attributional style in depressives (Sweeney, Anderson, & Bailey, 1986). Non-depressives would tend to attribute negative events rather to external, variable and specific factors ("The circumstances have been unfortunate recently"). This is called an optimistic explanatory style. Optimists would attribute good events rather to internal, stable and global causes, i.e., optimists would make self-serving attributions.

In many studies, optimistic explanatory style has been positively related to health and negatively to illness (Peterson & Bossio, 1991; Peterson & Seligman, 1987). But the causal link between this kind of optimism and health is not well established. One assumption is that people with an optimistic explanatory style take control of their life and adopt healthy practices that, in turn, lead to positive health outcomes in the long run. Another assumption is that optimists are physiologically different from pessimists. Kamen-Siegel, Rodin, Seligman, and Dwyer (1991) have studied the relationship between explanatory style and immune response in older adults. They found that pessimistic explanatory style was related to poorer immune function. This finding held even after several health behaviors were partialled out. Health behaviors were almost uncorrelated with explanatory style. This result points to the possibility that the missing link between optimism and health might be rather of a physiological than a behavioral nature. However, this finding was based only on a small sample of elderly people, although it was in line with earlier studies that found a compromised immune status among humans and animals who had been made helpless or who were hopeless and depressed (Peterson & Seligman, 1984).

Explanatory style is a useful construct, in particular in the interpretation of past stress events. However, optimistic explanatory style does not do justice to one's own behavioral potential and motivation to counteract challenges or threats. It does not explicitly refer to one's perception of personal coping resources.

Dispositional Optimism

The common-sense notion of optimism can be expressed in statements such as "I'm always optimistic about my future," which is an example item of a psychometric scale developed by Scheier and Carver (1985). In contrast to explanatory style, this view of optimism explicitly pertains to expectancies and reflects a positive outlook on the future. The scientific concept is derived from a comprehensive theory of behavioral self-regulation that uses outcome expectancies as major ingredients (Carver & Scheier, 1981). According to this theory, people strive for goals as long as they see them as being attainable and as long as they believe that their actions will produce the desired outcome. Expectancies can be generalized across a variety of situations and can be stable over time. Therefore, the label "dispositional optimism" has been chosen (Scheier & Carver, 1985, 1987, 1992). It is defined as the relatively stable tendency to believe that one will generally experience good outcomes in life. People who have a favorable outlook on life are considered to cope better with stress and illness, to invest more effort to prevent harm, and to enjoy better health than those with negative generalized outcome expectancies.

Indeed, there is ample evidence that dispositional optimism is associated with improved coping. Litt, Tennen, Affleck, and Klock (1992) have found that optimistic women who tried in vitro fertilization unsuccessfully, adapted better to this failure than pessimistic women. Scheier et al. (1989) have followed up a group of male heart patients who underwent bypass operation. At four points in time, optimists were compared to pessimists, having been identified before surgery. In the first week after surgery, the optimists recovered faster and were quicker to leave the bed and to ambulate. After six months, the life of the optimists had almost normalized in terms of work and exercise, whereas this process took longer for the pessimists. After five years, optimists reported superior quality of life, better sleep, less pain, and more frequent health behaviors. The authors explain these benign effects of optimism with a more adaptive coping style. Already before the operation, the optimistic patients made plans and set goals for the time to come, whereas the pessimists paid more heed to their current emotions.

A second study, conducted with breast cancer patients, yielded similar results (Carver et al., 1993). Dispositional optimism turned out to be a good predictor for recovery and adaptation. Most studies report positive associations between optimism and psychological as well as physical well-being, and preliminary data also point to a relationship with health habits (see Scheier & Carver, 1992).

Some concerns arise when examining the potential role of dispositional optimism in the health behavior adoption process. According to expectancy-value theories, there are two kinds of outcome expectancies: Action-outcome expectancies and situation-outcome expectancies (Bandura, 1986). The first refers to "The behavior will get me what I want", and the second to "The circumstances will get me what I want." If the situation itself leads to positive health outcomes, there is no need to invest effort. For example, if one believes that scientists would discover the right antidotes before a disease can hit one day, there would be no need to take precautions. If, however, only instrumental actions would lead to positive health outcomes, one has to adopt them in time to be prepared to face the health risks.

The eight-item Life Orientation Test (LOT; Scheier & Carver, 1985) contains statements such as "In uncertain times, I usually expect the best" and "I rarely count on good things happening to me," but it remains undetermined why the best is expected or why good things should happen or not. Scheier and Carver do not make the explicit distinction between action-outcome and situation-outcome expectancies, but instead conceptualize optimism as more global, including them both. Their theoretical focus is mainly on action-outcome expectancies by stating that people strive for desirable consequences. Thus, the instrument may not reflect exactly what the theory suggests. The authors argue that optimists view "the positive outcomes as at least partially contingent on continued effort" (Scheier & Carver, 1992, p. 218). Optimists do not "simply sit and wait for success to happen." Instead, "positive expectancies cause the person to continue to work toward the attainment of goals." Although this notion is not well reflected in the item content, the respondents seem to recognize the implicit considerations; otherwise, the scale could not operate the way it does. Those who fill out the test seem to make their own inferences about the causal underpinnings of these items. Some may respond with situations in mind, others with actions in mind. Due to the empirical evidence indicating positive associations between dispositional optimism and adaptive coping or preventive action, most people seem to respond with their actions or efforts in mind that would cause good things in the future.

Perceived Self-Efficacy

Coping with stress is facilitated by a personal sense of control. If people believe that they can take action to solve a problem instrumentally, they become more inclined to do so and feel more committed to this decision. While outcome expectancies refer to the perception of the possible consequences of one's action, perceived self-efficacy pertains to personal action control or agency (Bandura, 1992, 1994). A person who believes in being able to cause an event can conduct a more active and self-determined life course. This "can do"-cognition mirrors a sense of control over one's environment. It reflects the belief of being able to master challenging demands by means of adaptive action. It can also be regarded as an optimistic view of one's capability to deal with adversity.

Self-efficacy makes a difference in how people feel, think and act. In terms of feeling, a low sense of self-efficacy is associated with depression, anxiety, and helplessness. Such individuals also have low self-esteem and harbor pessimistic thoughts about their accomplishments and personal development. In terms of thinking, a strong sense of competence facilitates cognitive processes and academic performance. Self-efficacy levels can enhance or impede the motivation to act. Individuals with high self-efficacy choose to perform more challenging tasks. They set themselves higher goals and stick to them (Locke & Latham, 1990). Actions are preshaped in thought, and people anticipate either optimistic or pessimistic scenarios in line with their level of self-efficacy. Once an action has been taken, high self-efficacious persons invest more effort and persist longer than those low in self-efficacy. When setbacks occur, they recover more quickly and maintain the commitment to their goals. Self-efficacy also allows people to select challenging settings, explore their environments, or create new situations. A sense of competence can be acquired by mastery experience, by vicarious experience, by verbal persuasion, or by physiological feedback (Bandura, 1977). Self-efficacy, however, is not the same as positive illusions or unrealistic optimism since it is closer to experience and usually does not lead to unreasonable risk taking. Instead, it leads to venturesome behavior that is within reach of one's capabilities.

While self-efficacy has been defined by Bandura (1977) as a behavior-specific construct that is tailored to a narrow situation, other authors have later introduced trait-like versions of it that may be called dispositional or generalized perceived self-efficacy (Sherer & Maddux, 1982). It refers to a global confidence in one's coping ability across a wide range of demanding situations. Snyder et al. (1991) suggested such a construct that they coined "hope." They defined hope as a cognitive set that is composed of a reciprocally derived sense of successful agency and pathways. Agency pertains to self-efficacy expectancy, and pathway equals the action-outcome expectancy. Skinner, Chapman, and Baltes (1988) had earlier made a similar distinction between agency beliefs and means-ends-beliefs (see also Skinner, 1992). Another scale has been introduced by Wallston (1989, 1992), who has labeled it "generalized self-efficacy" or "perceived competence" (Smith, Dobbins, & Wallston,

1991; see also Smith & Wallston, 1992). In analogy to the above-cited work of Snyder et al. (1991), he combines an outcome expectancy ("The behavior will get me what I want") with a self-efficacy expectancy ("I am capable of doing the behavior").

In the 1980s, an equivalent German agency scale of 10 items was designed to measure dispositional optimistic self-beliefs and perceived coping competence (Jerusalem & Schwarzer, 1986, 1992; Schwarzer, 1993), then labeled "General Self-Efficacy." Typical items are "When I am confronted with a problem, I usually find several solutions" or "I remain calm when facing difficulties because I can rely on my coping abilities." The scale has been used in more than twenty German studies that have demonstrated generalized self-efficacy to be a better predictor of subjective well-being, self-reported illness, and coping than other concurrent measures, such as self-esteem or trait anxiety.[1]

We believe that the approaches chosen by Snyder et al. (1991), Wallston (1989, 1992), and ourselves have a theoretical advantage because they make explicit assumptions about the causal underpinnings of a positive outlook on life. The construct includes optimistic resource beliefs and optimistic action beliefs, and it excludes the naive situation-outcome beliefs that constitute the optimistic bias. A characteristic feature of this construct lies in its generality, which is in contrast to Bandura's claim that self-efficacy should be measured in a behavior-specific manner. We do believe, in agreement with Bandura, that specific behaviors are best predicted by specific cognitions. However, there are many situations where one wants to make predictions across a variety of situations, and for that purpose the Generalized Self-Efficacy scale had been developed.

In the following study, this measure was applied to assess optimistic resource beliefs in East German migrants after their stressful transition to the West. In contrast to health behavior change (e.g., smoking cessation) or academic stress (e.g., preparing for an exam), migration represents a major life transition that affects a variety of domains of human functioning. Relocation usually includes the loss of loved ones, of valuable resources, and of familiar environments. It requires the search for housing, employment, and social contacts. Thus, a globally defined self-efficacy construct seems to be the most appropriate for the prediction of overall readjustment. An optimistic outlook on the general consequences of migration would motivate to invest more effort and to persist when difficulties arise.

Adjusting to Life Stress After Migration From East to West Germany

During the revolutionary events in East Germany in 1989, more than 300,000 citizens left that country and moved to West Germany. As a result of this exodus,

---

[1] The scale is being used in various cultures. It can be obtained from the authors in English, German, Spanish, French, Hebrew, Hungarian, Turkish, Czec, and Slovak.

over 50,000 migrants settled in West Berlin. Some came via the West German embassies in Warsaw, Prague or Budapest, or fled the country under other dubious and dangerous conditions. A larger number crossed the border after the fall of the Berlin Wall on November 9, 1989. The aim of our research program was to investigate the coping and adaptation processes of these migrants and the long-term effects (Mittag & Schwarzer, 1993; Schwarzer, Hahn, & Jerusalem, 1993). Readjustment after migration is probably reflected by emotional well-being and health. Thus, depression and physical symptoms were chosen as dependent variables measured at three points in time. The research focus was to examine the direct or moderating effect of self-efficacy on these variables. As a second resource factor, social integration was considered by making a distinction between those who had a partner and those who had not. As an additional stress factor, unemployment was considered.

Major Factors That Influence Readjustment

The decision to leave one's country and home has far-reaching and severe consequences. According to stress theory, this step can be considered as the onset of a non-normative critical life transition. As with other critical events (such as accidents, losses, divorce, or illness) the resultant psychological crisis may have a tremendous impact on personality development, psychosocial functioning, and well-being (Cohen, 1988; Johnson, 1986; Montada, Filipp, & Lerner, 1992). It is not only necessary to cope with daily hassles, especially crowded living conditions in camps or gyms, but also with the threat of long-term unemployment and the need to find or cultivate new social networks. Thus, the migrants are disadvantaged not only by higher demands than previously, but also by their heightened individual vulnerability to stress because they have to deal with the loss of their jobs and social support from former colleagues, friends, and relatives.

Since employment and social integration serve as protective resource factors in coping with stressful demands, a lack or impairment of these resources create personal vulnerabilities to the adverse effects of unfavorable environmental conditions. Employment provides income for one's living and the basis for being respected in a Western society characterized by high material and economical values. Thus, the impact of unemployment goes beyond direct economic costs. Lack or loss of job creates insecurity regarding one's future life perspective. Although unemployment can produce variable effects, studies generally report an impairment of psychological and physical well-being for the majority of the unemployed, especially those in long-term unemployment (Dooley & Catalano, 1988; Feather, 1990; Schwefel, Svensson, & Zöllner, 1987; Warr, 1987). The stressful quality of unemployment can be attributed mostly to a weakened ability to exercise control over one's life due to financial hardships or social network disruption, fewer aspirations, too much time without meaningful activities to break up the day, and reduced opportunities for social contacts. An enduring status of unemployment requires continuous adaptational efforts--instrumental actions to eliminate the jobless state as well as emotional coping to alleviate distressing experiences of unemployment (Lazarus, 1991). For migrants, unemployment following relocation appears to be a universal phenomenon hardly under personal control. Thus, problem-focused behaviors such as searching or qualifying for a job may be seen as being of limited value only. Instead, efforts are focused more on coping strategies for managing emotional states, particularly in the case of extended unemployment. Long-term psychological consequences of unemployment may be feelings of discouragement, hopelessness and despondancy as well as impairments of self-worth and somatic health. Kelvin and Jarrett (1985) argue that these adverse effects are exacerbated by social comparison processes because working people may perceive long-term unemployed persons as a negative reference group whose members cope inadequately with life.

Another major factor in the readjustment process is social integration, which refers to the mere number of social relationships, such as relatives, friends, and colleagues, and the frequency of contacts with them. A well-established social network is a structural prerequisite to feeling socially integrated and emotionally accepted (Duck, 1990; Lin, Dean, & Ensel, 1986; Sarason, Sarason, & Pierce, 1990; Schwarzer & Leppin, 1992; Veiel & Baumann, 1992). The most common and important source of support is an intimate partner with whom one shares one's dwelling and everyday life. Partnership can expand social networks and create stronger social embeddedness because two people usually have more social ties than one. Moreover, a stable partnership might produce higher confidence in the trustworthiness in the supportiveness of an intimate partner. Interpersonal commitments to support each other may also lead to an actual increase in the amount of help actually given when needed. For these reasons, partnership should make a difference when it comes to stress, emotions, and health. People living with an intimate partner should suffer less from distressing experiences than those who are alone and have no one to turn to in time of need.

Resource factors may influence psychological and physical well-being through different mechanisms. Self-efficacy, employment, and partner support, respectively, may each have either a general benign effect on well-being, or, may alleviate stress and its consequences. In the former case, resources have a main effect, whereas in the latter instance, resources serve as a buffer or moderator between stressful events and their consequences. Strong efficacy beliefs might buffer stress effects caused by unemployment or a lack of a close partner. Employment and partner support may have a positive long-term influence by strengthening perceived efficacy or at least alleviate some of the negative effects of a weak sense of efficacy. Resources can differ in psychological significance making perceived efficacy a dominant predictor and environmental conditions subordinate, or vice versa. Moreover, beneficial and detrimental effects may depend partly on gender since both the importance of employment and social support may differ for men and for women (Feather, 1990; Schwarzer & Leppin, 1992).

In accord with these theoretical considerations, the present research examines individual differences in adjustment as a function of perceived self-efficacy, employment status, and partner support. The question is to what degree these major factors influence depression and physical symptoms over time.

Study Design and Variables

In early November 1989, before the opening of the Berlin Wall, a longitudinal study was launched to gain better understanding of the adaptation processes of refugees and migrants from East Germany. The longitudinal study consisted of assessments at three points in time. The first wave took place from fall 1989 to winter 1990, data for the second wave were obtained in summer 1990, and the third wave assessment was conducted in summer 1991. The participants were East German migrants who left their country between August 1989, and February 1990. Complete data are available of a sample of 235 migrants. These 126 men and 109 women had a mean age of 31 and 32 years, respectively. Of the men, 63 were married or had a partner, and of the women 72.

Employment status was assessed at the three points in time by a single item on whether the person was employed or unemployed. Employment status was categorized in two groups: (a) jobless at all points in time, (b) jobless at the beginning but employed at Time 3, or always employed.

Based on a differentiated family status measure (married, single with or without partner, etc.) the participants were categorized into two partnership groups: migrants who had a partner at all points in time contrasted to migrants who were without a partner at all points in time.

Depression was measured by a 16-item German depression scale (Zerssen, 1976), with items such as "I feel miserable" or "I feel blue and downhearted". The correlations between anxiety and depression were .62, .71, and .67 at the three points in time, respectively.

Health complaints were assessed by 24 items referring to physical symptoms, such as exhaustion, heart and gastric complaints, and rheumatic pains (Brähler & Scheer, 1983).

Generalized self-efficacy was measured by a German 10-item self-efficacy scale (Jerusalem & Schwarzer, 1986). Sample items are "I always manage to solve difficult problems if I try hard enough," and "I remain calm when facing difficulties because I can rely on my coping abilities."

Results

Analyses of variance with repeated measures were computed to examine the effects of gender, self-efficacy, employment, and social integration on the dependent variables depression and health complaints. Women obtained higher mean levels in depression and health complaints than men, which is in line with the literature. Moreover, an interaction between sex and time emerged, with men's scores remaining at the same low level while women's scores declined significantly over the two-year period. The men were on average healthy, stable and optimistic, which was corroborated by narrative interviews and some other psychometric variables. They appraised the migration as a challenge, and had usually been the moving force in leaving adverse circumstances behind. In contrast, the women were more often pushed or drawn by others, e.g., they followed their spouses reluctantly to the West, and they experienced the migration as threatening and troubling. After a while, however, they adjusted to the novel situation, as reflected by the decline of their depression and illness levels, which dropped almost to those of the men.

In terms of the hypothesized determinants of readjustment, gender did not play a role. There were no interactions with self-efficacy, employment, or social integration. Therefore, gender is no longer considered in the following section. Figure 1 displays the effects of self-efficacy, employment, and time on depression.

There is a significant descent of depression over two years, which is due to changes in the women. There are also main effects of the two other factors. The highest levels of depression are obtained by those who are jobless and do not feel self-efficacious. The lowest levels are acquired by those who harbor optimistic self-beliefs and who have found a job. The other two groups are located at intermediate levels. There were no interactions.

In the next analysis, the employment factor was replaced by social integration. These step-by-step computations were done to secure sufficiently large cell sizes. A similar pattern of results emerged. Figure 2 displays the effects of self-efficacy, social integration, and time on depression.

Those who are not efficacious and who live alone show the highest levels of depression at all three points in time, whereas their counterparts show the opposite pattern. At Wave 3, there were also differences between the two intermediate groups, since socially integrated individuals feel quite well even if they are not considered to be self-efficacious. Having no partner appears to be worse than having low self-efficacy.

The next series of results aims at the prediction of health complaints. There were no time effects because the migrants did not change in their average reporting of symptoms. Figure 3 shows the effects of self-efficacy and employment on health complaints.

Being jobless and not believing in one's competence results in the highest reporting of physical symptoms. The least symptoms were accounted for those working and cultivating a sense of mastery. The two lines indicating unemployment are the two highest ones in the Figure reflecting that employment is the superior determinant of health complaints. This is also indicated by their higher F values in the analysis of variance.

Finally, the employment factor is replaced by the social integration factor. Figure 4 displays the effects of partnership and self-efficacy on health complaints.

The above pattern replicates well. Those with no partner and no sense of competence report the most frequent physical symptoms. Their counterparts show the opposite. Again, social integration is the superior factor in this analysis as can be seen by the location of the two intermediate groups.

Discussion: The Adaptive Role of Personal Efficacy and External Coping Resources

This research investigated the adaptation processes of East German migrants and refugees during a stressful life transition over two years after their move to the West as a reaction to the collapse of the communist system. A key issue concerned the role of a generalized sense of efficacy to exercise control over the new and stressful life conditions in this adaptational process. Social resources in the form of employment and close partnership were also considered to influence readjustment. High self-efficacious migrants perceived the demands in their new life probably more as challenges and less as threats or losses. They reported lower depression and fewer health complaints than low self-efficacious migrants. A firm sense of <u>personal efficacy</u> seems to reduce the likelihood of negative appraisals of stressful life demands, and, as a consequence, it provides protection against emotional distress and health conditions (Jerusalem, 1990a, 1990b, 1993).

With regard to environmental factors, <u>employment</u> status seems to play an important role in the process of psychological adaptation. Particularly migrants who remained jobless over two years felt more depressed and reported more health complaints than those who were employed. Thus, long-term unemployment represents a risk factor that increases vulnerability to stress. This adverse effect applies particularly to migrants since they have to start from scratch, secure means to earn their living, and become accepted within the new society. Employment is central to fulfilling these aims. To be without a job means to remain an outsider. <u>Partnership</u> is a social factor that accounted also for interindividual differences in readjustment. Migrants who had an intimate partner reported less depression and physical symptoms than those who lived alone.

Considering all three predictors simultaneously deepens our understanding of the psychological dynamics. Not only were different risk groups of migrants identified, but developmental trends and mutual buffer mechanisms also become evident. When ranking the subgroups according to their appraisals of stressors, the most unfavorable adjustment at all points in time was found for low self-efficacious subjects who had no partner or were unemployed. In contrast to the conspicuous vulnerability of this high-risk group, migrants characterized by multiple strong resources, i.e., those with high perceived self-efficacy, a job and a partner, benefitted substantially from their resources. The remaining groups characterized by different patterns of resources experienced intermediate levels of stress and impairment of well-being.

The empirical findings are in accord with the theoretical expectations. However, certain limitations of this research should be acknowledged. Assessment of health status relied on subjective reports.

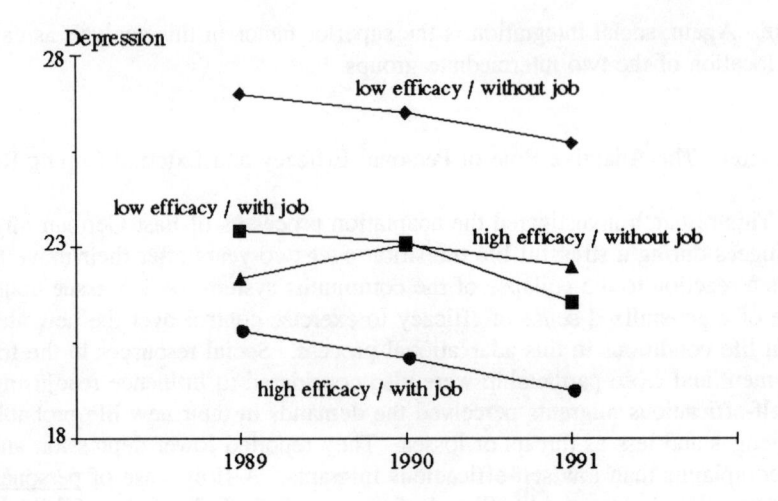

Figure 1. Effects of self-efficacy, employment, and time on depression

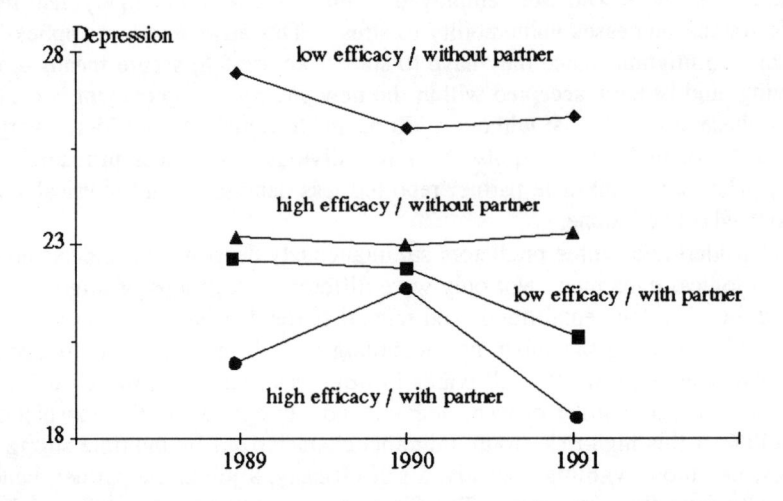

Figure 2. Effects of self-efficacy, social integration, and time on depression

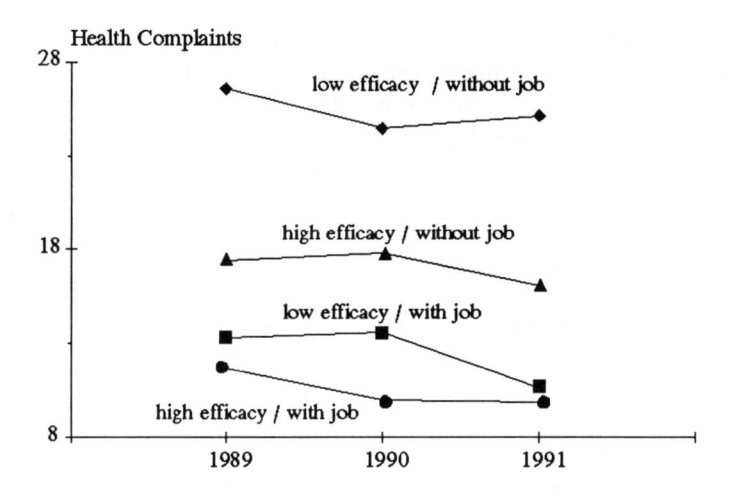

Figure 3. Effects of self-efficacy and employment on health complaints

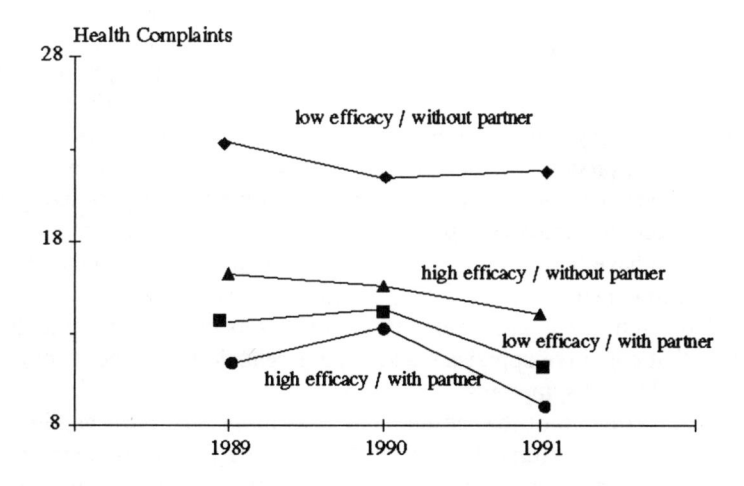

Figure 4. Effects of self-efficacy and social integration on health complaints

Also, the design implicitly assumes a causal influence of environmental constraints on adjustment. Although this direction is highly reasonable, it cannot be ruled out that the causality operates in the opposite direction. For example, feeling depressed or sick can be a justification for not searching for a job, or can be a reason for not being hired. On the other hand, healthy and psychologically stable individuals usually have a better chance of finding a job and of staying employed. Employment was assessed only as a dichotomous variable that does not consider job quality, job satisfaction, contract conditions, and other conditions of work. In the case of partnership, its psychological relevance might become more evident if indicators such as perceived and received social support, its subjective evaluation, size of the social network, and the qualitative character of social relationships or social support were considered as well. The measure of generalized self-efficacy taps a broad concept of optimism and perceived overall coping competence (Schwarzer, 1994). It would have been interesting to assess in addition situation-specific self-efficacies to cope with a variety of particular demands that arise typically after migration.

Another theoretical issue lies in the causal chain that leads from coping antecedents, to cognitive stress appraisal, coping, emotions, and health. Conceptual problems arise when coping is being separated from coping resources such as hardiness, dispositional optimism, self-efficacy, sense of coherence, social support, etc. Resources can be personal, social or other antecedents of appraisals and coping. An optimistic attitude towards life may result in a less disastrous appraisal of a taxing situation, in the adoption of an efficient problem-solving strategy, or in the creation of optimistic coping self-talk; the existence of a social network may result in successful support seeking behaviors when a situation of need arises. Although in reality coping resources and actual coping may be difficult to disentangle, it is important to make this distinction in theory and research. Resources are relatively stable antecedents, whereas coping is a process that depends on these resources. If, for example, an optimistic statement is made by a coper, it may mainly reflect a personality trait, or it may have just been generated as a product of effortful stress management. In the present study, we have not observed actual coping behaviors or thoughts, but were limited to the assessment of stable coping resources. Thus, there is a missing link in the causal chain from these antecedents to the indicators of readjustment. It is our interpretation that cognitive appraisals and coping behaviors resulted in more or less depression and physical symptoms.

The major strength of the present study lies in its ecological validity in assessing adaptation in a natural life setting longitudinally. It also is the only available panel study of psychological changes in East German migrants. It is necessary, however, to take into account some peculiarities of the East Germans observed here which make their psychosocial situation quite different from that of migrants in other cultural settings. With regard to West Germans, East German immigrants have the same language, cultural heritage, and perhaps even close relatives. Compared with this, migration presents more formidable problems to migrants who confront barriers of language, cultural patterns, ethnic differences and hostility as intruders. It certainly requires a very resistant sense of efficacy to surmount these multiple barriers. For that reason, the generalizability of the findings needs to be examined with other ethnic groups of refugees adapting to different cultures. Since we have chosen three basic resources we believe that their effects would be prevalent in all kinds of adaptation processes, even beyond those of migration.

References

Abramson, L. Y., Seligman, M. E. P., & Teasdale, J. (1978). Learned helplessness in humans: Critique and reformulation. Journal of Abnormal Psychology, 87, 49-74.

Alloy, L. B., & Abramson, L. Y. (1988). Depressive realism: Four theoretical perspectives. In L. B. Alloy (Ed.), Cognitive processes in depression (pp. 223-265). New York: Guilford.

Bandura, A. (1977). Social learning theory. Englewood Cliffs, NJ: Prentice Hall.

Bandura, A. (1986). Social foundations of thought and action. Englewood Cliffs, NJ: Prentice Hall.

Bandura, A. (1992). Exercise of personal agency through the self-efficacy mechanism. In R. Schwarzer (Ed.), Self-efficacy: Thought control of action (pp. 3-38). Washington, DC: Hemisphere.

Bandura, A. (1994). Self-efficacy. The exercise of control. New York: Freeman.

Brähler, E., & Scheer, J. (1983). Gießener Beschwerdebogen (GBB) [Health Complaints Rating Scale]. Bern, Switzerland: Huber.

Carver, C. S., Pozo, C., Harris, S. D., Noriega, V., Scheier, M. F., Robinson, D. S., Ketcham, A. S., Moffat, F. L., & Clark, K. C. (1993). How coping mediates the effect of optimism on distress: A study of women with early stage breast cancer. Journal of Personality and Social Psychology, 65 (2), 375-390.

Carver, C. S., & Scheier, M. F. (1981). Attention and self-regulation: A control-theory approach to human behavior. New York: Springer.

Cohen, L. (Ed.). (1988). Life events and psychological functioning. Theoretical and methodological issues. London: Sage.

Dooley, C. D., & Catalano, R. A. (Eds.). (1988). Recent research on the psychological effects of unemployment. Journal of Social Issues, 44 (4), 1-12.

Duck, S. (Ed.). (1990). Personal relationships and social support. London: Sage.

Feather, N. T. (1990). The psychological impact of unemployment. New York: Springer.

Hobfoll, S. E. (1988). The ecology of stress. Washington, DC: Hemisphere.

Hobfoll, S. E. (1989). Conservation of resources: A new attempt at conceptualizing stress. American Psychologist, 44 (3), 513-524.

Jerusalem, M. (1990a). Persönliche Ressourcen, Vulnerabilität und Streßerleben [Personal resources, vulnerability, and stress experience]. Göttingen, Germany: Hogrefe.

Jerusalem, M. (1990b). Temporal patterns of stress appraisals for high- and low-anxious individuals. Anxiety Research. An International Journal, 3, 113-129.

Jerusalem, M. (1993). Personal resources, environmental constraints, and adaptational processes: The predictive power of a theoretical stress model. Personality and Individual Differences, 14, 15-24.

Jerusalem, M., & Schwarzer, R. (1986). Selbstwirksamkeit [Self-Efficacy-Scale]. In R. Schwarzer (Ed.), Skalen zur Befindlichkeit und Persönlichkeit (pp. 15-28). Berlin, Germany: Freie Universität Berlin, Institut für Psychologie.

Jerusalem, M., & Schwarzer, R. (1992). Self-efficacy as a resource factor in stress appraisal processes. In R. Schwarzer (Ed.), Self-efficacy: Thought control of action (pp. 195-213). Washington, DC: Hemisphere.

Johnson, J. H. (1986). Life events as stressors in childhood and adolescence. Beverly Hills, CA: Sage.

Kamen-Siegel, L., Rodin, J., Seligman, M. P. E., & Dwyer, J. (1991). Explanatory style and cell-mediated immunity in elderly men and women. Health Psychology, 10, 229-235.

Kelvin, P., & Jarrett, J. E. (1985). Unemployment: Its social psychological effects. Cambridge: Cambridge University Press.

Lazarus, R. S. (1991). Emotion and adaptation. London: Oxford University Press.

Lin, N., Dean, A., & Ensel, W. (Eds.). (1986). Social support, life events, and depression. New York: Academic Press.

Litt, M. D., Tennen, H., Affleck, G., & Klock, S. (1992). Coping and cognitive factors in adaptation to in vitro fertilization failure. Journal of Behavioral Medicine, 15, 171-188.

Locke, E. A., & Latham, G. P. (1990). A theory of goal setting and task performance. Englewood Cliffs, NJ: Prentice Hall.

Mittag, W., & Schwarzer, R. (1993). Interaction of employment status and self-efficacy on alcohol consumption: A two-wave study on stressful life transitions. Psychology and Health, 8, 77-87.

Montada, L., Filipp, S.-H., & Lerner, M. J. (Eds.). (1992). Life crises and experiences of loss in adulthood. Hillsdale, NJ: Erlbaum.

Peterson, C., & Bossio, L. M. (1991). Health and optimism. New research on the relationship between positive thinking and well-being. New York: The Free Press.

Peterson, C., & Seligman, M. E. P. (1984). Causal explanations as a risk factor for depression: Theory and evidence. Psychological Review, 91, 347-374.

Peterson, C., & Seligman, M. E. P. (1987). Explanatory style and illness. Journal of Personality, 55, 237-265.

Sarason, B. R., Sarason, I. G., & Pierce, G. R. (Eds.). (1990). Social support: An interactional view. New York: Wiley.

Scheier, M. F., & Carver, C. S. (1985). Optimism, coping, and health: Assessment and implications of generalized outcome expectancies. Health Psychology, 4, 219-247.

Scheier, M. F., & Carver, C. S. (1987). Dispositional optimism and physical well-being: The influence of generalized outcome expectancies on health. Journal of Personality, 55, 169-210.

Scheier, M. F., & Carver, C. S. (1992). Effects of optimism on psychological and physical well-being: Theoretical overview and empirical update. Cognitive Therapy and Research, 16, 201-228.

Scheier, M. F., Matthews, K. A., Owens, J., Magovern, G. J. Sr., Lefebre, R. C., Abbott, R. A., & Carver, C. S. (1989). Dispositional optimism and recovery from coronary artery bypass surgery: The beneficial effects on physical and psychological well-being. Journal of Personality and Social Psychology, 57, 1024-1040.

Schwarzer, R. (1993). Measurement of perceived self-efficacy: Psychometric scales for cross-cultural research. Berlin, Germany: Freie Universität Berlin, Institut für Psychologie.

Schwarzer, R. (1994). Optimism, vulnerability, and self-beliefs as health-related cognitions: A systematic overview. Psychology and Health, 9, 161-180.

Schwarzer, R., Hahn, A., & Jerusalem, M. (1993). Negative affect in East German migrants: Longitudinal effects of unemployment and social support. Anxiety, Stress, and Coping: An International Journal, 6, 57-69.

Schwarzer, R., & Leppin, A. (1992). Social support and mental health: A conceptual and empirical overview. In L. Montada, S.-H. Filipp & M. J. Lerner (Eds.), Life crises and experiences of loss in adulthood (pp. 435-458). Hillsdale, NJ: Erlbaum.

Schwefel, D., Svensson, P. G., & Zöllner, H. (Eds.). (1987). Unemployment, social vulnerability, and health in Europe. Berlin, Germany: Springer.

Seligman, M. E. P. (1991). Learned optimism. New York: Knopf.

Sherer, M., & Maddux, J. E. (1982). The Self-Efficacy Scale: Construction and validation. Psychological Reports, 51, 663-671.

Skinner, E. (1992). Perceived control: Motivation, coping, and development. In R. Schwarzer (Ed.), Self-efficacy: Thought control of action (pp. 91-106). Washington, DC: Hemisphere.

Skinner, E. A., Chapman, M., & Baltes, P. (1988). Control, means-ends, and agency beliefs: A new conceptualization and its measurement during childhood. Journal of Personality and Social Psychology, 54, 117-133.

Smith, C. A., Dobbins, C., & Wallston, K. A. (1991). The mediational role of perceived competence in adaptation to rheumatoid arthritis. Journal of Applied Social Psychology, 21, 1218-1247.

Smith, C. A., & Wallston, K. A. (1992). Adaptation in patients with chronic rheumatoid arthritis: Application of a general model. Health Psychology, 11, 151-162.

Snyder, C. R., Harris, C., Anderson, J. R., Holleran, S. A., Irving, L. M., Sigmon, S. T., Yoshinobu, L., Gibb, J., Langelle, C., & Harney, P. (1991). The will and the ways: Development and validation of an individual-differences measure of hope. Journal of Personality and Social Psychology, 60, 570-585.

Sweeney, P. D., Anderson, K., & Bailey, S. (1986). Attributional style in depression: A meta-analytic review. Journal of Personality and Social Psychology, 50, 974-991.

Veiel, H. O. F., & Baumann, U. (1992). The many meanings of social support. In H. O. F. Veiel & U. Baumann (Eds.), The meaning and measurement of social support (pp. 1-9). Washington, DC: Hemisphere.

Wallston, K. A. (1989). Assessment of control in health-care settings. In A. Steptoe & A. Appels (Eds.), Stress, personal control, and health (pp. 85-105). Chicester,UK: Wiley.

Wallston, K. A. (1992). Hocus-pocus, the focus isn't strictly on locus: Rotter's social learning theory modified for health. Cognitive Therapy and Research, 16, 183-199.

Warr, P. (1987). Work, unemployment, and mental health. Oxford: Clarendon.

Zerssen, D. V. (1976). Depressivitäts-Skala [Depression scale]. Weinheim, Germany: Beltz Test.

STRESS AND SOCIAL SUPPORT

Irwin G. Sarason and Barbara R. Sarason
University of Washington
Seattle, Washington USA
Gregory R. Pierce
Hamilton College
Clinton, New York USA

Although there are differences in how stress is conceptualized, there is agreement that challenge and threat, key features of community cataclysms, are among its most active ingredients. A major task for stress researchers is identifying pertinent individual difference variables regarding how people respond to particular types of challenge and threat. Another major task for stress researchers concerns the development of intervention programs that increase the likelihood of personal effectiveness under challenging circumstances. One intriguing finding of stress research is that, whereas some people seem to deteriorate rapidly under stress, others show only minimal or moderate deterioration; still others seem unaffected. Stress can be a catastrophe, but it can also be an opportunity for personal growth. It brings forth coping efforts that vary in effectiveness.

Social support, either elicited or provided spontaneously, can play an important role in how people deal with challenges and threats. This chapter reviews research and theory concerning the role social support plays in preparing for and coping with stress. It considers how supportive interventions might promote adaptive coping when communities face widespread stress as, for example, when a natural disaster occurs.

The Social Support Concept

Research on social support has focused attention on three topics: (1) the idea that differences in interpersonal connectedness influence how people respond to various types of situations; (2) identification of supportive components of the environment; and (3) the individual's sense of being supported. This research has three aspects. The first concerns assessing social support and relating it to significant clinical and adjustment outcomes; the second concerns the relationship of assessed social support to behavior and cognitions in social interactions; and the third has to do with the relative contributions to a variety of outcomes of both global and relationship-specific support (B. Sarason, Pierce, & Sarason, 1990). Global perceptions of the forthcomingness of the social environment and perceptions of the supportiveness of particular relationships are not the same thing and each may play distinct and important roles in adjustment and health. While over the years, writers have described both these types of perceptions, they have rarely been compared. We will provide a thumbnail sketch of current work on conceptualizations and operationalizations of social support with special attention to how social support functions, the distinction between the perception of social support availability and the actual receipt of support, and the types of interpersonal relationships that provide support.

Social Networks

Definitions of social support that emphasize interpersonal connectedness have led to inquiries concerning the structure of individuals' social networks, for example, their size and correlates. Network analysts often base their studies on the assumption that structural features of a social network (for example, the density or interconnectedness of network members) influence the impact that social interactions have on network members. This approach calls attention to differences in the patterns of social interaction characterizing different support networks. Measures of network size and availability or adequacy of support have been shown to be only weakly associated (Seeman & Berkman, 1988). This may be because neither the size of the network nor the size of the group of network members to whom the person feels close can indicate how much support he or she actually receives. In general, the evidence of network measures' usefulness in studying the relationship between dependent measures (e.g., health) and social support has not been impressive compared with the more easily administered measures of social support that simply ask for the number of relationships (House & Kahn, 1985).

The Functions of Support

Researchers who are especially concerned with how social support functions have sought to specify those aspects of social support that are beneficial to individuals in specific types of stressful events. This approach was stimulated by Weiss's (1974) hypothesis that there are six specific provisions of social relationships: attachment, social integration, opportunity for nurturance, reassurance of worth, sense of reliable alliance, and guidance. Cohen and Wills (1985) have theorized that the buffering effect of social support, which serves to insulate or partially protect those who are vulnerable to the effects of stress, is a function of the match between the particular need engendered by the stressor and the type of support given. A problem with existing instruments measuring specific functions of support is that the scales representing the different functions tend to be highly correlated. The intercorrelations often are as high as the scale reliabilities. This suggests that the scales are not measuring distinct constructs. For this reason, some researchers have expressed dissatisfaction with the functional approach as it is currently operationalized.

Received and Perceived Support

An important question concerns the relative contributions to adjustment of support received and support perceived to be available. Typically, information on support received from others is gathered from the self-report of the recipient with the focus on the recipient's account of what he or she regarded as helpful. In using this information it is important to note that the agreement between givers and recipients on the support given often is only moderate (50-60%) (Antonucci & Israel, 1986; Shulman, 1976). It would probably be a mistake, however, to view this finding as an indication simply of a lack of validity regarding received support measures. Instead, this result underscores the need to consider both the evaluative aspects of social support (that is, how recipients evaluate supportive efforts) and the objective features of supportive transactions.

The finding that a recipient's evaluation of supportive activity does not necessarily match reports by others suggests that an individual's report of social support reflects at least two elements: objective properties of supportive interactions and the respondent's interpretation of the interactions. The importance of the subjective side of social support is reflected in the consistent finding that it is the perception of social support that is most closely related to adjustment and health outcomes (Antonucci & Israel, 1986; Blazer, 1982; Sandler & Barrera, 1984; Wethington & Kessler, 1986). A focus on perceived social support meshes with and is reinforced by the current emphasis in psychology on cognitive appraisal and the influence over behavior of cognitive schemata. It also fits well with the early conceptualizations of social support by Cobb (1976) and Cassel (1976). Cobb hypothesized that social support's major role is to convey information to the individual that others care about and value him or her. Thus, the support emanates not so much from what is done but from what that indicates to the recipient about the relationship. In a similar vein, Cassel argued that conveying caring and positive regard to the recipient is more responsible for positive outcomes than is any specific behavior. Evidence concerning the importance of perceptions of support suggests the need to consider both the intrapersonal and the interpersonal contexts in which supportive provisions become available (I. Sarason, Pierce, & Sarason, 1990). The intrapersonal context emphasizes personal perceptions of social relationships. Internal cognitive representations of self, important others, and the nature of interpersonal relationships influence perceptions of social support. The interpersonal context refers to the transactional quality of relationships (for example, to what degree they are marked by conflict). Perceived support instruments usually inquire about the adequacy and availability of support. They tend to be only moderately intercorrelated, but the correlations are higher than those for measures based on other definitions, such as, those that derive from the network or received support concepts.

Global and Relationship-Specific Perceptions of Support

Research on social support suggests that people have a set of general expectations and attributions about their personal relationships that reflect their ideas about how approachable and forthcoming people within the social environment are likely to be. This aggregate is what measures of perceived social support seem to be tapping. They may be assessing people's beliefs about whether others, in general, are likely to provide assistance and emotional support when needed (B. Sarason, Shearin, Pierce, & Sarason, 1987).

Person-specific expectations and attributions are not necessarily just instances of general or global perceptions of available support. In addition to these generalized beliefs concerning social support, people also develop expectations and attributions about the availability of support in specific significant relationships. For example, a person who generally sees the social environment as far from benign and forthcoming, might still have some specific relationships marked by warmth, caring, and reciprocity. While general and relationship-specific expectations for social support may be correlated, they reflect different facets of perceived support. Global and relationship-based perceptions of support each probably play an important and unique role in personal adjustment. Pierce, Sarason, and Sarason (1991) investigated this issue by relating measures of both global and relationship-based expectations to personal adjustment. They found that perceptions of available support from specific relationships added to the prediction of loneliness after accounting for the contribution made by global perceived available support and concluded that an independent link exists between relationship-specific perceptions of available support and loneliness (Pierce et al., 1991). We need to know more about this type of linkage. Research is needed to explore the processes involved in shaping the distinctiveness of support associated with specific interpersonal relationships, and also the mechanisms by which both aspects of perceived support (global and relationship-specific) relate to outcomes. Global perceptions and relationship-based perceptions of support might impact personal adjustment through quite different pathways. If so, theories of social support will be needed to encompass these pathways.

Other aspects of personal relationships, besides the support they provide, probably play important roles in influencing outcomes. A feature of the Quality of Relationships Inventory, the relationship-specific measure employed by Pierce, Sarason, and Sarason (in press), is its assessment of perceived conflict, as well as support, in individual relationships. The fact that a relationship is supportive does not mean that it is without conflict. B. Sarason, Pierce, Bannerman, and Sarason (1993) investigated how parents' assessments of their children's positive and negative characteristics are related to each child's global and relationship-specific perceptions of social support and found that family environments can be conceptualized in terms of specific relationships within the family that differ with regard to support and conflict. They showed that, while mothers whose children saw their relationships as either conflictual or not conflictual were equally likely to help their children, fathers with whom children perceived conflict were less likely to be helpful. Generally, parents' descriptions of their children's positive and negative characteristics were more strongly related to their children's perceptions of the supportiveness of their parental relationships than to the children's general perceptions of the supportiveness of the social network of their peers.

An Interactional-Cognitive View of Social Support

The various approaches that have been taken in social support research can seem puzzling. They often focus attention on promising but different, aspects of the social support equation. Problems can arise when the available findings are lumped together without regard for the methodology employed. When this happens the literature can appear to be inconsistent and even contradictory. Differences in the operationalization and assessment strategies associated with each approach limit the generalizability of research findings. For example, as we have seen, an important difference in assessment strategies concerns whether instruments focus on objective events (what actually happened) or subjective evaluations of supportiveness (e.g., perceptions of others' willingness to help).

While there are many methodological questions that surround social support, its assessment, pertinent interventions, and validation procedures, it is important to focus attention on questions related to the nature of support, factors that pertain to it, and the support process. We recently developed a model that emphasizes the interactive roles of the situational, intrapersonal and interpersonal contexts of social transactions (I. Sarason et al., 1990). The situational context encompasses the event to which relationship participants are responding. The event could range from minor to major and from simple to complex--a bruise from a minor fall, a disappointing academic grade, the breakup of a romantic relationship, the loss of a job, and the death of a loved one are only a few illustrations. Many of these events involve a complex of pertinent considerations. For example, losing a job is likely to involve how much money is in the bank account of the person who loses a job; whether the job loss resulted from poor performance, product phase-out, or company move; and the current state of the job market. The aspect of the situational context that has received most attention concerns whether or not situations are stressful, However, a broader perspective of situations might be productive.

The intrapersonal context refers to the individual's unique, stable patterns of perceiving self, important others, and relational expectations. Bowlby's (1988) attachment theory has influenced studies of the intrapersonal context of social support because of its emphasis on the role of working or cognitive models in the formation of an individual's expectations, appraisals, and responses to the potentially supportive behavior of others, and the provision of support to others (B. Sarason et al., 1990). Working models are cognitive representations of self, important others, and the nature of relationships that are linked to self-esteem, feelings of self-worth, and perceptions of being loved, valued, and cared for by others. Working models of others and of relationships with them lead to distinctive types of expectations and interpretations of others' behavior that interact with situational and social processes. Research using the Social Support Questionnaire and other perceived social support measures has shown that attributions and expectations concerning the global availability of social support reflect a stable personality characteristic, the sense of support (B. Sarason et al., 1990). The sense of support is linked to an additional feature of personality, the sense of acceptance that grows out of inferences about the self that are related to, but not necessarily implied in, the sense of support (B. Sarason et al., 1990; I. Sarason, Pierce, & Sarason, 1990). The sense of acceptance is the belief that others love and care for us and that they accept us for what we are, including our best and worst points. It is strengthened when we observe the support that others willingly provide to us along with their unconditional acceptance. The sense of acceptance may be part of a coherent personality constellation that includes a positive self-image, a favorable view of social relationships and an expectation that others value us as we are. People who are confident that others will meet their needs for support may be able to undertake challenging tasks without excessive preoccupation about failure because they anticipate sufficient support and resources to meet potential demands.

The interpersonal context not only includes the distinctive qualitative and quantitative (e.g., support, conflict, network size, density) features of specific relationships but also those of the larger social networks in which these relationships takes place. There are several features of relationships that in all likelihood strongly influence the impact of social support on health and well-being. These include interpersonal conflict, the sensitivity with which one participant responds to the support needs of the other participant, and the structure of their interpersonal connections. Cohen and Lichtenstein (1990) recently showed that the context of a close relationship mediates the impact of specific supportive or nonsupportive behaviors. Accumulating evidence indicates that the impact of social support is influenced (reduced) strongly by the presence of interpersonal conflict (Coyne & DeLongis, 1986; Zavislak & Sarason, 1991). Support received in the context of conflictual relationships may lead to feelings of indebtedness and ambivalence in the recipient that increase rather than decrease stress (Pierce, Sarason, & Sarason, 1990). Another aspect of the interpersonal context is the extent to which a support provider is aware of and sensitive to the needs of the recipient.

Supportive efforts are successful under certain conditions but not necessarily others and these conditions interact with the nature of the relationship between the provider and recipient. For example, Dakof and Taylor (1990) found that the effectiveness of a supportive intervention depends upon its context, with particular actions being perceived to be helpful from some but not other network members. Dakof and Taylor suggested that future investigations of social support might benefit from identifying the source as well as the type of support. Simons, Lorenz, Wu, and Conger (1993) found that spouse support is a more powerful determinant of quality of parenting when social network support is low. Bristol, Gallagher, and Schopler (1988) also found that spousal support plays an important role in quality of parenting. The recipient, the provider, and their relationship, need to be studied in an effort to better understand the give and take of social support processes.

The effect of support given to individuals varies as a function of the providers and recipients' histories of reciprocal supportive relationships. The study by B. Sarason et al. (1993) mentioned earlier investigated how parents' assessments of their children's positive and negative characteristics are related to each child's generalized and relationship-specific perceptions of social support and the status of the parent-child relationship. The results of this study were consistent with an interactional view of social support according to which characteristics of both the recipient and support provider are important determinants of perceptions of social support and outcome measures. The family environment would appear to be a productive setting in which to study the support process. While general family environmental factors play important roles in perceptions of support availability, specific family relationships make significant contributions (Gurung, Sarason, Keeker, & Sarason, 1992). For some types of questions, relationship-specific measures of social support might be better predictors than measures of general perceived support.

We see great potential in a broadened theoretical perspective of social support that includes life-long units like the family. Such a perspective calls for attention to, not only contemporaneous interactional processes, but also their origins and development. As Newcomb (1990) has pointed out, social support is a personal resource that evolves throughout life. He argues for abandonment of the conception of social support as a unidirectional provision of resources from the external social environment to the individual.

Social Support and Coping

Whether experienced at a personal and idiosyncratic or a community-wide level, stress calls forth efforts to reach an acceptable or satisfying resolution to the problem that created the stress. Coping refers to how people deal with difficulties in an attempt to overcome them. It is a complex process that involves personality characteristics, personal relationships, and situational parameters. Discussions of coping often take as their starting point the time at which a specified event occurs. Lazarus' model of coping, with its emphasis on primary and secondary appraisals, falls into this category (Lazarus, 1991). Temporality also plays a role in the buffering hypothesis according to which social support is beneficial primarily at the time individuals are coping with stress (Cohen & Wills, 1985). However, putting the focus on events when they happen ignores the role that various factors play in whether unwanted life events to which an individual must respond actually occur. Researchers have devoted little attention to the question of why some individuals experience certain types of difficulties while others do not (see Bandura, 1986, for an exception).

Both social relationships and personality characteristics play a role in the way individuals construct their environments. Life events are not randomly assigned to individuals, and people--and their social networks--play important roles in how they experience and respond to stressful life events.

Perceived social support influences coping through appraisal of situations and the personal characteristics of the important actors in them. B. Sarason, Pierce, Shearin, Sarason, Waltz, and Poppe (1991) found that individuals high in perceived social support were more accurate in estimating the personal characteristics of their peers than were others. They also found that high perceived support subjects attribute to themselves more positive and less negative attributes than do other subjects and that these attributions are positively related to their parents' and peers' perceptions of them. Perceived social support may foster more accurate and more positive appraisals of self and others and this, in turn, may enable individuals to develop more effective and realistic coping strategies for dealing with particular situations.

Besides strengthening appraisals of personal resources and exploratory behavior, perceived social support may also enable individuals to confront challenges more effectively because they believe others will help them if the challenge exceeds their personal resources. In one study, subjects high in perceived social support experienced fewer distracting cognitions while completing intellective tasks, and correctly solved more problems, than did other subjects (I. Sarason & Sarason, 1986). Other research suggests that individuals who perceive themselves as having good support are more interpersonally effective than others (e.g., they are better able to assume a leadership role and more considerate in their interactions with others) (I. Sarason, Sarason, & Shearin, 1986). Thus, perceived social support may serve to promote self-confidence and personal effectiveness that enhances the individual's coping repertoire.

Interactions with others are based in part on expectations about how those others will respond. While high perceived support individuals approach others for support based on their expectation that others are likely to provide help, those low in perceived social support may avoid asking others for assistance because they fear it will not be provided. One reason for this difference may be that high perceived support individuals have higher self-esteem, feel they are valued by others, and therefore are less concerned about how others might perceive them should they need to request assistance (Hobfoll & Freedy, 1990). Other evidence supporting this idea comes from an experimental study of social support in which subjects interacted with a confederate trained to provide one of two types of social support to subjects who were preparing to give a speech (Pierce & Contey, 1992). Despite the extensive training given to confederates (who were blind to subjects' level of perceived social support), when randomly assigned to subjects low in perceived social support, confederates provided fewer acts of emotional (e.g., positive feedback) or instrumental (i.e., advice) support than they did to subjects high in perceived social support. People high in perceived social support may provide potential support providers with more opportunities to administer support. Perceived social support influences coping in three ways. It could lead individuals to (a) structure situations so that stressful life events are relatively unlikely to occur, (b) develop effective personal coping skills, and (c) seek and obtain assistance when it is needed.

Supportive Relationships

While people have relatively well-formed expectations and attributions about available support in general, they also have specific expectations about the availability of support from particular significant people in their lives. Evidence reported by Pierce et al. (1990) and I. Sarason et al. (1990) suggests that relationship-specific cognitions are not simply the building blocks for general perceptions of available support. While a person's global and relationship-specific expectations for social support may be related, they reflect different aspects of perceived support and each may play an important and unique role in coping and well-being. Perceived support grows out of a history of supportive experiences, especially with family members (e.g., parents). The general expectations one has about the forthcomingness of others, in turn, influence whether and how an individual approaches others to form new potentially supportive relationships. Perceived social support, as a working model of relationships, may be especially influential in the formative stages of a relationship before individuals have developed clear ideas about how they would like their relationship partner, as opposed to others in general, to respond in particular situations. As a relationship progresses and relationship-specific expectations develop, each person's global expectations may become less influential in the relationship.

It is also possible for expectations developed within a specific relationship to influence general perceptions of social support. For example, one of the goals of psychotherapy is to provide the client with an interpersonal context in which to revise general working models regarding the nature of personal relationships. By developing a therapeutic alliance, the client and therapist are able to interact so as to help the client create healthier, more positive views of relationships. This work is often made possible by analysis of the transference relationship which results in the client's revision of previously established working models of personal relationships.

Support can play a role, not only in coping with events once they have occurred, but also avoiding or preventing the occurrence of stressful events. More attention needs to be paid to preventative coping, coping that reduces the likelihood of occurrence of unwanted, undesirable events. Social support can influence coping either by (a) rendering an individual less vulnerable to experiencing a specific life event or (b) facilitating coping before a situation reaches a maximum point of stressfulness. This could happen as a product of a process that begins with perceptions of support that leads to a problem-solving orientation and willingness to explore the environment and culminates in an enhanced coping repertoire. This view of social support and coping meshes with Bowlby's (1988) theory of attachment according to which a secure attachment enhances a child's exploratory behavior from which coping skills develop. These skills, in turn, enhance feelings of personal effectiveness or self-efficacy.

What Social Support Provides

As mentioned earlier, the term social support has been an umbrella term that covers a variety of diverse phenomena. A large percentage of research studies on the topic deal with associations between assessed support and particular aspects of life, including health status, illness, recovery from illness, adjustment and psychological functioning, and performance. A review of this research leads to the confident conclusion that social support is a good thing to have. People with satisfying levels of support seem to cope better with stress, are healthier and recover from illness more quickly, are better adjusted, and perform better--especially in the domains of social interaction and interpersonal social skills. Thus, perceived social support functions in many ways as an individual difference variable. It remains stable over time, even during periods of developmental transition (I. Sarason et al. 1986).

If it is a good thing to have and if it inheres within the individual, what is it that is doing the inhering? We think it is a set of working models of one's self, the social forthcomingess of others, and relationships with particular people. These working models lead a person to conclusions about the degree to which he or she is valued--not for surface characteristics, such as mathematics ability, but as someone who is worthy of being loved, valued and unconditionally accepted. This conclusion influences (1) the development of current relationships with others, (2) the acquisition of feelings of self-efficacy that are both generalized and related to specific tasks, (3) the perceived availability of social support, and (4) effectiveness in stress-coping and the ability to maintain a task focus.

Providing Support

Much research on social support has been directed toward two topics: social support as a stress moderator and the assessment of social support. If the lack of social support is a factor in negative health and adjustment outcomes, more needs to be known about how support is, or can be, provided in an effective manner. Surprisingly, the topic of the provision of social support (how it is provided, by whom, and under what circumstances) has been barely touched on. The provision of support has been widely discussed in terms of its role in personal development, clinical processes, and behavior observed in laboratory settings; however, we need much more empirical information about support provision in everyday life. What types of support are most helpful? Do some have negative side effects? Is the outcome of support the same for all people? Should interventions be directed mainly at high-risk groups? More knowledge is also needed about how to help individuals raise their own overall support level, as well as how they might obtain support in particular types of situations.

All of these questions lend themselves to inquiry within the laboratory and in field studies. Supportive interventions exist for a variety of problems including bereavement in adults and children, divorce, cancer, and unemployment (Gottlieb, 1988). Lehman, Ellard, and Wortman (1986) investigated the impact on bereaved individuals of the kinds of supportive comments offered to them by friends after bereavement. Gottlieb (1985) studied the effective elements of group interventions on children of divorcing parents and the effects of supportive involvements on both members of adult-child/elderly-dependent-parent duos. I.G. Sarason (1981) found that social support positively influenced subjects' performance in an evaluative situation. Heller and his coworkers (Heller, 1979; Heller & Swindle, 1983; Procidano & Heller, 1983) investigated the effects of the presence of others, either intimates or strangers, on performance in stressful laboratory situations in which overall support was analyzed as an individual difference variable.

When the social support concept first became of interest, its preventative or curative potentials were recognized. Support can be provided at various levels ranging from the community, as a stabilizing force in a troubled individual's life, to the empathy a loved-one feels and expresses toward someone facing real or imagined difficulties. Rather than sapping self-reliance, strong ties with others--particularly family members--seem to encourage it. Reliance on others and self-reliance are not only compatible but complementary to one another. While many examples could be given of social support's role as a buffer against stress, how to communicate support in a way that does not unduly tax the communicator and nurturer needs to be better understood. Lehman et al's. (1986) findings concerning the counter-productive effects of friends' "supportive" utterances to bereaved parents underlines the importance of this need, as do studies in the area of chronic illness. For example, Coyne and DeLongis (1986) found that inappropriate, poorly-timed or over-solicitous support from the spouse may prove to be quite stressful for chronically ill patients. Revenson and Majerovitz (1990) studied supportive interactions between rheumatoid arthritis patients and their spouses and found that, while spouses are important sources of support for the patients, the amount and quality of extra-familial support available to the spouses influenced how supportive they were able to be toward the patients.

It is important to analyze the experience or situation concerning which an individual needs support. For example, Jacobson (1990) analyzed stress and support in step-family formation and found that a central task in the process is family members' reorganization of their assumptions concerning family interactions and responsibilities. The process of remarriage calls for revision and disassembly of the microculture of the first marriage and the creation of a new social system. From this perspective, support includes information and motivation that enables individuals to undertake a process of cognitive restructuring. Such support offers feedback that alters the way in which a person views and experiences the world and enables him or her to achieve a better "fit" between the assumptive world and the self or environment. Self-help groups provide contexts in which individuals can reflect on the ideas that shape their behavior and then begin developing alternative perspectives from which to evaluate and establish the meaning of the circumstances in which they find themselves.

Strong evidence that support can be beneficially provided in real world settings comes from the areas of health and medical intervention. Kennell, Klaus, McGrath, Robertson, and Hinkley (1991) studied the effects of emotional support given by a companion while a woman is undergoing labor and delivery. They found that the presence of a supportive companion (another woman) had a significant positive effect on clinical outcomes. The companion met the study participant for the first time after hospital admission. Each companion stayed at her assigned patient's bedside from admission through delivery, soothing and touching the patient and giving encouragement. In addition, she explained to the patient what was occurring during labor and what was likely to happen next. The provision of social support had a number of effects including fewer Caesarian sections being necessary in the supported as contrasted with the control group. The supported group also had significantly fewer forceps deliveries than did the control group and fewer infants born to mothers in the supported group required a prolonged hospital stay.

Relatedly, Bertsch, Nagashima-Whalen, Dykeman, Kennell, and McGrath (1990) found significant differences in clinical outcomes when either male partners of obstetrical patients or female companions (who were strangers) were present. Male partners chose to be present for less time during labor and to be close to the mother less often than the female companions. Further study is needed of the most active ingredients of the supportive process in this type of situation. Answers are needed to such questions as: Does a supportive companion reduce catecholamine levels? Does this happen because maternal anxiety is reduced and uterine contractions and uterine blood flow are facilitated? A companion's constant presence, physical touch, reassurance, explanations, and anticipatory guidance, all probably play roles and may contribute to the laboring woman feeling safer and calmer and needing less obstetrical intervention for labor to proceed smoothly.

Provided support has been shown to play significant (but not necessarily simple) roles in several medical areas besides obstetrics. Coyne and Smith (1991) found that wives' ability to help their husbands cope with a heart attack depended on several factors: the character of the infarction, the couples' interactions with medical personnel, and the quality of their marital relationship. In a study of recovery from coronary artery surgery, King, Reis, Porter, and Norsen (1993) found that patients' perceptions of general esteem support was the only type of support that consistently accounted for a unique share of the relationship between social support and surgery outcome. These researchers concluded that the influence of general esteem support on feelings of well-being most probably derived from its enabling the person to feel valued, loved, and competent.

The evidence concerning the relationship between social support, mental health, physical health, and recovery from illness suggests that, while social support alone may play an important role, it also may interact with other individual difference and environmental variables which need to be identified and evaluated.

Social Support and Community Stress

Most of what we know about stress and social support comes from various types of clinical assessment, laboratory, and field studies. However, most of these studies do not directly deal with community-wide stress. Are there lessons and leads in the available evidence applicable to community interventions?

Residents of communities experiencing stress have many needs. They often require direct aid (e.g., food, housing), and will almost always need information, advice, and guidance. In addition, they usually need support in the form of acceptance, empathy, and expressions of reality-based hope. As the evidence reviewed in the last section shows, the mere presence of an interested other, or even better, physical contact with that person can have significant benefits. A support provider can be helpful through her/his effort to aid persons experiencing stress in cognitively reframing their post-stress lives. The ultimate goal of support is to enable the victim of stress to achieve the highest level of self-sufficiency and social integration possible under the existing or expected circumstances. Available psychological research provides a basis for highlighting two outcomes that relate well-being and effective coping. These are (1) anxiety reduction, and (2) increased ability to attend to the task at hand and, as a consequence, to cope realistically with problematic situations.

Anxiety Reduction

Stress induces high levels of anxiety with its various physiological and psychological concomitants. Studies of the effects of companions on the labor process and obstetrical complications suggest the important role the presence of a caring person can play in bodily processes under stressful situations. Along the same line, Kamarck, Manuck, and Jennings (1990) investigated the effects of a nonevaluative social interaction on cardiovascular responses to psychological challenge. In one condition, a friend accompanied a college student who participated in two laboratory tasks. In the other condition, the subject came to the laboratory unaccompanied. Subjects who were accompanied by a friend showed reduced heart-rate reactivity to both tasks relative to the alone condition. The results suggested that interpersonal support reduces the likelihood of exaggerated cardiovascular responsivity.

Many studies indicate that social support can reduce the anxiety and panic often experienced by disaster victims. Most of the evidence supporting this conclusion comes from naturalistic and correlational studies. However, the evidence from these studies is consistent with controlled research that has shown that supportive interventions reduce feelings of anxiety and personal insecurity and increase self-confidence (I. Sarason & Sarason, 1986). Supportive interventions may exert their anxiety-reducing influence by reducing impersonality and diminishing concerns about the unavailability of people on whom the individual can rely. Effective social support interventions reduce perceptions of social isolation (Jones, Hobbs, & Hockenbury, 1982; Peplau & Perlman, 1982).

Attentional and Coping Processes

If providing social support accomplished no more than anxiety reduction and enhanced well-being, its contribution would be substantial. However, support also may play an important role in facilitating attention to important factors in a stressful situation and enabling effective coping efforts. There is considerable evidence that cognitive interference, often in the form of self-preoccupation, reduces the ability to be task-focused under challenging conditions (I. Sarason, Sarason, & Pierce, 1990). This happens because concerns about real and potential threats, and self-preoccupations interfere with task-relevant thought. Thoughts about off-task matters and a general wandering of attention from the task function as cognitive intrusions in problem-solving. Sarason (1981) showed that an opportunity for social association and acceptance by others improves performance and reduces cognitive interference. Lindner, Sarason, and Sarason (1988) also found that a supportive intervention positively affects cognitive functioning and performance. Although there have been relatively few studies of the effects of supportive interventions, as the number increases, paths to community applications of techniques for reducing self-preoccupation and increasing the ability to be task-oriented may emerge.

In their review of research on war-related stress, Milgram and Hobfoll (1986) noted the negative impact on soldiers' performance of low levels of support from their commanding officers and the positive contributions of strong leadership support to perseverance, morale, and group cohesiveness. In reviewing research on factors in human responses to disasters, Solomon (1989) observed that victim's social networks and the supportiveness of the immediate social environment are powerful mediators of individual outcomes following exposure to disaster. These outcomes include the ability to maintain a task focus and to filter out intrusive thoughts.

What we know about social support suggests the need for two types of field studies. One is demonstration projects that build supportive elements into stress-relief programs. Serious community-wide stress often is unexpected and time to prepare for and confront it may be minimal. Under these circumstances, neatly controlled research cannot be expected. Yet, much can be derived from demonstration projects about the effectiveness of interventions as judged by victims, service-providers, and independent observers and evaluators. The judgments of victims, service providers, and observers can provide meaningful dependent measures concerning the effectiveness of interventive elements, such as the training provided to service-providers can be regarded as independent variables. Similarly, outreach and information dissemination programs are intervention elements whose contributions to victims' return to normal lives can be evaluated. Following suggestions made by Solomon (1989) concerning the methodology of research on community cataclysms, social support, as an individual difference variable and as an intervention, is a concept relevant to both theories of interpersonal relationships and how people cope with stress.

Conclusions

Social support theories need to incorporate the complexity of those situational, interpersonal, and intrapersonal processes that shape individuals' perceptions of their social interactions with the significant people in their lives. The study of social support requires a focus, not only on general perceptions of social support, but also on the diversity of cognitions, emotions, and behaviors associated with specific personal relationships that shape behavior and well-being under diverse circumstances.

A theoretical perspective that encompasses situational, interpersonal and intrapersonal processes has implications for the research agenda of the future. What are the cognitive models that lead people to relate to others as they do? Can these models and the behavior that flows from them be influenced--for example, by particular interventions? How do relationships between people and the personal meanings attached to them change over time? The realization that neither social support nor personal relationships are invariant or guaranteed for life has implications for a systems view of the individual. While the individual is, at any point in time, part of a system that includes situational, interpersonal and intrapersonal vectors, this multidimensional system undergoes changes over time. We need to improve our ability to describe these processes and their outcomes.

It is now clear that social support is not simply assistance that is exchanged among network members, nor is it solely an appraisal of that assistance, nor is it only one's perceptions of network members. Instead, social support reflects a complex set of interacting events that include behavioral, cognitive and affective components. Despite this complexity, one finding emerges consistently: personal relationships are an active, crucial ingredient in the social support equation. An adequate understanding of social support processes must specify the role of personal relationships in the provision, receipt and appraisal of support.

References

Antonucci, T. C., & Israel, B. A. (1986). Veridicality of social support: A comparison of principal and network members' responses. Journal of Consulting and Clinical Psychology, 54, 432-437.

Bandura, A. (1986). Social foundations of thought and action: A social cognitive theory. Englewood Cliffs, NJ: Prentice-Hall.

Bertsch. T. D., Nagashima-Whalen, L., Dykeman, S., Kennell, J.H., & McGrath, S. (1990). Labor support by first-time fathers: Direct observations. Journal of Psychosomatic Obstetric Gynecology, 11, 251-260.

Blazer, D. (1982). Social support and mortality in an elderly community population. American Journal of Epidemiology, 115, 684-694.

Bowlby, J. (1988). Developmental psychiatry comes of age. American Journal of Psychiatry, 145, 1-10.

Bristol, M. M., Gallagher, J. J., & Schopler, E. (1988). Mothers and fathers of young developmentally disabled and nondisabled boys: Adaptation and spousal support. Developmental Psychology, 24, 441-451.

Cassel, J. (1976). The contribution of the social environment to host resistance. American Journal of Epidemiology, 104, 107-123.

Cobb, S. (1976). Social support as a moderator of life stress. Psychosomatic Medicine, 38, 300-314.

Cohen, S., & Lichtenstein, E. (1990). Partner behaviors that support quitting smoking. Journal of Consulting and Clinical Psychology, 58, 304-309.

Cohen, S., & Wills, T. A. (1985). Stress, social support, and the buffering hypothesis. Psychological Bulletin, 98, 310-357.

Coyne, J. C., & DeLongis, A.M. (1986). Going beyond social support: The role of social relationships in adaptation. Journal of Consulting and Clinical Psychology, 54, 454-460.

Coyne, J. C., & Smith, D.A.F. (1991). Couples coping with a myocardial infarction: A contextual perspective on wives' distress. Journal of Personality and Social Psychology, 61, 404-412.

Dakof, G. A., & Taylor, S. E. (1990). Victims' perceptions of social support: What is helpful from whom? Journal of Personality and Social Psychology, 58, 80-89.

Gottlieb, B. H. (1985). Social support and the study of personal relationships. Journal of Social and Personal Relationships, 2, 351-375.

Gottlieb, B. H. (1988). Marshaling social support: The state of the art in research and practice. In B. H. Gottlieb (Ed.), Marshaling social support. Newbury Park, CA: Sage.

Gurung, R. A. R., Sarason, B. R., Keeker, K. D., & Sarason, I. G. (1992). Family environments, specific relationships, and general perceptions of adjustment. Paper presented at the annual meeting of the American Psychological Association, Washington, D.C.

Heller, K. (1979). The effects of social support: Prevention and treatment implications. In A. P. Goldstein & F. H. Kanfer (Eds.), <u>Maximizing treatment gains: Transfer enhancement in psychotherapy</u>. NY: Academic Press.

Heller, K., & Swindle, R. W. (1983). Social networks, perceived social support, and coping with stress. In R. D. Felner, L. A. Jason, J. N. Moritsugu, & S. S. Farber (Eds.), <u>Preventive psychology: Theory, research and practice</u>. Elmsford, NY: Pergamon.

Hobfoll, S. E., & Freedy, J. R. (1990). The availability and effective use of social support. <u>Journal of Social and Clinical Psychology, 9</u>, 91-103.

House, J. S., & Kahn, R. L. (1985). Measures and concepts of social support. In S. Cohen & S.L. Syme (Eds.), <u>Social support and health</u> (pp. 83-108). Orlando, FL: Academic Press.

Jacobson, D. (1990). Stress and support in stepfamily formation: The cultural context of social support. In B. R. Sarason, I. G. Sarason, & G. R. Pierce (Eds.), <u>Social support: An interactional view</u> (pp. 199-218). NY: John Wiley & Sons.

Jones, W. H. Hobbs, S. A., & Hockenbury, D. (1982). Loneliness and social skills deficits. <u>Journal of Personality and Social Psychology, 42</u>, 682-689.

Kamarck, T. W., Manuck, S. B., & Jennings, J. R. (1990). Social support reduces cardiovascular reactivity to psychological challenge: A laboratory model. <u>Psychosomatic Medicine, 52</u>, 42-58.

Kennell, J., Klaus, M., McGrath, S., Robertson, S., & Hinkley, C. (1991). Continuous emotional support during labor in a U.S. hospital: A randomized controlled trial. <u>Journal of American Medical Association, 265</u>, 2197-2201.

King, K. B. Reis, H. T., Porter, L. A., Norsen, L. H. (1993). Social support and long-term recovery from coronary artery surgery: Effects on patients and spouses. <u>Health Psychology, 12</u>, 56-63.

Lazarus, R. S. (1991). Emotion and adaptation. NY: Oxford University Press.

Lehman, D. R., Ellard, J. H., & Wortman, C. B. (1986). Social support for the bereaved: Recipients' and providers' perspectives on what is helpful. <u>Journal of Personality and Social Psychology, 54</u>, 438-446.

Lindner, K. C., Sarason, I. G., & Sarason, B. R. (1988). Assessed life stress and experimentally provided social support. In C. D. Spielberger, I. G. Sarason, & P. B. Defares (Eds.), <u>Stress and anxiety</u> (Vol. 11). Washington, DC: Hemisphere.

Milgram, N., & Hobfoll, S. (1986). Generalizations from theory and practice in war-related stress. In N.A. Milgram (Ed.), <u>Stress and coping in time of war: Generalizations from the Israeli experience</u> (pp. 316-352). NY: Brunner/Mazel.

Newcomb, M. D. (1990). Social support and personal characteristics: A developmental and interactional perspective. <u>Journal of Social and Clinical Psychology, 9</u>, 54-68.

Peplau, K. A., & Perlman, P. (Eds.) (1982). Loneliness: A sourcebook of current theory, research, and therapy. NY: John Wiley.

Pierce, G. R., Sarason, I. G., & Sarason, B. R. (in press). Coping and social support. In M. Zeidner and N. Endler (Eds.). Handbook of Coping. NY: Wiley.

Pierce, G. R., Sarason, B. R., & Sarason, I. G. (1990). Integrating social support perspectives: Working models, personal relationships, and situational factors. In S. Duck (Ed.), Personal relationships and social support. Newbury Park, CA: Sage Publications.

Pierce, G. R., & Contey, C. (1992). An experimental study of stress, social support, and coping. Clinton, NY: Hamilton College. Unpublished research.

Pierce, G. R., Sarason, I. G., & Sarason, B. R. (1991). General and relationship-based perceptions of social support: Are two constructs better than one? Journal of Personality and Social Psychology, 61, 1028-1039.

Procidano, M. E., & Heller, K. (1983). Measures of perceived social support from friends and from family: Three validation studies. American Journal of Community Psychology, 11, 1-24.

Revenson, T. A., & Majerovitz, D. (1990). Spouses' support provision to chronically ill patients. Journal of Social and Personal Relationships, 7, 575-586.

Sandler, I. N., & Barrera, M., Jr. (1984). Toward a multimethod approach to assessing the effects of social support. American Journal of Community Psychology, 12, 37-52.

Sarason, B. R., Pierce, G. R., Bannerman, A., & Sarason, I. G. (1993). Investigating the antecedents of perceived support: Parents' views of and behavior toward their children. Journal of Personality and Social Psychology, 65, 1071-1085.

Sarason, B. R., Pierce, G. R., & Sarason. I. G. (1990). Social support: The sense of acceptance and the role of relationships. In B.R. Sarason, I.G. Sarason, & G. R. Pierce (Eds.), Social support: An interactional view. NY: John Wiley.

Sarason, B. R., Pierce, G.R., Shearin, E.N., Sarason, I.G., Waltz, J.A., & Poppe, L. (1991). Perceived social support and working models of self and actual others. Journal of Personality and Social Psychology, 60, 273-287.

Sarason, B. R., Shearin, E. N., Pierce, G. R., & Sarason, I. G. (1987). Interrelationships among social support measures: Theoretical and practical implications. Journal of Personality and Social Psychology, 52, 813-832.

Sarason, I. G. (1981). Test anxiety, stress, and social support. Journal of Personality, 49, 101-114.

Sarason, I. G., Pierce, G. R., & Sarason, B. R. (1990). Social support and interactional processes: A triadic hypothesis. Journal of Social and Personal Relationships, 7, 495-506.

Sarason, I. G., & Sarason, B. R. (1986). Experimentally provided social support. Journal of Personality and Social Psychology, 50, 1222-1225.

Sarason, I. G., Sarason, B. R., & Pierce, G. R. (1990). Anxiety, cognitive interference, and performance. Journal of Social Behavior and Personality, 5, 1-18.

Sarason, I. G., Sarason, B. R., & Shearin, E. N. (1986). Social support as an individual difference variable: Its stability, origins, and relational aspects. Journal of Personality and Social Psychology, 50, 845-855.

Seeman, T. E., & Berkman, L. L. (1988). Structural characteristics of social networks and their relationship with social support in the elderly: Who provides support. Social Science and Medicine, 26, 737-749.

Shulman, N. (1976). Network analysis: A new addition to an old bag of tricks. Acta Sociologica, 23, 307-323.

Simons, R., Lorenz, F. O., Wu, C-I, & Conger, R. D. (1993). Social network and marital support as mediators and moderators of the impact of stress and depression on parental behavior. Developmental Psychology, 29, 368-381.

Solomon, S. D. (1989). Research issues in assessing disaster's effects. In R. Gist and B. Lubin (Eds.), Psychosocial aspects of disaster (pp. 308-340). NY: Wiley & Sons.

Weiss, R. S. (1974). The provisions of social relationships. In Z. Rubin (Ed.), Doing unto others (pp. 17-26). Englewood Cliffs, NJ: Prentice-Hall.

Wethington, E., & Kessler, R. C. (1986). Perceived support, received support, and adjustment to stressful life events. Journal of Health and Social Behavior, 27, 78-89.

Zavislak, N., & Sarason, B. R. (1991, August). Predicting parent-child relationships: Influence of marital conflict and family behavior. Paper presented at the annual meeting of the American Psychological Association, Washington, DC.

SECTION IV: BRIDGES TO COMMUNITY STRESS (OVERVIEW)

Stevan E. Hobfoll, Kent State University, Kent, Ohio, USA
Rebecca P. Cameron, Kent State University, Kent, Ohio, USA
Marten W. deVries, University of Limburg, Maastricht, the Netherlands

In Section Four, the challenges of conducting intervention and research at the community level are further explored, with particular attention to appropriate and comprehensive methodologies. With regard to both of these enterprises, a need for methodological flexibility and creativity is clearly established. In addition, the authors in this section incorporate temporal and cultural factors into their thinking about community stress, thus modeling the application of ecological concepts such as adaptation and succession.

De Jong (Chapter Nine) begins with a reminder of the impossibility of treating all the victims of disaster on an individual basis, given the large numbers of victims and the limited supply of clinicians available to engage in dyadic treatment modalities. With that in mind, he presents the IPSER (Institute for Psycho-social and Socio-ecological Research) program currently being implemented in collaboration with the World Health Organization. It consists of a multimodal, multilevel public health approach to prevention and intervention with war-related community stress. The IPSER-WHO program utilizes a diverse assortment of data collection methods to gather qualitative and quantitative information at the level of society, community, and the individual. This approach generates cultural, contextual, and temporal data. The program is provided to governments upon request, and is implemented primarily by local personnel. Evaluations are built in, allowing for ongoing adjustments to be made.

De Jong then reviews the concepts of primary, secondary, and tertiary prevention, and relates these to new terminology and subclassifications presented by the U.S. Committee on Prevention of Mental Disorders in 1994. Primary prevention is divided into universal, selective, and indicated preventive interventions. Universal preventive interventions are targeted to the population as a whole, whereas selective preventive interventions are targeted to subgroups with higher risk of morbidity, and indicated preventive interventions are geared towards high-risk individuals already showing signs of their vulnerability. Secondary prevention, according to this new system, is called treatment, and consists of two subcategories: case identification and standard treatment of known disorders. Case identification emphasizes the need for widespread knowledge of, and access to, early intervention. Tertiary prevention is reconceptualized as maintenance, and is also divided into two subcategories: compliance with long-term treatment and after-care.

Next, de Jong discusses three levels of prevention: the (inter)national level, the community level, and the family and individual level. He presents a wide variety of preventive strategies, along with illustrations of those strategies that have been or are being investigated. He stresses the importance of dispelling myths about human aggression if prevention is to be carried out effectively. Instead of presenting aggression as an inevitable part of human behavior, de Jong outlines the situations that increase the probability of aggression. He argues that our vulnerability to war stems, in part, from our deep-seated identification with group memberships, and stresses the role that our leaders play in defining our stance towards other groups as aggressive or non-aggressive.

Some of the preventive or intervention strategies that de Jong suggests at the (inter)national level include forms of recognition such as the Nobel peace prize, prosecution of war criminals, politically-negotiated solutions to issues of migration and repatriation, arms control, human rights advocacy, reparations to victims, adequate building standards, alarm systems, and evacuation plans.

Previous work on community-level prevention that de Jong reviews includes efforts such as providing culturally-appropriate rituals in programs for refugees, prejudice reduction, empathy training, increasing prosocial behavior, and reducing aggressive behavior. The importance of two IPSER-WHO strategies for intervention is stressed. They are: gathering data before intervening with survivors in a particular cultural context, and establishing mutual training between professional providers and local healers.

Universal preventive interventions that the IPSER-WHO program emphasizes include the provision of security for survivors relocated into refugee camps, strategies to decrease the learned helplessness of survivors suddenly dependent on external sources of aid, and rural development initiatives that restore a sense of control, provide income, and increase the future orientation of refugees. In addition, rural development can serve to provide soldiers with alternatives to their military occupations, contributing to the demobilization of forces.

Universal and selective preventions are also aimed at children and families. These include family reunification and establishing supportive extended family networks, or providing foster care as needed. Group-based interventions are designed to allow children to deal with intensely traumatic experiences. Again, culturally-appropriate forms of healing are applied. Interventions often occur within schools, and involve both professionals and paraprofessionals. An important feature of this approach is attending to the recovery of service providers who have been traumatized before having them intervene with others. Universal preventive interventions for families and individuals include establishing living environments that provide for basic physical and social needs, including providing for constructive activities, decreasing overcrowding in refugee camps, and ensuring a varied diet.

Although individualized treatment cannot be provided to all survivors of war or other trauma, prevention strategies will not suffice for severely traumatized individuals. Treatment strategies will be needed and should be able to address the problems of repeatedly traumatized victims. Compromises can be utilized to maximize the availability of treatment, through the implementation of self-help groups and by training primary health-care workers to disseminate basic mental health care. Similarly, maintenance needs are built into community interventions through increased training of primary health care workers that focuses on the needs of the mentally ill and explains the psychiatric consequences of trauma.

Solomon (Chapter Ten) reviews evidence of the pathological consequences of war as experienced by Israelis, with careful consideration of the temporal issues involved in the manifestation and assessment of pathology. Solomon's discussion of the negative effects of combat-related psychopathology lends support to de Jong's call for prevention of aggression at the international level. She and her colleagues have conducted a comprehensive research program on war-related stress, and she draws on this rich source of data to review five categories of effects of war stress.

First, Solomon discusses the clinical manifestations and prevalence of acute stress. One striking finding that she reports regarding reactions to the Gulf War air raids is that more civilians died as a direct or indirect result of fear than died as a result of wounds inflicted by missiles. However, civilians habituated somewhat over time to the threat of missile attack. In general, evacuees from bombed homes showed initially high levels of distress that tended to lessen over time. Research on soldiers' acute responses focuses on combat stress reaction (CSR), which is a frequent cause of casualties in any war.

The long term psychological sequelae of war stress can be demonstrated through Solomon and her colleagues' research comparing soldiers who experienced CSR during war with matched controls. Many CSR casualties go on to suffer from post-traumatic stress disorder (PTSD), as do a smaller number of those who were not treated for CSR. A history of CSR constitutes a significant risk factor for increased severity and duration of PTSD. Solomon discusses the contextual features of Israeli conflict that may contribute specifically to long-term outcomes for Israeli soldiers. In addition, she discusses the tendency for CSR to be associated with multiple losses, including lowered self-efficacy and impaired social functioning, that could be understood as part of the loss cycle phenomenon conceptualized by COR theory.

Solomon next discusses delayed onset post traumatic stress reactions, which occur when an individual at first appears to function adaptively following traumatic stress, but then develops symptoms at a later point. This could potentially reflect one of several patterns: the exacerbation of subclinical PTSD; delayed help seeking for chronic PTSD; delayed onset PTSD; other psychiatric disorders that are triggered or exacerbated by wartime stress; or reactivation due to a new stressor or due to accumulated stressors. Solomon and her colleagues have found that genuinely delayed onset of traumatic stress reactions is relatively rare, whereas delayed help seeking is relatively common, at least among their sample of Israeli soldiers.

Another manifestation of combat-related stress is the reactivation of previous war stress reactions. This can take the form of either uncomplicated reactivation (i.e., war stress reactions that occur following symptom-free functioning between wars) or exacerbated PTSD. Exacerbated PTSD can occur to those who suffer from specific sensitivity, moderate generalized sensitivity, or severe generalized sensitivity to stress. Victims of reactivated stress reactions have generally put a lot of effort into functioning well, before the reactivation of war-related stress causes them to break down.

The final major type of combat-related distress that Solomon discusses is the secondary traumatization of people close to directly traumatized individuals. This has been studied with spouses and children of traumatized individuals. The finding that stress reactions cause ongoing difficulties for the intimates of veterans again highlights the need for prevention of the original trauma and the development of interventions that are geared towards family members of traumatized individuals. In this chapter, Solomon has shown us that trauma can have an impact beyond the acute phase of the stressor and the initial period of adjustment and beyond the traumatized individual her- or himself.

McFarlane (Chapter Eleven) makes the case for increased specificity in the assessment of extreme stress, but also notes methodological and conceptual problems with quantifying the experience of stress. He initially presents two major issues: the need to conduct longitudinal research and the importance of considering the role of individual-level, internal psychological processes in the experience of stress.

Next, McFarlane presents the rationale for quantifying the stress of disasters. First, in order to demonstrate and quantify the nature of the relationship between disaster stress and psychological outcomes, adequate measures of stress must be developed. This requires clarification of the exact nature of the stress under consideration as well as attention to reliability and validity of measures. Acute responses and their relationship to long-term adjustment, including the mediating links between these two phenomena need to be studied. In addition, it is important that we be able to differentiate the immediate impact of the trauma from the impact of long-term loss of resources and declines in psychological well-being.

Explicit attention to measuring the phases of disaster is an important ingredient in developing a meaningful longitudinal approach to disaster stress. In addition, attending to the phases of disaster facilitates an understanding of the interactions between victims and the traumas they experience. Phases of disaster that need to be taken into account at community, family, and individual levels of analysis include: planning (risk appraisal and management); threat (anticipatory anxiety and its adaptive management); impact; inventory and rescue (the process of assessing impact and re-establishing communication with the family and community); and remedy and recovery phases. Each phase has its own particular issues that need to be specified in a thorough measure of disaster stress.

Using the phase of impact as an example, it becomes clear that the exact impact of a disaster depends on a number of things: the type of event; unequal impact within a particular event; individual losses relative to community patterns of loss; differing combinations of threat, property loss, or loss of life; and the behavior of victims during impact. One problem in measurement is the difficulty of scaling and comparing disaster experiences, especially since neither victims nor outsiders can provide measures of impact that are necessarily valid. This is due to the effects of memory and the differences in appraisal that may occur when one has experienced an event versus having considered it hypothetically. In addition, it is difficult to conceptualize meaningful ways to measure cumulative impact, to differentiate objective and subjective components of impact, and to measure and combine such dimensions as duration, awareness, control, the role of chance outcomes, and the intensity of impact.

Our current understanding of the relationship between acute responses and long-term effects of extreme stress is limited due to the use of retrospective rather than prospective data. Although initial experiences of intrusive memories and avoidance are thought to be of primary importance in differentiating successful and unsuccessful adaptations, prospective data suggest that affect and arousal processes may be more central.

An additional issue in research that attempts to link extreme stress and psychological outcomes is the nature of the outcomes under consideration. McFarlane suggests that the stressor criterion used in diagnosing PTSD according to DSM-IV limits understanding by its emphasis on a particular acute reaction. Another concern is that other outcomes than PTSD may be equally important to consider, such as resilience and comorbidity. Sampling strategies will affect the outcomes that are studied. A complicating factor in research on outcomes of disaster is the possibility of secondary trauma that is caused by the experience of powerlessness or threat of disintegration associated with PTSD itself.

McFarlane's chapter raises a number of questions and considerations for researchers interested in the impact of extreme stressors. Measurement strategies need to be developed that more fully and clearly account for the complexities of the disaster context and its course over time if we are to make significant progress in an ecological understanding of disaster impact.

Bromet (Chapter Twelve) provides a contextually-grounded discussion of the compromises involved in designing feasible research on a major community event, the Chernobyl nuclear disaster. She discusses the relevance of epidemiologic strategies, such as representative sampling, appropriate control groups, reliable measurements, and multivariate analyses, to the study of community stress. She then proceeds to illustrate the difficulties of conducting optimal research on disaster-stricken communities. She critiques common sources of bias found in disaster research, including recall bias, selective mortality from either the stress exposure or the study, investigator bias due to funding from special interest groups, and failure to adequately note study limitations.

In order to fully understand the process of designing research on the Chernobyl catastrophe, Bromet provides background information on the incident. Important features of this disaster are its lack of clear spatial or temporal boundaries, resulting in ongoing concerns among and effects on a large number of people scattered throughout a large geographic region. Many secondary traumas have occurred since the actual explosion of the nuclear reactor at Chernobyl, including misinformation from the government, evacuations, abortions conducted on a large scale, hostility from residents of communities receiving large numbers of refugees, and government failure to provide needed services. These traumas have occurred in the context of a nation with inadequate resources, poor record-keeping, other environmental problems, and ongoing economic problems, all of which contribute to difficulties in teasing apart the nature and impact of Chernobyl-related stress.

Bromet goes on to discuss the methodological adjustments that were needed to design a cohort study on children of evacuees from a particular village, given the practical limitations of the Chernobyl context. Judging that a random sample would be difficult to obtain due to the uncertain quality of the available registries of evacuees, she decided to utilize a convenience sample of refugees living in Kiev. Due to the large number of coexisting stressors in the Soviet Union that were not specific to Chernobyl, she decided to include a comparison group of children originally from Kiev.

Next, Bromet considered measurement issues, including the necessity of relying on self-report, some of which would of necessity be retrospective. Again, this was due to limitations imposed by the context: pre-existing records had been abandoned in the contaminated village. In order to disentangle somatic from psychosomatic disorders to the degree possible, Bromet and her colleagues decided to incorporate a medical assessment of each child. Multiple measures of objective and subjective stressors were also incorporated into the study design. Since parental alcoholism presents a significant additional risk factor to children, and since it is frequently found in Russia, priority was assigned to developing measures of alcohol abuse that would be valid cross-culturally. A final issue of study design that Bromet presents is that of obtaining informed consent from a group of people who have learned to distrust authorities and who might view an elaborate explanation of possible negative results of study participation with suspicion.

Bromet concludes that there are methodological problems inherent in almost any study of extreme stress conditions. However, she illustrates how research planned with thoughtful consideration of the limitations of a data set and appropriate awareness of flaws that compromise generalizability could result in productive additions to our knowledge base.

Finally, Norris, Freedy, DeLongis, Sibilia, and Schönpflug (Chapter Thirteen) articulate the need for research that is theoretically and ecologically sound, and provide examples of research endeavors that are both. They include frequent references to the other chapters in this volume in order to demonstrate the ways in which their concepts can be and are being applied.

First, Norris et al. discuss the need to establish conceptual definitions and an ecological context for community research. They define a community as "an aggregated group of people that exists for the function of providing for the physical, social, psychological, and spiritual or philosophical needs of community members." Community members are associated with functional subgroups, and are generally obligated to be involved in give-and-take relationships with the larger community and its members. Communities tend to be characterized by geographic, physical, and functional stability over time. Comprehensive theoretical models are advocated that provide a basis for systematic research that incorporates attention to historical and developmental dimensions of the community, that focus on a wide range of outcomes of community stress, and that allow for a community-level conceptualization of variables such as resources.

With regard to ecological context, Norris et al. advocate a consideration of the dynamic interplay between researchers and community members and how that relates to the validity and relevance of data that is collected. Entry into the community of interest needs to be handled appropriately, collaborative relationships need to be built, and community members need to understand that researchers are committed to them. Methods of generating qualitative data, such as focus groups and key informant interviews, are particularly useful at the beginning stages of a research endeavor. Thus, both comprehensive theory and familiarity with the target community are essential to conducting good community research.

Next, Norris et al. present three strategies for conceptualizing communities in research designs: single community studies, subcommunity studies, and studies of multiple communities. Single community studies may overemphasize the role of individual-level variables due to the fact that the stressor is held constant, in a broad sense, for the community. Describing contextual features of the affected community helps to make such research more generally relevant. Subcommunity research focuses on groups within the targeted community that are expected to show differential effects of the stressor. This approach highlights political issues such as access to resources. Subcommunity strategies should attend to the possibility that patterns of relationships between variables may differ more than global outcomes. Multiple community studies allow for empirical analysis of the role of community-level variables. As such, they provide a uniquely useful avenue to understanding communities under stress.

Norris et al. conclude with an overview of productive avenues for future research. Longitudinal studies could be designed to examine possible non-linear relationships between variables, as well as to determine the relationships between acute stress responses and long-term outcomes. Studies of children and of intervention programs are especially sparse and would add to the available literature in important ways. Attention to the clinical and social significance of findings would add depth and relevance to the literature. Finally, Norris et al. call for an creative and activist stance on issues related to community stress.

The authors of the following chapters are all concerned with the question of how to thoroughly operationalize our inquiries into communities under stress. Through consideration of these authors' suggestions and experiences, intervention and research programs can be designed and implemented that meet the standards of a rigorous scientific approach, yet that remain practical and community-oriented. Although individual-level factors remain important, they become only one level of a multilevel understanding of extreme stress. An integral component of doing community research is acknowledging that decisions are made in a value-laden, real-world context. Authors throughout this section reiterate the need to adopt a stance of involvement rather than passive or detached observation, even when conducting scientifically rigorous research.

PREVENTION OF THE CONSEQUENCES OF MAN-MADE OR NATURAL DISASTER AT THE (INTER)NATIONAL, THE COMMUNITY, THE FAMILY AND THE INDIVIDUAL LEVEL

Joop TVM de Jong
International Institute for Psychosocial and Socio-Ecological Research (IPSER)
University of Maastricht, and Free University of Amsterdam, the Netherlands

It is possible by definition to prevent a posttraumatic stress syndrome by eliminating the traumatic event or by reducing its consequences. However, the psychotraumatic sequelae of a man-made or natural disaster often affect so many people that they cannot be addressed with current models of clinical psychology and psychiatry. These models are often based on dyadic curative care such as crisis intervention or brief psychotherapy, sometimes complemented with a systemic approach. Instead it is necessary to resort to a public mental health approach based on community action in order to deal with the enormous size of the problems in a number of war and postwar situations, or after natural disasters. The mere figures make this public mental health approach necessary. In the Nineties the number of refugees and displaced persons alone is estimated at 18 million refugees covered by the 1951 UN Convention relating to the status of refugees and there are twice that number of internally displaced persons (De Jong et al. 1994). Most mental health professionals have limited training or experience working at the broader community, national, or international levels, although war, political repression, human rights violations and natural disasters have direct mental health consequences that can eventually come to the attention of mental health professionals (Punamäki, 1989; Westermyer, 1987; Williams & Berry, 1991).

This chapter reviews a number of preventive initiatives and proposes a model that deals with prevention on several levels, descending from the (inter)national level to communities of displaced persons and refugees, families, and individuals. The model integrates concepts from the fields of public health, psychology, anthropology and psychiatry. It has a matrix structure, i.e. it proposes multi-modal preventive interventions in relation to the different societal levels involved. Moreover, the model can be used in an eclectic way by applying a specific preventive principle in a specific post-disaster situation. Some of the current ideas regarding primary prevention such as the de-escalation of conflicts may seem Utopian. Regarding the containment or prevention of armed conflicts, this chapter only aims at sensitizing colleagues to some of the current international discussions. Other preventive interventions are quite feasible and are currently being tested in a large international collaborative program among refugee populations in a number of African and Asian countries. In addition, preparations are under way for initiatives in Europe.

This chapter emphasizes the prevention of psychosocial and mental health consequences and only briefly mentions political and polemic issues that are left to the experts in that field. After a brief outline of the international multi-site program, the chapter reviews preventive experiences elsewhere and describes the preventive principles and guidelines that are being implemented to deal with massive community stress among refugees and other victims of man-made or natural disaster. When the word disaster is used, it implies both man-made disaster (such as war, civil war, genocide, autogenocide, nuclear disasters), and natural disasters (such as hurricanes, vulcano eruptions). Although the model can be applied in both types of disaster, the IPSER-WHO program is only active in situations of organized violence such as wars.

Figure 1 shows the different multi-modal preventive interventions in relation to the different societal levels.

Outline of the IPSER-WHO Program

Over the last three years, the Cross-Cultural Division of IPSER (Institute for Psycho-social and Socio-ecological Research) in the Netherlands, in collaboraton with the World Health Organization, has developed an intervention and research program addressing the psychosocial and mental health problems of refugees in Africa, Asia and Europe. The program has developed a pragmatic step-wise model to collect data descending from the population level to the level of the society, the community, and the individual. This multimethod hierarchical model uses a combination of qualitative and quantitative ethnographic, epidemiological, and psychometric methods such as participant observation, focus groups, key informant interviews, snowball sampling, experience sampling, and surveys with psychodiagnostic and psychometric instruments. These techniques provide information on context, culture, and time perspective. Ethnographic material is collected to design or adapt research instruments that can then be transformed into culturally valid psychometric or psychodiagnostic instruments. Simultaneously, the ethnographic and epidemiological data are used for a pilot intervention phase, and later on for the extension of the interventions to larger populations and other areas or countries. In order to evaluate the progress of the program, a cybernetic monitoring strategy has been developed enabling the program to assess its efficacy and to adapt its objectives and methods.

Countries or organizations that wish to participate can apply and the program reacts to their request. The program is carried out by local personnel, and if a country or organization requires professional expertise from abroad, the program recruits international professionals who support the national staff. The program has been active or is going to be implemented through government agencies in countries such as Cambodia, Ethiopia, Mozambique, and Uganda, or through governments in exile, international agencies, Non-Governmental Organizations or other organizations, among the Tibetans in India, the Palestinians in Gaza, or the Bhutanese in Nepal.

Figure 1. Preventive interventions at the (inter)national, the community, the family and the individual level.

	(INTER) NATIONAL	COMMUNITY	FAMILY & INDIVIDUAL
PREVENTION (PRIMARY)	Universal preventive interventions Deescalation of conflicts Diminish hostility Reconciliation Reinforce peace-initiatives Persecution perpetrators Voluntary repatriation Arms control Natural disaster: quality standards for constructions, alarm systems, evacuation plans, land distribution **Selective preventive interventions** Human rights advocacy **Indicated preventive interventions** Disclose the truth	Universal preventive interventions Security measures Decreasing dependency Empowerment: management and multisectoral activities Rural development (initiating gain cycles) **Universal/selective interventions** Family reunion Group activities with children **Selective interventions for children** Supporting network Strengthening coping skills **Selective/indicated interventions** Engaging teachers	Universal Improvement physical aspects Involving professionals Interpreter services
TREATMENT (SECONDARY)	Reparation and compensation	Restore a sense of control Create a perspective for the future Fostering self-reliance Self-help groups for rape victims, children & mothers Dealing with substance abuse	Indivual & family therapy

Prevention: Reformulation of Basic Concepts

According to Kaplan and Sadock (1985) primary prevention aims to eliminate a disease or disordered state before it can occur. In order to do so, one must know the etiology of the disorder. In the case of post-traumatic stress syndromes (or PTSD, according to the more culture-bound concept of DSM-IV or ICD-10), knowledge about the etiology is a condition to qualify for the diagnosis. Hence, since the cause of post-traumatic stress syndromes can often be eliminated, they are among the few psychological disturbances amenable to primary prevention. Williams and Berry (1991) indicated the need to develop prevention programs for refugees using a systematic approach. They recommended that prevention programs for refugees be group or population based (cf. Turshen, 1989) and that groups that are at risk for disorders are especially appropriate. Their ideas fit the new definitions for prevention as formulated in the recent volume Reducing Risks for Mental Disorders: Frontiers for Preventive Intervention Research by the U.S. Committee on Prevention of Mental Disorders (1994). The committee has adapted the terms used by Gordon (1983) and makes the following distinction that I will use throughout this chapter:
Universal preventive interventions for mental disorders are targeted to the general public or a whole population group that has not been identified on the basis of individual risk. Such interventions have advantages when their cost per individual is low, the intervention is effective and acceptable to the population, and there is low risk associated with the intervention. Selective preventive interventions are targeted to individuals or a subgroup of the population whose risk of developing mental disorders is significantly higher than average. The risk may be imminent, or it may be a lifetime risk. Indicated preventive interventions are targeted to high-risk individuals who are identified as having minimal but detectable signs or symptoms foreshadowing mental disorder.

According to Kaplan and Sadock (1985) the goal of secondary prevention is to shorten the course of the illness by early identification and rapid intervention or crisis intervention. In the aforementioned book the U.S. Committee on Prevention of Mental Disorders has relabeled the term secondary prevention as Treatment, subdivided into Case Identification and Standard Treatment of Known Disorders. Thus Case Identification is the equivalent of the previous secondary prevention. The Case Identification involves a network of community resources that aid in early identification, prompt treatment, or referral. If Case Identification is to be useful, the people who need help must be trained to seek it. Most of all, it depends on wide knowledge of the availibility of prompt and early intervention. After a disaster this means that, for example, a network of relief workers should be able to recognize traumatized persons and that the victims are informed of where they can get support. Accessibility is an important aspect of Treatment. For victims this implies that the threshold to get help should be low, both from a geographic, an economic, and a cultural point of view.

The goal of tertiary prevention is to reduce chronicity through the prevention of complications and through active rehabilitation. Usually, the concept of tertiary prevention in psychiatry is applied to the problem of institutionalization of patients, which results in the disruption of social skills and rejection by family members and by others in the patient's usual social support network. Tertiary prevention has been relabeled by the U.S. Committee as Maintenance, subdivided into Compliance with Long-term Treatment with the goal of reducing relapse and recurrence, and After-care including rehabilitation. The relabeling of the terms secondary and teriary prevention as Treatment and Maintenance may increase the goodness of fit between these terms and the Western-style mental health care systems. For technologically less developed countries, however, I regard this redefinition as an impoverishment of the original concepts. This holds a fortiori for situations of massive trauma. To prevent confusion, I will use the new nomenclature of the U.S. Committee as shown in Figure 2.

Figure 2. The mental health intervention spectrum for mental disorders (from: Reducing risks for mental disorders, 1994).

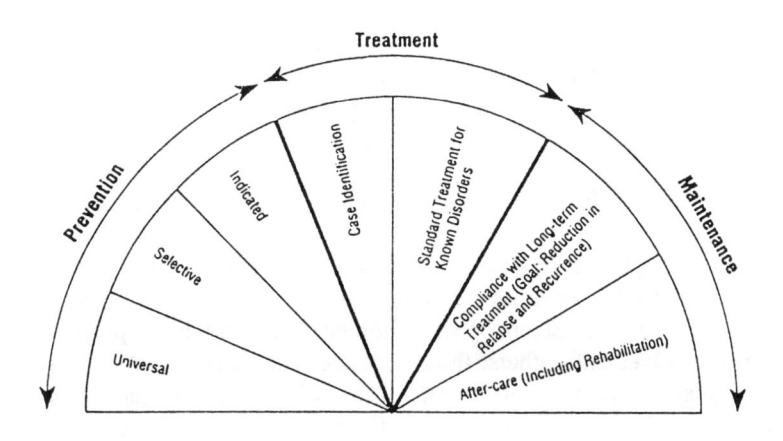

Prevention on the (Inter)national Level: General Considerations

In Aggression and War (Groebel & Hinde, 1991) a number of scholars express their concern about two beliefs that, although erroneous, are commonly held in our society. The first is that, because aggressive behavior is in some sense part of human nature, humans inevitably behave aggressively. The second is that international war is closely related to, and even a direct consequence of, the aggressiveness of individuals. It is often suggested that violence can only be reduced by providing harmless outlets for aggressive propensities, or by segregating offenders, which distracts us from attempting to build a world where aggressive behavior is less likely. The authors challenge a number of commonly held viewpoints and criticize the misuse of the theory of evolution to justify not only war, but also genocide, colonialism, and suppression of the weak. They challenge alleged biological findings that have been used to justify violence and war. They criticize the statement that we have inherited a tendency to make war from our animal ancestors or that it is genetically programmed into our human nature. They also challenge the view that humans have developped a 'violent brain' or that war is caused by 'instinct' or any single motivation.

Like genocide, war is often the outcome of steps along a continuum of antagonism (Staub, 1993). Hostile acts by one party or acts of self-defense that are perceived as hostile, cause retaliation, which evokes more intense hostility. A progression of mutual retaliation may start with small acts that escalate, resulting in a 'malignant social process' (Deutsch, 1983). The escalation of conflict is often the result of "us"-"them" differentiation, negative evaluation and mistrust, or a societal self-concept (e.g. Black-White, Aryan-Jew, Tutsi-Hutu, Israeli-Palestinian, Indian-Pakistani). If the societal self-concept is based on superiority or self-doubt or their combination, it may give rise to war-generating motives (e.g. Germany after WW-I, the Khmer Rouge dreaming of restoring the old Khmer empire).

A societal self-concept often designates the territories that are part of a nation and may include some that the nation has not possessed for a long time (China claiming Tibet, Jews claiming Jerusalem, Iraq claiming Kuwait, Argentina reclaiming the Falklands), or, as an alternative, one part of the territory may want to split off from a country to which it 'belongs' (Rhodesia from South Africa, Biafra from Nigeria, East from West Pakistan, Erythrea from Ethiopia, Kurdistan from Turkey, Iran and Iraq).

Since belonging to groups is of profound significance for human beings, nations and their leaders have a tremendous capacity to enlist the loyalty and self-sacrifice of their citizens (Staub, 1993). Groups, like individuals, project unacceptable aspects of themselves onto others; those who are repudiated become "bad": they possess the rejected and renounced parts of the self which remains pure and good (Pinderhughes, 1979) (as happened e.g. in the genocide of the Armenians in Turkey; the tensions between Xosa and Zulu leading to witchcraft accusations and necklace murders; the 'set up' accusations of 'parasitism' as happened to the Jews in pre-WW-II Europe, with Indians in Uganda under Amin, or the Chinese in Indonesia in 1994; or Mozambique's Renamo claiming to restore traditional values that were felt to be derogated by Frelimo).

Leaders have great power to shape relations between nations, but they are also the products of their societies. The leaders' power is enlarged by their capacity to initiate a cycle of hostility. Citizens rarely criticize hostile acts of their own country, but they are aroused to patriotic fervor by hostile acts against their country, even retaliatory ones (Staub, 1993). The process of leadership may also produce faulty decision making, such as groupthink (e.g. in ex-Yugoslavia). Heterogeneity in society is essential for diminishing the chance of war or genocide because it contributes to a balance of power and to discussions on war-generating motives. However, heterogeneity can be counterbalanced by a yearning for a larger unity in order to 'face external threat'. In addition to the UN, there are only a few institutions whose purpose is to restrain hostile acts against another nation. Those who do speak out may have to face the wrath of the rest of the society. For example, a president in the U.S. still cannot be a Vietnam-deserter; until today a Nazi-deserter is still often regarded as a deserter in his German village; a deserter of the Netherlands' colonial war against Indonesia - euphemistically called a 'police action' - still does not get permission to visit the Netherlands.

Prevention on the (Inter)national Level: Illustrative Cases

Based on these considerations, a number of preventive interventions can be outlined. I will use the terms "universal," "selective," and "indicated" preventive interventions as described earlier. Since these interventions belong to the realm of politicians and decision-makers, they will only be briefly mentioned here.

One universal preventive intervention (defined as an intervention for the general public or a whole population group) is the deescalation of conflicts that may lead to war, genocide, or civil war. Leaders are able to diminish hostility (as was done by Gorbachev and Reagan, by Sadat's trip to Jerusalem, or by Mandela and de Klerk) and can be stimulated by the international or the local community to decrease a hostile atmosphere. This attitude of leaders is paramount for a process of reconciliation among the population and a prerequisite for the prevention of further retaliation. In addition to reinforcement of peace-increasing initiatives such as the Nobel prize for peace, the (inter)national community should see to it that perpetrators of gross violations of human rights or war criminals are brought to justice (as happened in the war tribunal on ex-Yugoslavia). Another important universal preventive activity is to work towards political solutions that allow for voluntary migration or repatriation to the place of origin. This has recently been achieved for hundreds of thousands of refugees in Cambodia and Mozambique, and less successfully in Afghanistan.

In the coming decades arms control may become one of the most important universal preventive interventions of the UN. The decrease of the nuclear threat can be paralleled by a prohibition on possession of large stocks of conventional arms that cannot be justified as means for self-defense. The international community could start with banning 'innocent' arms such as anti-personnel land mines. Despite the 1981 Land Mines Protocol designed to protect civilians, the tens of millions of anti-personnel mines placed worldwide results in tens of thousands of victims a year, mostly mothers and children. One out of every 236 Cambodians and one out of 1250 Vietnamese is handicapped as a result of the war, and for every mine victim who makes it to a hospital, another will die in the fields or on the way to hospital (Asia Watch, 1991).

In the context of prevention, human rights advocacy is regarded as a form of selective and indicated prevention (selective preventive interventions are targeted to individuals or a subgroup at risk; indicated preventive interventions are targeted to high-risk individuals). An international forum on this issue concluded that every state has the responsibility to redress human rights violations and to enable victims to exercise their right to reparation (Van Boven et al., 1992). The UN and other intergovernmental organizations at the global and the regional level should support and assist a proper consideration and management of reparation at national levels. Compensation is a form of reparation that is to be paid in cash or to be provided in kind. The latter includes health and mental health care, employment, housing, education and land (Van Boven et al., 1992). The IPSER-WHO program is a means of providing reparation for victims of gross violations of human rights. Moreover, since the program engages in epidemiological studies of traumatic events and their psychological and psychopathological consequences, it verifies facts and helps to disclose the truth. This is in itself a form of non-monetary reparation serving the moral and social welfare of the victims. It is to be hoped that further disclosure of the impact of regular or low intensity warfare on individuals and families may have some preventive effect in the future.

With regard to the prevention of the consequences of natural disaster, it is obvious that a number of (inter)national initiatives can have a preventive effect. For example, higher quality standards for building in earthquake-prone areas or for the construction of nuclear power stations, accessibility of land in areas with land slides, better alarm systems for floods, and sheltered areas or evacuation plans in areas which are hit by vulcano eruptions or typhoons would be (inter)national preventive iniatives.

Prevention on the Level of the Community

Previous Initiatives

Duncan and Kang (1985) developed a mental health promotion program for the resettlement of Khmer refugee children in a Catholic area in the U.S. All children reported sleep disturbances, frequently characterized by dreams or nightmares about lost family members, and many reported disturbing visits of spirits, including parents and grandparents. The authors recognized the tremendous acculturative stress these young people were likely to experience given their migration to the U.S. The main components of their prevention program included three Theravada Buddhist ceremonies and rituals honoring the children's dead family. The unaccompanied refugee minor was the central figure in one of these ceremonies. In addition to working through loss and grief, the child was able to begin seeing the foster family, their friends, and the agency's caseworkers as sources of support. These preventive interventions reinforced the integration mode of acculturation by retaining important Buddhist values and traditions within a Catholic resettlement agency's program (Williams & Berry, 1991).

Based on his work with Indo-Chinese children in the U.S., Eisenbruch (1991) launched the term cultural bereavement which he defines as "the experience of the uprooted person or group resulting from loss of social structures, cultural values and self-identity: the person or group continues to live in the past, is visited by supernatural forces from the past while asleep or awake, suffers feelings of guilt over abandoning culture and homeland, feels pain if memories of the past begin to fade, but finds constant images of the past (including traumatic images) intruding into daily life, yearns to complete obligations to the dead, and feels stricken by anxieties, morbid thoughts, and anger that mar the ability to get on with daily life." Within the framework of prevention, this somewhat elusive concept of cultural bereavement has the advantage of offering an approach to grief and posttraumatic stress on the level of the group or the community. In an empirical study Eisenbruch (1991) examined the differences in cultural bereavement between two groups of unaccompanied and detached refugee adolescents fostered in Cambodian group care in Australia and in foster families in the U.S.. He found that the cultural bereavement among those in the U.S. was significantly greater than that found among their counterparts in Australia, where there was somewhat less pressure to leave the old culture behind, and where the children were encouraged to participate in traditional ceremonies. The ceremonies helped the survivors to come to terms with their losses; make the world a safer place for them; reduce the tension between life in "this world" of the host society and the "Khmer" other world which is internalized in the person; and consolidate their sense of self. Ceremonies were culturally coded "corrective emotional experiences," that many children in need were otherwise denied.

Regarding prevention, a number of authors have mentioned the importance of attitude change, prejudice reduction, empathy training, and increase of prosocial behavior, as well as aggression reduction. For example, Ilaz (in Williams & Berry, 1991) used a multidimensional approach to changing children's attitudes toward people with origins in India. Among other activities, students were encouraged to literally step into the shoes of a child from India and to sense and express their feelings and thoughts. Using a pretest-posttest design, significant changes in attitudes were found immediately after, and again three months after the completion of the program. Such a school-based demonstration of attitude change is encouraging for those who seek to prevent psychological problems from arising for acculturating groups and individuals that result from their experience of negative attitudes, prejudice, and discrimination (cf. Williams & Berry, 1991).

Feshbach (1993) reviewed data indicating that empathy is a meaningful psychological attribute associated with lesser degrees of aggression in children and in adults. Empathy is also associated with prosocial behaviors, more consistently for adults than for children. The data further indicate that empathy is linked to significant developmental experiences of the child. Physical abuse, family conflict and lack of cohesion impede empathy in boys and girls. In contrast, a non-competitive paternal focus facilitates empathy in boys and a positive accepting maternal attitude that permits independence is conducive to the development of empathy in girls.

Goldstein (1993) regards the ways in which currently employed interventions designed to reduce human aggression, (i.e. belief in control, catharsis and cohabitation in the sense that aggression is "human nature"), are ineffective and hold little potential for successful outcomes. In his view, intervention planning and implementation must become much more complex, prescriptive, situational and learning based. Regarding complexity of cause and solution he provides the example of school violence: in order to reduce school violence, to have even a modest chance of enduring success, interventions must not only be oriented towards the aggressor, but also at the levels of the teacher, school administration and organization, and the larger community context. With regard to learning, Goldstein (1993) shows that a major source of aggressive behavior is human learning. Applying some behavioral principles to the situations of soldiers in countries such as Bosnia, Kroatia, Liberia, Mozambique, Angola and Uganda shows the explanatory value of Bandura's theory that behavior such as aggression is learned in two ways, directly or vicariously. Direct learning follows from reinforced practice where the behavior is tried and brings the direct result. For example, walking into a village and demanding at the point of a gun may not only provide food or sex, but also a sense of mastering of a potential life-threatening war situation. Vicarious learning occurs by observing others behave aggressively and receive reward from doing so. The inter-generational transmission of abusive parental child rearing practices stands in empirical support of the aggression-as-vicariously-learned theme that can play a role in adult life. In the case of the soldier, if he sees the success of his colleague's aggression towards the villagers, by vicarious learning he learns the principle of "might makes right." Vicarious learning partially explains what Niebuhr (1932) argues in his classic Moral Man and Immoral Society, that there is "a basic difference between the morality of individuals and the morality of collectives." Goldstein (1993) has developed an Aggression Replacement Training that fits the concept of secondary prevention on the community level. His multi-method, multi-channel interventions are designed to decrease the likelihood of antisocial behaviors and increase the likelihood of prosocial, alternative behaviors. They consist of structured learning (modeling of lacking skills, role playing, performance feedback, transfer training of skills to the real world), anger control training (teaching what not to do in anger-instigating situations), and moral education (which is cognitive in nature). A few preventive intervention programs using a randomized controlled trial design have successfully tried to influence aggressive and antisocial behavior. Examples are the program of Kellam and Rebock (1992) using Mastery Learning and the Good Behavior Game as interventions, and the programs of Olweus (1991) and Shure and Spivack (1982).

An Approach to Prevention of Community Stress

The IPSER-WHO methodology functions as a blueprint for disaster-stricken areas that should be tailored to local circumstances. One of the main objectives of our model is to identify problems and stressors in the specific socio-cultural setting in order to define preventive targets. In order to decrease the distance to the target population, the first step is to contact male and female government officials from every administrative level. A discussion is held on the character and the scope of the problems they confront due to the consequences of the disaster. Subsequently, focus groups of key informants are formed on the level of the community (De Jong et al., 1994). They are interviewed on the following topics: (1) their opinion about the consequences of the man-made or natural disaster as perceived by the community; (2) opinions about positive coping strategies and protective modifiers (e.g. mutual help, cultural bereavement, religious beliefs/possession cults, the creation of social networks and/or political movements); (3) help-seeking behavior of victims (e.g. whether support was sought from the head of the family, village chief, health worker, healer, priest); and (4) information about health care facilities, relief organizations, local or allopathic practitioners, healing cults, and other formal and cultural help providers.

Simultaneously, an anthropologist or sociologist engages in participant observation among healers and healing cults in order to obtain insight into the problems of the community, families and children, about trauma related folk illnesses and idioms of distress and about rituals. The latter include healing, purification, reconciliation and mourning rituals as well as processes of cultural bereavement related to these rituals. The information collected by the social scientist serves both to adapt the program and the training materials to the local culture, as well as to engage the healers in the program. The healers are requested to share part of their knowledge with the program representatives, while being offered complementary training on the psychological effects of man-made or natural disaster and the possibilities to deal with these consequences.

Preventive Interventions at the Community Level: Current Iniatives

Based on the information collected, psychosocial preventive interventions are designed and implemented on the level of the community. Within the IPSER-WHO program, universal preventive interventions focus on security and empowerment, in the sense of decreasing dependency, of stimulating rural development, and of strengthening social support. These interventions lead to communal pride and a psychological sense of community (Sarason, 1974), and initiate what Hobfoll calls resource gain cycles (Hobfoll, Briggs, & Wells, this volume).

Universal prevention: Security

After having survived a natural diaster or after a successful escape from a war zone, survivors are often re-traumatized by robbers or gangs of armed bandits, shelling, ambushes or land mines. In refugee camps the relief workers and expatriates often live in designated areas, wherein the refugees often have to protect themselves. A simple preventive measure is to create as safe an environment as possible, especially in camps with a majority of women and children.

From a medical point of view, security measures can reduce the neuropsychiatric consequences of head trauma. Head trauma is common among victims of war or torture victims, and its consequences often are hard to differentiate from post-traumatic stress syndromes.

Universal prevention: Decreasing dependency

Most programs for refugees or victims of disasters are emergency-oriented in material and logistic terms. In addition to priorities such as food and shelter, the victims are often reduced to people without a psyche, an attitude partially due to the fear that their problems may be endless. Therefore, most relief agencies do not regard psychological problems as an issue. In a sense they contribute to the "conspiracy of silence" as it has been described in the literature on the post-Holocaust era. Both in developing countries and in the West, refugee camps easily become "total institutions" in Goffman's (1961) sense. Subsequently, a dependency syndrome may develop that reinforces the learned helplessness that quickly emerges in the wake of war or natural disaster. This can happen especially in those camps that reproduce the authoritarian regimes from which the refugees escaped, often articulated by the rather militarist approach of many relief agencies.

To complete the vicious circle, after imposing learned dependency the international donor agencies complain about the dependent and inert behavior of the refugees. After the previous impact of the trauma, this process easily results in a form of secondary traumatization.

To prevent the secondary traumatization from taking place, one may take another stance by seeing refugees as resilient people living in cultures that have often developed ingenious coping strategies. By empowering the refugees, our program tries to break the vicious circle of disempowerment by eliciting domains of preventive activities. For example, wherever possible women and men are engaged in the management and administration of the area; they are involved in the organization of tasks in the camp (helping in PHC-activities such as filling in vaccination cards, implementing hygiene, helping with health education; distributing food; and helping in education). These acivities are one aspect of empowerment and restoring a sense of control.

Universal prevention: Rural development. As is well known, traumatized people are not only confronted with a sense of hopelessness, helplessness and a feeling of loss of control, but they are also damaged in their basic sense of invulnerability which we all need in order to be able to carry on our lives. Therefore, another important example of universal prevention at the community level is the stimulation of rural development, especially among populations that are being displaced for long periods of time. Rural development helps to restore a sense of control and to create a perspective for the future. The IPSER-WHO program as such does not carry final responsibility for rural development. Collaboration with different levels of the community, the government and international organizations such as Non-Governmental

Organizations (NGOs) are sought to implement this part of the program. Rural development is not only a priority in order to prevent economic deprivation, it also fosters self-reliance by stimulating a sustainable agricultural system and by generating income for refugees. This can be realized by setting up small-scale technological projects and by vocational skills training (palm oil presses, leather handicraft, fishing, pottery, blacksmithing), improving the water supply, diversifying food crops and cash crops, or reforestation. One of our motives to choose East-Moyo in North-Uganda as an intervention area to work among Sudanese refugees was the presence of a range of rural development initiatives. Another aspect that we consider of utmost importance to prevent a return of war, is a proper demobilization of soldiers by providing them a possibility for income generation either by distributing land or by teaching them vocational skills. In Mozambique our program has been involved in advising the government on how to demobilize its army using these methods.

Rural development also has a selective preventive effect in a physical sense by decreasing malnutrition which may develop into pellagra and subsequently into dementia.

Universal and Selective Prevention Aimed at Children and the Family

A third area of prevention at the community level is family reunion. Children and their mothers constitute about 50 to 70% of the world's refugee population, especially in technologically less advanced countries (UNHCR, 1990). In Mozambique about two thirds of the children were abducted over the last ten years, 77% of the children witnessed murder, 51% have been physically abused, 28% were trained for combat, and about half of the children witnessed other atrocities such as cutting off the hands, penis, ears, nose or mouth of adults (Boothby, 1991; Geffray, 1990; Minter, 1989; Richman et al., 1989). Similar events took place in Cambodia in the period 1975-1979. A study of 3-9 year olds in Lebanon discovered that war was the major topic of conversation for 96% of the children, of play for 80%, and of drawing for 80% (Abu Nasr, 1985). The drawings of Ugandan refugee children show their preoccupation with their experiences of violence, death and starvation; pictures of soldiers shooting their mothers, infants lying bleeding to death, decapitations, dogs eating human corpses, and other grotesque subjects. A year later these children were still drawing like this (Harrel-Bond, 1986).

A universal preventive intervention for children, akin to health promotion, tries to promote the wellbeing of children who have suffered intense trauma. In our program non-professionals have to play an important role, especially in technologically less developed countries, where one often has to resort to less trained persons in order to compensate for a lack of an elaborate therapeutic potential. Working in groups is the most effective course because of the importance of contact and the mutual support from fellow-sufferers (Paardekoper, 1994; Udwin, 1993). We are starting up a program for children, using a variety of activities. These include games, role playing, drawing, writing and telling stories, music, puppet theatre and feasts. A pilot program with these activities has taken place in Croatia (Trapman, 1994).

Another aim of our program is the selective prevention of disturbed personality development among children. By taking away damaging factors that result in developmental interference among children, the children are able to regain their natural development or at least to reduce the long-term negative effects on their personalities. The program also aims at indicated preventive interventions for high-risk children with potentially chronic disorders such as dumb silent withdrawal and mutism, hyperactivity with violent behavior, or chronic regression to an earlier devlopmental stage. On the community level we try to achieve this by supporting the social network, by strengthening existing coping skills, by training school teachers, and by various activities that I will breifly review.

As a guidepost, we assumed that supportive network, preferably a family network is an important protective variable for traumatized children. Our program disapproves of western-style orphanages that in several technologically less advanced countries have created additional problems such as being a breeding place for banditism and prostitution. Orphans or children from disrupted families are instead accomodated within their extended families or within foster families, while simultaneously trying to assess whether one or both parents or other first or second grade family members are still alive. The same approach is often used by relief agencies. For example, during the pilot phase of our program in North-Kenya, the camp was split up in areas with large signs that indicated names of cities in South-Sudan from where most of the refugees originated. By choosing a living place in an area that assembled people from their place of origin, the refugees were often able to trace family members.

Another method used in the same camp is the regrouping of about twelve thousand boys and adolescents-who wandered about five years from Sudan to Ethiopia and Kenya-in groups of about 50 youngsters under the supervision of an adult or a foster family. In Mozambique, during the last years a successful program for family reunion has been implemented. Sometimes family reunification has to be realized with precaution. In Cambodia, women who were victims of rape were so ashamed that at the time of reunion with their family, they were unable to pluck up courage to describe their misfortune to their husbands-even years after separation from their family and children-or preferred to commit suicide (Hiegel & Landrac, 1990).

With the already mentioned method of focus groups or with the help of participant observation we try to get insight into existing coping skills in order to strengthen them. Among the Dingka from South-Sudan, the adolescent boys with whom we worked in North-Kenya not only make poems for their initiation bull, but they also write poems about the traumatic events they experienced during the war in Sudan or during the time they tried to escape the circumscription by one of the armed factions in South-Sudan. They also tell each other dreams and analyze them in the group, which they consider as a way of healing the wounds of the past. In addition, they compose songs, also about severe problems, because song making plays an important role in Dinka culture (Deng, 1972).

One of the categories of professionals trained by our program are school teachers. We utilize a prevention and treatment system incorporating triage, evaluation, and involvement of a network of community resources that aid in early identification and referral for prompt treatment. Since teachers have daily contacts with the children, they get additional training to identify children with serious problems and to develop skills to support these children, to prevent scapegoating, and to refer them when necessary. A number of teachers also learn basic counseling techniques to assist children to cope with their trauma. By the training of teachers the program provides orphans and ex-boy soldiers (e.g., in Mozambique) with a person who is willing and able to listen to their story without condemning the child. So far, the general tendency is to deny the child's trauma and to press the child to continue living without mourning the past. This imposed coping strategy often originates in the coping style of the adult. Since teachers, and often health workers as well, themselves are often so seriously traumatized that they have difficulties in supporting their pupils, the participants of the training program first learn to work through their own trauma in order to be able to help the children.

Prevention on the Level of the Family and the Individual

Universal Preventive Interventions

One preventive intervention that simultaneously has an important physical preventive effect is the improvement of the basic physical aspects of the camp. This includes developing acceptable amounts of water, decreased overcrowding, alloting some land to grow vegetables, more varied diets, and drainage of the terrain. In addition, we try to empower the disaster victims by tracing professionals from the administration of the camp or by snow ball sampling among the camp inhabitants. We involve them in the camp and allow them as much employment as possible. For example, they may provide interpreter services for management, community development, or somatic and psychosocial consultations. Similarly, we involve teachers in education programs for children and adults, engage primary health care-workers in basic health care and traditional birth attendants in deliveries and birth control. We encourage religious leaders and healers to do ceremonies and rituals, and we stimulate musicians, dancers, story tellers and comics to organize leisure activities.

Treatment

Especially after man-made disasters such as wars, many people suffer from type II trauma (i.e. repetitive serious traumatic events). Among Cambodian, Hmong, Laotian and Vietnamese psychiatric patients in the USA, Mollica (1987) found that

50% of the patients suffered from PTSD. On average these refugee patients had experienced 10 traumatic events such as lack of food, water, or shelter, imprisonment, war injury, sexual abuse, or witnessing death or murder. During a pilot study among displaced persons in Mozambique (de Jong & Mandlhate, 1992) we found that on average they had experienced six traumatic events, especially lack of food, lack of shelter, forced separation from their family, being close to death, being in a combat situation and murder of family members or friends. Thirteen percent of the women told they had been sexually violated. About 70% of the respondents told the most gruesome stories about the things they had experienced or seen happening before their eyes: people being beaten to death, people dying after bajonetting their abdomen while their intestines are hanging outside, men bleeding to death after their genitals have been cut off, or the cutting off of breasts, ears, or noses. One person saw a house that was set on fire with a child inside. Several people had to kill others. One very depressed woman told that after having been kidnapped and taken to a Renamo area, she was forced to kill two other persons otherwise she would have been shot. She was raped and conceived a child with a Renamo soldier. When she finally succeeded in escaping she was rejected by her husband.

It is not naive to think that our professions can assist in providing some sort of relief in these circumstances, although it surely is naive to think that community-oriented preventive measures alone are sufficient to deal with this kind of multiple traumatization. Our program therefore provides support to set up self-help groups and trains and supervises hundreds to thousands of primary health care-workers, teachers, healers and other community workers. The aim of these efforts is treatment (formerly secondary prevention). This implies empowering people to help themselves, to teach them to identify, manage or refer psychosocial problems once they occur, and to train PHC-workers and other community workers to treat a number of priority conditions.

Self-Help Groups. Rape victims are supported by teaching relief workers to identify and assist victims of rape. The workers get instructions on respecting confidentiality, on the possibility that the victim has contracted a venereal disease, on ending the social isolation of the victim, and on organizing support groups (Wali, 1992). For each age group of children, groups are set up in which both the mothers and the children participate. The groups learn how to protect the mental health of the children in the artificial environment in which they live, and how to practice culturally appropriate child stimulation exercises (Williamson, 1992).

Training primary health care-workers. Our program uses a training-the-trainer-approach (de Jong et al., 1994). The trainees who gradually become trainers themselves, learn how to set up a public mental health program, how to design a program for psychosocial and rural development interventions, and how to adapt the program to the local culture. In order to identify and manage psychosocial problems among disaster-survivors, the training courses consist of:

(1) An introduction to counseling, stress and psychotrauma. The training is based on the elicitation of the participants' own experience with dislocation,

disruption of their social network, their acculturation to another culture, and the other traumas which they experienced being a disaster victim.

(2) The assessment of the seriousness of the participants' own stress responses with the help of two instruments. This assessment is conducted before and after the training course. A similar before-after assessment is used for various interventions on families and individuals.

(3) Common stress responses and how to deal with them. During this part of the course the trainees learn counseling techniques and eclectic directive psychotherapeutic techniques. Simultaneously, the trainees exercise their acquired psychosocial skills with each other, and deal with their own traumas. This part of the course follows the WHO/UNHCR Refugee Mental Health Manual (De Jong & Clarke, 1992) and includes group and individual support regarding: (a) stress and the use of relaxation techniques; (b) the recognition and management of functional complaints; (c) traumatized children with their parents; (d) community support in dealing with alcohol and drug problems; (e) self-help groups for women who are victims of rape trauma; (f) torture victims and victims of serious violence; (g) the collaboration with healers.

Maintenance (Formerly Tertiary Prevention)

A number of persons who are hit by a disaster or who had prior psychiatric problems need psychiatric assistance. After the earthquake in Managua, postdisaster admissions for neurosis rose by 209% in the first three months, new cases of psychosis declined 17%, while readmissions of psychosis jumped 49% in the postearthquake year (Ahearn & Riza Castellón, 1978). This increase was attributed to the social disorganization after the earthquake, both on the level of the family and on the level of services.

In order to reduce chronicity and prevent complications among people with more serious psychopathology, in the IPSER-WHO program a large number of primary health care-workers receive training which is similar to the training provided within the framework of a WHO-study (Harding et al., 1983; Sartorius & Harding, 1983; de Jong, 1987). The training focuses on the psychiatric consequences of trauma. Participants receive training on the treatment of the mentally ill and on the integration of mental health into their primary health care-activities. During this part of the training they learn how to identify and manage serious stress responses and psychiatric disorders. For health care workers who only received limited training, basic flow charts are most appropriate. For those with more training the corresponding section in the WHO/UNHCR Refugee Mental Health Manual is used. In addition to theory, practical exercises play an important role.

Conclusions

Posttraumatic stress syndrome can be prevented by eliminating the traumatic event or by reducing its consequences. The multi-modal preventive interventions mentioned in this chapter involve different societal levels, descending from the (inter)national level to communities of traumatized people, families and individuals. The preventive interventions can be applied in an eclectic way in accordance with the specific man-made or natural post-disaster situation.

Mental health professionals often feel that in public they should refrain from any political stance when war or (auto)genocide occurs. Many prefer to provide therapy instead of raising their voice to the national or international community. Although this attitude may be professionally and politically correct, simultaneously many colleagues have painful and precious information on human right violations or the consequences of wars. In combination with their insight into the psychological mechanisms of escalating conflicts, they possess a powerful resource to sensitize politicians or the community at large. Although this chapter mentions some of the current major political and polemic themes, it emphasizes the prevention of psychosocial and mental health consequences. Following the new definitions for prevention that have recently been formulated by the U.S. Committee on Prevention of Mental Disorders, it distinguishes Universal, Selective and Indicated Preventive Interventions (formerly called primary prevention), Case Identification and Standard Treatment (formerly called secondary prevention), and Maintenenace (formerly called tertiary prevention). Applying these concepts to the (inter)national level, the level of the community, the family and the individual yields a variety of preventive interventions that are currently tested out in an international program in post-war situations. Our experience shows that prevention is a feasible necessary option, especially in technologically less advanced countries. Training primary care workers, teachers or relief workers alone cannot compensate for the lack of psychosocial and mental health professionals that still exists in most post-war situations.

References

Abu-Nasr, J. (1985). Unpublished paper. Institute for Women's Studies in the Arab World. Beirut University College. Beirut.
Ahearn, F.L., R.S. Castellón (1978). Problemas de salud mental despues de una situación de desastre. Boletin, 85, 1-15.
Asia Watch & Physicians for Human Rights (1991). Land Mines in Cambodia. The Coward's War. USA. ISBN 1-56432-001-4.
Boven, van T., Flinterman, C., Grünfeld, F., & Westendorp, I. (1992). Seminar on the right to restitution, compensation and rehabilitation for victims of gross violations of human rights and fundamental freedoms. SIM Special no. 12. University of Limburg. Maastricht.
Cowen, E.L. (1982). Primary prevention research: Barriers, needs and opportunities. Journal of Primary Prevention, 2, 131-137.
de Jong, J.T.V.M. (1987). A descent into African psychiatry. Amsterdam: Royal Tropical Institute.
de Jong, J.T.V.M., Mandlhate, C. (1992). Proposal to the Netherlands Government for a public mental health program on the management and prevention of psychosocial and mental health problems of displaced persons, refugees and returnees within primary care in Mozambique. Maastricht: International Institute for Psychosocial and Socio-Ecological Research.
de Jong, J.T.V.M., L. Clarke (1992). Refugee mental health manual. WHO/UNHCR. Geneva.
de Jong, J.T.V.M., Kaplan, C. D., Ketzer, E., Mandlhate, C., Muller, M., & de Vries, M. W. (1994). Bringing order out of chaos: The identification and prevention of public mental health problems of refugees and victims of organized violence. Submitted to the American Journal of Public Health.
Deng, F.M. (1972). The Dingka of Sudan. New York: Holt, Rinehart & Winston.
Deutsch, M. (1983). The prevention of WW-III: A psychological perspective. Political psychology, 4, 3-31.
deVries, M. W. (this volume). Culture, community and catastrophe: Issues in understanding communities under difficult conditions. In S. E. Hobfoll & M. W. deVries (Eds.), Extreme stress and communities: Impact and intervention. Dordrecht, the Netherlands: Kluwer.
Duncan, J. & Kang, S. (1985). Using Buddhist ritual activities as a foundation for a mental health program for Cambodian children in foster care. J. Duncan, 6920 220nd Street, SW, Mount Lake Terrace, WA 98043, USA.
Eisenbruch, M. (1991). From post-traumatic stress disorder to cultural bereavement: Diagnosis of Southeast Asian refugees. Social Science and Medicine, 33 (6), 673-80.
Fesbach, S. The bases and development of individual aggression. In: Groebel, J, & Hinde, R.A. (eds.) (1993). Aggression and War. New York: Cambridge University Press.

Geffray, C. (1990). La cause des armes au Mozambique. Anthropologie d'une guerre civile. Paris: Karthala.

Goffman, E. (1961). Asylums: Essays on the social situations of mental patients and other inmates. Garden City, NY: Doubleday.

Goldston, S.E. (1986). Primary prevention: Historical perspectives and a blueprint for action. American Psychologist, 41, 453-460.

Gordon, R. (1983). An operational classification of disease prevention. Public Health Reports, 98, 107-109.

Harding, T.W., Climent, C.E., Diop, Mb., Giel, R., Ibrahim, H.H.A., & Srinivasa Murthy, R. et al. (1983). The WHO Collaborative Study on Strategies for Extending mental Health Care, II: The Development of New Research Methods. American Journal of Psychiatry, 983, 140, 1474-1480.

Harrell-Bond, B. (1986). Imposing aid: emergency assistance to refugees. Oxford: Oxford University Press.

Hiegel, J.P., & Landrac, C. (1990). Suicides dans un camp de réfugiés khmers. Nouvelle Revue d'Ethnopsychiatrie, 15, 107-138.

Hobfoll, S. E., Briggs, S., & Wells J. (this volume). Community stress and resources: Actions and reactions. In S. E. Hobfoll & M. W. deVries (Eds.), Extreme stress and communities: Impact and intervention. Dordrecht, the Netherlands: Kluwer.

Kaplan, H.I., & Sadock B. J.(1985). Comprehensive Textbook of Psychiatry, IV. Baltimore. Williams & Wilkins.

Kellam, S. G., & Rebok, G. W. (1992). Building developmental and etiological theory through epidemiologically based preventive intervention trials. In: J. McCord and R. E. Tremblay, Eds. Preventing antisocial behavior: Interventions from birth through adolescence. New York, NY: Guilford Press; 162-195.

Minter, W. (1989). The Mozambican National Resistance Renamo as described by ex-participants. Research report submitted to Ford Foundation and SIDA

Niebuhr, R. [1932] (1960). Moral man and immoral society: a study in ethics and politics. Reprint. New York. Charles Scribner's Sons.

Olweus, D. (1991). Bully/victim problems among schoolchildren: Basic facts and effects of an intervention program. In: K. Rubin and D. Pepler, Eds. The development and treatment of childhood aggression. Hillsdale, NJ: Lawrence Erlbaum Associates.

Paardekoper, B. (1994). A study for a culturally sensitive psychosocial intervention program for South Sudanese refugee children. Utrecht.

Pinderhughes, C. A. (1979). Differential bonding: toward a psychophysiological theory of stereotyping. American Journal of Psychiatry, 136- 33-37.

Punamäki, R. (1989). Political violence and mental health. International Journal of Mental Health, 17, 3-15

Reducing risks for mental disorders: Frontiers for Preventive Intervention Research (1994). National Academy Press, 2101 Constitution Avenue, N.W., Box 285. Washington, D.C.

Richman, N., A. Ratilal, A. Aly (1989). The effects of war on Mozambican children: preliminary findings. Ministry of Education. Maputo.
Sarason, S. B. (1974). The psychological sense of community: prospects for a community psychology. Washington, DC: Jossey-Bass.
Sartorius, N., & Harding, T. W. (1983). The WHO Collaborative Study on Strategies for Extending Mental Health Care, I: The Genesis of the Study. American Journal of Psychiatry, 140, 1470-1473.
Shure, M. B. & Spivack, G. (1982). Interpersonal problem-solving in young children: A cognitive approach to prevention. American Journal of Community Psychology, 10, 341-356.
Trapman, M. J. (1993). Suggestions on the structuring of games and activities for Suncokret. Preliminary draft. Zagreb.
Turshen, M. (1989). The politics of public health. New Brunswick, NJ: Rutgers University Press.
Udwin, O. (1993). Annotation: Children's reactions to traumatic events. Journal of Child Psychology and Psychiatry, 2, p. 115-127.
UNHCR (1990). Report for 1989-1990 and proposed programmes and budget for 1991. Geneva: UN Centre for Documentation on Refugees.
Wali, S. (1992). Helping victims of rape in their communities. In Jong, de J.T.V.M., & Clarke, L. (eds.) Refugee mental health manual. Geneva: WHO/UNHCR.
Westermeyer, J. (1987). Prevention of mental disorders among Hmong refugees in the U.S.: lessons from the period 1976-1986. Social Science and Medicine, 25, 941-947.
Williams, C. L. & Berry J. W. (1991). Primary prevention of acculturative stress among refugees. American Psychologist, 6, 632-641.
Williamson, J. (1992). Helping refugee children. In Jong, de J.T.V.M., & Clarke, L. (eds.) Refugee mental health manual. Geneva: WHO/UNHCR.

THE PATHOGENIC EFFECTS OF WAR STRESS: THE ISRAELI EXPERIENCE

Zahava Solomon
Mental Health Department, Medical Corps, Israel Defense Forces
The Bob Shapell School of Social Work, Tel Aviv University
Tel Aviv, Israel

Israel is a small, stress-ridden country that has known seven full-scale wars and countless hostilities during its 46 years of existence. Our national history over 2000 years has been beset with persecution, pogroms and deportations, culminating in the Nazi Holocaust. The establishment of the State of Israel brought with it the hope for a secure existence, which unfortunately has not been achieved. Israel is a natural laboratory of war stress.

Over the past 12 years, with Israeli Army colleagues at the Army Medical Corps and Tel Aviv University, we have conducted a series of studies of three wars, the 1973 Yom Kippur War, 1982 Lebanon War, and the 1991 Gulf War. We studied men and women, civilians and soldiers, combat stress reaction casualties, heroes and POWs, children, adolescents, adults, and the elderly. We assessed the social, psychological, and physiological outcomes of war-related stress in periods of hours, days, and many years after exposure, and examined the implication of a host of psychological, social, and cultural factors in the genesis of and recovery from war-induced psychopathology.

In this chapter I shall present some of the results of our studies, attesting to the heavy toll of war on civilians and soldiers. More specifically, the following five issues will be presented and discussed:

(1) The clinical manifestations and prevalence of acute psychological reactions during or shortly after exposure to war.
(2) The long term psychological sequelae of war stress.
(3) Delayed onset post traumatic stress disorder.
(4) Reactivation of previous war stress reactions.
(5) Secondary traumatization of people close to traumatized individuals.

Acute Reactions

Very few of the many studies on war stress have focused on real time, immediate reactions. Wartime is obviously a most difficult time to conduct research, as both subjects and researchers are inevitably engrossed in their own survival. With the exception of Rachman's study of the Blitz in London (Rachman, 1990) and Saigh's study of students in Beirut (Saigh, 1984), very little has been done in this area.

These works dispelled three prevalent myths about people's behavior in mass catastrophes: the myth of panic, the myth of looting, and the myth of shock (Drabek, 1986). They showed that most people remain calm and keep their wits about them and that there is generally very little looting. We examined these and other aspects of civilian behavior during the recent Gulf War.

Reactions of Civilians During the Gulf War

In the midst of the crisis, and for months prior to this war, the threat of chemical attack hung over Israelis' heads. Although chemical attacks never materialized, the threat was imminent. Conventional missile attacks, 18 in all, caused destruction of property, bodily injury, and some loss of life. Through it all, the government policy of restraint meant that the army was kept tightly leashed, leaving the civilian population feeling vulnerable and defenseless. My colleagues and I (Bleich, Dycian, Koslowsky, Solomon & Wiener, 1992) examined the reactions of the general civilian population to these stressors as reflected in emergency hospital admissions, and the reactions of persons who were evacuated from their homes after attacks.

Throughout the war there were 1,059 war-related hospital emergency room admissions. Of these, only 22% were direct casualties, who were injured by the missiles or flying debris. 78% were indirect casualties, whose "injuries" stemmed from their fear when the air raid alerts were sounded. Of these, 11 died: 7 by suffocation due to faulty use of the gas masks and 4 due to heart attack. That is, more people died from fear than from actual exposure to the missiles. Evidently, under certain circumstances fear may be not only distressing, but also fatal. A quarter of all emergency hospital admissions had suffered physical injuries while rushing to safety at the sound of the warning siren, or had needlessly injected themselves with Atropine (the nerve gas antidote that was distributed to all residents of Israel before the outbreak of the war). An astonishing number of admissions, 554, 51% in all, came with symptoms of acute psychological distress.

We examined patterns of indirect injuries according to different stages of the war. As can be seen from Figure 1, most of the admissions for acute stress or for self-injected Atropine came right after the first missile attack. Thereafter the numbers dropped sharply. This, along with other measures (Solomon, 1995), points to progressive habituation to the threat and perhaps a quick learning process.

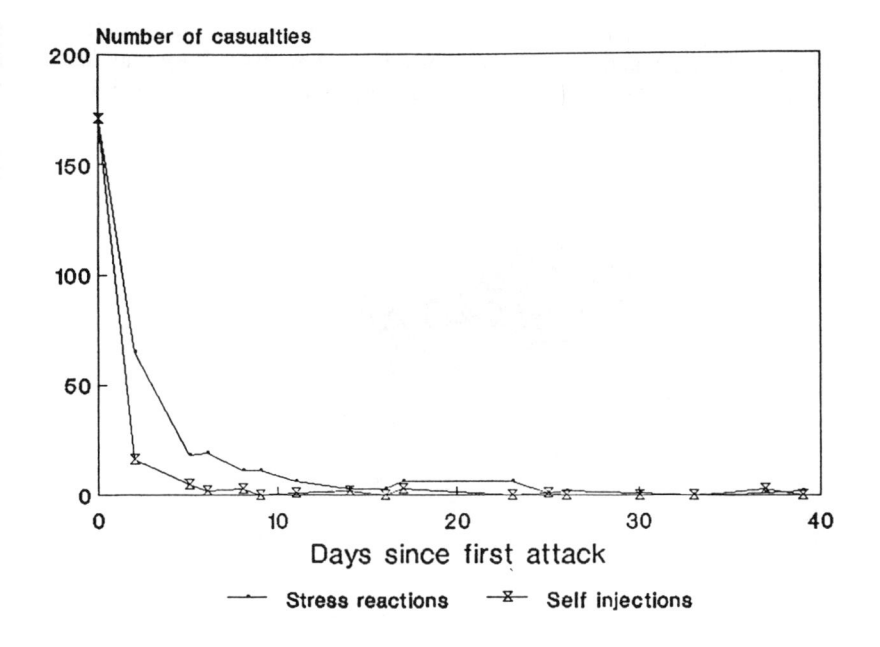

Figure 1: Stress reactions and injections by time

Evacuees During the Gulf War

Acute reactions were also assessed among evacuees whose homes were damaged or destroyed in the missile attacks. Our findings showed that one week after the missile strike that forced them to leave their homes, most evacuees manifested a very high level of distress (Solomon et al., 1993). Their state and trait anxiety scores exceeded those reported among Lebanese one week after heavy shelling of Beirut (Saigh, 1988). As many as 80% of those assessed displayed a constellation of symptoms consistent with DSM-III-R criteria (APA, 1987) for diagnosis of PTSD (Solomon et al., 1993). While it is of course impossible to consider a formal diagnosis of PTSD so soon after a traumatic event, this finding suggests that most people who were directly affected by the attacks initially respond with a fairly predictable pattern of distress symptoms, even if, in most cases, these abate with time.

Combat Stress Reaction Among Combatants

These acute stress symptoms are displayed most frequently and strongly by soldiers who break down in battle. They form what is today known as "combat stress reaction" or CSR; sometimes termed "battle fatigue" or "battle shock" (Kormos, 1978). CSR encompasses a variety of combat induced polymorphous behavioral, cognitive and affective responses, that impair the soldier's functioning. The symptoms may include dissociative states, confusion, disorientation, overreaction or inappropriate response to minor threat, restlessness, agitation, stupor, motor retardation, uncontrolled affects, conversion symptoms, and somatic manifestations of anxiety. They may also include diminished interest in things that were commonly meaningful to the soldier, reduced social interaction and mistrust (Solomon, 1993).

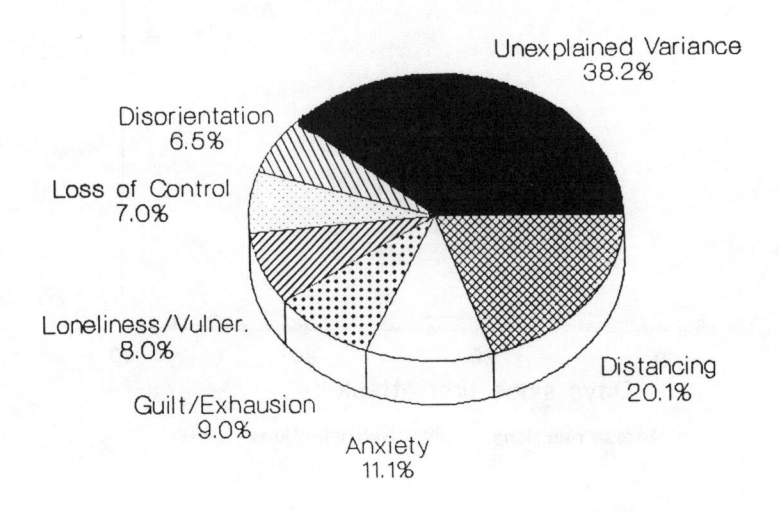

Figure 2: CSR Factors

- Unexplained Variance 38.2%
- Disorientation 6.5%
- Loss of Control 7.0%
- Loneliness/Vulner. 8.0%
- Guilt/Exhausion 9.0%
- Anxiety 11.1%
- Distancing 20.1%

Israeli clinicians who treated the CSR casualties of the Lebanon War, like their colleagues in other countries in other wars, observed a wide range of symptoms. For the most part, the CSR manifestations observed in the Lebanon War were quite similar to those observed in other wars and other armies (e.g., Bailey, Williams, Komora, Salmon & Fenton, 1929). In the past, several taxonomies of CSR were proposed, all based on clinical impressions (e.g., Cavenar & Nash, 1976; Grinker, 1945). Inspection of clinical features of CSR in Lebanon War revealed that 17 manifestations were reported in 10% or more of casualties. Several of them were particularly widespread: acute anxiety (48%), fear of death (26%), psychic numbing (18%), and helplessness (17%). In an attempt to systematically study this clinical entity we subjected the manifestations with prevalence of more than 10% to factor analysis. As can be seen in Figure 2, six main factors explaining 62% of the variance were derived. These included: distancing-psychic numbing, anxiety, guilt and exhaustion, loneliness and vulnerability, and loss of control and disorientation (Solomon, 1993; Solomon, Mikulincer & Benbenishty, 1989). In general, the taxonomy obtained here is consisted with the one proposed by the U.S. Army (Bartmeier, 1946).

In the Lebanon War, combat stress reaction casualties constituted 23% of all Israeli casualties (Solomon, 1993). In the 12 years after the war, the number of CSR casualties <u>tripled</u> due to the emergence of delayed reactions (Solomon, Singer & Blumenfeld, in preparation). In the Yom Kippur War, estimated CSR rates ranged between 10% and 30% of all casualties (Noy, 1991). The Israeli experience is consistent with repeated evidence from other armies the CSR is an inevitable consequence of any war.

The Long Term Sequelae of War Stress

To examine the long term effects of combat stress, we conducted two extensive multi-cohort longitudinal research projects: one followed the Yom Kippur War (Solomon, Neria, Ohry, Waysman & Ginzburg, 1994), the other following the Lebanon War (Solomon, 1993).

In each study we examined two groups: CSR casualties, consisting of soldiers who were diagnosed and treated for CSR during the war, and matched controls. Veterans of the Yom Kippur War were followed 18 years after the Yom Kippur battles. Veterans of the Lebanon War were studied for three consecutive years after the war ended. Both studies assessed a wide range of possible outcomes, including posttraumatic residues, psychiatric symptomatology, somatic complaints, illness and health related behaviors, cognitive schemata, positive and negative changes and a host of physiological outcomes. The same measures were employed in both studies to allow comparison.

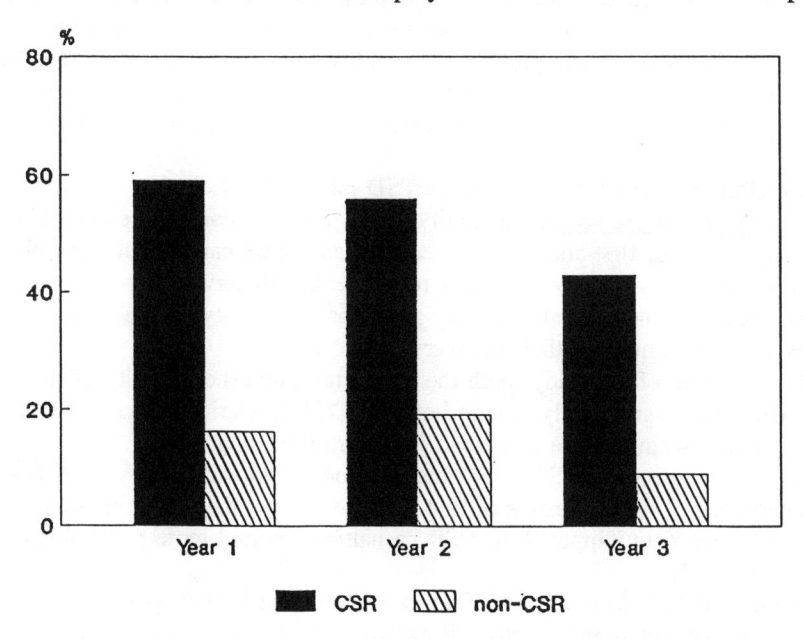

Figure 3: PTSD Rates by Study Group and Time

Since the posttraumatic stress syndrome is the most common and conspicuous long-term consequence of trauma, we first assessed the rates, type, and intensity of PTSD among CSR casualties and compared non-CSR controls (Solomon, 1993). Figure 3 presents the findings of the Lebanon follow-up.

Inspecting these figures it becomes clear that for a large proportion of Israeli combatants, the trauma of war left enduring and disruptive sequelae. Among the identified CSR casualties, PTSD rates were quite high in all three years of the study: 59% one year after Lebanon; 56% two years later; and 43% three years later. In other words, nearly half of the soldiers who sustained a CSR on the battlefield were still suffering from a full-blown <u>diagnosable</u> disorder three years after their participation in battle. Clearly, for a large proportion of combatants, war does not end when the shooting stops. For many CSR casualties of the Lebanon War, the wartime breakdown was not a transient episode, but crystallized into chronic PTSD from which recovery, if and when it came, was slow.

The control group also showed substantial, if not nearly as dramatic PTSD rates. Sixteen percent of controls were diagnosed with PTSD the first year after Lebanon, 19% the second year, and 9% the third year. It is important to note, that this is a diagnosable disorder, yet these afflicted men did not seek help. These figures point to the detrimental impact of war on men who weathered the immediate stress of combat without a visible breakdown and resumed their lives without applying for assistance. Undoubtedly, many were not aware that they had a diagnoseable disorder or believed that their symptoms were a natural and inevitable outcome of their harrowing experiences on the front. Others probably did realize their plight, but were reluctant to seek help. It is all too likely that these silent PTSD veterans are a mere fraction of a much larger number of psychiatric casualties of war whose distress is similarly unidentified and untreated.

If we accept the assessment that these PTSD rates in the Lebanon War were high, the question: <u>why they are so high</u> naturally arises. Here, of course, we can only offer speculations. When our first and second measurements were carried out, the Lebanon War had not completely ended. All of our respondents still served in Israel's reserve forces and could have been recalled at any point for active duty on the front. This threat may well have impeded their recovery.

By the third year of the study, both the PTSD rates and the intensity of the syndrome decreased significantly among both the CSR casualties and controls. Time and circumstances seem to have combined in fostering healing.

Similar amelioration of PTSD over time was found following the Yom Kippur War (Solomon et al., 1994). Results of that follow-up show that 18 years after their participation in the Yom Kippur War, CSR casualties reported more psychological distress than controls.

Although a gradual decline in PTSD rates was evident in both groups, the decrease was faster among the controls. Rates among controls dropped from 13% to 3% over time, while rates among former casualties dropped from 37% to only 13%.

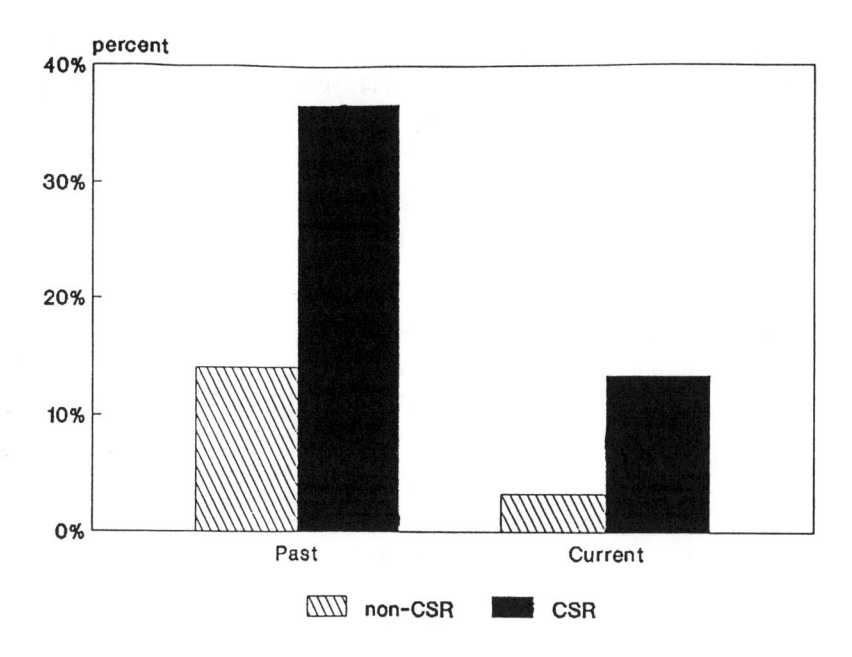

Figure 4: PTSD Rates by Study Group and Time

Results of both studies clearly demonstrate the strong association between acute CSR sustained during war and subsequent PTSD and the stress impact of war for those who do not have a CSR. We know of no other studies that directly assessed the connection between CSR and PTSD. Nevertheless, studies of Vietnam veterans (without reference to whether or not they had a CSR episode) found rates of PTSD ranging from 15% to 48% (Egendorf, Kadushin, Laufer, Rotbarth & Solan, 1981; Kulka et al., 1988; Walker & Cavenar, 1982), indicating a similar risk factor in combat exposure.

The differences in PTSD in the CSR and control groups were not only quantitative but also qualitative. The groups differed qualitatively in the number and duration of their symptoms, with the CSR group reporting a larger number of symptoms and longer duration of symptoms than the controls (Solomon et al., 1994).

There are several possible explanations for the greater prevalence, intensity, and duration of PTSD among CSR casualties. First, CSR veterans probably suffered more profound injury than the controls. They were emotionally overwhelmed and experienced profound helplessness that left them with a deep imprint of vulnerability. Second, both the CSR and the labeling it entails severely undermine the afflicted soldiers' self-esteem and social adjustment. This is especially true in Israel, where masculine identity is strongly associated with army service.

The psychological consequences of trauma are not limited to PTSD (e.g., Ohry et al., 1994; Solomon, 1993). Our findings showed that, years after the fighting, CSR casualties of both the Yom Kippur and Lebanon wars similarly reported:
(1) wider and more severe generalized psychiatric symptomatology than controls.
(2) more impairment in social functioning.
(3) more somatic complaints and changes in health-related behaviors such as increased smoking, and
(4) lower self-efficacy.

Interestingly, neither alcohol nor drug consumption increased after the war. This, however, may be due to the low rates of substance abuse in Israel. In addition, despite the great differences in the two wars, the CSR casualties of both wars suffered from similar co-morbidity including elevated levels of anxiety, depression, hostility, and obsession-compulsion.

Delayed PTSD

The manifestations of the trauma sometimes are, or seem to be, delayed. Delayed onset occurs when an individual at first appears to respond adaptively to traumatic stress, but then develops psychopathology after an asymptomatic latency period. As mentioned before, the number of psychiatric casualties stemming from the Lebanon war tripled in the 12 years that followed it (Solomon et al., in preparation). This issue raises a considerable amount of interest.

Delayed PTSD was described among WWII veterans (Archibald & Tuddenham, 1965) and survivors of the Holocaust (Neiderland, 1968). Yet, it became a major issue after the Vietnam War. At the same time, the validity of this diagnosis was questioned as some clinicians claimed that malingering, factitious symptoms, drug abuse, and pre-combat psychopathology (e.g., Atkinson, Henderson & Sparr, 1982; Sparr & Pankratz) were mistakenly diagnosed as delayed PTSD.

Assessment of several hundred veterans who sought treatment between six months and five years after the end of the Lebanon War revealed five categories of combat-related PTSD (Solomon, 1993; Solomon, Kotler, Shalev & Lin, 1989).

1. Exacerbation of Subclinical PTSD (33% of cases). These individuals were traumatized on the front in 1982 and suffered uninterruptedly from mild residual PTSD symptoms until accumulated tensions or exposure to subsequent adversity, either military or civilian, resulted in a full-blown PTSD syndrome. Reserve duty was the major military trigger. Other triggers included life events such as marriage and the birth of a child. The veterans in this group sought professional help when their subclinical symptoms were exacerbated.

2. Delayed Help seeking for Chronic PTSD (40% of cases). These veterans were already suffering from chronic PTSD, which DSM-III defines as PTSD

having a six month or longer duration, when they sought psychiatric help. Unlike the soldiers in the previous group who had mild, subclinical symptoms throughout the so-called latency period, these veterans suffered from the full-blown syndrome right from around the time they fought in Lebanon. They sought help not when an external trigger exacerbated their symptoms, but when they could no longer bear their distress usually during reserve duty. These soldiers put a great deal of effort into containing a relatively severe and disruptive disturbance before they finally gave up trying to cope with it on their own. Not infrequently, treatment was initiated by a family member who could no longer endure the pressure that the casualty's symptoms created.

3. Delayed Onset PTSD (10% of cases). These individuals included soldiers who came through the Lebanon War with no apparent psychiatric disturbance, and were asymptomatic and functioned well during and for some time after the war. The latency period lasted from several weeks to several years. Then following exposure to stressful stimuli, their latent disturbance surfaced and they applied for treatment.

4. Other Psychiatric Disorders (4% of cases). This group consisted of veterans who had mild, transient pre-war psychiatric disturbances. They sought help for underlying problems that were either triggered or colored by their war experiences, but that were not originally induced by military events.

5. Reactivation (13% of cases). These veterans were also asymptomatic for a certain period following their participation in the Lebanon War. Most of them experienced a reawakening of their earlier trauma in connection with threatening military stimuli, such as a call-up to the reserve or a change in military unit. In other cases there was no single trigger, but rather the accumulated stress of repeated military exposure to both actual warfare and periodic reserve duty.

In general, our results show that the genuinely delayed onset of CSR was quite rare in our sample. By far the most prevalent phenomenon was delayed help-seeking for ongoing combat-induced disorders of various degrees of severity. The relatively low rates of delayed PTSD can be attributed to the relatively short follow-up period. It is possible that a longer follow-up of our sample would reveal a higher rate of delayed PTSD following a longer latency period and with aging.

These findings should be considered in light of the social context in which the traumatic event took place. In Vietnam, where the highest rates of delayed PTSD were reported (e.g., Boulanger, 1985; Laufer, Gallops & Frey-Wouters, 1984), the wide use of drugs and alcohol may have masked immediate CSR symptoms. In Lebanon, however, substance abuse was relatively rare among Israeli troops and so would not have played a significant role in masking or delaying distress.

Another major contextual difference has to do with the dead and the consolation of the bereaved, which bring comfort and relief that help survivors to complete the mourning process. In the Holocaust, the Nazis pointedly disallowed these rites as part of their overall attempt to dehumanize their victims. In Vietnam, the rites of mourning were not observed on account of the relatively long tours of duty (one year) and the fact that the soldiers were far from home. It might be that the unresolved grief of both Holocaust survivors and Vietnam veterans contributed to their subsequent vulnerability wherein reminders of their loss or other stressors would more readily trigger a reaction at a later date.

In Lebanon, on the other hand, as in other Israeli wars, the IDF made a concerted and well organized effort to encourage the full mourning process. Every possible effort was made to evacuate the dead and bring them to burial in Israel; soldiers knew that nobody would be abandoned on the battlefield; and a special Rabbinical unit was in charge of seeing to the proper rites. Soldiers were routinely given leave to attend funerals and pay consolation calls. The ability to mourn and resolve their grief may have made the soldiers in our sample less vulnerable to the triggering effect of subsequent stressors. These rites may have also served as a reattachment to what S. Sarason (1974) called a psychological sense of community for the soldier.

From a different point of view, Horowitz and Solomon (1978) have suggested that delayed onset may occur only after circumstances allow the individual to sufficiently relax his defenses. Both the long, one-year tours of duty in Vietnam and the constant, unalleviated danger of the Holocaust made it extremely unsafe for people to let down their guard during the events themselves. In Israel, on the other hand, wars are fought very close to home, allowing soldiers frequent home leaves. It may be that the warmth, comfort, and security of the home environment enabled repressed traumatic contents to surface, and be addressed, while the soldiers were still serving in the army.

Furthermore, for the veterans of Lebanon, homecoming at the end of the war was by and large a positive event. Although public opinion on the war was divided, the men who had fought it were welcomed back with respect and affection as brave sons who had risked their lives in defense of the country. For both Vietnam veterans and Holocaust survivors, in contrast, the post-war periods continued to be traumatic. Not only were Vietnam veterans denied a hero's welcome, but they came back to a country that had disowned them, to mass anti-war demonstrations. As for Holocaust survivors, they had no place to come back. Most of their families and communities had been exterminated, their homes and property had been appropriated, and the communities where they had once lived were hostile and rejecting. Then, when many of them finally immigrated to new countries, they had to overcome substantial adversity in rebuilding their lives. In both these groups, the accumulation of stress may have eventually led to the delayed onset of their latent disorder.

Reactivation of Stress Response

The Reactivation of CSR

We became attentive to the subject of reactivation when we repeatedly heard older CSR veterans of the 1982 Lebanon War spontaneously refer to their prior experiences at the front in the 1973 Yom Kippur War. Although many of them had not sought help or were identified as CSR casualties during the earlier war, it became evident that their Lebanon reactions, in fact, brought back to their consciousness their experiences of nine years earlier. We found 4 distinct types of reactivation (Solomon, Garb, Bleich, & Grupper, 1987):

1. Uncomplicated Reactivation. These veterans seemed to have completely recovered from their 1973 Yom Kippur CSR. They were virtually symptom-free between the wars. The first indication that all was not well came with their breakdown in the 1982 Lebanon War, which was generally precipitated by a threatening incident directly reminiscent of their Yom Kippur experience.

The rest of the cases are more aptly termed exacerbated PTSD. Here the earlier CSR left more visible residuals, and veterans continued to suffer from residual symptoms. Moreover, these men were sufficiently vulnerable so that their second reaction could be triggered by an incident unrelated to the earlier trauma and, in many cases, one that did not pose a direct or immediate danger. The exacerbated PTSD cases were subdivided into three groups:

2. The Specific Sensitivity group consisted of men who suffered from mild, diffuse PTSD symptoms that did not interfere with their day to day functioning, and from heightened sensitivity to military stimuli. During reserve duty they tended to be tense and withdrawn and to have stress related symptoms, but so long as their tours of duty were uneventful, they functioned adequately. Their residual or sub-clinical PTSD developed into a full blown syndrome during the Lebanon War.

3. The veterans in the third group showed Moderate Generalized Sensitivity in both their civilian and military lives. They suffered from sleep disturbances, nightmares, irritability, and uncontrollable outbursts of anger that sometimes impaired their functioning. To cope with their distress, a few resorted to drugs, and alcohol; whereas others developed phobic reactions. Some did everything in their power to avoid contact with weapons, even while they were in active reserve duty. During the Lebanon War these men went to the front, but soon developed CSR in response to relatively minor military stimuli and some were discharged even before they saw actual combat.

4. The fourth group, the Severe Generalized Sensitivity group, consisted of the most seriously ill veterans who suffered from severe generalized sensitivity throughout the entire period between wars. For such veterans, the mere arrival of the call-up order to Lebanon brought on an immediate and severe stress reaction. Many of these men never saw combat before having their second breakdown.

What should be emphasized is that all the casualties who had reactivated or exacerbated PTSD in Lebanon had put a great deal of effort into their functioning--especially in the military--in the nine years between the Yom Kippur and the Lebanon wars, and generally succeeded. By selectively utilizing such coping mechanisms as repression, denial and avoidance, most of them married, started families, and held jobs. None were hospitalized. All continued to serve in the reserves, despite the fact that their symptoms were intensified in the presence of military stimuli. Many hid their symptoms from their friends, family, and army commanders.

Their second reaction revealed and deepened the psychological damage that the first breakdown had created. In general, there were more symptoms following the second reaction than the first, and the symptoms were more intense and debilitating (Solomon, 1993; Solomon, Oppenheimer, Elizur & Waysman, 1990a).

Soldiers who experience a reactivated episode of CSR manifest a more severe clinical syndrome than those who experience a single episode. Even though some soldiers participate in battle after a CSR episode without further breakdown, the debilitating effects of the earlier CSR episode are still detectable a decade later (Solomon, 1993; Solomon, Oppenheimer, Elizur & Waysman, 1990b).

Reactivation of Stress Responses Among Holocaust Survivors in the Gulf War

The same phenomenon of reactivation was also evident among a different population, in a different war, namely, Holocaust survivors during the Gulf War. Clinical impressions suggest that the Gulf War was indeed an especially painful reminder for the Holocaust survivors. The feeling of being "sitting ducks," the sense of impending doom, the threat to use gas and the rows of decontamination showers positioned at the entrance to every hospital (which reminded the survivors of the entrance to the gas chambers in the concentration camps) all made this war particularly stressful for the Holocaust survivors. In a study conducted during the Gulf War, we assessed the psychological effects of the war on 192 elderly civilians, both with and without a Holocaust background (Solomon & Prager, 1992).

Results showed that elderly Holocaust survivors perceived significantly higher levels of danger, experienced more emotional distress, and had higher levels of both state and trait anxiety than subjects without a Holocaust background (Solomon & Prager, 1992). Therefore, our findings indicate that Holocaust experience rendered the elderly more vulnerable. In fact, we found that more than half of the Holocaust survivors were at risk for a degree of psychological distress that would require intervention. The variability in the Holocaust survivors' reaction was related to their prior experiences. Among the Holocaust survivors, those who had undergone prior similar war-related experiences were found to be more vulnerable than other Holocaust survivors (Hantman, Solomon & Prager, 1994).

Secondary Traumatization

The final issue to be presented is secondary traumatization. The term "Secondary Traumatization" (Figley, 1983) has been used to convey the idea that traumatic events may effect not only the survivors, but also their significant others -

their spouses, their children, and even their therapists. People can be traumatized without actually having been physically harmed or threatened. It is enough that they are intimate with people who were in fact traumatized.

Two studies of secondary traumatization, one involving offspring and the other with spouses of traumatized individuals will be discussed.

The Transgenerational Impact of PTSD

The long arm of posttraumatic sequelae also stretches into the next generation. We assessed the possible implication of a trauma experienced by many of the parents of the present generation of Israeli soldiers: The Nazi Holocaust.

The literature suggests that many Holocaust survivors suffer from PTSD residuals decades after their ordeal (e.g., Eitinger, 1980), and that many of their children suffer from a milder version of similar symptoms (Barocas & Barocas, 1979; Danieli, 1980). Offspring of Holocaust survivors have been found to be highly anxious, manifest excessive narcissistic vulnerability, survival guilt, and more than usual ambivalence about aggression (Danieli, 1980). On the battlefield, these traits might exacerbate the anxiety and fear that all soldiers experience and at the same time create more than the usual qualms about killing to secure one's survival.

To examine the implication of the Holocaust in PTSD in the second generation, we asked our Lebanon CSR subjects to indicate whether either of their parents were Holocaust survivors and compared their responses on the PTSD inventory (Solomon, Kotler & Mikulincer, 1988).

The comparison confirms the transgenerational impact of trauma. Two and three years after their participation in the Lebanon War, second generation CSR casualties had significantly higher rates of PTSD than casualties without Holocaust background: 73% vs. 52% two years later, and 64% vs. 39% three years later. In other words, the PTSD of second generation survivors was more likely.

There was also a difference in the number of symptoms. For the first two years after their CSRs, the two groups had essentially the same average number of symptoms. Between the second and third years, however, that number declined among non-second generation casualties, but not among PTSD casualties whose parents had gone through the Holocaust. In other words, while the PTSD in many veterans was abating by the third year, in second generation Holocaust survivors it remained as severe as it had been at its onset.

The exposure to combat of the second generation seems to have unmasked a latent vulnerability that was not activated by more run-of-the-mill life events. Their PTSD is suggestive of reactivated PTSD, which is also more severe and enduring than a first episode.

A CSR breakdown may have a particular meaning for children of survivors. Almost every CSR casualty feels that he has failed, and most suffer agonies of shame and reduced self-esteem. But among the second generation the sense of failure cuts deeper. Children of Holocaust survivors see themselves in their uniforms and bearing their weapons as guardians and protectors of their parents. The second generation was raised to undo the damage that the Holocaust had brought to their parents' lives. The magnitude of this expectation probably intensifies the failure implicit in a combat breakdown. Finally, recovery might be impeded by the excess of secondary gains to be had from the survivors' parents well-documented overprotectiveness. It is also possible that survivor parents may have unconsciously discouraged the recovery of their CSR sons so as to avert the very real danger of their being sent back to the front.

Secondary Traumatization Among wives of CSRs

Many of the debilitating PTSD symptoms are not only stressful for the casualties, but may also have direct bearing on the casualty's most intimate companion--his spouse (e.g., DeFasio & Fascucci, 1984; Hendon & Law, 1986). Especially relevant are the symptoms that interfere with the casualty's intimate relationship. These include reduced involvement, diminished interest, feeling of detachment, alienation and constricted affect. PTSD veterans are often withdrawn, edgy, depressed and may have unpredictable outbursts of rage and aggression. These severe symptoms may have considerable implications for the well-being of the spouses.

In a study involving families of traumatized veterans we examined the implications of combat-related psychopathology among veterans on the psychosocial status of their wives (Solomon et al., 1992; Solomon, Waysman, Avizur & Anoch, 1991; Waysman, Mikulincer, Solomon & Weisenberg, 1993). Two groups of subjects were included: wives of CSR casualties, and wives of regular combatants who served as a control group. The two groups were queried about their mental and physical health, their social functioning, and their satisfaction in marital relationship.

CSR casualties' wives reported higher levels of psychiatric symptomatology, and more somatic complaints than the controls. In addition, wives who perceived their husbands as suffering from PTSD, tended also to display social dysfunction in a broad range of contexts, ranging from inner-feelings of loneliness through impaired marital and family relations. This was also evident in lack of satisfaction with the wider social network.

These high levels of distress manifested by the CSR casualties' wives may be explained in one of two ways: close and prolonged contact with a person who had experienced a severe trauma may serve as a chronic stressor, that leads over time to both somatic and psychiatric impairment. The second explanation relates to the concept of "secondary traumatization." The wives may also be contending with some stressors that are unique to spouses of trauma victims. Identification with their husbands may be so strong that they may have actually internalized their stressor imagery, and learned to feel and behave in ways similar to their husband.

Contrary to expectations, however, we found a surprisingly low divorce rate in our sample. This contrasts sharply to the divorce rate for Vietnam veterans, for example: an estimated 38% of the marriages of Vietnam veterans broke up within half a year of their return from Southeast Asia. The very low divorce rate in our sample suggests that in Israel, wives of traumatized veterans tend to remain with their husbands, possibly due to social pressure not to abandon casualties who had made sacrifices for their country. Israeli wives may therefore not only suffer considerable distress in their marriages, but may also feel that they are trapped and do not have the option to leave. Lower divorce rates, in general, in Israel also make this generally less acceptable alternative.

Conclusion

War stress is a highly potent pathogenic agent. While most individuals experience elevated distress the overall immediate response is in the majority of cases quite contained. Under moderate levels of war stress progressive habituation is observed.

At the same time, traumatized individuals following extreme stress often continue for extended periods to suffer from diagnosable psychiatric disorders, well after the disappearance of the external threat. Their distress has many different manifestations including PTSD, other psychiatric disorder, impaired functioning, somatic complaints and illness, and alteration of their world view.

The pathogenic effects of trauma are in some cases delayed and emerge only after an asymptomatic latency period, although we generally found low rates of delayed PTSD. In contrast, reactivated PTSD is more intense and debilitating than a first time breakdown.

Finally, the damages caused by war-trauma are so great that they are not contained within the survivors but create a ripple effect and have detrimental implications for significant others including offspring and spouses.

References

American Psychiatric Association. (1987). Diagnostic and statistical manual of mental disorders (DSM-III-R), (third edition, revised). Washington, D.C.: Author.

Archibald, H., & Tuddenham, R. (1965). Persistent stress reactions after combat: A twenty-year follow-up. Archives of General Psychiatry, 12, 475-481.

Atkinson, R.M., Henderson, R.G., & Sparr, L.F. (1982). Assessment for Vietnam veterans for post-traumatic stress disorder in Veterans Administration disability claim. American Journal of Psychiatry, 139, 1118-1121.

Bailey, P., Williams, F.E., Komora, P.O., Salmon, T.W., Fenton, N. (1929). The medical department of the United States Army in the World War: Vol. X. Neuropsychiatry. Washington, DC: Government Printing Office.

Barocas, H., & Barocas, C. (1979). Wounds of the fathers: The next generation of Holocaust victims. International Review Psychoanalysis, 5, 331-341.

Bartemeier, L.H. (1946). Combat exhaustion. Journal of Nervous and Mental Disease, 104, 359-425.

Bleich, A., Dycian, A., Koslowsky, M., Solomon, Z., & Weiner, M. (1992). Psychiatric implications of missile attacks on civilian population. JAMA, 268, 613-615.

Boulanger, G. (1985). An old problem with a new name. In S.M. Sonnenberg, A.S. Blank, & T.A. Talbott (Eds.), The trauma of war: Stress and recovery in Vietnam veterans. Washington, DC: American Psychiatric Press.

Cavenar, J.O., & Nash, J.L. (1976). The effects of combat on the normal personality: War neurosis in Vietnam returnees. Comprehensive Psychiatry, 17, 647-653.

Danieli, Y. (1980). Families of survivors of the Nazi Holocaust: Some long and short term effects. In N. Milgram (Ed.), Psychological stress and adjustment in time of war and peace. Washington D.C.: Hemisphere.

DeFasio, V.J., & Pascucci, N.J. (1984). Return to Ithaca: A perspective on marriage and love in posttraumatic stress disorder. Journal of Contemporary Psychotherapy, 14, 76-89.

Drabek, T.E. (1986). Human system responses to disaster: An inventory of sociological findings. New York: Springer Verlag.

Egendorf, A., Kadushin, C., Laufer, R.S., Rotbarth, G., & Solan, L. (1981). Legacies of Vietnam: Comparative adjustment of veterans and their peers. New York: Center for Policy Research.

Eitinger, L. (1980). The Concentration Camp Syndrome and its late sequelae. In, J. Dimsdale (Ed.), Survivors, victims and perpetrators, Washington DC: Hemisphere.

Figley, C.R. (1983). Catastrophes: An overview of family reactions. In C.R. Figley & H.I. McCubbin (Ed.), Stress and the family, vol. 2: Coping with catastrophe (pp. 3-20). New York: Brunner/Mazel.

Grinker, R.P. (1945). Psychiatric disorders in combat crews overseas and in returnees. Medical Clinics of North America, 29, 729-739.

Hantman, S., Solomon, Z., & Prager, E. (1994). How the Gulf War affected aged Holocaust survivors? Clinical Gerontologist, 14, 27-37.

Hendon, A.G., & Law, J.G. (1986). Post-traumatic stress and the family: A multimethod approach to counseling. In C.R. Figley (Ed.), Trauma and its wake, Vol 2: Traumatic stress, theory, research and intervention (pp. 264-279). New York: Brunner/Mazel.

Horowitz, M.J., & Solomon, G.F. (1978). Delayed stress response syndromes in Vietnam veterans. In C.R. Figley (Ed.), Stress disorders among Vietnam veterans. New York: Brunner/Mazel.

Kormos, H.R. (1978). The nature of combat stress. In C.R. Figley (Ed.), Stress disorders among Vietnam veterans (pp. 3-22). New York: Brunner/Mazel.

Kulka, A.R., Schlenger, W.E., Fairbank, J.A., Hough, R.L., Jordan, B.K., Marmar, C.R., & Weiss, D.C. (1988). Contractual report of findings from the Vietnam veterans readjustment study. NC: Research Triangle Institute.

Laufer, R.S., Gallops, M.S., & Frey-Wouters, E. (1984). War stress and post-war trauma. Journal of Health and Social Behavior, 14, 215-216.

Neiderland, W.G. (1968). The problem of the survivor. In H. Krystal (Ed.), Massive Psychic Trauma. New York: International University Press.

Noy, S. (1991). Combat stress reaction. Tel Aviv: Ministry of Defense Publications [Hebrew].

Ohry, A., Solomon, Z., Neria, Y., Waysman, M., Bar-On, Z., & Levy, A. (1994). The aftermath of captivity: An 18-year follow-up of Israeli ex-POWs. Behavioral Medicine, 20, 27-33.

Rachman, S. (1990). Fear and courage, New York: Freeman & Co.

Saigh, P. (1984). Pre- and postinvasion anxiety in Lebanon, Behavior Therapy, 15, 185-190.

Saigh, P. (1988). Anxiety, depression and assertion across alternating intervals of stress, Journal of Abnormal Psychology, 97, 338-341.

Sarason, S. B. (1974). The psychological sense of community: Prospects for a community psychology. San Francisco: Jossey-Bass.

Solomon, Z. (1993). Combat stress reaction: The enduring toll of war. New York: Plenum Press.

Solomon, Z. (1995) Coping with war-induced stress, Forthcomoing in Plenum Press.

Solomon, Z., Garb, R., Bleich, A., & Grupper, D. (1987). Reactivation of combat related post-traumatic stress disorder. American Journal of Psychiatry, 144, 51-55.

Solomon, Z., Kotler, M., & Mikulincer, M. (1988). Combat related post-traumatic stress disorder among the second generation of Holocaust survivors: Preliminary findings. American Journalof Psychiatry, 145, 865-868.

Solomon, Z., Kotler, M., Shalev, A., & Lin, R. (1989). Delayed onset PTSD among Israeli veterans of the 1982 Lebanon War. Psychiatry, 52, 428-436.

Solomon, Z., Laor, N., Weiler, D., Muller, U.F., Hadar, O., Waysman, M., Koslowsky, M., Ben Yakar, M., & Bleich, A. (1993). The psychological impact of the Gulf War: A study of acute stress in Israeli evacuees. Archives of General Psychiatry, 50, 320-321.

Solomon, Z., Mikulincer, M., & Benbenishty, R. (1989). Combat stress reaction: Clinical manifestations and correlates. Military Psychology, 1, 35-47.

Solomon, Z., Neria, Y., Ohry, A., Waysman, M., & Ginzburg, K. (1994). PTSD among Israeli former prisoners of war and soldiers with combat stress reaction: A Longitudinal study, American Journal of Psychiatry, 151, 554-559.

Solomon, Z., Oppenheimer, B., Elizur, Y., & Waysman, M. (1990a). Trauma deepens trauma: The consequences of recurrent combat stress reaction. Israel Journal of Psychiatry and Related Sciences, 27, 233-241.

Solomon, Z., Oppenheimer, B., Elizur, Y., & Waysman, M. (1990b). Exposure to recurrent combat stress: Can successful coping in a second war heal combat-related PTSD from the past? Journal of Anxiety Disorders, 4, 141-145.

Solomon, Z., & Prager, E. (1992). Elderly Israeli Holocaust survivors during the Persian Gulf War: A study of psychological distress. American Journal of Psychiatry, 149, 1707-1710.

Solomon, Z., Singer, Y., & Blumenfeld, A. Clinical characteristics of delayed and immediate onset combat induced PTSD. In preparation.

Solomon, Z., Waysman, M., Avizur, E., & Enoch, D. (1991). Psychiatric symptomatology among wives of soldiers following combat stress reaction: The role of social network and marital relations. Anxiety Research, 4, 213-223.

Solomon, Z., Waysman, M., Levy, G., Fried, B., Mikulincer, M., Benbenishty, R., Florian, V., & Bleich, A. (1992). From front-line to home front: A study of secondary traumatization. Family Process, 31, 289-302.

Sparr, L., & Pankratz, L.D. (1983). Factitious post-traumatic stress disorder. American Journal of Psychiatry, 140, 1016-1019.

Walker J.I., & Cavenar, D. (1982). Vietnam veterans: Their problems continue. Journal of Nervous and Mental Disease, 170, 174-180.

Waysman, M., Mikulincer, M., Solomon, Z., & Weisenberg, M. (1993). Secondary traumatization among wives of post traumatic combat veterans: A family typology. Journal of Family Psychology, 7, 1-17.

STRESS AND DISASTER

Alexander C McFarlane
Rehabilitation and Community Psychiatry
University of Adelaide
Australia

The Paradoxical Interest in Disasters

Disasters capture the attention of the media and the mind of the researcher alike because of the horror and the threat which they embody. They confront the individual with the most basic challenge of life: survival against the odds and in the face of danger and devastation. They epitomise the external nature of destruction and the threat which lies outside the self, in a world of uncontrollable forces. In natural disasters it is men and women versus the natural world with its ebbs and flows, the extremes against which many engineering projects and much technology aim to protect us. Man-made disasters involve the externalisation of evil and responsibility into those to blame.

This focus on the threat of the external world stands in striking contrast to the clinical focus of psychologists and psychiatrists that typically addresses the inner workings of the mind; the idiosyncratic behaviors, thoughts, and feelings of patients. Sufferers of psychological disorders are people who face an internal sense of disintegration, who feel that they have lost control of aspects of the self that are central to their sense of identity. Many mental disorders leave sufferers in a state where their perception of and affective reactions to the external world are changed. Familiar and unthreatening tasks and environments become unpredictable and frightening; they demand much greater effort and new strategies to manage them.

Paradoxically, psychological disorders are a predictable consequence of traumatic events. The setting of disaster and trauma provides a meeting of the inner and external worlds that makes it such a fruitful area of investigation and one of fascination for clinicians and researchers alike. It is an area where those who are interested in the workings of the mind can also be involved in the struggle against external threat.

Against this background this paper aims to address several issues about the nature of the stress of disaster. First, I will examine the demands and consequences of dealing with the immediate threat and loss and the prolonged social disruption. This is an important area of investigation because of the need for valid measure of the intensity of exposure to the disaster. To date many of the complexities of this issue have not been addressed. *There is a need to examine the stress of disaster from a longitudinal perspective, beginning before the event.*

Second, the nature of the internal psychological process in the trauma response will be described. *For some this is potentially the most damaging aspect and change that a disaster can cause.* The individual's sense of safety and capacity to relate to family and friends can be severely disrupted. The disaster can lead to a sense of constant threat where the individual's sense of reality is changed to a state of continuing vulnerability and over reaction to minor threats. Ultimately, it can be the scars of trauma, the development of a posttraumatic stress disorder which can be the critical consequence of the disaster.

The Rationale For Quantifying the Stress of Disasters

In many regards, the stress involved in disasters is obvious and needs little elaboration. However, this issue requires examination for several reasons. Firstly, the need to define the exact nature of the stress in disasters is an important issue in improving the sophistication of the measurement of severity of the trauma. This is a major methodological question that has been given little attention in disaster research.

This is a necessary concern for researchers who wish to quantify the relationship between disasters and the various patterns of adjustment that describe the trauma response. The failure to examine these issues in disaster research contrasts with the careful attention given to inter-rater reliability, scaling and contamination of the measures by the individual's psychological state in the measurement of stresses associated with everyday adversity. The exact methodology for developing valid and reliable measures of extremely traumatic events has been discussed little to date, an issue which will be addressed in this manuscript. For example, a series of practical questions arise about the quantification and scaling of any trauma related measure.

A second reason for considering this issue is that few studies have been done of the relationship between victims' acute patterns of response and their longer-term adjustment. The available data have often found that acute patterns of distress and subsequent psychological morbidity are not as closely linked as might have been anticipated. This suggests that the meaning structures and the cognitive reworking of these events needs to be seen as a process. The reality of the trauma is often not the critical issue. Rather, it is the perception of what occurred that may be the critical determinant of outcome. Thus, while the intensity of exposure is generally seen as the critical criterion in the aetiology of PTSD, the data demonstrates a more complex relationship (Solomon and Canino, 1990). The traumatic experience is a necessary but not sufficient contributor to many features of the post traumatic response. This necessitates an examination of the process and the secondary stresses that surround a disaster if the outcome is to be better understood as an environmentally determined process. This issue has taken on a new significance with the inclusion of the individual's response at the time of the trauma, specifically a the experience of a sense of powerlessness and loss of control, as one component of the new stressor criterion for PTSD in DSM IV (APA,1993) and ICD 10 (WHO,1992).

Finally, the question is seldom asked as to how the trauma of the disaster itself ranks in contrast to the suffering caused by the long term practical consequences such as the loss of the amenities of life and possessions. This issue is important both in the disaster setting and with the sufferers of psychological disorders generally. However, the distress associated with having a mental disorder has been largely ignored by those working with psychiatric patients (McFarlane, 1991). Hughes (1990) an orthopaedic registrar who served in the Falklands, subsequently developed a panic disorder and describes his experience in a graphic manner.

"For no obvious reason I had suddenly been overwhelmed by a crescendo of blind unreasoning fear, defying all logic and insight... nothing that General Galtieri's men had generated compared with the terrors that may own mind invented that night. Having looked death full in the eye on a windswept isthmus outside Goose Green and again, but two weeks later, on a barren hillside called Wireless Ridge, I think I can honestly say I no longer feared death or the things real and imagined that usually become the objects of phobias. I was afraid that night of the only thing that could still frighten me, myself. I was terrified of losing my control".

This suggests that the psychological consequences of trauma may be worse than the experience of the actual event. The paradox is that some people who experience the distress and trauma of disaster and survive, nevertheless undergo a secondary process whereby there is a primary shift in the psychological state that itself becomes a major threat to their survival and is a source of stress in its own right.

Measuring the Phases of Disaster

Current inventories of traumatic events have attempted to quantify the level of exposure, the risk and actual occurrence of injury, the extent of losses and the death and injury of relatives (Freedy et al, 1993; Raphael et al, 1989). These constitute the impact phase of a disaster. In general, disasters are seen as events that are independent of the victim's control. As such, the nature and components of the disaster experience are generally considered to be objective predictors of subsequent adjustment. This contrasts to life events research where in it has long been recognised that an event, such as loss of a job or breakdown of a marriage, may be the consequence of an individual's disorder rather than a cause.

There are, however, a variety of ways in which individuals may contribute to their disaster-related experiences. For example, in many disasters there is the potential for the victim to anticipate the threat and modify the impact of the event by their behaviour during the emergency. Equally, the resources available to the individual during and immediately after the disaster may significantly mitigate its effects.

It follows that, to fully understand the stress of disasters the events should be conceptualised as a longitudinal process both at the level of the community and the individuals. During this process there exist a variety of points at which victims can potentially modify the outcome. This implies that different issues and stresses are created by disaster at different points in their evolution and resolution, and these should perhaps be documented if the totality of the trauma is to be understood and those factors which are most toxic identified. The various phases of disaster have been documented extensively and are useful in examining the trauma process. Some of the issues that should be documented in relation to these various phases are described. The duration of these phases are variable according to the nature of the disaster, for example, the threat and impact phases may last for only seconds in an aircraft crash but days or weeks in a flood.

Planning

Disasters can be anticipated with varying degrees of accuracy. Disaster plans embody the collective knowledge and risk assessment for any particular region. Therefore one dimension of the stress response to disaster involves anticipation and a willingness to contemplate the possibility of disaster and to see that the provision of resources in the development of disaster plans is an adaptive strategy. This reflects an attitude of risk appraisal and management that can decrease the possibility of exposure in the event of a disaster. The effect of this preparation on outcome should be examined as Weisaeth (1989) has demonstrated that training is a predictor of post-disaster adjustment.

The effects of planning are relevant in the case of both communities and individuals. For example, families may choose to live in a particular site and in a particular type of dwelling because it takes account of various possible risks in the natural environment. This may include choosing not to live in a fire-prone suburb or to avoid a low-lying coastal district because of the risk of flooding in storms. Evidence about the role that inherited personality traits play in determining the level of exposure to traumatic events was found in a recent study of Vietnam veteran twins (True et al, 1993) and also that of Breslau et al (1991) of traumatic exposure in young adults. Thus, the anticipation and management of risk is an important determinant of the level of stress in a disaster. This is an issue that the insurance industry knows and exploits.

Threat

Once the possibility of a disaster emerges, a willingness to respond to the threat and take a variety of precautionary steps is important in modulating the stress of the event. With some disasters, (e.g., a plane crash) there will be no warning. However, with certain natural disasters, such as hurricanes and bush fires, authorities are able to make reasonably accurate predictions of risk. The community's response to warnings can play a very important role in improving survival-orientated behaviors. Thus, anticipatory anxiety and its adaptive management can further decrease the individual risks when the disaster strikes and should be documented. Hotel guests (e.g. conference attenders) should identify the site of the fire escapes when they first occupy their room and count the number of steps that it takes from their room so that they can negotiate the escape when the corridor is smoke filled and the lights are out.

Impact

The impact phase of disasters is extremely variable according to the type of event. There is also great variability within events. One house can be destroyed while the one next door is left unscathed. There is a need to compare the different types of disaster and identify the differing role of the components of threat, exposure, and loss in the patterns of adjustment (Fontana et al, 1992). In some regards, this question has been pre-empted by the definition of the stressor criteria for PTSD in DSM IV. However, the validation of this criteria was done in field trials that mainly examined the impact of crime and urban violence as determinants of PTSD, rather than disasters (Davidson and Fao, 1992). For example, the role of property loss, a major component of many disasters, may not strictly satisfy the DSM IV criteria, although studies of two disasters, one in Australia (McFarlane, 1989), the other in the People's Republic of China (McFarlane and Cao, 1993), property loss rather than the level of threat or exposure was the most powerful predictor of PTSD.

Disaster components. In a disaster there is also a need to compare the effect of individuals' direct experiences of the disaster and the effect of the disaster on the community in which victims live. For example, what is the relative psychological impact of losing one's home in a disaster when you are the only person to do so in neighbourhood, in contrast to the experience of living in an area where virtually all of the homes were destroyed. To date most disaster inventories have simply examined individuals' losses and have not examined the interaction with the community context (Freedy et al, 1993; Raphael et al, 1989). The characteristics of these different types of disasters are described (see Table 1) to highlight the issues involved in characterising both the individual and community experience.

First, some disasters affect a group of people who coincidentally happen to be together at a particular point in time, such as in an aircraft accident. In the aftermath of such a disaster, the survivors will be scattered over wide geographical areas. Such disasters are characterised by their very high levels of danger and threat to the individuals exposed as well as the substantial risk of death or being bereaved. These are events in which the individual's behavior can contribute relatively little to survival. Equally, the survivor's community is often left intact, except those who happen to live in the immediate proximity of the disaster.

Table 1: Differing role of threat, bereavement and property loss in disasters.

```
High loss of life:  High threat:  Low property loss
                -Industrial disasters
                -Transport disaster
                -Terrorist attack

High property loss:  High threat:  Moderate loss of life
                -Bushfires
                -Earthquakes
                -Wind storms  (Hurricanes etc)
                -Volcanoes

High property loss: Low threat: Low loss of life
                -Flood
                -Drought/Crop failure

High threat:  Low property loss:  Low life loss
                -Nuclear contamination/accident
                -Toxic waste spill
```

This contrasts to disasters that affect circumscribed geographical regions and generally involve very substantial property loss, such as bushfires and hurricanes. These disasters often involve high levels of threat but the main impact stems from the losses sustained. A third type of disaster, for example some floods and agricultural disasters, result in very substantial property loss but, because of their slow onset, carry relatively low threat to individuals and a low loss of life. It may be that these disasters, whilst extremely distressing, do not produce PTSD to the same degree, although they may trigger a variety of other psychological problems.

Finally, some disasters involve very little or no property loss or loss of life, but entail a very high level of threat. One such example would be the Three Mile Island disaster when there was a threatened meltdown of a nuclear reactor (Bromet, Schulberg, & Dunn, 1982). Given that no actual harm may have occurred, focusing on the potential threat may lead to a heightened sensitivity and exaggerate people's sense of danger and lead to inappropriate litigation. Thus, measures of trauma need to be able to reflect the individual characteristics of these events as they are likely to have different impacts on different groups.

<u>Victim's behavior and the impact of exposure.</u> The impact of extremely traumatic events on the victim's behavior and mental state during the event may also be important issues affecting the nature of exposure. This is a vexing issue to discuss as it can be seen to be blaming the victims of the event for their losses and injury. The issue of dissociative responses to trauma has primarily been raised by clinicians interested in the role of memory in the trauma response rather than empirical researchers. As van der Kolk and van der Hart (1991) have highlighted, this is not a new interest, but rather one that was at the core of nineteenth century concepts of the trauma response and general psychopathology. Before adopting his instinctual theory of the neuroses, Freud (1973) believed that trauma and the resultant dissociative response was a cornerstone of the psychopathological process.

Dissociation is an important issue for empirical researchers to consider because it is a common response during extremely traumatic events. Its significance is twofold in the measurement of the severity of the stress involved in disasters. First, dissociative amnesia and time distortion could potentially lead to the under-reporting of aspects of individuals' experiences and the misperception of various components of the trauma. Second, whilst major traumatic events are clearly events beyond individuals' control in the sense they cannot possibly have been caused by the individual, the individuals' mental states may have important effects on their experiences. People who panic, dissociate, or who respond in other maladaptive ways may effectively increase their exposure. For example, they may not use the safest escape route or fail to take other emergency action that would optimise their potential for survival. This is an important issue in the measurement of the stress associated with disasters as exposure can be a confounded measure of the individuals' mental state at the time and the severity of the trauma.

<u>The problem of scaling and comparing different disaster experiences</u>. How to assign relative stress scores to the different components of the experience is a major question in compiling a scale of the total stress of a disaster. In life events research, individuals who are being studied do not rate the comparative stressfulness of the events that they have experienced because it is believed that the ratings will be contaminated by their response to the event. In other words, the individual who develops depression following a loss will rank the event as more stressful than the individual who copes and does not become depressed.

This approach would suggest that the victims should not rate the severity of the stress associated with the different experiences they have suffered in the disaster. Brown and Harris (1978) developed a more sophisticated methodology where they get independent raters to define the contextual threat of a particular experience. There are good arguments for using similar methodologies for quantifying the effects of disasters. However, the ability of outsiders to judge the degree of stress involved in disaster exposure is arguable. One of the only populations who rated the stressfulness of the items in the Holmes and Rahe's (1967) life events scale in a significantly different way was a group of earthquake victims. Surprisingly, they rated the severity of the impact of major losses as less than populations unaffected by disaster (Janney, Masuda, & Holmes, 1977). This suggests that traumatised groups may have a different perspective of their experience from populations who have not confronted that particular event, and that the experience of disaster victims may not be correctly perceived by those who have not been through the event.

The cumulative impact of the various components of a disaster is also poorly understood. In the face of a disaster there are a variety of traumatic experiences that may befall individuals, such as the actual impingement of the event, including injury, as well as the events those involved witnessed (Green,1993). The disaster experience will have both objective and subjective components. People's mental states, for example did they panic or dissociate, and their perceptions of the risks and capacity to act adaptively are factors that will influence the stressfulness of the experience but are subjective. On one hand, there will be the more objective aspects of exposure such as seeing death and injury or actually being injured. Similarly the duration of exposure and awareness of destruction and loss are objective issues. In contrast, matters that might be equally important in determining individuals' traumatisation include survival by freak circumstances, being safe by chance, and having no control of the circumstances or their behavior.

Common sense suggests that there will be a gradation of experience with increasing distress and threat occurring with increasing intensity of exposure. There has been little systematic validation of the interrelationship of these phenomena or whether it is appropriate to construct composite scales. Composite scales imply that there is an additive effect of these different experiences, (i.e. that the death of two children is twice as bad as one and can be numerically compared in a consistent way with the loss of one's home). These examples immediately highlight the issues and complexity of the problem. Similarly how does one compare the effect of a close encounter with death and such losses? This an important issue for any researcher wishing to investigate the impact of disaster. It may be the case that once a certain level of loss or exposure has been reached that there is a threshold effect and that any further loss or impact does not modify the individuals' responses as their capacity to be distressed has been saturated (Hauff and Vaglum, 1993).

It would seem that the community of disaster researchers could perhaps more profitably address this issue rather than further adding to the increasing series of descriptive studies of small non-representative samples of disaster victims. Several strategies are available. These include getting the victims' impressions of the differing impact of the components of the disaster and the nature of the interactions. This could be done with scales where the threat and harm caused by the experiences is rated. Second, a series of scenarios could be put and comparative ratings obtained. Finally, Brown and Harris' (1978) interview for contextual threat could be adapted to the disaster setting as this may address the protean nature of human response to these situations.

Understanding the severity of individuals' traumatic exposure is a complex and difficult issue. Whether meaningful scales that combine a range of very different experiences can be developed needs careful theoretical and methodological examination. There has been little systematic examination of the assumptions (Wortman and Silver, 1989) and issues involved in constructing a valid quantitative representation of the experience of trauma.

Inventory and Rescue

The true impact of a disaster may not be apparent to the victims during the emergency, particularly if they are away from their homes and families at the time the threat strikes. During this phase of the disaster, there is an attempt to build up a picture of what has occurred and to re-establish contact with family and community. The effectiveness of the provision of basic services such as shelter, food and water by a range of authorities, including the military, is another factor that can determine the stressfulness of a disaster. These activities are obviously essential for survival but also have a powerful symbolic value in that they are critical to re-establishing the individual's sense of safety with the containment of the threat. However, if a disaster has not devastated an entire community the immediate response of the informal networks such as family and friends should not be underestimated and should be assessed as these are often preferred to relief provided by a disaster authority.

This is a period when many victims will have contact with a range of disaster relief workers and authorities. These encounters can play an important role in containing the distress of the victims and should be documented (Carr et al, 1992). For example, the way that victims are made aware of the death of a relative and the reasons given for why they should not view the body may have a critical role in determining their memories and perceptions of the death. This is also a time when many victims will be provided with some form of preventive counselling. The nature of the intervention, the offers received and their resultant satisfaction should be documented. In developed countries there are probably very few disasters where victims are not offered these interventions. Therefore, any study wishing to document the outcome of a disaster should report the nature of the interventions offered and whether these were utilised by the victims. The educational component of these interventions also has the capacity to modify the perceptions and memories the victims have of the disaster.

The reporting of the disaster in the media is an additional factor that can compound the trauma of the event if there has been misreporting or insensitive reporting of the extent of the losses. In the Ash Wednesday Bushfire disaster, the foreign media reported that whole areas of the city of Adelaide were destroyed, which caused great distress to those who heard the news but who were unable to validate the story because the communications system was overloaded. The impact of this misinformation on these people as well as on those who did lose homes and family members is an important question. The impact of media reports on relatives reactions is an issue of legal importance and was discussed at some length in the legal judgements after the Hillsborough soccer disaster (Pugh et al, 1993). This issue was a determinant of eligibility for compensation.

Remedy and Recovery Phases

The tasks of reconstruction and the long term impact of the disaster on the financial and material well being of the victims are critical in the rebuilding of their lives. The rapidity of the process and the ease of organisation are critical issues and should be systematically documented in the investigation of the impact of disasters. This stage can be complicated if there are major disputes in the payment of insurance money for damage to property or if here are disputes about liability. Profiteering can be an issue if the task of reconstruction overwhelms the available resources. Thus there is a need to develop scales that document the components of the reconstruction phase. If they are not measured, it might be assumed that the disaster is directly responsible as the difficulties at this stage are likely to be proportional to the severity of the losses in the disaster whereas it is not their direct effects which is the critical issue.

If financial compensation and litigation become involved, this adds a whole new level of trauma and distress to the disaster experience. As the prominent British disaster lawyer Napier (1991) stated:

"I have tried to understand the feelings of disaster victims and to be sensitive to what they expect from the legal system, which in my view is poorly designed to cope with disaster aftermath. The victims frequently feel that in the legal process their interests come well down in the list of considerations. We have learned that as soon as the victims suffer what they see as inadequacies in the legal system, they visit their resulting dissatisfaction on who else, their lawyers. The result is that the medical trauma of the disaster is worsened by further trauma to the victims as they battle with a confusing system that is often slow and ineffective in providing answers that they and the public reasonably seek".

Many claims are made about the effects of litigation on the outcome of disaster related trauma but there are very few systematic studies. This issue should be documented and examined so that the prejudicial statements that are made about victims involved in the legal process can be challenged where appropriate. In an unpublished study, many Ash Wednesday disaster victims commented that the litigation process was more distressing than the disaster itself. The duration and imbalance of power in the legal process were issues of particular distress for the victims.

The Acute Patterns of Response

The current formulations of the stress response are almost totally based on the retrospective reconstruction of the accounts of the event and the initial pattern of response of the survivors. There are very few prospective accounts that have systematically examined the survivors in the immediate aftermath and followed them until the long term pattern of adjustment can be judged. Such studies are likely to provide critical evidence about the elements of the trauma that are causes of acute distress rather than long-term adjustment. It is this state of acute distress that is the intermediary stage between the event and the onset of PTSD. This is an important question as the prevailing theories about the aetiology of PTSD are based on the observations of the established disorder. The possibility remains that the appraisal of the trauma that is thought to occur in PTSD is actually contaminated by the secondary appraisal generated by the need to cope with the symptoms of PTSD.

These investigations raise a series of issues about how the severity of the acute stress response should be judged. Most instruments used in the investigation of disasters are derived from the investigation of symptoms in patient populations. There has been insufficient study of the patterns of acute distress following traumatic events to know whether these instruments do adequately document victims' responses. The instrument developed by Spiegel (1993) is likely to make an important contribution in this regard, because it characterises the dimensions of the acute stress response.

Shalev (1992) studied the victims of a terrorist bomb attack during their hospitalisation and related their response to their long term outcome. This study failed to demonstrate that the early intensity of the intrusive affects and cognitions related to longer term outcome and challenges the theoretical proposition that the intensity of the response to the trauma is of primary aetiological importance (Foa et al, 1989). Thus the studies that have suggested that the intrusive reworking of the traumatic event is a central determinant of the emerging disordered arousal are not substantiated by this study during the immediate post-trauma period (Creamer, et al. 1992; McFarlane, 1992).

First, in the initial days after a traumatic event, the intrusive memories are a universal phenomenon and indicative of a normal process of reappraisal of the experience where various representations of the trauma are developed and an attempt is made to integrate these with existing psychological schemata. At this early stage, the intensity of these intrusions is unlikely to be an adequate measure of their psychopathological significance because their existence is virtually universal. It is unclear at which stage traumatic memories develop the typically fixed and irreconcilable quality with the associated sense of retraumatization often experienced in PTSD. The relatively inflexible quality of these more permanent memories represents the failure to resolve the issue of meaning.

An associated concern is the nature of the process that leads to the onset of the avoidance phenomena. One view is that they represent a defence that modulates the affect associated with the intense traumatic cognitions and images, and thus are manifest as part of the immediate trauma response (Horowitz 1986). Shalev's study found that the avoidance was not proportional to the intrusions in the immediate post accident period. It appeared that this phenomenon only emerged once the individual may not have been able to work through these phenomena.

The intensity of the affective disturbance and the pattern of arousal are the phenomena that particularly appear to separate the normal reprocessing of the event and PTSD. The factors that influence their recruitment and the definition of the nature of the underlying process are central to understanding the core of PTSD. From the beginning, clinicians such as Kardiner, who was attempting to define the characteristic features of combat related psychiatric disorder, focused on the unusual pattern of physiological arousal, the 'physioneurosis' (Freidman, 1988).

The inability of the initial levels of intrusion and avoidance to predict the onset of PTSD points to the role of some other process, such as the destabilisation of individuals' normal patterns of arousal which, in turn, has a feedback effect on patterns of cognitive and affective processing (Shalev, 1993). The focus on a cognitive processing model that has been very influential in determining the current conceptualisation of PTSD may have inadvertently hampered the need to investigate what differentiates adaptive and maladaptive trauma responses. The importance of the emerging pattern of arousal as a predictor of outcome was also suggested by Weisaeth's study (1989) of the victims of an industrial accident. He found that the failure of intense anxiety and sleep disturbance to settle in the first two weeks after the accident was a predictor of subsequent PTSD.

We need to increase our understanding of the stresses of disaster that are the most toxic determinants of PTSD, we need to further investigate the early stages of the trauma response and, we need to differentiate the distress response from the more enduring symptoms of PTSD.

The Stressor Criteria for PTSD

One of our foremost concerns is to understand and prevent the adverse health outcomes of disasters. The discussion of this issue has become dominated in the last 15 years by the focus on PTSD. However this is one of only a number a possible consequences of disaster. Thus, in discussing the stress of disaster, the focal issues are largely those associated with negative outcomes.

Hobfoll's (1991) conservation of resources (COR) model is attractive because it does not limit the focus on the development of PTSD, but considers a range of challenges and demands that a disaster presents to individuals' adaptational capacities. This implies that disasters can result in a variety of states, from becoming less able to manage and modulate the day to day demands of life, an undermining of normal coping strategies, the development of grief and the need to respond to the loss of attachments, through to the development of a range of psychological symptoms. These issues need to be judged in the context of the attributes and temperamental characteristics of individuals' lives, the groups' attributes, and the broader social context. The evidence of high levels of comorbidity in community civilian populations, on the one hand, and the fact that many people actually do quite well, on the other hand, demonstrate that the focus solely on PTSD is too narrow and does not adequately describe the range of responses. There is also the issue of the long term negative impact that these events have on physical health, which is not necessarily encompassed by a sole focus on PTSD.

The recent focus on PTSD has also had an important impact on the way the stress of disaster has been investigated. This is characterised by the definition of the stressor criterion, which not only defines the pathogenic elements of the trauma, but also the affective states that individuals must experience in response to the disaster if the event is considered to be the type that can cause a PTSD. The existence of the stressor criterion raises two concerns. First, there is a need in disasters to validate the strict boundaries of the criteria. How would a clinician conceive of those many victims who satisfy the other diagnostic criteria but who do not satisfy the stressor criterion? These may be people who have had a very high exposure but dissociated at the time of the disaster and therefore did not report the feelings of powerlessness, loss of control, and helplessness. In some regards the specificity of these criteria is premature and has the capacity to limit future research into this aetiological process. This may prevent and bias the understanding of the trauma response if researchers' enquiries are simply directed by the DSM IV diagnostic criteria.

Second, the criteria may have limited the scope of investigation into the quality and characteristics of the trauma that can lead to a range of other outcomes. It is also the case that the focus on PTSD has oversimplified the nature of the relationship between the stressor and PTSD. There are a series of well conducted studies that demonstrate that, while exposure is a necessary determinant of PTSD, it is not sufficient to explain the onset. The strength of the correlation between the severity of the trauma and the onset of disorder may not be any greater than with day to day life events. Thus, there are many victims of disasters who cope adequately and do not become symptomatic. The focus of mental health professionals on the negative outcome of these events may in itself have a detrimental effect on victimized communities. The few outcome studies on debriefing that have comparison groups suggest that these interventions may worsen the outcome of those participating, rather than having the desired effect of lessening the distress of those involved. This raises a series of critical ethical and theoretical issues because attempting to facilitate the psychological process presumed to be associated with coping may, in fact, have the reverse effect.

Conversely, focusing on the general issues of appraisal and coping and the more non-specific outcomes may deflect from a recognition of what are the most adverse outcomes. Given that even in most disaster studies PTSD has a prevalence of under 20%, most of the causal variance of non-specific distress may be determined by those stresses such as loss of property, the disruption of relationships and the undermining of a range of social resources (Freedy et al, 1993; Hobfoll, 1991). This might lead to an underestimation of the role of threat and horror as the determinant of the most pervasive and destructive long-term consequences of disaster for a small group of victims. Thus sampling can be a critical issue in developing an understanding of the particularly pathogenic element of the disaster, a question that is critical in determining whether the determinants of PTSD are different from the range of other adverse health outcomes that follow disasters.

It is therefore important to focus specifically on the elements of trauma that are thought to be critical in the aetiology of PTSD. The critical process appears to be the embedding of the trauma in victims' memory in a way that becomes frozen and unmalleable. The issue is whether there is specific quality of the experience of a traumatic event such as a disaster that can lead to this pattern of symptoms. Equally, disasters are events that often involve gradients of exposure and threat. It is unclear at what point the level of exposure ceases to have the quality that is necessary to trigger the typical traumatic stress response and the pattern of conditioned anxiety that is central to aspects of this syndrome. Unless the specific components of disasters are examined and if general theories of the stress response are utilised, these issues may not be identified.

The Secondary Trauma of PTSD

Several studies have now demonstrated that patients who have been psychotic can develop a series of symptoms identical to PTSD in response to the experience of the illness. Thus the experience of a psychological disorder can create the same sense of powerlessness and threat of disintegration that confronts the victims of disaster. What about the experience of PTSD? In contrast to the actual trauma, the symptoms of the illness seemingly have no apparent end for those with the more chronic form of the disorder. Sufferers have to cope with the constant recurrence of the memory of the trauma, particularly when they occur in the form of flashbacks having many of the qualities of the original trauma. Thus, while the realistic danger has ended, the affective reality can be that of ongoing retraumatisation. For those who develop the disorder, the internal sense of threat and loss of control may present a new dimension of trauma. The inability to control the content of their thoughts and feelings constantly revictimises sufferers.

It is generally assumed that the attitudes, appraisals and behaviors seen in PTSD sufferers are a consequence of the experience of the disaster. However, Spurrell and McFarlane (1993) found that the secondary appraisal caused by the onset of the disorder played a major role in determining the described pattens of coping behaviors. The presence of nightmares and sleep disturbance mean that even the safety of withdrawal into unconsciousness is lost. The irritability, emotional numbing and anhedonia mean that the relationships that are critical to individuals' sense of identity and attachments are equally threatened and undermined by the changed pattern of reactivation. Thus, the very attachments that can provide a powerful motivation for survival in the face of disaster can be threatened by the secondary changes in the responsiveness of PTSD sufferers. The disorder of attention and concentration means that they are no longer able to lock into their current environment with the same sense of energy and involvement. Simple activities, like reading, participating in conversation and watching television are no longer reflex activities but demand greater effort.

It is this world and the sense of being damaged that many of the victims of disaster describe as the worst aspect of the experience in the long term, not the immediate horror. Any measure of trauma and coping taken a significant period after the disaster is likely to be contaminated by this secondary process. This issue has not been addressed in the trauma area and is likely to be a particular issue in the Vietnam veteran literature which has examined this population long after combat.

The effect of having PTSD on the recall of the event is a related issue, particularly in studies of victim groups where there is a large delay between the trauma and its recall. There are two studies which demonstrate the differential recall of events by those with PTSD and those without. In a longitudinal study of firefighters, those without PTSD failed to report that they had been injured in over 50% of cases in contrast to the PTSD group who continued to recall accurately their injuries. A measure of exposure taken 12 months after the disaster would have identified incorrectly that the frequency of injury was a determinant of PTSD. This phenomenon has also been observed in holocaust survivors who gave evidence about their experience soon after the end of the war and then had to present evidence in war crimes trials many years later, at which time they give muted accounts of the trauma.

It is my conclusion that, the emergence of PTSD in some disaster survivors can be an equally traumatic experience to the disaster itself and this can then retrospectively modify their appraisal and recall of the disaster. This has a major potential to bias retrospectively collected data. This is a critical point in defining the valid window of observation for the effects of trauma and disaster and the importance of considering the appraisal and consequences of developing a PTSD in the aftermath of a disaster.

Conclusion

Defining the reality of a disaster is a much more complicated task than it appears at first glance. The issue of measurement is one that is needs to be confronted by the community of disaster researchers if the field is going to advance in the immediate future. The danger is that the stressor criterion for PTSD in DSM IV will artificially constrict and limit the examination of the issue because it imposes an unwarranted degree of certainty in a setting where some of the most basic questions remain to be answered.

Many of the propositions that are accepted in the trauma area are potentially distorted through the retrospective perceptions of the victims. There is a need to better understand the immediate distress response and the process of appraisal which occurs at this stage. The cognitive and affective distortions that are core components of PTSD subsequently become a secondary layer through which the disaster comes to be interpreted and defined. Equally the distress generated by the disorder comes to challenge the primacy of the trauma as the most threatening and damaging aspect of the experience.

References

American Psychiatric Association (1993). Diagnostic and statistical manual of mental disorders. (3rd ed.). Washington DC: American Psychiatric Association.

Breslau, N., Davis, G. C., Andreski, P., & Peterson, E. (1991). Traumatic events and posttraumatic stress disorder in an urban population of young adults. Archives of General Psychiatry, 48, 216-222.

Bromet, G. E., Schulberg, H. C., & Dunn, L. O. (1982). Reactions of psychiatric patients to the Three Mile Island nuclear accident. Archives of General Psychiatry, 39, 725-730.

Brown, G. W., & Harris, T. (1978). The social origins of depression: a study of psychiatric disorder in women. London, Tavistock.

Carr, Y. J., Lewin, T. J., Carter, G. L., & Webster, R. A. (1992). Patterns of service utilisation following the 1989 Newcastle earthquake: findings from phase 1 of the Quake Impact study. Australian Journal of Public Health, 16, 360-369.

Creamer, M., Burgess, P., & Pattison, P. (1992). Reaction to trauma: a cognitive processing model. Journal of Abnormal Psychology, 101, 452-459.

Davidson, J. T. R., & Foa, E. (1992). DSM-IV Trauma and Beyond. Washington: APA Press DC.

Foa, E. B., Steketee, G., & Rothbaum, B. O. (1989). Behavioral cognitive conceptualizations of post-traumatic stress disorder. Behavioral Therapy, 20, 155-176.

Fontana, A., Rosenheck, R., & Brett, E. (1992). War zone traumas and posttraumatic stress disorder symptomatology. Journal of Nervous and Mental Disease, 180, 748-755.

Freedy, J. R., Kilpatrick, J. R., & Resnick, H. S. (1993). Natural disasters and mental health: theory, assessment, and intervention. In Allen, R. (ed), Handbook of post-disaster interventions. (Special Issue). Journal of Social Behavior and Personality, 8, 49-63.

Freud, S. (1973). Introductory lectures on psychoanalysis: fixation to traumas - the unconscious. Translated by Strachey, James. Ringwood, Victoria: Penguin Books.

Freidman, M. J. (1988). Toward rational pharmacotherapy for posttraumatic stress disorder: an interim report. American Journal of Psychiatry, 145, 281-285.

Green, B. L. (1993). Identifying survivors at risk trauma and stressor across events. In J. P. Wilson, and B. Raphael (Eds), International handbook of traumatic stress syndormes, (pp. 135-144). New York, Plenum Press.

Hauff, E., & Vaglum, P. (1993). Vietnamese boat refugees: the influence of war and flight traumatization on mental health on arrival in the country of resettlement: a community cohort study of Vietnamese refugees in Norway. Acta Psychiatrica Scandinavica, 88, 162-168.

Hobfoll, S. E. (1991). Traumatic stress: a theory based on rapid loss of resources. Anxiety Research, 4, 187-197.

Holmes, T. H., & Rahe, R. H. (1967). The social readjustment of rating scale. Journal of Psychosomatic Research, 11, 215-218.

Horowitz, M. J. (1986). Stress response syndromes. New York, Jason Aronson.

Hughes, S. (1990). Inside Madness. British Medical Journal, 301, 1476-1478.

Janney, J. G., Masuda, M., & Holmes, T. H. (1977). Impact of a natural catastrophe on life events. Journal of Human Stress, 3, 22-35.

McFarlane, A. C. (1989). The aetiology of post-traumatic morbidity: predisposing, precipitating and perpetuating factors. British Journal of Psychiatry, 154, 221-228.

McFarlane, A. C. (1991). Victims and survivors. Current Opinions in Psychiatry, 4, 833-836.

McFarlane, A. C. (1992). Avoidance and intrusion in posttraumatic stress disorder. Journal of Nervous and Mental Disease, 180, 439-445.

McFarlane, A. C., & Cao, H. (1993). Study of a major disaster in the People's Republic of China: The Yunnan Earthquake. In Raphael, B. and Wilson, J. (Eds.). The International Handbook of Traumatic Stress Syndromes (pp. 493-498). New York, Plenum Press.

Napier, M. (1991). The medical and legal trauma of disasters. The Medical and Legal Traumas of Disasters, 59, 157-181.

Pugh, C., & Trimble, M. R. (1993). Psychiatric injury after Hillsborough. British Journal of Psychiatry, 163, 425-429.

Raphael, B., Lundin, T., & Weisaeth, L. (1989). PTSS-10: Reactions following an accident or a disaster. Acta Psychiatrica Scandinavica, Supplementum, 353 (80), 58.

Shalev, A. (1992). Posttraumatic stress disorder among injured survivors of a terrorist attack: predictive value of early intrusion and avoidance symptoms. Journal of Nervous and Mental Disease, 180, 505-509.

Shalev, A. Y. (1993). Post-traumatic stress disorder: a biopsychological perspective. Israeli Journal of Psychiatry and Related Science, 30, 102-109.

Solomon, S. D., & Canino, G. J. (1990). Appropriateness of DSM-III-R criteria for Post-traumatic Stress Disorder. Comprehensive Psychiatry, 31, 227-237.

Spiegel (1993). Standford Acute Stress Reaction Questionnaire. (Unpublished manuscript).

Spurrell, M., & McFarlane, A. C. (1993). Posttraumatic stress disorder and coping after a natural disaster. Social Psychiatry and Psychiatric Epidemiology, 28, 194-200.

True, W. R., Heath, A. C., Rice, J., Eisen, S. A., Goldberg, J., & Lyons, M. J. (1993, October). Multivariate analysis of genetic and environmental contributions to susceptibility to posttraumatic stress disorder. Proceedings of ISTSS Meeting, San Antonio, Texas, U.S.A.

van der Kolk, B. A., & van der Hart, O. (1991). The intrusive past: the flexibility of memory and the engraving of trauma. American Imago, 48, 425-454.

Weisaeth, L. (1989). The stressors and the post-traumatic stress syndrome after an industrial disaster. Special Issue: Traumatic stress: Empirical studies from Norway. Acta Psychiatrica Scandinavica, 80, 25-37.

World Health Organisation. (1992). Mental disorders: glossary and guide to their classification in accordance with the tenth revision of the International Classification of Disease. Geneva: World Health Organisation.

Wortman, C. B., & Silver, R. C. (1989). The myths of coping with loss. Journal of Consulting and Clinical Psychology, 57, 349-357.

METHODOLOGICAL ISSUES IN DESIGNING RESEARCH ON COMMUNITY-WIDE DISASTERS WITH SPECIAL REFERENCE TO CHERNOBYL

Evelyn J. Bromet, Ph.D.
State University of New York at Stony Brook
Stony Brook, New York, U.S.A.

Research aimed at elucidating the effects of community-wide or traumatic stress on the health and well-being of exposed populations represents a classic function of epidemiology. In this instance, the primary purpose is to delineate the distribution of illness or impairment in the population and the stress-related risk factors that are associated with both incidence (new onsets of disorder) and prevalence (recurrent episodes). As is true for any type of exposure, there are two basic approaches to investigating the effects of community-wide stressors. As Schlesselman and Stolley (1982) straightforwardly note: "One is to proceed from cause to effect; the other is to proceed from effect to cause" (p. 10).

Prior to the 1979 nuclear power plant accident at Three Mile Island, there were few disaster studies that incorporated the basic elements of epidemiologic research. Important among these are: representative sampling, appropriate control groups, systematic and reliable measurement of outcome variables, and multivariate analysis of exposure effects that takes into account the array of known risk factors, moderators, or mediators of the disorders under study. In epidemiologic terms, disaster and community stress research by and large represent a special case of the classic cohort paradigm (Henderson, 1988; Kelsey, Thompson, & Evans, 1986; Lilienfeld & Lilienfeld, 1980) in which a random sample, or stratified random sample, of exposed and unexposed individuals are assessed prospectively to determine the risk of disease attributable to the exposure. Because the study population in disaster research is usually selected <u>after</u> rather than <u>before</u> the occurrence of an exposure or traumatic event, as required by the classical cohort design, the paradigm is referred to as a "modified cohort" design.

Disaster studies utilizing a modified cohort design have been either cross-sectional or longitudinal. Cross-sectional studies can address short-term effects, such as Solomon's study of Israelis who evacuated from Tel Aviv during the 1991 Gulf War (Z. Solomon et al., 1993), or long-term effects. A noteworthy example of the latter is the National Vietnam Veterans study in which a randomly selected sample of Vietnam veterans were compared with veterans who served elsewhere during the same era, and with civilian controls (Kulka et al., 1990). The dependent measures encompassed an array of psychosocial and psychiatric sequelae, including post-traumatic stress disorder. The risk factors included specific data on the intensity and duration of combat exposure, as well as predispositional and social situational variables that could modify the effects of exposure to combat. A growing body of longitudinal studies of disaster victims have focused on the evolution of clinically-relevant as well as subclinical mental health effects of man-made (e.g., Dew & Bromet, 1993; Palinkas, Petterson, Russell, & Downs, 1993; Green et al., 1990) as well as natural catastrophes (e.g., Shore, Tatum, & Vollmer, 1986; Canino, Bravo, Rubio-Stipec, & Woodbury, 1990). Such research has also identified disaster-related factors, such as involvement and proximity, that can magnify the adverse effects of a disaster in both adults and children (Bromet & Schulberg, 1987). Several excellent substantive and methodological reviews of this research have recently appeared (e.g., Rubonis & Bickman, 1991; Saylor, 1993; S. Solomon, 1989; Vogel & Vernberg, 1993).

The modified cohort study design provides a powerful paradigm for understanding stress. However, because assessments usually take place after the target event, there are several intrinsic biases that constrain the inferences we can draw. These include selective mortality from the exposure itself (e.g., studies of earthquake victims or war veterans focus on survivors of these experiences); recall bias or faulty memory (e.g., women living near Three Mile Island who were recently depressed overreported prior episodes of major depression compared to women who were symptom-free at the time of interview [Bromet et al. 1986]; nonresponse -- especially in controls who are often less motivated to participate or exposed who are too preoccupied or angry to participate (Weisaeth, 1989); and interviewer bias, when raters are not blind to exposure status and also reside in the exposed area.

Another source of bias occurs when investigators, intentionally or not, try to prove that an exposure does or does not result in a particular set of outcomes. In some cases, this type of bias occurs when the research is funded by special interest groups, such as the tobacco industry or the lead industry. However, it is important to note that many investigations are undertaken without prejudice from a funding source. For example, the Nuclear Regulatory Commission sponsored a longitudinal study of stress following the Three Mile Island accident. In that study, Baum, Gatchel and Schaeffer (1983) reported significantly higher levels of chronic stress symptoms in residents living within five miles of the plant compared to controls living near another nuclear reactor, a fossil-fuel power plant, or in an area with no power plant. In other cases, biased conclusions are drawn when authors do not specify the study limitations or alternative explanations for the findings. To illustrate, the International Chernobyl Project (International Advisory Committee, 1991; Mettler et al., 1992) is the largest published epidemiologic study to date which compared the health status of five groups who remained in contaminated villages (2 year olds born in 1988; 5 year olds born in

1986; 10 year olds born in 1980; 40 year olds born in 1950; and 60 year olds born in 1930) with controls from "uncontaminated" villages. The investigators concluded that these populations were not significantly different from controls on hematological, thyroid, and general health problems (except abdominal problems), but that 3-5% of all children had health problems that required treatment. Psychological stress was the only variable described as more prevalent in the settlements contaminated by radiation, but the measures of psychological stress were rudimentary. The fact that the control sites were heavily contaminated by pesticides went unmentioned, and the possibility that the effects of radiation might not appear for two decades was minimized. More importantly, as a study of the effects of radiation exposure from Chernobyl, the design itself was inadequate because the sampling scheme did not include evacuees from the most exposed villages or clean-up workers who received the greatest exposure after the accident. Because these limitations were not well addressed by the investigators and might not be apparent to readers unfamiliar with the event and geographic area, a naive reader could easily conclude that Chernobyl had no immediate health consequences. In fact, other medical research has demonstrated increased rates of thyroid disease (Baverstock, 1993; Furmanchuk et al., 1992) and other radiation-related health problems (Brennan, 1990).

There have been several thoughtful discussions of the types of methodological problems noted above and the strategies that can be implemented to overcome potential weaknesses of the modified cohort design. In particular, S. Solomon (1989) identified several ways in which the modified cohort design could be strengthened, such as characterizing the disaster and its component parts, assessing the full range of relevant outcomes, and measuring appropriate predispositional and mediating factors. Most importantly, she urges investigators to take advantage of "natural experiments" arising during the course of a longitudinal investigation so that unbiased pre-event information can be utilized. Although there are precious few examples, this prospective method is the most powerful paradigm for understanding the health consequences of stress. Such an opportunity arose during our Three Mile Island research program when the comparison site in western Pennsylvania underwent a major recession in the steel industry and a large proportion of the husbands of these subjects were laid off from their jobs. Since the lay-offs occurred after we had obtained 2-3 waves of data, it was possible to evaluate the mental health effects of this community stress prospectively (Dew, Bromet, & Schulberg, 1987; Penkower, Bromet, & Dew, 1988). Another research example that deserves special mention in this context is Solomon's study of Israeli soldiers who fought in Lebanon for whom longitudinal pre-event evaluations had been routinely performed, enabling this investigator to determine the unique contribution of the war-stress experience on subsequent mental health (Z. Solomon, 1993).

Most disaster research has been conducted in the developed world even though most of the worst disasters have occurred in developing countries (Lima et al., 1990; Weisaeth, 1993). Moreover, modern disasters, such as Chernobyl, can arise without fixed temporal or spatial boundaries. In 1992, we were asked to design a study of the mental health effects of Chernobyl on children who were evacuated to Kiev from Pripyat, a town built to house Chernobyl workers and their families. In attempting to design such a study, it became apparent that the conceptual and methodological underpinnings of prior research could not be easily applied to this circumstance. This paper addresses the special methodological issues that arose and highlights the alternatives, compromises, and inferential limitations that evolved when we attempted to design a feasible, yet epidemiologically sound, mental health study.

Background: The Chernobyl Catastrophe

The catastrophe at the Chernobyl nuclear plant began on April 26, 1986, when one of the four reactors exploded. "An area of 1000 square kilometers, containing 98 villages and many farms, was heavily contaminated and evacuated and has since been deemed unsuitable for continuing human habitation" (Kidd, 1991, p. 765). The accident at the Chernobyl nuclear power station proved to be one of the worst long-term disasters in modern history. Thousands of families living near the Chernobyl plant were exposed to radiation, and their lives were permanently disrupted by relocation to new, often unreceptive environments and, for many, by unremitting fears about the long-term health effects of the exposure. Although incontestable statistics on exposure, mortality, morbidity, and evacuation are not available, the invisible threat of cancer is an omnipresent vestige of the Chernobyl catastrophe. A recent summary of the events ensuing from Chernobyl, written by Z. Medvedev (1994), indicates that an alarming increase in thyroid cancer has already occurred in highly exposed children, with 85 known cases in 1992-93 in Belarus compared to 2-3 known cases before 1986.

The environmental threats resulting from the Chernobyl accident have persisted, particularly since the sarcophagus built to contain the damaged reactor is eroding. There is continuing fear of further contamination from the damaged reactor, of a malfunction of the remaining reactors, and most importantly, of the unknown long-term health effects of the radiation exposure.

One of the larger towns to be evacuated was Pripyat (population 45,000) built adjacent to the reactors to house the workforce and their families. Almost half of the Pripyat families were evacuated to Kiev. Many of the women from Pripyat had organized themselves into a political action group called Children of Chernobyl. In a meeting with epidemiologists from the University of Pittsburgh who were conducting a study of cataract development (Day et al., 1994), they expressed strong concerns about the mental health of their children and indicated the need for a systematic evaluation of the effects of the stress from Chernobyl on the well-being of their children. Their ultimate goal was to obtain appropriate help for their children. Since these investigators were aware of the Pittsburgh study of the mental health effects of the Three Mile Island accident on mothers of young children (e.g., Bromet et al., 1982; Dew et al., 1987; Dew & Bromet, 1993), they contacted the present author about designing a similar study with these evacuees. With funding from the National Institute of Mental Health, Dr. Bromet, together with Dmitry Goldgaber, a molecular biologist from the former Soviet Union, conducted a feasibility study to determine the breadth and scope of a possible epidemiologic inquiry. After extensive meetings with key informants in Kiev, including local physicians, academicians, politicians, and psychiatrists, as well as with groups of mothers from Pripyat, we learned about several important issues that were to shape our research plans.

One group of issues centered around the traumatic events that occurred during the relocation period. The evacuation was extremely chaotic and traumatic. Most families were actually evacuated twice, first from Pripyat, and then from the village where they were relocated which turned out to be contaminated as well. Although people were told that nothing very serious had happened, pregnant women were strongly advised to have abortions. These abortions were performed on a massive scale in May at children's summer camp sites temporarily used during the resettlement.

A second set of issues emanated from the resettlement in Kiev. For years, the families evacuated to Kiev lived in a state of uncertainty because they were not given permanent residency papers. Instead, they were given temporary residency papers which meant that they could be relocated against their will at any moment. It took extensive efforts to obtain permanent residency papers for Kiev and decent apartments. In addition, in spite of the privileges granted to the evacuees in the form of social benefits and health care, actually obtaining these benefits was a constant struggle in the deteriorating economy of the country. Several evacuated mothers complained that doctors were often reluctant to treat their children because of the amount of paperwork required. At the same time, their neighbors, who incurred their own hardships because of the poor economic conditions, were initially hostile to the evacuees whom they perceived as privileged because of the social and financial benefits they were granted. Throughout this period, many evacuated women continued to grieve for Pripyat where life was objectively more pleasant and the community was close knit.

Another factor to be considered in designing the research was the wide range of somatic symptoms reported by mothers and local doctors. Some children were reportedly sick for long periods of time and missed a great deal of school. We were frequently told that the children's immune systems had been compromised. Consistent with findings from the few systematic studies of children exposed to severe, sustained traumas (Aptekar & Boore, 1990; Raphael, 1986), the women described a wide range of anxiety, mood, somatic, and externalizing symptoms in their children. The most common diagnosis we heard from local doctors was an illness unknown in Western medicine, namely, "vascular dystony," a syndrome believed to be associated with blood pressure changes. This syndrome encompassed a variety of symptoms, such as weakness, irritability, headaches, angina, and tiredness. These doctors also noted "unique changes in blood cells" in exposed children.

An issue of considerable importance was the general distrust of authorities. In fact, the truth about what happened at the Chernobyl nuclear plant was withheld from the public for more than two years. As a consequence, by 1992, official information was generally distrusted. We found that evacuees were also suspicious of government-sponsored studies, such as the International Chernobyl Project noted above, which showed no health differences between exposed and control populations.

Finally, and of crucial importance to planning our research, many mothers we met appeared to relive these traumatic experiences during our meetings as if they had happened very recently. Our encounters had the quality of "sitting Shiva," the Jewish process of ritualized mourning, as the evacuees expressed extreme distress and anxiety about the events unleashed by Chernobyl. Perhaps because of the continued threats and uncertainty, the ritualized grieving process never ceased.

In summary, the Chernobyl disaster shared some features with other man-made disasters. Similar to other disasters, the explosion led to a cascade of successive exposures and stressors that impacted on the community. Like other technological accidents, this event has unknown temporal boundaries. However, unlike previous technological accidents, including Three Mile Island, this event also had undefined spatial boundaries both with respect to the geographic areas affected, the disorganized evacuation of thousands of people from the 30 kilometer zone around the plant, as well as the dispersal of an estimated 600,000-1,000,000 clean-up workers, or "liquidators," many of whom remain anonymous to this day.

The remainder of this chapter describes the methodological challenges we faced in designing a cross-sectional comparative study of the Pripyat children.

Methodological Adjustments

To study the mental health effects of Chernobyl on children evacuated to Kiev from Pripyat, what types of modifications to the basic cohort design would be necessary? The challenges involved every issue inherent in designing a cohort study. These issues include (1) defining the population at risk, (2) selecting an appropriate control group, (3) choosing impairment measures that reflected unique cultural expressions of distress and had cross-national validity, (4) characterizing the array of stresses from the event and from everyday life and assessing them with minimal bias, and (5) identifying relevant dispositional and mediating variables; and (6) designing a culturally appropriate informed consent procedure.

Population at Risk

In order to have results that would be generalizable to all children from Pripyat, the ideal cohort is a random sample of these evacuated children. Theoretically, each of the three affected republics, Ukraine, Russia, and Belarus, maintains a registry of all families who were evacuated from the 30-kilometer area. The Division of Mental Health of the World Health Organization (WHO) drew samples from the three registries for a follow-up screening of neurological damage in children who were in utero at the time of the evacuation (World Health Organization,

1993). However, there is no published information on the completeness and accuracy of these registries. With the possible exception of the WHO, Western scientists were not given direct access to the registries to examine their integrity as a research sampling frame. Without the ability to investigate the adequacy of the registry, it was impossible to develop a complete sampling frame for the Pripyat population.

The second best cohort was the 20,000 Pripyat evacuees living in Kiev. Clearly, this sample includes fewer than half of the original population and contains its own, albeit unknown, biases. In addition, some families who moved to Kiev subsequently relocated to another nuclear plant town (Slavuta), and others moved abroad (some to seek better medical care). Since there were few Jewish families in Pripyat, emigration to Israel was not a major source of sample leakage. Within the boundaries of Kiev itself, however, there was no central listing of evacuee families. This left us with two options. One was to design a two-stage household sampling procedure in Kiev to assemble a sampling frame; the second was to identify a sample of convenience.

During our meetings in Kiev, we were presented with a convenience sample comprised of two schools in which 32% and 47% of the student bodies, respectively, were from Pripyat (N=1276 Pripyat-born children aged 9-18 in 1992). Of course, this school-based cohort contained all of the limitations of any school sample. That is, drop-outs, institutionalized, and very sick children were excluded. In Ukraine, a school-based sample has additional limitations. Children living in orphanages do not attend public school. In addition, after age 15, many adolescents leave school to attend vocational or technical school, and they would need to be located by other means.

In psychiatric epidemiology, there are some noteworthy precedents for selecting samples of convenience. Chief among them is the Epidemiologic Catchment Area project (Robins & Regier, 1991). This study involved samples drawn from selected catchment areas in five unique sites (New Haven, Connecticut; Raleigh-Durham, North Carolina; Baltimore, Maryland; Los Angeles, California; and St. Louis, Missouri). Much was learned about the occurrence and correlates of mental illness in these populations. However, because the catchment areas were neither randomly selected nor representative of census tracts in their communities, the resulting estimated rates of mental illness in the geographic areas from which the samples derived must be considered tentative at best. However, the range in prevalence estimates across the sites, and the differences in the demographic correlates of specific disorders across sites, served as useful information for subsequent planning of local and national mental health research. Some of the substantive findings, particularly the unexpectedly high rate of comorbidity of lifetime disorders, the inverse relationship between age and mental illness, and the underutilization of mental health services by community residents with diagnosable disorders, represented important advances in knowledge.

Thus, in spite of sampling limitations emanating from a sample of convenience, we decided that we could gain valuable information about the rates and correlates of mental disorder in a school-based sample of evacuated children. Although a two-stage sampling strategy potentially provides more generalizable data, a sample of convenience drawn from public schools is less costly and more efficient. Moreover, the high level of support from the teachers and administrators facilitated the inclusion of teacher ratings, which are an essential component of mental health research on children.

Comparison Groups

Because of the extreme social and economic turmoil that followed the dismantling of the Soviet Union, it was crucial to have a comparison group to disentangle the effects of socioeconomic stresses from those associated with the evacuation and exposure experiences. One desirable comparison group was exposed children who were not evacuated from their homes. Such a group would permit an analysis of the degree of risk associated with exposure independent of the evacuation. Unfortunately, the exposed populations who were not evacuated resided in small villages that received lower levels of radiation. Psychiatric disorders and educational problems have been found to be more prevalent in urban than rural children (e.g., Rutter et al., 1975) in part because of economic and cultural differences (Zahner, Jacobs, Freeman & Trainor, 1993). Thus, potential disparities between evacuees who grew up in Kiev and children living in contaminated villages could be explained by urban-rural differences.

Since the evacuee children moved to Kiev in 1986, they in fact were reared in the same general environment as their Kiev-born peers and shared many of the same life experiences. Evacuated families lived in the same housing projects, shopped in the same markets, and were subject to the same shortages of food, hot water, medicine, and other necessities, as their neighbors (e.g., for a three-day period in December 1991, no food was available in Kiev). Thus a reasonable comparison group were the Kiev-born school peers (N=1977) of the evacuated children. It is important to note, however, that in 1986, the children in Kiev were also exposed to radiation, albeit at lower levels. Our on-site collaborators described Kiev in the summer of 1986 as a city without children. Conceivably, the Kiev parents' perceptions of ensuing dangers could minimize the differences between these children's health and the well-being of the evacuated children. A method frequently used in epidemiology to dampen the effects that arise when controls are potentially influenced by the factor being investigated is to use sampling ratios of 1 exposed to 2-4 controls. Fortunately, in the two schools, there were more locally-born than evacuated children.

Thus, the exposed and comparison samples were to be drawn from two schools in Kiev. These samples were less than ideal from the perspective of an epidemiologically-oriented study. The evacuees were not only the tip of the iceberg with respect to exposed children, but also a potentially non-representative group. The comparison group endured more stress than children normally encounter growing up. Could we identify measures that offset the limitations of the design?

Measurement

It is not within the purview of this chapter to describe available interview schedules in detail or general guidelines for establishing reliability and validity in disaster or cross-cultural research on children. Asking direct questions about the impact of a disaster when there is the potential for monetary gain is obviously risky. Within the context of a disaster with no temporal boundaries, there may never be a time when exposure-connected gains are not sought. However, there were several measurement issues that merit special comment in the context of designing a study of the mental health effects of Chernobyl.

Limitations of self-report symptom data. In psychiatric epidemiology, particularly in studies of adult populations, researchers rely on self-report data typically without corroboration from records or from significant others. There has also been an unquestioned acceptance that a differential diagnosis can be formulated on the basis of data from 1-2 hour cross-sectional diagnostic interviews scored by a computer algorithm (Fennig & Bromet, 1992). In our view, this has been an extremely naive tradition perpetuated by convenience and shortsightedness in the same way that simple life event checklists, rather than detailed assessments of stress in its context, became the method of choice for measuring stress.

In children's mental health research, investigators routinely collect information from the child, the teacher, and a parent, thus obtaining rich albeit often contradictory and confusing, symptom reports. When mental health surveys are conducted in settings with no epidemiologic or social psychiatric research tradition and a general lack of understanding of Western psychiatry, as is the case in Kiev, the choice of assessment tools is limited. In the context of studying Chernobyl's mental health effects, it was not possible to use semi-structured diagnostic interview schedules, as in our TMI and other studies, because there were no master's level mental health professionals and few psychiatrists who understood and practiced Western psychiatry. In spite of their disadvantages, fully-structured interviews to assess children's psychopathology can be administered by educated non-professionals and were the instruments of choice. However, their sensitivity and specificity in non-western cultures were unknown.

A unique issue in the assessment of mental health after a disaster, such as Chernobyl, is the bias imposed when the disaster is viewed as a cause of poor health. As a result of our meetings with a variety of local informants, it was clear that many mothers and teachers firmly believed that evacuated children had a greater than expected level of physical morbidity. Thus, methods for detecting and calibrating such bias would need to be employed. Since retrospective reports about mental health are influenced by current status (Bromet et al., 1986), objective medical and school records can serve as a valuable resource in children's research. However, when the families were evacuated from Pripyat, they were not allowed to remove their belongings because everything they owned was contaminated. Original medical and school records that might have provided objective historical information were left behind. Thus, the pre-event competence and well-being of the exposed children and their parents could only be assessed retrospectively.

One of the most common symptoms in both children and adults are phobias. The findings from the ECA (Robins & Regier, 1991) and from the National Comorbidity Study indicated that the diagnosis of phobias was also the most prevalent of the psychiatric disorders evaluated (Kessler et al., 1994). After the Chernobyl accident, many medical professionals regarded people's fears as an indicator of "radiophobia" (Giel, 1991). This opinion was promulgated even though it was illogical to consider such fears as `irrational' when radioactive contamination was widespread. It was thus important to design an assessment of the full range of phobias without raising suspicions about the integrity of the research.

Disentangling somatic from psychosomatic disorder. The Pripyat mothers expressed overwhelming concerns about their children's physical health. Because they frequently kept them home from school, the local teachers also regarded the evacuees as a physically ill population. Findings from a survey of high school students by social psychologists in Kiev indicated that somatic symptoms were significantly elevated in evacuees compared to Kiev controls. There was also evidence from Western physicians that exposed children were not healthy. For example, Kidd (1991) reported that 42 children sent to Australia from orphanages in Ukraine were suffering from "the effects of chronic radiation exposure and malnutrition, such as anemia and mild thyroid disorders" as well as chronic fatigue, headaches, and recurrent respiratory and skin infections (p. 766). As in other non-western societies, physical complaints are also a common means of expressing psychological distress (Rueck & Porter, 1965). Recent data gathered by a psychiatric genetics research group showed that children outside of Moscow had elevated rates of somatic complaints compared to children in other countries (Pauls, 1992).

A study of the effects of Chernobyl should have the ability to separate somatic symptoms with a functional etiology from somatic symptoms resulting from psychological stress. Even under the best conditions, this task is extremely difficult. In a cross-sectional study conducted in setting with inadequate medical services, disentangling somatic from psychosomatic symptoms poses a special challenge. At the time of our visit to Kiev, there was a single Western medical clinic in Kiev. Funded by governmental agencies in France, this clinic was established to examine children from the 30-kilometer zone. Because the clinic was mandated only to make diagnoses and not to provide treatment, there was some suspicion among the evacuees about its "real purpose." Nevertheless, we incorporated a diagnostic evaluation of each study child by the French clinic in order to identify serious medical problems, such as thyroid disease, that could account for somatic complaints. However, in the absence of physical findings, reported somatic complaints cannot confidently be attributed to psychological stress.

Chernobyl-related stress. While some stressors were differentially experienced (e.g., some women were pregnant at the time, and among them, most but not all had government-recommended abortions), other stresses from Chernobyl were universal.

Moreover, the sample received a triple exposure - first from the radioactivity before evacuating, second from the evacuation, and third from relocation. It therefore is difficult if not impossible to disentangle the effects of these co-existing stresses. Furthermore, because the study would take place several years after the event, the cumulative impact encompassed both objective Chernobyl-induced stressors and stress deriving from ineffective coping with Chernobyl-related problems. The children themselves weathered stress through their own experiences as well as through the reactions of their parents. McFarlane, Policansky, and Irwin (1987) suggested that in some cases, maternal response to a disaster is a better predictor of posttraumatic phenomena in children than direct exposure. Thus, multiple measures of objective and subjective stress occurring within and outside the family setting would be needed. Even so, the retrospective accounts of stressful experiences associated with Chernobyl would be colored by the resolutions that occurred over time.

Disaster researchers have described the deleterious effects of social network disruptions that ensue when members of communities are relocated without regard to existing bonds (Raphael, 1986). During the Chernobyl evacuation, many Pripyat children were separated from their families. In Kiev, they had difficulty becoming integrated into their new neighborhoods and schools where other children regarded them as contaminated and objects of fear. Raphael (1986) commented: "The loss of home, a strange environment, ... separation from parents, from familiar neighborhood and environment... the loss of toys and treasures, and crowded and strange accommodations are all likely to be stressful for children in the post-disaster period" (p. 165). Evacuated children had all of these experiences. Was it possible for these children or their mothers to recall, several years later, each relevant stressor and the associated distress that ensued? In the absence of specific information, was the global picture a suitable alternative?

Other risk factors. In children's mental health research, including studies of children under stress, the most important risk factor for psychopathology is parental mental health (Rutter, 1988). It has been well established that Russian men have a high rate of alcoholism (Grant, 1992). After the Chernobyl accident, there were widespread rumors that consumption of vodka and red wine counteracted the effect of radiation. It was also reported that evacuated adults, especially Chernobyl workers, expressed their distress by engaging in heavy drinking and alcohol abuse. Thus, parental alcohol abuse stands out among the more prominent variables that might moderate or mediate the relationship between Chernobyl-related stress and children's mental health. Prevailing definitions of what constitutes alcoholism derive from Western conceptualizations of substance abuse and dependence. Establishing the reliability and validity of alcohol abuse scales in Kiev would thus have to become a priority among the many cross-national measurement issues at hand.

Informed consent. The final data collection issue that arose in attempting to design a study of Chernobyl was obtaining informed consent. The American procedure involves parent and child signatures on a sometimes elaborate consent form detailing all of the untoward possibilities that could arise from being interviewed as well as release forms allowing the researcher to review medical and school records. We were told that in Kiev, many people might view these forms with suspicion and worry that their signatures could have unknown adverse consequences. As American investigators, we needed to consider culturally appropriate methods for implementing the spirit and intent of informed consent procedures in this setting which had no similar tradition and in which these practices might be perceived with distrust.

Conclusion

A series of compromises were necessary in designing a feasible cohort study of the mental health effects of Chernobyl on children. These concessions included selecting a school-based sample, selecting a comparison group that was also exposed to radiation, relying on retrospective data without corroborative evidence from records, and possibily not being able to disentangle the various stresses emanating from the accident. In order words, many epidemiologic principles would be violated. Is such a study still worth undertaking? The answer, of course, depends on the values of the individual investigator, or in our case, the review committee. If one believes that an epidemiologically flawed descriptive study can be worthwhile if the results are useful for generating new clinical knowledge and meaningful clinical interventions, then the answer is yes. In our view, the effects of Chernobyl cannot be understood without a descriptive mental health study, imperfect though it might be, and such data are sorely needed by residents and health care providers in Kiev to identify the types and sources of problems experienced by children evacuated to that community. Such a study could be the first-stage in a series of larger prevalence studies with more representative samples of evacuated children from the 30-kilometer zone or from non-evacuated, highly contaminated areas in Ukraine, Belarus and Russia.

On the other hand, if one holds the opinion that the only worthwhile study is one that provides results that are truly unbiased and generalizable, then the compromises needed to be made to undertake a study of Chernobyl's effects would seriously undermine the value of such a project. Funding sources typically take such a purist perspective.

In conclusion, technological disasters such as Chernobyl offer the opportunity to examine short-term as well as long-term consequences of persistent disasters. Conceptual models of the stress process refer primarily to consequences of acute life events occurring to adults, particularly events with end points that lend themselves to resolution (Turner & Avison, 1992). For children and adolescents, progress is required with respect to developing strategies to understand the effects of stress constellations that have an acute onset and persistent sequelae. This involves advances in both conceptualizations of the stress process as well as multi-measurement methodological procedures that fully capture their psychological experiences.

References

Aptekar, L., & Boore, J.A. (1990). The emotional effects of disaster on children: A review of the literature. International Journal of Mental Health, 19, 77-90.
Baum, A., Gatchel, R.J., & Schaeffer, M.A. (1983). Emotional, behavioral, and physiological effects of chronic stress at Three Mile Island. Journal of Consulting and Clinical Psychology, 51, 565-572.
Baverstock, K.F. (1993). Thyroid cancer in children in Belarus after Chernobyl. World Health Statistics Quarterly, 46, 204-208.
Brennan, M. (1990). USSR: Medical effects of Chernobyl disaster. Lancet, 335, 1086.
Bromet, E.J., Dunn, L.O., Connell, M.M., Dew, M.A., & Schulberg, H.C. (1986). Long-term reliability of diagnosing lifetime major depression in a community sample. Archives of General Psychiatry, 43, 435-440.
Bromet, E.J., Parkinson, D.K., Schulberg, H.C., Dunn, L.O., & Gondek, P.C.(1982). Mental health of residents near the Three Mile Island reactor: A comparative study of selected groups. Journal of Preventive Psychiatry, 1, 225-276.
Bromet, E.J., & Schulberg, H.C. (1987). Epidemiologic findings from disaster research. In R. Hales, & A. Frances (Eds.). American Psychiatric Association Annual Review: Vol. 6. (pp. 676-689). Washington, DC: American Psychiatric Press, Inc.
Canino, G., Bravo, M., Rubio-Stipec, M., & Woodbury, M. (1990). The impact of disaster on mental health: Prospective and retrospective analyses. International Journal of Mental Health, 19, 51-69.
Day, R., Gorin, M.B., Eller, A.W., & the Pittsburgh-Chornobyl Study Group. (1994). Prevalence of lens changes in Ukrainian children residing around Chornobyl. Under editorial review.
Dew, M.A., & Bromet, E. (1993). Predictors of temporal patterns of psychiatric distress during 10 years following the nuclear accident at Three Mile Island. Social Psychiatry and Psychiatric Epidemiology, 28, 49-55.
Dew, M.A., Bromet, E.J., & Schulberg, H.C. (1987). A comparative analysis of two community stressors' long-term mental health effects. American Journal of Community Psychology, 15, 167-1884.
Dew, M.A., Bromet, E.J., Schulberg, H.C., Dunn, L.O., & Parkinson, D.K. (1987). Mental health effects of the Three Mile Island nuclear reactor restart. American Journal of Psychiatry, 144, 1074-1077.
Fennig, S., & Bromet, E. (1992). Issues in memory in the Diagnostic Interview Schedule. Journal of Nervous and Mental Disease, 180, 223-224.
Furmanchuk, A.W., Averkin, J.I., Egloff, B., Ruchti, C., Abelin, T., Schappi, W., Korotkevich, E.A. (1992). Pathomophological findings in thyroid cancers of children from the Republic of Belarus: a study of 86 cases occurring between 1986 ('post-Chernobyl') and 1991. Histopathology, 21, 401-408.
Giel, R. (1991). The psychosocial aftermath of two major disasters in the Soviet Union. Journal of Traumatic Stress, 4, 381-392.

Grant, M. (1992). International perspectives on alcoholism and the family: an overview of WHO activities. In S. Saitoh, P. Steinglass, & M. Schuckit. (Eds.). Alcoholism and the family (pp. 97-116). NY: Brunner/Mazel.

Green, B.L., Lindy, J.D., Grace, M.C., Gleser, G.C., Leonard, A.C., Korol, M., & Winget, C. (1990). Buffalo Creek survivors in the second decade: stability of stress symptoms. American Journal of Orthopsychiatry, 60, 43-54.

Henderson, A.S. (1988). An introduction to social psychiatry. NY: Oxford University Press.

International Advisory Committee. (1991). The International Chernobyl Project: An overview . Vienna: International Atomic Energy Association.

Kelsey, J.L., Thompson, W.D. & Evans, A.S. (1986). Methods in observational epidemiology. NY: Oxford University Press.

Kidd, M. (1991). The children of Chernobyl. Medical Journal of Australia, 155: 764-767.

Kulka, R.A., Schlenger, W.E., Fairbank, J.A., Hough, R.L., Jordan, B.K., Marmat, C.R. & Weiss, D.S. (1990). Trauma and the Vietnam war generation. NY: Brunner/Mazel.

Kessler, R.C., McGonagle, K.A., Zhao, S., Nelson, C.B., Hughes, M., Eshleman, S., Wittchen, H-U., & Kendler, K.S. (1994). Lifetime and 12-month prevalence of DSM-III-R psychiatric disorders in the United States. Archives of General Psychiatry, 51, 8-19.

Lilienfeld, A.M. & Lilienfeld, D.E. (1980). Foundations of epidemiology: Second edition. NY: Oxford University Press.

Lima, B.R., Santacruz, H., Lozano, J., Chavez, H., Samaniego, N., Pompei, M.S., & Pai, S. (1990). Disasters and mental health: Experience in Colombia and Ecuador and its relevance for primary care in mental health in Latin America. International Journal of Mental Health, 19, 3-20.

McFarlane, A., Policansky, S., & Irwin, C. (1987). A longitudinal study of the psychological morbidity in children due to a natural disaster. Psychological Medicine, 17, 727-738.

Medvedev Z. (1994). Chernobyl: 8 years later. Novoye Russkoye Slovo pp. 11-12, April 22 (translated by Dmitry Goldgaber).

Mettler, F., Williamson, M., Royal, H., Hurley, J., Khafagi, F., Sheppard, M., Beral, V., Reeves, G., Saenger, E., Yokoyama, N., Parshin, V., Griaznova, E., Taranenko, M., Chesin, V. & Cheban, A. (1992). Thyroid nodules in the population living around Chernobyl. Journal of the American Medical Association, 268(5): 616-619.

Palinkas, L.A., Petterson, J.S., Russell, J., & Downs, M. (1993). Community patterns of psychiatric disorders after the Exxon Valdez oil spill. American Journal of Psychiatry, 150, 1517-1523.

Pauls, D., personal communication, 1992.

Penkower, L., Bromet, E. & Dew, M.A. (1988). Husbands' layoff and wives' mental health. Archives of General Psychiatry, 45, 994-1000.

Raphael, B. (1986). When Disaster Strikes. NY: Basic Books, Inc.
Rueck A, & Porter R. (Eds). (1976). Transcultural psychiatry. Boston: Little, Brown & Co.
Robins, L. & Regier, D. (1991). Psychiatric disorders in America: The Epidemiologic Catchment Area study. NY: The Free Press.
Rubonis, A., & Bickman, L. (1991). Psychological impairment in the wake of disaster: The disaster-psychopathology relationship. Psychological Bulletin, 109, 384-399.
Rutter, M. (1985). Resilience in the face of adversity: Protective factors and resistance to psychiatric disorder. British Journal of Psychiatry, 147, 598-611.
Rutter, M., Cox, A., Tupling, C., Berger, M., & Yule, W. (1975). Attainment and adjustment in two geographical areas: I. The prevalence of psychiatric disorder. British Journal of Psychiatry, 126, 493-509.
Saylor, C. (Ed.) (1993). Children and disasters. NY: Plenum Press.
Schlesselman, J.J., & Stolley, P.D. (1982). Research strategies. In J.J. Schlesselman, Case-control studies (pp. 7-26). NY: Oxford University Press.
Shore, J.H., Tatum, E.L., & Vollmer, W.M. (1986). Psychiatric reactions to disaster: The Mount St. Helens experience. American Journal of Psychiatry, 143, 590-595.
Solomon, S.D. (1989). Research issues in assessing disaster's effects. In R. Gist and B. Lubin (Eds.). Psychosocial aspects of disaster (pp. 308-340). NY: Wiley & Sons.
Solomon, Z. (1993). Combat stress reaction: The enduring toll of war. NY: Plenum Press.
Solomon, Z., Laor, N., Weiler, D., Muller, U.F., Hadar, O., Waysman, M., Koslowsky, M., Ben Yakar, M., & Bleich, A. (1993). The psychological impact of the Gulf War: A study of acute stress in Israeli evacuees. Archives of General Psychiatry, 50, 320-321.
Turner, R.J. & Avison, W.R. (1992). Innovations in the measurement of life stress: Crisis theory and the significance of event resolution. Journal of Health and Social Behavior, 33, 36-50.
Vogel, J. & Vernberg, E.M. (1993). Children's psychological responses to disasters: Part I. Journal of Clinical and Child Psychology, 22, 464-484.
Weisaeth, L. (1989). Importance of high response rates in traumatic stress research. Acta Psychiatrica Scandinavica Supplement 355, 80, 131-137.
Weisaeth, L. (1993). Disasters: Psychological and psychiatric aspects. In L. Goldberger & S. Breznitz (Eds.). Handbook of stress (pp. 591-616). New York: The Free Press.
World Health Organization. (1993). International programme on the health effects of the Chernobyl accident: Brain damage in utero pilot project. Geneva: Division of Mental Health, World Health Organization (unpublished manuscript).

Zahner, G.E.P., Jacobs, J.H., Freeman, D.H., & Trainor, K.F. (1993). Rural- urban child psychopathology in a Northeastern U.S. state: 1986-1989. Journal of the American Academy of Child and Adolescent Psychiatry, 32, 378-387.

RESEARCH METHODS AND DIRECTIONS: ESTABLISHING THE COMMUNITY CONTEXT

Fran H. Norris, Georgia State University, Georgia, USA
John R. Freedy, Medical University of South Carolina, South Carolina, USA
Anita DeLongis, Arizona State University, Tempe, Arizona, USA
Lucio Sibilia, Universita degli Studi di Roma "La Sapienza", Rome, Italy
Wolfgang Schönpflug, Freie Universitat Berlin, Berlin, Germany

Overview

Whereas the larger focus of this four-day meeting was community stress, our working group was given the responsibility of discussing and developing ideas concerning research methods and directions. The working group initially struggled in deciding the appropriate purpose for this chapter. Initially, we discussed the possibility of writing a technical chapter that discussed the fine points of research methodology as applied to stress occurring within community settings. However, the working group decided that a number of excellent reviews of research methods concerning disaster research or other applied research are available (Baum, Solomon, & Ursano, 1987; Kazdin, 1992; Raphael, Lundin, & Weisaeth, 1989; Solomon, 1989). Another chapter covering the same ground seemed redundant. Alternatively, the working group decided to focus on

---

The ideas in this chapter were developed in consultation with a small group of colleagues: Evelyn J. Bromet, Ph.D., Anita DeLongis, Ph.D., John R. Freedy, Ph.D., Bonnie L. Green, Ph.D., Vijaya L. Melnick, Ph.D., Fran H. Norris, Ph.D., Prof. Dr. Wolfgang Schönpflug, Prof. Dr. Ralf Schwarzer, Lucio Sibilia, M.D., Susan D. Solomon, Ph.D., and Zahava Solomon, Ph.D. This *working group* met in June 1994 at the NATO Advanced Research Workshop at Chateau de Bonas in southern France. To give the group a starting point, members of the working group corresponded with the first two authors (co-leaders for this working group) prior to the NATO conference. At the conference, our group met on several occasions to discuss a range of research issues. Although members of our working group did not universally agree on all topics, we did agree on many things. This chapter presents a balanced account of the consensus achieved within the working group. All participants in the working group made meaningful contributions to our discussions.

developing a set of practical recommendations and examples that might be helpful to researchers as they attempt to establish the community context of their work. The idea was to model a thinking process for researchers who wish to conduct research of maximum relevance to community settings. Generally, the members of the working group agreed that quantitative approaches to research alone were insufficient in establishing the community context. The working group advocated the need to incorporate more qualitative forms of research borrowed from such fields as social anthropology (e.g., ethnographic methodologies). That is, they believed established quantitative methods need to supplemented by innovative and alternative qualitative methods.

To be clear, the working group believed that both quantitative and qualitative forms of research have a useful role in the study of community stress. However, a tendency has developed among social scientists to view more qualitative approaches as unacceptable or inferior to more rigorous quantitative methodologies. A key point of agreement within the working group was to challenge this position as harmful to optimal efforts to understand community level stress. Qualitative strategies hold the promise of guiding us to key points for intervention and represent a crucial preliminary step in developing an understanding of how the community affects individuals, how individuals shape the community, and how disastrous events may impact the community and individuals. Both qualitative and quantitative approaches have a role to play in the development of knowledge concerning community level stress. Inspired by these discussions, we decided to offer researchers a guide for use in thinking through research projects concerned with community stress.

The purposes of this chapter are (a) to highlight some of the major issues in conducting research on community stress and (b) to illustrate different ways that researchers can operationalize *community context* in their studies of community stress. For the sake of convenience, the rest of this chapter is divided into three sections. The first section is titled *Conducting Community Research*. This section defines *community* as a construct, suggests the importance of broad theoretical models, and illustrates how researchers can begin to think in ecological terms on an *a priori* basis. The second section is titled *Examples of Community Research*. This section discusses three different research situations that require unique ways of accounting for the community context. The final section is titled *Concluding Comments*. This section provides a discussion about needed directions for future research on community level stress. We trust that this chapter will provide a useful stimulus towards creative thinking by researchers interested in studying stress within the context of communities.

Conducting Community Research

Establishing Conceptual Definitions

Two major themes emerged in the context of working group discussions. The first theme concerned the importance of developing conceptual definitions. The second theme concerned importance of defining and illustrating the process by which researchers can conduct research that is relevant to the community context. We will first present our ideas regarding conceptual definitions.

We initially attempted to develop a basic definition of the term *community*. This was surprisingly more difficult than we anticipated. After all, what are the relevant dimensions that go into defining what constitutes a community (e.g., size, geographic location, functional relationships)? Members of the working group thought that this complexity, in part, may be part of the reason that the broader field of social science has struggled to account for community level factors in research concerning stress. Based upon lively discussions, the working group settled on a basic definition that will be used for the purposes of this chapter.

We define community as an aggregated group of people that exists for the function of providing for the physical, social, psychological, and spiritual or philosophical needs of community members. Community members usually participate in several functional subgroups (e.g., families, peer networks, work groups, church groups) as a method of meeting personal and collective needs. Except in special circumstances (e.g., physical or mental incapacitation) it is generally expected that individuals have an obligation both to contribute energy, resources, and assistance to others and likewise to receive from other individuals and subgroups with whom a functional relationship exists (e.g., even children are expected to assist with age-appropriate chores within a family). Though subject to change, communities are characterized by relatively stable boundaries with regard to location, physical proximity, function, and continuity over time.

Consistent with an effort to define the term community, the working group discussed the importance of using comprehensive theoretical models as a basis for conducting community-based stress research. In the existing literature, there is a great degree of variability in the degree to which studies operationally define various aspects of stress theory. This is understandable, as many community wide events are of a catastrophic nature (e.g., natural disasters) and thus are difficult to study. It is common for researchers to select a limited number of measures and to contact convenient samples (i.e., small non-representative samples) in an effort to collect data. Indeed, such an approach is reasonable if the alternative is to gather no data whatsoever (Bromet, this volume). Our argument is simply that research, even under these difficult circumstances should be guided by comprehensive theoretical models. The field needs to go beyond *post hoc* interpretations of data and move towards the *a priori* statement and testing of theoretical models (Freedy, Kilpatrick, & Resnick, 1993; Freedy et al., 1994). A basis of a common language in studying community-level stress can only be facilitated if we think about stress in common terms.

Prior theoretical understandings of community stress have been too limited in scope. Time is a dimension that is often oversimplified (Green, this volume; McFarlane, this volume). Longitudinal studies are relatively rare, in large part due to practical restraints (e.g., environmental chaos, funding restraints, available baseline data). Also, many studies fail to assess prior or subsequent factors to a community stressor that may be important determinants of adjustment within the community (e.g., mental health history, trauma history, social support, chronic life stressors). Another concern with current conceptual models lies in the narrow conceptualization of outcome. Extant models tend to emphasize pathological outcomes heavily (e.g., physical illness, mental illness), while ignoring more positive adjustment possibilities (Lyons, 1991; Meichenbaum, this volume).

Beyond issues of accounting for developmental influences and considering a full range of outcomes, current theoretical models seldom conceptualize community level variables. Hobfoll, Briggs, and Wells (this volume) offer an advance in this regard by extending Conservation of Resources (COR) theory from the individual to the community level in order to provide a theoretical framework for research on community stress. The framework enumerates community resources using the same topology developed for individuals. Resource categories include *objects* (roads, shelter), *conditions* (employment opportunity, service availability), *characteristics* (communal pride, competence), and *energies* (finances, reserves). On a basic level, COR theory (Hobfoll, 1988; 1989) proposes that stress occurs in the wake of resource loss, and that such loss also makes the system (individual, group, or community) more vulnerable to further loss. For example, following a catastrophic natural disaster the loss of basic goods and services (e.g., shelter, food, water, clothing, health care, police and fire protection) renders a community more vulnerable to subsequent problems (e.g., spread of disease, substance abuse, familial discord). By highlighting baseline resources, COR theory focuses attention both on what causes subsequent problems and on what can be done to reduce subsequent problems within the community (i.e., the replenishment of depleted resources).

The breadth of COR theory makes it a potentially useful template for studying community level stressors. This fact is illustrated by two studies that have applied COR stress theory in studying adult adjustment following natural disasters. Following Hurricane Hugo (September 1989; Charleston, South Carolina, USA) it was found that high levels of hurricane related resource loss were associated with clinical levels of psychological distress. Among three blocks of predictor variables (demographics, resource loss, and coping behavior), resource loss accounted for the lion's share (34.1%) of variance in predicting psychological distress (Freedy, Shaw, Jarrell, & Masters, 1992). Following the Sierra Madre earthquake (June 1991; Los Angeles, California, USA) high earthquake related resource loss was related to elevated psychological distress. Resource loss accounted for 11.2% of psychological distress variance *even after* the variance due to the following variables was partialled out: demographics, prior trauma exposure, exposure to non-traumatic life events in the past year, and perceived life threat during the earthquake (Freedy et al., 1994). Promising findings from these two studies suggest that COR theory should be extended to studies of other community level stressors.

Establishing An Ecological Context

We now turn attention to the second major theme that emerged during the deliberations of our working group. Specifically, many working group members endorsed the importance of illustrating the process by which researchers can develop studies that account for the community context. Several group members strongly endorsed the modeling of this process as the most important contribution we could make to this book and to the broader field of social science research.

A theoretical framework is only the starting point for conducting ecologically meaningful community research. The spirit of ecological inquiry is one of improvisation and flexibility (Trickett, Kelly, & Vincent, 1985) because it relies on a changing understanding and an ongoing interplay between the researcher and community members. Beyond knowledge of theory, researchers need to understand the concrete issues and dynamics involved in particular ecological contexts.

This volume provides several meaningful examples of how researchers can integrate theoretical and other scientific aspects of research within the context of particular ecological boundaries. For example, Bromet (this volume) discusses the decision making processes involved in developing a study of children impacted by the Chernobyl nuclear catastrophe. She carefully describes the trade offs between purist scientific rigor and attempting to conduct research that is timely, meaningful, and relevant to the members of the impacted community. Weisaeth (this volume) describes an effort to study factors predicting adjustment among Norwegian nationals called to serve as United Nations (UN) soldiers. Beyond theoretical understanding, this study attempts to find factors (e.g., prior maladjustment, improper training, inadequate time between mobilization and deployment) that may contribute to negative outcomes during or following UN military service.

An ecological perspective has implications for how research is conducted as well as for what information is collected. These implications are perhaps better characterized as values than as methods, but they influence the research process nonetheless. A central tenet of ecological inquiry is that the relationship between the data gatherer and the data provider affects both the reliability and the ecological validity (range, trustworthiness, use) of the data (Trickett et al., 1985). Often it is important for the target community to be involved in the conduct of the research that is done on its behalf. What is most critical for research to be successful in bringing about change in communities is the community's perception that the researchers have a real interest in the community and are there for the long haul. Any initiative to improve matters must fully involve the community residents from planning the research to collecting the data to implementing interventions based on that research. Involving the community first to identify the major problems and designing data collection with the cooperation and active participation of community activists will increase both the success and quality of data collection. The perceptions of the local community may lead the field to broaden its perspective regarding what outcomes are important. When thinking at the community level, we need to consider outcomes other than psychopathology of selected individuals. It is even possible to argue that community members would not identify mental health as their sole or primary concern to researchers.

According to Trickett et al. (1985), the task of the researcher is to become a knowledgeable and credible collaborator. He or she must take the time and effort to relate to the local culture. The research needs to find out how the setting has traditionally coped with and adapted to outsiders, how the very notion of scientific inquiry is defined by the local culture, and how the entry process is managed. The research must also learn how to manage the tension between the research project and the host environment. Thus the first step in conducting research on community stress is the systematic exploration of the setting and situation. Theories are the starting point but the community is the ending point. Theoretical models must be adapted to events that take place in the context of a *specific community setting*. The idea is to let the research agenda emanate from the needs of the community as perceived by members of the community.

It is at the formative stage of the research that quantitatively oriented researchers may feel most at a loss, for traditional survey research methods do not achieve these goals very well. Focus groups, participant observation, and key informant interviews may be useful additions to our more traditional research tools. Hughes and DuMont (1993) recently presented a very useful discussion of both how to conduct and analyze data from focus group research to which readers interested in more detailed information are referred.

It should also be recognized that the need to establish the community context is not specific to formative research. Distinctions are often made among different types of research: formative versus hypothesis testing; descriptive versus explanatory versus intervention. Ideally, a range of research approaches are incorporated into research programs on community stress. In keeping with this *zeitgeist*, schemes for conducting multi-method research are beginning to appear in both the public health and community psychology literature. These frameworks appear to share the goal of pushing the researcher to alternate between inductive and deductive thinking.

One excellent model of ecologically sensitive research is presented by deVries in this volume (see also deVries, 1987). He advocates for a "cascade approach," which is a step-wise method for gathering information at the multiple levels that exist between the population and the person. The approach begins with the identification of risks and problems, using epidemiological survey methods, then moves to a problem clarification stage in which focus groups constitute the primary method. Then, a small number of individuals are studied as intensively and naturalistically as possible. Laboratory testing of hypotheses and clinical trials complete the five-stage cascade approach.

As is described by deJong in this volume, a similar strategy is advocated by the World Health Organization (WHO). The WHO model for prevention research functions as a blueprint that has to be tailored to local circumstances and culture. The recommended procedures incorporate: (a) interviews with governmental officials about the scope of the problem; (b) focus groups with key informants, who are asked to give their opinions about the consequences of the disaster or stressor and the protective factors available in the local community or culture; (c) participant observation with important groups such as healers to obtain insight into rituals and culture; and, (d) interventions that are designed, implemented, and monitored at the community level.

Though not specifically related to community stress, Maton (1993) has presented one of the most useful examples of how ethnographic and empirical methodologies may be linked in conducting culturally anchored research. Maton became involved with a religious community for a number of months as a participant observer before selecting the specific questions to be asked in the empirical phase of the research. He believed his initial experiences as a member of the community helped to ensure both the cultural and theoretical relevance of the topics subsequently chosen for study.

Overall, our working group endorsed the importance of integrating comprehensive theory with the surrounding community context. Some members of our group spoke most strongly in favor of an emphasis upon stating definitions and theory on an *a priori* basis. Other group members believed that developing the ecological context was the most important priority for researchers. On balance, there was consensus that comprehensive theory in the absence of community knowledge (or visa versa) was inadequate. Therefore, we recommend that researchers give attention to both of these important areas in developing programs of research.

Examples of Community Research

It is, of course, crucial that we operationalize the ideas from our working group. This is a challenge that presses traditional scientific thinking to its borders. How do we operationalize environmental context and culture? How do we link community level phenomena to individual outcome variables? The extent to which these links can be established empirically depends upon the nature of the study. For illustrative purposes, we will discuss three broad research situations that require different ways of operationalizing the community context: studies of a single community, studies of subcommunities within a larger community, and studies of multiple communities.

Single Community Studies

The first and most common research plan involves studying a particular population within a particular setting at a particular point in time (or across several time points). Most disaster studies can be characterized in this manner as most disasters (e.g., floods, hurricanes, tornadoes, earthquakes, wild fires) occur within defined geographic boundaries. The fundamental problem in this situation is that post-disaster community level variables are constant (for that community) and thus cannot be empirically analyzed. An analogy can be made to research on homelessness; empirical studies that were conducted within particular communities were destined to discover individual determinants of homelessness (e.g., education, mental illness) because structural determinants (e.g., housing availability) did not vary within a particular community.

The consideration of context in the study of community stress may involve data collection at the extra-individual level, the individual level, or both. At the extra-individual level, the intent is to describe the event and the setting in which observed effects occurred. Deciding what constitutes "context" is aided by taking an ecological perspective. Simply stated, ecology means that behavior both shapes and reflects the environment in which it occurs. The ecological perspective requires the researcher to attend to four key principles: adaptation, cycling of resources, interdependence, and succession (Kelly, 1966). These principles have been described in more detail elsewhere (Trickett, this volume), so will only be briefly summarized here.

Adaptation refers to the structures, norms, attitudes, and policies that, taken together, constitute the demand characteristics of the setting. Of the four principles, adaptation may come closest to representing what we mean by "context;" it is the backdrop against which individual behavior occurs. The *cycling-of-resources* principle reminds us that communities develop, distribute, and use resources. This principle gives rise to the research question of what resources are present in and necessary for the community under study. Hobfoll's COR theory expands upon this point nicely (Hobfoll et al., this volume). *Interdependence* points to the interactive nature of component parts of an ecological system; we will return to this principle when we turn to the second broad research situation (subcommunities). Finally, the *succession* principle references the time dimension. Communities have histories and traditions both about how they face stressful circumstances and about how they deal with outsiders. The researcher who has given attention to each of the principles in describing a setting will have gone a long way toward understanding the community context in which the research takes place. Ideally, as previously discussed, one should conduct this descriptive research first so that the findings can shape subsequent hypotheses to be tested. That is, does the context have implications for what psychological outcomes may be observed or not observed in the specific setting?

Because community *stress* research involves events and change as well as settings, the context is all the more important and complex. As Green (this volume) notes, disasters in some areas may be more devastating that the same type of event in a different region. The world sees strong evidence of this when earthquakes cause thousands of deaths in less developed nations (e.g., Armenia, Colombia, India, Mexico), though an earthquake of the same magnitude would cause minimal loss of life in the United States. Features of a setting more idiosyncratic than its economic status may be just as important.

Similarly, the nature of the event or stressor is an important part of environmental context. Disaster researchers have long noted the importance of describing any studied event in terms of its trauma potential. The following types of catastrophic stressors have been emphasized: threat to life, physical injury, receipt of intentional harm, exposure to grotesque sights, deaths, and information regarding exposure to toxic substances (Green, 1990). In addition, global distinctions have been made between disasters of natural origins, such as hurricanes and earthquakes, and those of technical origins, such as nuclear accidents, toxic spills, and airplane crashes (Baum, 1987; Green, 1982). Other features believed to be important are the centrality of the affected population, the proportion of the community that is affected, the threat of recurrence and predictability, and the adequacy of the recovery environment (see Bolin, 1985; Lindy & Grace, 1985; Quarantelli, 1985).

These considerations lead to the minimum requirement that when studying a single setting it is necessary to provide a descriptive account of the context in which observed effects occur. Green, in this volume, provides an excellent example of providing such a rich context because she and her colleagues have consistently reminded us that findings from studies of the Buffalo Creek Dam collapse are not interpretable without considering the disaster's Appalachian location, the relationship of the stricken community with the mining company that caused the disaster, and the litigation efforts that further split the community apart.

Subcommunity Studies

The second broad research situation occurs when a study takes place within a specific setting, but that setting encompasses distinct subcommunities. From an ecological perspective, this is important because of the principle of interdependence. As noted earlier, interdependence points to the interactive nature of component parts of an ecological system; the principle implies that community-level events will *differentially* affect various subcommunities. Social psychological theories will often generate specific hypotheses about which subcommunities will be more or less affected by community-level events. COR theory predicts that subcommunities will vie for protection of their own resources and act to limit their losses. Because different subcommunities have different resources available to invest in this process, they do not stand to lose or gain the same resources to the same extent. Kaniasty and Norris (1994), for example, documented differential receipt of help across subcommunities defined by race, age, and education following Hurricane Hugo. Hobfoll and colleagues (this volume) likewise remind us that disasters and other major community stressors are inherently political events. As such, political processes and the competition for resources can be expected to emerge. Leaders will act to limit resource loss of their constituencies at the expense, if necessary, of other subgroups in the community. As Hobfoll et al. also note, we need more research on how leaders act under conditions of community stress and on how to improve the decision making process.

A question of particular interest for community stress research is how change in one place ripples through the community. For example, how does stress proliferate in a community? How do the effects of disaster spread from primary victims (those with personal losses) to secondary victims (others who live in the affected area)? Perhaps the best example of the interdependence principle is Jackson and Inglehart's reverberation model, which also is described in this volume. According to this model, minority (subordinate) group members are more adversely affected by community stress than majority (dominant) group members because stress leads to increased racism that "reverberates" through the community.

Though seldom driven as clearly by theory, the most prevalent approach to subcommunity research is to differentiate between cultural or ethnic groups within a larger geographic community. These distinctions are often important, but bring with them a host of thorny research issues. Birman (in press) discussed the difficulties in defining the boundaries and distinctions between the constructs of culture, race, and ethnicity and noted that cultural identity and manifest behavior may not be one and the same. Demographic variables (e.g., race) at best serve as markers that stand in for other variables and imply a degree of within-group homogeneity that may not be justified (Hughes, Seidman, & Williams, 1993; Jackson, 1993; Sasao & Sue, 1993). After discussing the utility of within-group versus between-group (comparative) designs for understanding various cultural phenomena, Hughes et al. (1993) argued that the important question is whether two or more groups differ from one another in the *pattern of relationships* among variables rather than in the level of those variables.

The research difficulties grow even larger when the subcommunities under study speak different languages. In cross-cultural research, it is imperative to establish both the conceptual equivalence and the linguistic equivalence of the instruments to be used. Even when linguistic equivalence is established via methods such as back-translation, conceptual equivalence is still not assured. Hines (1993) recently described several techniques from cognitive science that may be useful in this regard.

Studies of Multiple Communities

A third broad research situation occurs when a study takes place across multiple communities. Here, community-level factors vary and can be measured and analyzed empirically. Sources of community level data are many -- official records, social indicators (e.g., census data, infant mortality), key informants, focus groups, and newspapers.

An example of a study that encompassed multiple communities was conducted by Norris and her colleagues (see Norris, Phifer, & Kaniasty, 1994 for a review) following the Kentucky Floods of 1981 and 1984. This study explored the effects of community destruction by incorporating the "impact ratio" of respondents' counties of residence into the data set. This measure was the number of homes that were damaged or destroyed relative to the population size of that county and was collected from administrative records kept by the Kentucky Division of Disaster and Emergency Services. Across the 10 flooded counties and 5 adjacent non-flooded counties included in the study, values ranged from 0 (for non-victims residing in non-flooded counties) to 15.6 homes damaged per 1000 population. Tested was the extent to which this community-level measure of disaster impact explained variance in psychosocial functioning *over and above* that accounted for by individual-level measures of disaster impact (e.g., personal loss). There were numerous interesting distinctions between the effects of measures of personal loss and the effects of this measure of community destruction. Personal loss was associated most strongly with *increases* in *negative* affect, i.e., sadness, anxiety, worry. Community destruction, in contrast, was associated most strongly with *decreases* in *positive* affect, reflecting a community wide tendency for people to feel less positive about their surroundings, less enthusiasm, less energy, and less enjoyment of life. These effects could still be observed two years after the flood. Similarly, high levels of community destruction were related to decreases in social participation and lowered expectations concerning the helpfulness of non-kin networks. These declines were also observable two years post-flood. Destruction of the physical environment may have altered usual patterns of social interactions -- disrupting daily activities such as visiting, shopping, recreation, and church-going. While no one would characterize such effects as psychopathology, there was ample evidence from this study that the floods impaired the community's quality of life for quite some time.

A second study that incorporated multiple communities was conducted by Freedy and his colleagues (Freedy et al., 1994). This study compared disaster responses of two adult samples. One sample was exposed to Hurricane Hugo (September 1989; Charleston, South Carolina, USA), whereas the other sample was exposed to the Loma Prieta earthquake (October 1989; San Francisco, California, USA). The study was guided by a multivariate risk factor model that encompassed a range of *pre-disaster* (e.g., previous traumatic events, mental health history), *within-disaster* (e.g., threat to life, injury), and *post-disaster* (e.g., initial distress level, disruption of basic goods and services) factors. Both samples completed 40 minute interviews approximately two years post-event. Relative to one another, the South Carolina sample had experienced greater life threat, greater damage to property, greater deprivation of services (water, electricity, transportation), and greater loss of resources. The California sample, on the other hand, had experienced greater fear over separation from family and greater acute anxiety because of the surprise element entailed in an earthquake. Despite these differences in the nature of the stressor, there were no setting-level differences in psychological symptoms two years post-event. However, there were strong individual-level differences in symptoms, which were explained by such factors as prior traumatic exposure, prior mental health problems, disaster related resource loss, and past-year life events. The applicability of the proposed risk factor model to diverse events in separate communities is a particular strength of this approach. Overall, the findings confirm the complexity of mental health adjustment patterns and remind us that an increased focus on community-level forces does not imply that individuals will not exhibit varying needs within those stricken communities.

Concluding Comments

We will close this chapter with a few comments regarding future research directions. At least with regard to natural disasters, we now have sufficient studies to indicate that disasters are a mental health risk. We also have excellent studies of risk factors for negative outcomes among community populations. We are beginning to have a data base on the longitudinal course of responses to disaster, although this is a newer area and additional sophisticated research on the nature of these reactions, including testing for non-linear relationships, would add to our theoretical understanding of what drives initial emotional reactions and adaptation over time. This is especially true if we can gain early access to exposed populations and follow them over time. More studies are also needed about children, who are not sufficiently represented in research on representative samples in the community.

As in other areas of mental health research, the study of interventions lags behind more descriptive work. There are good reasons for this. Intervention research is extremely difficult even in an ongoing stable setting, let alone in the chaotic atmosphere surrounding disasters. Despite the sparsity of research efforts, a great deal of intervention work is occurring (Green, this volume; McFarlane, in press). Debriefing efforts, for example are very common following catastrophic events and yet we have little information concerning the efficacy of debriefing procedures. Though it is clear that intervention efforts will be necessary following catastrophic events, more research is needed to quantify the potential efficacy of various approaches.

This volume describes several relevant intervention approaches. Orner (this volume) discusses the practice of Critical Incident Stress Debriefing (CISD). He points out the lack of efficacy data and goes on to challenge the field to consider more carefully the proper goals of CISD efforts (in his view the goal should be to provide a healing ritual that promotes group cohesion and functioning). Pynoos, Goenjian, and Steinberg (this volume) describe a comprehensive school-based intervention model for children and their families. A variety of intervention sites are identified (e.g., the school, family, the community) and a range of examples are offered. Joop de Jong (this volume) describes a prevention-intervention model that spans from the level of international communities, through local communities, and down to the level of individual community members.

Another issue related to the significance of the findings we report. Although it is interesting that stress-exposed groups usually differ significantly from non-exposed groups on symptom measures, and on some diagnoses, and that there are certain factors that predict this minority of individuals who are distressed, it is difficult to ascertain from most studies the clinical or social significance of these differences. We need to be able to ground our findings in estimates of the magnitude of the problems relative to other things going on. For example, if having access to a range of basic goods and services (e.g., shelter, food, water, clothing, health care) is the strongest factor impacting emotional recovery from disaster, then perhaps we should spend substantial amounts of money to provide basic goods and services with the aim of minimizing emotional stress.

In closing it should be noted that community oriented research does not occur in a political vacuum. Different subgroups within a community may have a vested interest in particular findings (e.g., HIV research, research on sexual harassment). Under such conditions, how does the researcher protect the integrity of the research? To what extent can or should a researcher allow their personal beliefs whether consistent or inconsistent with some agenda within the community guide what research questions are addressed? Despite such tensions that impact community oriented research, it is believed that its benefits will outweigh its costs. Ability to achieve true partnership between researchers and members of the community will be key to studying, understanding, and influencing areas of community life that impact the welfare of thousands of community members. Long term social change, for the better or worse, will occur with or without the input of community oriented researchers. We believe that any changes in social policy will assist the greatest number of people for the greatest amount of good when community oriented researchers add their voices and skills to the debate that typically proceeds long term social change.

In closing, consistent with the sentiments of the working group, this chapter advocates for the adoption of more innovative and community-oriented strategies than have typically been used in studies of community level stress. Just repeating the same studies, with a slight improvement in methodology on yet another sample, does not seem like an appropriate way to spend our scarce resources. We need to push research into new areas that will really add to our understanding of human reactions and adaptation to stress and traumatic stress. The study of community stress has both the potential to make a contribution to mainstream behavioral science if it is well-done and can aid our timely reactions to victimized communities and enhance their recovery, well-being, and quality of life.

References

Baum, A., Solomon, S., & Ursano, R. (1987, September).Emergency/disaster research issues: A guide to the preparation and evaluation of grant applications dealing with traumatic stress. Proceedings of the Workshop of Research Issues: Emergency, Disaster, and Post-traumatic Stress, Uniformed Services University of the Health Sciences, Bethesda, MD.

Baum, A. (1987). Toxins, technology, and natural disasters. In G.R. VandenBos & B.K. Bryant (Eds.), Cataclysms, crises, and catastrophes: Psychology in action (pp. 9-53). Washington, DC: American Psychological Association.

Birman, D. (in press). Acculturation and human diversity in a multicultural society. In E. Trickett, R. Watts, & D. Birman (Eds.), Human diversity: Perspectives on people in context. San Francisco, CA: Jossey Bass.

Bolin, R. (1985). Disaster characteristics and psychosocial impacts. In B. Sowder (Ed.) Disasters and mental health: Selected contemporary perspectives (pp. 3-28). Rockville, MD: National Institute of Mental Health.

Bromet, E. J. (this volume). Methodological issues in designing research on community-wide disasters with special reference to Chernobyl. In S. E. Hobfoll and M. W. deVries (Eds.), Extreme stress and communities: Impact and intervention. Dordrecht, The Netherlands: Kluwer.

de Jong, J. T. V. M. (this volume). Prevention of the consequences of man-made or natural disaster at the (inter)national, the community, the family, and the individual level. In S. E. Hobfoll and M. W. deVries (Eds.), Extreme stress and communities: Impact and intervention. Dordrecht, The Netherlands: Kluwer.

deVries, M. W. (1987). Investigating mental disorders in their natural settings. The Journal of Nervous and Mental Disease, 175, 509-513.

deVries, M. W. (this volume). Culture, community, and catastrophe: Issues in understanding communities under difficult conditions. In S. E. Hobfoll and M. W. deVries (Eds.), Extreme stress and communities: Impact and intervention. Dordrecht, The Netherlands: Kluwer.

Freedy, J.R., Addy, C.L., Kilpatrick, D.G., Resnick, H.S., & Garrison, C.Z. (1994). Examination of a multivariate risk factor model for predicting post-traumatic stress disorder following two major natural disasters. Manuscript submitted for publication.

Freedy, J.R., Kilpatrick, D.G., & Resnick, H.S. (1993). Natural disasters and mental health: Theory, assessment, and intervention. Journal of Social Behavior and Personality, 8(3), 49-103.

Freedy, J.R., Saladin, M., Kilpatrick, D.G., Resnick, H.S., & Saunders, B.E. (1994). Understanding acute psychological distress following natural disaster. Journal of Traumatic Stress, 7(2), 257-273.

Freedy, J.R., Shaw, D., Jarrell, M.P., & Masters, C. (1992). Towards an understanding of the psychological impact of natural disaster: An application of the conservation of resources stress model. Journal of Traumatic Stress, 5(3), 441-454.

Green, B.L. (1982). Assessing levels of psychological impairment following disaster: Consideration of actual and methodological dimensions. Journal of Nervous and Mental Disease, 170, 544-552.

Green, B.L. (1990). Defining trauma: Terminology and generic stressor dimensions. Journal of Applied Social Psychology, 20, 1632-1642.

Green, B.L. (this volume). Long-term consequences of disasters. In S. E. Hobfoll and M. W. deVries (Eds.), Extreme stress and communities: Impact and intervention. Dordrecht, The Netherlands: Kluwer.

Hines, A. (1993). Linking qualitative and quantitative methods in cross-cultural survey research: Techniques from cognitive science. American Journal of Community Psychology, 21, 729-746.

Hobfoll, S. E., Briggs, S., & Wells, J. (this volume). Community stress and resources: Actions and reactions. In S. E. Hobfoll and M. W. deVries (Eds.), Extreme stress and communities: Impact and intervention. Dordrecht, The Netherlands: Kluwer.

Hobfoll, S.E. (1988). The ecology of stress. New York: Hemisphere Publishing.

Hobfoll, S.E. (1989). Conservation of resources: A new attempt at conceptualizing stress. American Psychologist, 44(3), 513-524.

Hughes, D., Seidman, E., & Williams, N. Cultural phenomena and the research enterprise: Toward a culturally anchored methodology. American Journal of Community Psychology, 21, 687-704.

Hughes, D., & Du Mont, K. (1992). Using focus groups to facilitate culturally anchored research. American Journal of Community Psychology, 21, 775-806.

Jackson, J. (1993). African American Experiences through the adult years. In R. Kastenbaum (Ed.) Encyclopedia of Adult Development (pp. 18-26). Phoenix, AZ: Oryx Press.

Jackson, J. S., & Inglehart, M. R. (this volume). Effects of racism on dominant and subordinant groups: A reverberation model of community stress. In S. E. Hobfoll and M. W. deVries (Eds.), Extreme stress and communities: Impact and intervention. Dordrecht, The Netherlands: Kluwer.

Kaniasty, K., & Norris, F. (1994). In search of altruistic community: Received and provided social support following Hurricane Hugo. Manuscript submitted for publication.

Kazdin, A.E. (1992). Methodological issues and strategies in clinical research (Ed.). Washington, DC: American Psychological Association.

Kelly, J. (1966). Ecological constraints on mental health services. American Psychologist, 21, 535-539.

Lindy, J., & Grace, M. (1985). The recovery environment: Continuing stressor versus a healing psychosocial space. In B. Sowder (Ed.) <u>Disasters and mental health: Selected contemporary perspectives</u> (pp. 137-149). Rockville, MD: National Institute of Mental Health.

Lyons, J.A. (1991). Strategies for assessing the potential for positive adjustment following trauma. <u>Journal of Traumatic Stress</u>, 4(1), 93-111.

Maton, K. (1993). A bridge between cultures: Linked ethnographic empirical methodology for culture anchored research. <u>American Journal of Community Psychology</u>, 21, 747-775.

McFarlane, A.C. (in press). Helping the victims of disaster. In J.R. Freedy & S.E. Hobfoll (Eds.), <u>Traumatic stress: From theory to practice</u>. New York: Plenum.

McFarlane, A.C. (this volume). Stress and disaster. In S. E. Hobfoll and M. W. deVries (Eds.), <u>Extreme stress and communities: Impact and intervention</u>. Dordrecht, The Netherlands: Kluwer.

Meichenbaum, D. (this volume). Disasters, stress, and cognition. In S. E. Hobfoll and M. W. deVries (Eds.), <u>Extreme stress and communities: Impact and intervention</u>. Dordrecht, The Netherlands: Kluwer.

Norris, F., Phifer, J., & Kaniasty, K. (1994). Individual and community reactions to the Kentucky floods: Findings from a longitudinal study of older adults. In R. Ursano, B. McCaughey, and C. Fullerton (Eds.) <u>Individual and community responses to trauma and disaster</u> (pp. 378-402). Cambridge: Cambridge University Press.

Omer, R. J. (this volume). Intervention strategies for emergency response groups: A new conceptual framework. In S. E. Hobfoll and M. W. deVries (Eds.), <u>Extreme stress and communities: Impact and intervention</u>. Dordrecht, The Netherlands: Kluwer.

Pynoos, R. S., Goenjian, A., & Steinberg, A. M. (this volume). Strategies of disaster intervention for children and adolescents. In S. E. Hobfoll and M. W. deVries (Eds.), <u>Extreme stress and communities: Impact and intervention</u>. Dordrecht, The Netherlands: Kluwer.

Quarantelli, E. (1985). What is disaster? The need for clarification in definition and conceptualization in research. In B. Sowder (Ed.) <u>Disasters and mental health: Selected contemporary perspectives</u> (pp. 41-73). Rockville, MD: National Institute of Mental Health.

Raphael, B., Lundin, T., & Weisaeth, L. (1989). A research method for the study of psychological and psychiatric aspects of disaster. <u>Acta Psychiatrica Scandinavia</u>, 80(353), 1-75.

Sasao, T., and Sue, S. (1993). Toward a culturally anchored ecological framework of research in ethnic-cultural communities. <u>American Journal of Community Psychology</u>, 21, 705-728.

Solomon, S.D. (1989). Research issues in assessing disaster's effects. In R. Gist & B. Lubin (Eds.), <u>Psychosocial aspects of disaster</u> (pp. 308-340). New York: John Wiley & Sons.

Trickett, E. J. (this volume). The community context of disaster and traumatic stress: An ecological perspective from community psychology. In S. E. Hobfoll and M. W. deVries (Eds.), Extreme stress and communities: Impact and intervention. Dordrecht, The Netherlands: Kluwer.

Trickett, E., Kelly, J., & Vincent, T. (1985). The spirit of ecological inquiry in community research. In E. Susskind & D. Klein (Eds.), Community Research: Methods, paradigms, and applications, (pp. 5-38). New York: Praeger.

Weisæth, L. (this volume). Preventive psychosocial intervention after disaster. In S. E. Hobfoll and M. W. deVries (Eds.), Extreme stress and communities: Impact and intervention. Dordrecht, The Netherlands: Kluwer.

SECTION V: LONG-TERM EFFECTS OF COMMUNITY STRESS (OVERVIEW)

Stevan E. Hobfoll, Kent State University, Kent, Ohio, USA
Rebecca P. Cameron, Kent State University, Kent, Ohio, USA
Marten W. deVries, University of Limburg, Maastricht, the Netherlands

Section Five seeks to address the need for a far-reaching longitudinal approach to trauma that captures the interwoven processes of community stress, community support, cultural change, and individual adaptation across the lifespan. These chapters provide novel perspectives on theory and methodology. As such, they serve as exciting beginnings of answers to issues of complex interactions, and even more, as sources of promising lines of questioning that should be pursued.

Green (Chapter Fourteen) reviews research findings regarding the long-term consequences of disasters, drawing especially on her work studying the survivors of the Buffalo Creek dam collapse. Her data indicate that risk factors for negative psychological outcomes of disasters change over time, and may be linked in some ways to developmental issues.

Green begins her review of the literature on long-term adaptation to disaster with a presentation of her and her colleagues' model for understanding the psychological processes affecting responses to extreme stress events. She proposes that disaster exposure is accompanied by cognitive appraisals and emotional responses, both of which are shaped by personal characteristics and ongoing aspects of the recovery setting. These factors combine to produce outcomes in many domains of functioning.

Studies of adults and children tend to reveal negative mental health effects of disasters that can last for extended periods of time, although the limited data available on children are more equivocal than the data on adults. Reported rates of diagnosable disorders in both disaster-exposed adults and children vary widely depending on the criteria used in a particular study, but most studies show that victims of disaster experience improvement in their symptoms over time. Relevant outcomes range from self-reported psychological symptoms of anxiety, post-traumatic stress disorder (PTSD), depression, and somatization, to objectively measured phenomena, such as health care utilization, encounters with the legal system, and altered physiological processes.

A commonly-found risk factor for more severe outcomes is having been exposed to more profound levels of the initial stressor. Gender influences the risk associated with specific outcomes: women report more psychological consequences and men evidence more somatic or physiological symptoms, higher levels of aggression, and more alcohol abuse. With respect to age, middle-aged individuals experience the highest level of risk, presumably due to life stage issues involving a greater number of non-disaster-related stressors in multiple domains, and a relative imbalance in the ratio of support received to support provided. Prior exposure to trauma and previous psychological problems are related to increased risk, at least under certain circumstances. Finally, children's adaptation is affected to a large degree by their family's level of functioning.

Green goes on to explore the relative risk associated with features of the larger community setting: disasters are not random occurrences, but rather disproportionately affect developing nations and socioeconomically stressed communities. Thus, the overwhelming nature of some disasters in relatively less developed regions of the world may be qualitatively different from the more circumscribed disasters typically experienced by developed nations. This possibility calls into question the generalizability of disaster research conducted in developed settings to the vast majority of disaster victims, who live in less developed settings.

Next, Green discusses her findings on the outcomes associated with the Buffalo Creek disaster. She carefully characterizes many of the factors that help to contextualize this particular event, including the nature of the losses experienced by the community, the filing of a lawsuit against the company responsible for the event, and the limits on generalizability of her sample. Her research is highly unusual in the length of time of followup, which extends up to seventeen years post-disaster. A major issue that she raises is whether there is continuity or non-continuity of risk groups over time, a question that has implications for both theory and methodology. Her data suggest that survivors of the disaster improve over time, with those who were children at the time of the disaster becoming relatively indistinguishable from a non-exposed comparison group at seventeen years followup. Adults, on the other hand, continued to show elevated symptom levels when compared to a non-exposed group at fourteen years followup.

Gender differences in types of symptoms reported were found at both a two-year and the fourteen-year followups. However, gender and age show complicated patterns of association with risk that indicate there may be discontinuity of risk over time. Currently being middle aged was associated with higher risk, regardless of age at the time of the disaster, and the differential risk associated with gender decreased over time. Long-term risk was predicted by pre-disaster psychological difficulty, whereas relatively short-term risk (two years followup) was not associated with pre-disaster functioning, again indicating a need to account for changing risk factors over time. Retrospective reports of symptoms tended to reflect more stable assessments of functioning than did concurrent reports of symptoms, and thus had more predictive value.

Green's discussion of changes in risk factors and relative risk indicates a need for more research that assesses these processes using longitudinal designs. In addition, her research calls attention to the rarity of truly long-term followup studies. Developmental perspectives are likely to be useful in informing the conceptualizations of researchers and theorists. Green closes with a call for additional research on children and on interventions, noting that few of the newly-developed intervention strategies have been empirically evaluated.

Lomranz (Chapter Fifteen) continues the discussion of the long-term impact of extreme community stress with a focus on Holocaust survivors in Israel. He articulates a broad theoretical orientation that combines levels of analysis ranging from the larger culture to the individual with multiple temporal levels of analysis, including historical timeframes and personal developmental timeframes. In relating this perspective to the experiences of Holocaust survivors in Israel, the reader is struck by the enormity and complexity of the impact of the Holocaust and the inadequacy of research methods applied to date in providing more than a glimpse into what Holocaust survivorship means on an ongoing basis.

Lomranz critiques the existing Holocaust stress literature on a number of levels. Of profound significance is the focus in most of the literature on pathology, rather than adaptation. Lomranz provides eloquent arguments for the need to understand that Holocaust survivors are not simply "damaged". In addition to the concrete experiences of the Holocaust, survivors suffered profound disruptions to normal developmental processes, including the development of intimacy, the establishment of a career identity, the identification with a particular culture, and the development of systems of meaning, including religious meanings, personal meanings, and relational meanings. Many of these issues are resolved through seeming paradoxes. Survivors exhibit strength, despite their extreme vulnerability. They have developed inconsistent meaning systems. They are both completely unable to articulate their experiences and at the same time, increasingly motivated to bear witness. As Lomranz points out, they may utilize coping strategies that are constructive on one level and destructive or inefficacious on another. And, despite the ongoing trauma associated with the Israeli culture's ambivalent reception of them, the Holocaust and Holocaust survivors have become central to the cultural identities of Israelis.

Lomranz provides several suggestions for improving the work that is conducted in an effort to understand Holocaust survivors. He suggests replacing pathology-oriented conceptualizations with life-span adaptational conceptualizations. He suggests that research tools need to be particularly sensitive to pick up variations in outcome among a group that has demonstrated tremendous resilience, and that researchers need to examine demographic factors from pre- and post-Holocaust life. He advocates combining ideographic and nomothetic approaches to assessment. He proposes that theoretical attention be paid to interactive effects between stages of trauma and stages of development that may increase or change the nature of risks. And he characterizes the unique cultural context that Holocaust survivors have helped to shape, and that continues to affect them. Lomranz emphasizes the complexity of the issues affecting Holocaust survivorship, but also provides suggestions for researchers interested in tackling that complexity. His conceptual framework offers an approach that would be extremely useful in guiding future research.

In Chapter Sixteen, Jackson and Inglehart present their reverberation theory of racism in hierarchically structured communities. This theory represents a significant advance in the study of racism through its conceptualization of the interrelationships between racism, stress, and health, and through its consideration of the impact of racism on both the subordinate and the dominant groups in hierarchically organized societies.

Jackson and Inglehart review the current world context of racism: racism that appears to have lessened on the surface of communities may simply be dormant; ongoing immigration and refugee flight continue to present major challenges to dominant groups' ability to be tolerant; diplomatic and historical issues complicate issues of immigration and racism; and the increasing availability of weapons of mass destruction makes racist conflict an ongoing source of concern to the international community. Jackson and Inglehart suggest that an analysis of root causes of racism is essential to developing interventions into racist processes.

Next, Jackson and Inglehart review the inadequacy of individually-based theoretical ideas to provide coherent and useful insights into racist processes. Attempts to focus on psychopathology as the source of racism have been unable to explain large-scale episodes of racism, such as the Holocaust. Explorations of more general personality factors and national identities, although suggestive, have failed to comprehensively answer the important questions related to large-scale racism. The theoretical model being proposed in this chapter asserts that personal and community stress affect both the dominant group and the subordinate group(s) in a society, that these stresses result in increased racism and conflict, that in turn lead to increased stress, and that the combined effects of racism and stress affect the well-being of individuals at all levels of the hierarchy.

Using African-Americans as an example, Jackson and Inglehart discuss some of the stressors that affect this particular subordinate group's functioning: urban environments, low socioeconomic status, stressful lifestyle factors, perceptions and experiences of crime, high levels of community and personally-experienced violence, and resulting losses in social support networks. They note that, despite the widely-cited impact of racist processes on African-American well-being, stress scales do not tap stressors of relevance to the poor in general and the black poor in particular. All of the factors outlined above may result in qualitative as well as quantitative differences in the experience of stress by members of a subordinate group as compared to the experience of stress by members of a dominant group. A complicating factor they cite is African-Americans' use of denial and passivity when confronted with racist treatment, that reflects the reality of low levels of control over those situations, but results in demonstrable negative health effects.

According to this theory, dominant group members also experience significant effects of racism. Racist attitudes are associated with poor psychological health, including increased hostility, which is associated with poor physical health. Poor physical health, in turn, has negative practical and psychological ramifications. In addition, stress and stereotyping can combine into a perpetuating feedback loop as a result of the decrease in cognitive complexity that results from stress. Intergroup conflict also results in lost opportunities for social interaction and social support, thus deepening the negative cycle.

Jackson and Inglehart develop two models based on their theory. One links community stressors, within-group experiences of stress, racist processes, and their effects on the health and well-being of each group's members. The other links financial stress to racism and well-being within the dominant group, with resulting impacts on experienced racism, financial stress, and well-being among subordinate groups. They draw on data from large-scale surveys of dominant and subordinate groups in the United States and of dominant groups in Europe to test some of the hypotheses proposed by these models. Results provide initial support for the proposed links between financial stress and racism and racism and well-being, among both dominant and subordinate groups and in both U.S. and European cultures.

It is clear that Jackson and Inglehart have provided a well-conceived and novel approach to conceptualizing the interplay between stress and culture with particular reference to racism. Their work models the ability of stressors and stress processes to be conceptualized at a community level, and should be utilized as a valuable source of hypotheses for future research.

DeVries (Chapter Seventeen) begins his chapter with review of the multiple, interacting processes that are relevant to individual and community stress. For individuals, major life events and daily hassles are important; stress has biological effects; social support exerts moderating influences; and individual, community, and environmental contexts interact to affect the experience of stress. For communities, social contexts, cultural rules, and community life are important variables in the stress process. DeVries outlines three stages of the community response to stress: inducing and legitimizing the communication of distress, and beginning to mobilize resources; facilitating resource mobilization, including cultural coping mechanisms; and maintaining support processes after the crisis has ended, including such resources as self-help healing strategies.

DeVries discusses the role of culture in coping with stress: it organizes and provides meaning in stressful circumstances; maintains itself through rules, roles, and rituals; and, especially within traditional cultures, utilizes symbols to conceptualize the relationships between individuals, religious beliefs, body, and mind.

Next, deVries illustrates the three processes of inducing, facilitating, and maintaining community-level support systems with examples from traditional and developed cultures. He illustrates the ritualization of social communication and coping responses through the example of Digo trance states. These emerged as an expression of extreme anxiety about border disputes, and became a legitimized illness resulting in community rallying of support for the afflicted individual. DeVries relates this to the legitimization of Vietnam veterans' Agent Orange complaints and the resulting increase in financial and medical resources allocated to sufferers of this trauma. Similarly, indigenous social security systems are creatively utilized to understand and treat problems in individuals and families. Self-help approaches are found in traditional African societies as well as modern American society, and represent a significant long-term source of support for members.

The cascade approach to studying health and illness, and the relationships of these concepts to the multiple levels of population, community, and individual are presented next. The cascade approach represents a systematic way of gathering data, moving from clinical, ethnographic, and interview techniques at Stage 0 to studies of clinical field trial outcomes at Stage V. In between are: Stage I, which utilizes epidemiological surveys to identify population-specific problems and risks; Stage II, which emphasizes the use of social network techniques such as snowball sampling and focus groups, in order to identify increasingly specific and relevant variables of interest; Stage III, which utilizes intensive small-size field sampling techniques, that can include data on the time-sequences of processes of interest; and Stage IV, which involves laboratory testing of specific hypotheses derived at Stages II and III.

These research techniques can also serve as interventions. For example, snowball sampling and focus groups can lead to self-help initiatives. The advantages of the cascade approach are its outline of a clear methodological sequence that, by its nature, increases the relevance of research to the population on which it is conducted, and its dual function as a research tool and a means of intervention and prevention. The cascade approach is another model of research that offers clarity even while addressing complex and intertwined social processes.

Section Five provides insight into some of the compelling questions associated with the long-term impact of community stress, and highlights the need for continued longitudinal research. Of particular note for theorists and researchers are issues related to the changing nature of risk over time, the association between life-span development and disaster adjustment, and the mutually-impactful interactions between the victims of extreme stress and the societies in which they live. In addition, this section highlights a methodology for studying long-term community support processes, through deVries' cascade approach. As the field of traumatology develops, the increasing sophistication of the conceptual issues brought to bear on community stress must be addressed through corresponding methodological advances.

LONG-TERM CONSEQUENCES OF DISASTERS

Bonnie L. Green
Department of Psychiatry/Georgetown University
Washington, D.C., USA

It has become clear that disasters have a negative impact on mental health. To date, virtually all studies using control groups have found that disaster exposed individuals fare more poorly than their non-exposed peers, at least in the short run. Negative effects have also been shown with regard to general health and the use of services in the community. Risk factors for negative responses to these events have also been well-studied. The present report briefly summarizes this literature, as well as the literature addressing the impact of these events over time in adults and children. The review will focus on studies which have examined the impact of these events for at least a year. While this is actually a short follow-up, compared to, for example, the events of World War II, it likely captures more chronic, as opposed to acute, effects. Next, I will note the importance of the context in which the event occurs, and that disasters in some areas may be more devastating than the same type of event in a different region. My and my colleagues' work in the Buffalo Creek disaster, including two second decade follow-ups, will be briefly described, and some beginning hypotheses about the shift in risk for negative outcomes over time, depending on one's subgroup, will be offered. Finally, I will suggest areas where research is needed to better understand the impact of these events on mental health over time.

Long-term Impact of Disasters on Mental Health:
An Overview

While the distinction between events of human origin and those originating in "nature" is sometimes missed by those outside of this field of investigation (all events are often referred to as "natural disasters"), in the disaster literature this distinction has been more salient theoretically, although it is difficult to study. Natural disasters are "acts of God" that can't be prevented, while technological events are mishaps, that, by definition, could have been prevented (Baum, Fleming & Davidson, 1983). These latter events highlight that we are not in control of technology, and that someone has erred (and can be blamed). Because of this characteristic, such events may be more difficult to process psychologically. Neither of the two types of events would fall at the upper end of an hypothesized dimension of "deliberateness" (Green, 1993), as would some other events covered in this publication (i.e., the Holocaust, racism) and might therefore be expected to have somewhat better outcomes in the long-run. Some data on disaster outcomes suggest that the "natural" versus "technological" distinction may be a useful one to maintain, although, as noted, it is nearly impossible to study, since, for a true comparison, one would have to study a series of events with the same instruments, in the same timeframes, which varied only by the origin of the event.

A model for studying the psychological impact of these events was proposed a number of years ago by myself and colleagues (Green, Wilson & Lindy, 1985). In slightly modified form, it begins with the person's exposure to the disaster or other traumatic events (eg., loss, life threat, exposure to grotesque sights), which leads to the immediate appraisal of the event, and one's initial emotional reactions, as the person tries to process the event psychologically and cognitively. This processing takes place in the context of personal characteristics (eg., past history with similar or other traumatic events, mental health history, characteristic coping styles, maturity) and characteristics of the recovery environment (eg., continued disruption, disaster aid, community response, social support). Outcomes may be positive or negative, general or specific, acute or prolonged, and can cut across domains (psychological, physical, social).

Controlled studies of adults following disaster events have indicated the presence of negative mental health effects lasting a year or longer in a number of studies of natural disasters (Bravo, Rubio-Stipec, Canino, Woodbury & Ribera, 1990; Goenjian, 1994; Murphy, 1984; McFarlane, 1987; Norris, Phifer & Kaniasty, 1994; Phifer & Norris, 1989; Shore, Tatum & Vollmer, 1986). Lasting effects in adults have also been noted in most studies of technological events (Baum, Schaffer, Lake & Collins, 1986; Bromet, Parkinson & Dunn, 1990; Davidson, Fleming & Baum, 1986; Green et al., 1990a; Holen, 1991; Palinkas, Downs, Patterson & Russell, 1993; Smith, Robins, Przybeck, Goldring & Solomon, 1986), although a study of workers in the leaking TMI plant showed no effects (Bromet et al., 1990). The most studied event has been the nuclear leak at Three Mile Island (TMI) in which no one was killed or immediately injured, although the likelihood of later physical effects may have been increased.

Few studies of children have followed them for periods of longer than a year, and the results of such studies have been mixed. A study of a bushfire (McFarlane, Policansky & Irwin, 1987) showed continued negative impacts of a natural disaster at about two years, and a study of child survivors of an earthquake in Armenia showed impacts at the 18 month follow-up point (Pynoos et al., 1993). With regard to technological events, only investigators of nuclear leaks have followed children for more than a year, generally with negative findings (Cornely & Bromet, 1986; Bromet, Hough & Connell, 1984; Korol, 1990), although the latter study showed that children who were very close (within 1 1/2 miles) to the leaking plant did differ from controls at five years. It is not clear whether the lack of findings in these events was related to the time frame assessed, the proximity to the leak, or the nature of the event.

Rates of "disorder" (i.e. PTSD diagnoses or symptoms reaching a cut-off identified for screening probable "cases" needing psychiatric treatment) vary considerably in these studies. Diagnosable pathology is the exception rather than the rule, and rates rarely go beyond a quarter of the sample studied (Green, in press), especially at periods of one year or more after the disaster. Rates of disorder in children are similar at these later periods (Green et al., 1991; McFarlane, et al., 1987); however, Pynoos et al. (1993) found PTSD rates (by clinical interview) of 91% in a community sample of children at 18 months after the devastating Armenian earthquake, and Goenjian et al. (1994) found rates of 67% in adults for the same time period in the same setting.

The types of outcomes documented have also indicated a range of types of symptoms, with consistent effects found for PTSD symptoms, other anxiety symptoms, depression, and somatization (Green, in press). In addition to self-reported distress and diagnoses based on interviews, these longer (and shorter) effects were also noted in visits to health providers, and in the legal system, as well as in physiological indicators. Thus the findings are quite robust across domains and do not depend solely on the individual's perception of the impact (Green, in press).

The longevity of impact of these events has been studied longitudinally and in long-term cross-sectional studies. While most studies show improvement in subjects over time, some studies of natural disasters have detected continuing negative impacts for over a year (Galante & Foa, 1986; McFarlane, 1989; McFarlane et al., 1987; Murphy, 1984; Norris et al., 1994; Phifer & Norris, 1989; Pynoos et al., 1993; Shore et al., 1986). Technological disasters may produce even longer effects. For example, following the Three Mile Island disaster, where a nuclear facility leaked radioactivity, negative psychological effects were detected up to five years later (Davidson, et al., 1986); and survivors of an oil rig collapse showed elevated sick leave and psychiatric problems for eight years (Holen, 1991). Green et al. (1990a, 1990b) showed continuing effects of a dam collapse disaster for 14 years in the adults. The children of this disaster (Buffalo Creek) were not different from controls at 17 years (Green et al. 1994), although retrospective diagnoses indicated that differences existed at two years.

Most studies in the disaster literature have attempted to determine which subgroups of individuals were most at risk for developing disaster-related symptoms, diagnoses or other outcomes. Such information suggests the processes by which these events may lead to the various outcomes, and may be useful in targeting interventions to those most in need. The most often studied risk factor for negative outcomes following disaster events is the severity of the exposure to the event (eg., extent of life threat, loss, injury). The association between the presence and severity of disaster exposure and negative psychological consequences has been demonstrated across a myriad of events in both adults and children (Bromet et al, 1990; Freedy, Shaw, Jarrell & Masters, 1992; Freedy, Kilpatrick, Resnick & Saunders, 1994; Galante & Foa, 1986; Gleser, Green & Winget, 1981; Goenjian et al., 1994; Green, Grace & Gleser, 1985; Green et al., 1991; McFarlane, 1987; Murphy, 1984; Palinkas et al., 1993; Pynoos et al., 1993; Shore et al., 1986; Thompson, Norris & Hanacek, 1990; Weisaeth, 1989). Not all exposure differences were associated with all outcomes, but a consistent pattern has emerged. The few studies which do not show this trend have tended to include mostly highly exposed subjects, and may suffer from a restriction of range.

The remaining risk factors are not as well studied or as easily reported on in a brief format. For more details about the findings on the various risk factors described below, see Green (in press), and Green & Solomon (in press). Studies on the effects of gender on outcome following disaster have been mixed, although when differences are found, more symptoms are usually reported in women and girls. Usually, the symptoms studied have been PTSD, anxiety or depression, symptoms and disorders more prevalent in women (cf. Kessler et al., 1994). It may be that males and females express their distress in different ways, as a few studies with a broad range of outcomes suggest (eg., Bennett, 1970; Gleser et al., 1981). These studies showed women to have higher/increased psychological symptoms, anxiety and depression, while men had higher/increased physician visits, physical symptoms, hospital referrals, belligerence, and alcohol abuse.

The most thorough study of age differences following disaster was done by Thompson et al. (1993). These investigators studied the effects of a hurricane in the USA and found that younger people exhibited the most distress in the absence of disaster, but middle-aged people did so in its presence. The variable most associated with this differential age-related risk was "burden", meaning the additional stresses that are associated with this life stage. These authors found that burden peaked in middle age, i.e. that parental stress, filial stress, financial stress, occupational stress, and ecological stress were all higher for the middle-aged subjects. Middle-aged persons also provided support to others in amounts greater than received. This differential risk in middle-age is consistent with another review of this literature and a study by Green et al. (in press; and see below). Age effects in children are not completely consistent but tend to be related to the nature of the outcomes assessed, along a developmental line (Green et al., 1991; Green, in press) so that more regressive symptoms (general fears, distractibility, regressive toileting habits) are found in younger children, while older children show more overall disturbance. However, few studies have used the same instruments or measured the same constructs, so no firm conclusions can be drawn. It is clear, however, that even quite young children may develop symptoms of PTSD following disaster events, so this syndrome is not limited to older children and adults. Only recently has PTSD been routinely assessed in child disaster studies.

Pre-existing psychological symptoms have now been shown to predict disaster-related distress in a number of studies, both in retrospective and in prospective designs (Green, in press). However, there is some evidence that this effect may be less powerful with regard to PTSD symptoms per se (Smith et al., 1990), and that it may make less difference in the acute post-disaster phase (Smith, North & Spitznagel, 1993) for individuals with high exposure. Studies of personality traits as they relate to post-disaster pathology have all collected the trait data <u>following</u> the events, and need to be interpreted cautiously until these findings can be replicated in prospective studies. Prior disaster exposure and previous exposure to other traumatic events have been shown to increase the risk for post-disaster symptoms (Freedy et al., 1992, Freedy, et al., 1994).

The effects of the family and parents on the mental health of children following disaster have been clearly demonstrated. Parental life events, and parental pathology or parental disaster response have been shown to be good predictors of how the child will respond (Bromet et al., 1984; Cornely & Bromet, 1986; Gleser et al., 1981; Green et al., 1991; Korol, 1990; McFarlane, 1987). Family atmosphere over and above parental symptoms has been shown to predict child outcome as well (Green, et al., 1991; McFarlane, 1987).

The Impact of Setting on Disaster Effects

Disasters, even "acts of God", do not strike randomly, and their physical impact may vary considerably, depending on the setting in which they occur. A recent report by the International Federation of Red Cross and Red Crescent Societies (1993) reported that between the years of 1967 and 1991, nearly 8000 disasters were reported worldwide. These events killed over seven million people, and affected nearly three trillion (affected being defined as those needing immediate or long-term assistance as a direct consequence of the disaster). It was the poorest countries, and those with the largest populations, which sustained the most deaths during this period, and the people in the least developed countries continue to run the greatest risk of dying from disaster. An earlier report (US Agency for International Development, 1986) found that 86% of disasters occurred in developing nations, and 78% of all deaths occurred in these settings, where over 97% of affected individuals are located. Further, the ratio of affected to killed individuals was calculated to be 2.9 in developed countries, but tenfold in developing countries, so that each disaster in a developing country left more affected individuals in need of disaster relief and other services, likely under conditions of fewer available resources.

It is almost difficult to imagine the level of devastation connected with some of these events. For example, a disaster studied by Lima and his colleagues (eg., Lima, Pai, Santacruz, Lozano & Luna, 1987; Lima et al., 1993), was a volcanic eruption in Armero, Columbia which destroyed that town and killed 22,000 people, or 80% of the area inhabitants. Two small neighboring towns of about 3000 people each had to assimilate approximatley 6000 homeless victims. Survivors were mostly unskilled workers with limited possibilities for alternative gainful employment (Lima, Santacruz, Lozano & Luna, 1988). The Armenian earthquake of 1988 (cf. Goenjian et al., 1994) was estimated to have killed between 25,000 and 100,000 people, and left over half a million homeless. Entire cities were destroyed. These events have tended not to be studied systematically, but the few studies that have been done indicate high levels of mental health problems over extended periods of time (Goenjian et al., 1994; Lima et al., 1993; Pynoos et al., 1993). Disasters of this scope are difficult to imagine in more developed settings, where events that are considered severe, and which tax resources significantly (e.g., Hurricane Andrew in the USA), are of much lower magnitude. Individuals who live in the less developed settings may have a qualitatively different overall experience than that which occurs in most events studied to date, both with regard to initial exposure severity, and with regard to ongoing disruption.

A related issue is the populations which such events may effect. Disasters may strike populations that are differentially vulnerable to begin with. Seaman (1984, cited in Lima et al., 1988) noted that disasters are more likely to affect socioeconomically disadvantaged populations, as the fast rise in some city populations, the pressure on the land, and deteriorating economic conditions have forced underprivileged populations into more hazardous areas where they are more likely to encounter disasters. Oliver-Smith (1993) also suggested that low income groups, even if they have information that certain areas are more prone to hazards, may not have a choice about where they live, since more dangerous areas may be all that they can afford. These points suggest that the settings in which these events take place are extremely important in determining the degree of exposure to stress, and consequently, the mental health outcomes that may be found. This is important in conceptualizing disaster as a stressor in the first place, and conplicates cross-cultural comparisons, since disaster events may be confounded with the populations they effect. Even research in the USA suggests that events do not occur randomly to individuals, but may effect those most vulnerable at the outset. For example, Smith et al. (1986) found that those directly exposed to disaster were younger, had less often completed high school, had lower incomes, and were more often separated or divorced, than those who were not exposed to tornados, floods and the toxic chemical dioxin in Missouri. These confounds, and qualitative differences in the disaster experience, make it difficult to generalize from research in more developed countries to other settings where little research has been conducted.

The Buffalo Creek Disaster:
Long-term Consequences of a Human-Caused Event

The research group from the Traumatic Stress Study Center at the University of Cincinnati Psychiatry Department did several studies over two decades focusing on the long-term effects of disaster events. We were interested in the impact of these events over time, especially in the very long term. Two studies examined outcomes in the adult and child survivors of the Buffalo Creek dam collapse, following these individuals into the second decade post-disaster. Since my focus is on the long-term, rather than the more immediate, effects of stressful events, I will focus on these disaster studies as a way of highlighting the potential for disasters to have negative impacts over long periods, and to indicate some of the problems inherent in doing this type of research. Of particular focus is the continuity or non-continuity of risk among individuals and subgroups across such a long time period (and how difficult this is to study). The sample itself was not a random one, and likely does not represent the community at large. All 588 individuals originally studied were participants in a lawsuit, although the follow-up studies recruited comparison samples not involved in legal proceedings, and other samples not exposed to the disaster. However, the overall proportions of individuals affected are not likely to be accurate estimates of general community responses. On the other hand, the initial sample was quite large, and allowed the exploration of prediction of risk for psychological symptoms at a time when this had rarely been studied. And the long-term follow-up of these samples extends our information about the longevity and predictability of risk over a longer time period than heretofore investigated in the aftermath of disasters.

Event Description

In February of 1972, a dam, built from coal mining waste without attention to safety standards, collapsed and unleashed millions of gallons of black water and sludge, which had collected behind it, onto the small community below. The wall of water careened from side to side down the narrow valley, killing 125 people, making it one of the most deadly disasters of the decade in the United States, and leaving thousands homeless. Nearly everyone knew someone who died, although since it was Saturday morning, families tended to be together, and die together, so few survivors lost nuclear family members. The coal company was sued for wrongful death, property damage and "psychic impairment," brought about by the substandard construction of the dam. Psychiatric teams from the University of Cincinnati examined all of the plaintiffs for the prosecution, and a psychiatrist from West Virginia, where the collapse occurred, examined all of the same plaintiffs for the defense. The original research findings were based on both sets of reports, which were done between 18 months and two years following the dam collapse. The UC team examined individuals in their homes, while the defense psychiatrist had subjects come to his office, about two hours away by car. Although the diagnosis of post-traumatic stress disorder (PTSD) did not exist at the time, the prosecution psychiatrists were examining subjects for symptoms of "traumatic neurosis," and the defense psychiatrist for symptoms of "gross stress reaction," so most PTSD symptoms could be rated, along with other symptoms.

Methodology

All original psychiatric diagnostic reports were rated by the research team (with funding from NIMH) using the Psychiatric Evaluation Form (PEF; Spitzer, Endicott,

Mesnikoff & Cohen, 1968; Endicott & Spitzer, 1972) along 19 dimensions of psychopathology, and the scales were combined into clusters using rational and empirical methods. Clusters covered symptoms related to depression, anxiety, and belligerence. The scales of alcohol abuse and overall severity were used separately. The scales showed good interrater agreement and scores for the two sides of the lawsuit were significantly correlated, although attributions for the symptoms usually varied by side of the suit (Gleser et al., 1981). The average scores from the two sides were used in the analyses. Some adult subjects also filled out a modified version of the Hopkins symptom checklist (Lipman, Rickles, Covi, Derogatis & Uhlenhuth, 1969). At the time of rating the psychopathology, extent of exposure to the disaster was also rated along the dimensions of bereavement (loss, including by death, in the disaster), life threat (eg., proximity to flood waters, extent of warning), extended trauma in the form of exposure to the elements and other experiences, and displacement from original homesite. Family atmosphere (violent, irritable, depressed, supportive) in the home was rated from the reports for each family.

The lawsuit was settled out of court the summer after the initial data collection. Several follow-up trips were made between 1975 and 1977 to interview subsamples of survivors, but the major follow-ups were conducted under separate funding from NIMH at 14 years post-disaster (adults), and 17 years post-disaster ("children", [now adults]). 120 of the original adult plaintiffs were located and re-interviewed (39% of living survivors). Of the 61% not interviewed, 36% of were refusers (Green & Grace, 1988). Based on the 1974 reports, adult survivors who participated in the follow-up had significantly less personal loss through death than those who refused, but there were no initial differences in any of the psychopathology scores. At follow-up, 80 individuals who were in the dam collapse but not the lawsuit were also recruited, as well as a culturally and demographically similar comparison sample who had not been exposed to the event.

Of the original 207 children, 99 were located and re-interviewed at 17 years post-disaster, with 76% of those approached agreeing to participate. Those followed-up were rated as significantly less impaired in 1974 on overall severity, belligerence, alcohol abuse, and suspicion. Since most of the children in the area eventually sued the coal company, only a non-exposed comparison sample was recruited (Green et al., 1994). Thus, the participants in the follow-up were either less exposed to the disaster (adults) or healthier (children) at the earlier time point than those who were lost to follow-up, a finding similar to that for other longitudinal studies we have done (Green, Grace, Lindy, Titchener & Lindy, 1983). The findings may therefore present a somewhat more optimistic picture than if all initial participants had been re-interviewed.

Data collected at follow-up for both adults and children included the Structured Clinical Interview for DSM III-R (SCID; Spitzer & Williams, 1986; Spitzer, Williams, Gibbon & First, 1989; both draft versions of the III-R version of the DSM) for past and current diagnoses. At the end of the interview, subjects were rated on the PEF, filled out the SCL-90 (Derogatis, 1983), and the Impact of Event Scale (Horowitz,

Wilner & Alvarez, 1979), in addition to a number of other measures. Disaster experiences were reviewed to help fill in details missing from some of the earlier reports.

Summary of Findings

The findings at two years are described in the context of the follow-up data. Complete findings on both the adults and the children at the earlier time point are described in Gleser et al. (1981).

The early adult follow-ups had shown some decrease in the psychopathology ratings 1-3 years after the settlement. At 14 years, scores on the PEF and the SCL had continued to decline; significant decreases were noted for both men and women for all symptom types except alcohol abuse, which was relatively low initially. The reports from 1974 were rated for "probable PTSD" diagnoses at the time of the follow-up. Based on this information, and the figures for current diagnoses from the SCID, the proportion of PTSD went down from 44% to 28% for the men and women combined, a significant change for the women (52% to 31%) but not the men (32% to 23%) (Green et al., 1990b) While the overall improvement was clear-cut, survivors continued to show significant impairment in the areas of anxiety and depression symptoms relative to a non-exposed sample. However, they were not different from a comparison group of exposed non-litigants who lived in the valley at the time of the disaster and had similar exposure scores (Green et al., 1990a). Men and women did not differ from each other at the long-term follow-up, although they had differed significantly by type of pathology at two years.

At the time that the "children" (ages 2-15 at the time of the disaster) were followed up, they were between the ages of 19 and 33. Over this period, ratings on the PEF generally declined. Anxiety, belligerence, somatic concerns, agitation (separate scales of the PEF) and Overall Severity all decreased significantly. Conversely, symptoms of substance abuse and suicidal ideation, absent in the original sample, increased significantly. Post-disaster rates of PTSD and Major Depression (retrospectively from the SCID), which were 32% and 33% for a post-disaster diagnosis, were down to current rates of 7% and 13%. While these latter rates were higher than general norms, they were quite similar to those found in the comparison community. SCL-90 and PEF scores were also nearly identical for the Buffalo Creek and comparison samples, suggesting that the specific impact of the disaster was no longer detectable in these subjects (Green et al., 1994). Older children, who had shown the highest levels of symptoms of most types at two years, continued to show more symptoms, but the difference was not significant. The PTSD rate in the oldest group was 14% compared to 3-4% in the younger groups, and the number of PTSD symptoms was marginally higher in this group (p <.06). Gender differences, however, were quite notable, although they were circumscribed. Women had higher scores than men on rated anxiety, social isolation, and self-reported PTSD symptoms on the

Impact of Event Scale. PTSD and depression rates were marginally higher (Green et al., 1994).

To summarize the longitudinal findings, clear-cut improvement was noted in both samples by the second decade post-disaster. However, for the adults, the exposed survivors continued to be more impaired than their non-exposed neighbors. Gender differences (present in both samples at two years) had disappeared in the adult sample at the long-term follow-up. Conversely, in the child sample, the subjects were not different than their non-exposed neighbors on any of the current follow-up measures. However, gender differences continued to be detected in stress-related symptoms.

Risk Factors and Shifting Risk

As noted in the earlier summary of disaster studies, the two year data from Buffalo Creek found severity of exposure (life threat loss, displacement, prolonged exposure) to be predictive of outcome in both the adult and the child samples. Prediction was somewhat different for men and women, but less educated individuals had higher impairment ratings. Race, marital status and post-disaster life events also added to the prediction. About 32% of the variance of Overall Severity (the global rating from the PEF) in the women and 40% in the men was predicted by exposure, demographics (including age [see below]), and subsequent life events (Gleser et al., 1981). For the children, the functioning of the parent and the atmosphere in the home explained additional variance over and above exposure and demographics, explaining about one third of the variance in Overall Severity, and slightly less of the variance (28%) in PTSD (Gleser et al., 1981; Green et al., 1991).

A number of analyses were done to examine the effects of age within the adult sample. Initially, at two years, significant curvilinear trends were found for the adult sample, with middle-aged survivors doing the worst. This included the groups spanning the ages of 25 to 54, with some specific differences between the group aged 25-39 and the group aged 40-54. Generally, women in the younger of the two age groups were more at risk, while men in the older group were more at risk (Gleser et al., 1981). Re-analysis of this earlier data indicated that the group aged 36-45 at the early follow-up were rated as most impaired on the PEF. Data at follow-up were analyzed in several different ways (Green et al., in press a; Green et al., in press b). These analyses indicated that the oldest groups (combining plaintiffs and non-plaintiffs) were doing the best. At long term follow-up, subjects who were aged 36-45 at that time also showed the most risk for self-reported and clinically-rated symptoms (PTSD differences were not significant). Thus, risk for symptoms was associated with "middle-age" regardless of the age at which the person was exposed to the disaster. This fits well with the findings of Thompson et al. (1993), described earlier, as this is likely the group with the most "burden" and the least reciprocity of support. As noted, older children were more at risk at both points in time although this difference was not significant in the follow-up sample. However, there was no age overlap in the child sample to compare cross-sectional and longitudinal data.

Putting the adult and child samples together showed that risk increased with age, up to the middle-age period noted above, then decreased (Green et al., in press a). The oldest group of children looked similar to the youngest group of adults, although their anxiety ratings and their PTSD rates were lower than the adults (PTSD: 14% compared to 23%).

These findings suggest that the risk associated with age, and perhaps with gender (see earlier findings of decreasing gender differences in the aging adult sample) change over time, so that the groups at most risk at one point may differ from those at risk at another point. We also examined this directly by exploring the relationship of the outcome measures over time. Scores in 1974 for the adults and children were not highly predictive of later functioning. For the adults, the highest relationship was for the Symptom Checklist total score ($r=.43$). Overall Severity on the PEF at the two points in time was correlated only .17, and PTSD was correlated .18 at the two points. While these figures were all significant, they are relatively low. Specific subscale scores were not correlated between 1974 and 1986 (Green et al., 1990b). With regard to PTSD, 61% of the adult sample had the same diagnosis at both points (17%, PTSD; 44%, no PTSD). Twenty-eight percent (28%) of the sample changed from having the diagnosis in 1974 to not having it in 1986, while 11% carried the diagnosis only at the later time point (Green et al., 1990b). The low correlations are due in part to the reduction of variability at follow-up, and the actual changes in many individuals. Further, some of the discontinuity may be due to inconsistancy in the rating criteria. However, the risk for negative outcomes clearly shifts over time. The findings were similar for the children: correlations between the same scales on the PEF in 1974 and in 1989 were non-significant (Green et al., 1994), suggesting no prediction between the two time periods. The number of past PTSD symptoms measured in 1974 was correlated .21 ($p<.05$) with the number of current PTSD symptoms in 1989.

Methodologic Issues

Comparing predictors at the two time points for the same survivors also proved to be interesting. Using only those individuals on whom we had complete data at the two points in time, we examined the prediction of 1974 scores and 1986 scores (for the adults) using the same variables. With regard to the PTSD diagnosis, pre-flood education and marital status predicted outcome at both points in time (PTSD was associated with lower education and being married rather than single). Stressors predicted outcome at both points as well. However, having any pre-flood diagnosis (according to retrospective report on the SCID) did not predict the 1974 outcomes, but did predict the 1986 outcomes. Further, the number of moves (an indicator of disruption) also predicted later but not earlier outcome. Both of these variables were significant in the 1986 prediction equation on the larger (plaintiff and non-plaintiff) sample combined. Stressors predicted only PTSD at the later follow-up, and not more general pathology. It would appear that these variables were more potent at the later point in time. This makes some sense in that one's prior vulnerability may indeed influence who continues to have chronic symptoms, compared to who recovers. However, both of these variables were measured in 1986, so their relationship with other measures at that time could be due to this measurement strategy, and not reflect the actual variables (or some combination of the two explanations).

A related finding compares the relationship of current (at second decade follow-up) PTSD symptoms to past PTSD symptoms. As noted, the longitudinal data from the "child" sample indicated a relationship of .21 for these two sets of symptoms. However, if one compares the current number of symptoms in 1989 with the number of past symptoms remembered in 1989 on the SCID, the correlation is .68. Although there are real reasons why the longitudinal data might actually be less correlated (e.g., the 1974 data was for a particular point in time, while the lifetime SCID assessed symptoms at any point post-disaster), the retrospective data give a more stable picture of risk prediction than the data collected at the two periods. The data for the adults was not as good for comparing the longitudinal to the retrospective findings; however, we did find that, of those individuals who were rated as never having had PTSD according to the SCID in 1986, 34% were rated to have had the diagnosis in 1974.

Conclusion

With regard to the substantive findings, it is clear that disasters have the potential to impact mental health over long periods of time in an untreated sample. This was amply demonstrated by the adult follow-up data, which showed continuing effects in a subset of the survivors at 14 years. Both adults and children showed some prediction of current PTSD-related symptoms from the initial exposure (life threat, loss, prolonged exposure) variables, while more global pathology was not predictable from stressors. However, the individuals at risk shifted somewhat over time, and the early (two year) indicators of adaptation were not good predictors of adaptation in the second decade. Age-related risk appeared to be associated with middle-age regardless of the age at disaster exposure. Further, the adult sample continued to have disaster-related mental health problems while the child sample had essentially recovered at follow-up. Gender differences continued in the younger adults, but disappeared in the adult sample. We have speculated about the reasons for these differential outcomes elsewhere (Green et al., 1994; Green et al., in press b), but primarily want to make the larger point here. It would appear that developmental issues are important in understanding disaster responses. While most studies show a "dose-response" relationship between exposure and outcome, even over extended periods, the other variables that determine risk may not be as clear-cut.

This study is not the ideal one for examining methodologic issues in studying disaster survivors, since it was not meant to be a longitudinal study. However, it likely shares a number of problems with studies that follow individuals over long periods, while methodologies are constantly changing and diagnoses are being invented. Tentatively, however, our findings suggest that some of what we accept as risk factors from disaster studies may in part be due to how we study these events. In particular, retrospective reports of symptomatology may overestimate the link between prior and current symptoms. Fortunately, we have now have a number of studies that have pre-disaster data on large samples (Bravo et al., 1990; Phifer & Norris, 1989; Robins et al., 1986) and these indicate that pre-disaster functioning indeed predicts post-disaster functioning. However, these studies are assessing individuals in the relatively short-term. A longer, more developmental perspective may indicate periods of risk for exposed individuals that shift over time, so that risk may be non-continuous. This may or may not be best conceptualized as relating to the disaster event.

Research Directions

Research directions growing out of the general thrust of this paper include more longitudinal and prospective studies. While assessments at any point in time may be quite helpful in describing current status, risk factors may be more difficult to assess from a distance. For human-caused disasters and more devastating disasters of natural origin (along with other types of traumatic events), which are likely to have extended effects, a more developmental perspective might be helpful in conceptualizing long-term effects, and the investigation of differential risk over time should be systematically pursued. Cross-sectional epidemiologic and risk factor studies of individual responses to disaster events have likely told us as much as they can, and should not be encouraged. A possible exception is studies of children, which have been scarce. However, the same comments apply generally to child studies as well.

Aspects of responses to traumatic disaster events which have not been well-studied include biological and physiological outcomes and processes, as well as studies in developing countries and those with a cross-cultural perspective. Disasters may also provide a mechanism for studying more basic human processes like memory, or the role of external stressors on family processes, etc. From this perspective, disaster may be a good operationalization of stressors that are less confounded with outcome than more common life events or traumas that originate within the family or indicate ongoing family disruption.

Finally, intervention studies are needed. A great deal of intervention is presently going on, as crisis counseling and debriefing, without any empirical support for its efficacy. Much of disaster research is done in the name of contributing to the identification of survivors at risk, and to the development of treatment modalities. Now we need to take the next step. Many treatments have been designed but few have been tested. This is a challenge, to be sure, but is not impossible. As resources for treatment become more scarce, allocation will proceed with or without empirical information. It would be helpful to have data to bring to bear on these questions.

References

Baum, A., Fleming, R., & Davidson, L. (1983). Natural disaster and technological catastrophe. Environment and Behavior, 15, 333-354.

Baum, A., Schaeffer, M., Lake, R., Fleming, R., & Collins, D. (1970). Psychological and endocrinological correlates of chronic stress at Three Mile Island. Perspectives on Behavioral Medicine, 2, 201-217.

Bennet, G. (1970). Bristol floods 1968. Controlled survey of effects on health of local community disaster. British Medical Journal, 3, 454-458.

Bravo, M., Rubio-Stipec, M., Canino, G., Woodbury, M.A., & Ribera, J.C. (1990). The psychological sequelae of disaster stress prospectively and retrospectively evaluated. American Journal of Community Psychology, 18, 661-680.

Bromet, E., Hough, L., & Connell, M. (1984). Mental health of children near the Three Mile Island reactor. Journal of Preventive Psychiatry, 2, 275-301.

Bromet, E., Parkinson, D., & Dunn, L. (1990). Long-term mental health consequences of the accident at Three Mile Island. International Journal of Mental Health, 19, 8-60.

Cornely, P., & Bromet, E. (1986). Prevalence of behavior problems in three-year-old children living near Three Mile Island: A comparative analysis. Journal of Child Psychology and Psychiatry, 27, 489-498.

Davidson, L., Fleming, I., & Baum, A. (1986). Post-traumatic stress as a function of chronic stress and toxic exposure. In C. Figley (Ed.). Trauma and its wake, Vol. 2 (pp. 57-77). New York: Brunner/Mazel.

Derogatis, L.R. (1983). SCL-90 R version: Manual I. Baltimore: Johns Hopkins University.

Endicott, J., & Spitzer, R. (1972). What! Another rating scale? The Pychiatric Evaluation Form. Journal of Nervous Mental Disease, 154, 88-104.

Freedy, J.R., Shaw, D.L., Jarrell, M.P., & Masters, C.R. (1992). Towards an understanding of the psychological impact of natural disasters: An application of the conservation of resources stress model. Journal of Traumatic Stress, 5, 441-454.

Freedy, J.R., Saladin, M.E., Kilpatrick, D.G., Resnick, H.S., & Saunders, B.E. (1994). Understanding acute psychological distress following natural disaster. Journal of Traumatic Stress, 7, 257-274.

Galante, R., & Foa, D. (1986). An epidemiological study of psychic trauma and treatment effectiveness for children after a natural disaster. Journal of the American Academy of Child Psychiatry, 25, 357-363.

Gleser, G.C., Green, B.L., Winget, C.N. (1981). Prolonged psychosocial effects of disaster: A study of Buffalo Creek. New York: Academic Press.

Goenjian, A.K., Najarian, L.M., Pynoos, R.S., Steinberg, A.M., Manoukian, G., Tavosian, A., & Fairbanks, L.A. (1994). Post-traumatic stress disorder in elderly and younger adults after the 1988 earthquake in Armenia. American Journal of Psychiatry, 151, 895-901.

Green, B.L. (1993). Identifying survivors at risk: Trauma and stressors across events. In J.P. Wilson, & B. Raphael (Eds.), International handbook of traumatic stress syndromes (pp.135-144). New York: Plenum.

Green, B.L. (in press). Traumatic stress and disaster: Mental health effects and factors influencing adaptation. In C.C. Nadelson & F. LiehMak (Eds.), International review of psychiatry (vol 2). Section on Traumatic stress: An international perspective (J.R.T. Davidson, & A.C. McFarlane, Eds.)

Green, B.L., & Grace, M.C. (1988). Conceptual issues in research with survivors and illustrations from a follow-up study. In J.P. Wilson, Z. Harel, & B. Kahana (Eds.), Human adaptation to extreme stress: From the Holocaust to Vietnam (pp. 105-124). New York: Plenum.

Green, B.L., Grace, M.C., Vary, M., Kramer, T.L., Gleser, G.C., & Leonard, A.C. (1994). Children of disaster in the second decade: A 17-year follow-up of Buffalo Creek survivors. Journal of the American Academy of Child and Adolescent Psychiatry, 33, 71-79.

Green, B.L., Gleser, G.C., Lindy, J.D., Grace, M.C., & Leonard, A.C. (in press-a). Age-related reactions to the Buffalo Creek Dam collapse: Second decade effects. In P.E. Ruskin, & J.A. Talbott (Eds.), Aging and posttraumatic stress disorder. Washington, DC: American Psychiatric Press.

Green, B.L., Grace, M.C., Lindy, J.D., Titchener, J.L., & Lindy, J.G. (1983). Levels of functional impairment following a civilian disaster: The Beverly Hills Supper Club fire. Journal of Consulting and Clinical Psychology, 51, 573-580.

Green, B.L., Grace, M.C., Gleser, G.C. (1985). Identifying survivors at risk: Long-term impairment following the Beverly Hills Supper Club fire. Journal of Consulting and Clinical Psychology, 53, 672-678.

Green, B.L., Grace, M.C., Lindy, J.D., Gleser, G.C., Leonard, A.C., & Kramer, T.L. (1990). Buffalo Creek survivors in the second decade: Comparison with unexposed and nonlitigant groups. Journal of Applied Social Psychology, 20, 1033-1050.

Green, B.L., Korol, M., Grace, M.C., Vary, M.G., Leonard, A.C., Gleser, G.C., & Smitson-Cohen, S. (1991). Children and disaster: Age, gender, and parental effects on PTSD symptoms. Journal of the American Academy of Child and Adolescent Psychiatry, 30, 945-951.

Green, B.L., Kramer, T.L., Grace, M.C., Gleser, G.C., Leonard, A.C., Vary, M.G., & Lindy, J.D., (in press-b). Traumatic events over the lifespan: Survivors of the Buffalo Creek disaster. In T.W. Miller (Ed.), Stressful life events II. New York: International Universities Press.

Green, B.L., Lindy, J.D., Grace, M.C., Gleser, G.C., Leonard, A.C., Korol, M. & Winget, C. (1990). Buffalo Creek survivors in the second decade: Stability of stress symptoms. American Journal of Orthopsychiatry, 60, 43-54.

Green, B.L., & Solomon, S.D. (in press). The mental health impact of natural and technological disasters. In J.R. Freedy & S.E. Hobfoll (Eds.), Traumatic stress: From theory to practice. New York: Plenum.

Green, B.L., & Solomon, S.D. (in press). The mental health impact of natural and technological disasters. In J.R. Freedy & S.E. Hobfoll (Eds.), Traumatic stress: From theory to practice. New York: Plenum.

Green, B.L., Wilson, J.P., Lindy, J.D. (1985). Conceptualizing post-traumatic stress disorder: A psychosocial framework. In C. Figley (Ed.), Trauma and its Wake: Vol 1. New York: Brunner/Mazel.

Holen, A. (1991). A longitudinal study of the occurrence and persistence of post-traumatic health problems in disaster survivors. Stress Medicine, 7, 11-17.

Horowitz, M.J., Wilner, N., Alvarez, W. (1979). Impact of Event Scale: A measure of subjective stress. Psychosomatic Medicine, 41, 209-218.

International Federation of Red Cross and Red Crescent Societies. (1993). World disaster report 1993. Dordrecht, The Netherlands: Martinus Nijoff. (Contact address, Geneva, Switzerland).

Kessler, R.C., McGonagle, K.A., Zhao, S., Nelson, C.B., Hughes, M., Eshleman, S., Wittchen, H., & Kendler, K.S. (1994). Lifetime and 12-month prevalence of DSM-III-R psychiatric disorders in the United States. Archives of General Psychiatry, 51, 8-19.

Korol, M. (1990). Children's psychological responses to a nuclear waste disaster in Fernald, Ohio. Doctoral dissertation, University of Cincinnati.

Lima, B.R., Pai, S., Santacruz, H., Lozano, J., & Luna, J. (1987). Screening for the psychological consequences of a major disaster in a developing country: Armero, Columbia. Acta Psychiatrica Scandinavica, 76, 561-567.

Lima, B.R., Pai, S., Toledo, V., Caris, L., Haro, J.M., Lozano, J., & Santacruz, H. (1993). Emotional distress in disaster victims: A follow-up study. Journal of Nervous and Mental Disease, 181, 388-393.

Lima, B.R., Santacruz, H., Lozano, J., & Luna, J. (1988). Planning for health/mental health integration in emergencies. In M. Lystad (Ed.), Mental health responses to mass emergencies. (pp. 371-393). New York: Brunner/Mazel.

Lipman, R.S., Rickles, K., Covi, L., Derogatis, L.R., & Uhlenhuth, E.H. (1969). Factors of symptom distress. Archives of General Psychiatry, 21, 328-338.

McFarlane, A. (1987). Family functioning and overprotection following a natural disaster: The longitudinal effects of post-traumatic morbidity. Australian and New Zealand Journal of Psychiatry, 21, 210-218.

McFarlane, A. (1989). The aetiology of post-traumatic morbidity: Predisposing, precipitating and perpetuating factors. British Journal of Psychiatry, 154, 221-228.

McFarlane, A., Policansky, S., & Irwin, C. (1987). A longitudinal study of the psychological morbidity in children due to a natural disaster. Psychological Medicine, 17, 727-738.

Murphy, S. (1984). Stress levels and health status of victims of a natural disaster. Research in Nursing and Health, 7, 205-215.

Norris, F.H., Phifer, J.F., & Kaniasty, K.Z. (1994). Individual and community reactions to the Kentucky floods: Findings from a longitudinal study of older adults. In R. Ursano, B. McCaughey, & C. Fullerton (Eds.), Individual and community responses to trauma and disaster. (pp. 378-400). Cambridge, Great Britain: Cambridge University Press.

Oliver-Smith, A. (1993). Anthropological perspectives in research literature. In E.L. Quarantelli & K. Popov (Eds.), Proceedings of the U.S.-Former Soviet Union seminar on social science research on mitigation for and recovery from disasters and large scale hazards: Vol. 1. The American participation (pp. 94-117). Newark, DE: University of Delaware, Disaster Research center.

Palinkas, L., Downs, M., Patterson, J., & Russell, J. (1993). Social, cultural, and psychological impacts of the Exxon Valdez oil spill. Human Organization, 52, 1-13.

Phifer, J., & Norris, F. (1989). Psychological symptoms in older adults following natural disaster: nature, timing, duration, and course. Journal of Gerontology: Social Sciences, 44, 207-217.

Pynoos, R., Goenjian, A., Tashjian, M., & Karakashian, M., Manjikian, R., Manoukian, G., Steinberg, A.M., & Fairbanks, L.A. (1993). Post-traumatic stress reactions in children after the 1988 Armenian earthquake. British Journal of Psychiatry, 163, 239-247.

Robins, L.N., Fischbach, R.L., Smith, E.M., Cottler, L.B., Solomon, S.D., & Goldring, E. (1986). Impact of disaster on previously assessed mental health. In J. Shore (Ed.), Disaster stress studies: New methods and findings (pp. 21-48). Washington, D.C.: American Psychiatric Press.

Shore, J., Tatum, E., & Vollmer, W. (1986). Psychiatric reactions to disaster: The Mount St. Helens experience. American Journal of Psychiatry, 143, 590-595.

Smith, E., North, C., & Spitznagel, E. (1993). Post-traumatic stress in survivors of three disasters. In R. Allen (Ed.), Handbook of post-disaster interventions. [Special Issue of the Journal of Social Behavior and Personality, 8(5)]. Corte Madera, CA: Select Press.

Smith, E.M., North, C.S., McCool, R.E., & Shea, J.M. (1990). Acute postdisaster psychiatric disorders: Identification of persons at risk. American Journal of Psychiatry, 147, 202-206.

Smith, E.M., Robins, L.N., Pryzbeck, T.R., Goldring, E., & Solomon, S.D. (1986). Psychosocial consequences of a disaster. In J.H. Shore (Ed.), Disaster stress studies: New methods and findings. Washington, D.C.: American Psychiatric Press.

Spitzer, R.L., Endicott, J., Mesnikoff, A.M., & Cohen, M.S. (1968). The Psychiatric Evaluation Form. New York: Biometrics Research Department, New York State Psychiatric Institute.

Spitzer, R.L., & Williams, J.W. (1986). Structured Clinical Interview for DSM-III: Non-patient version (11-1-86). New York: Biometrics Research Department, New York State Psychiatric Institute.

Spitzer, R.L., Williams, J.B., Gibbon, M., & First, M.B. (1989). <u>Structured Clinical Interview for DSM III-R: Non-patient version (5/1/89)</u>. New York: Biometrics Research Department, New York State Psychiatric Institute.

Thompson, M., Norris, F., Hanacek, B. (1993). Age differences in the psychological consequences of Hurricane Hugo. <u>Psychology and Aging, 8</u>, 606-616.

United States Agency for International Development, Office of U.S. Foreign Disaster Assistance. (1986). <u>Disaster history: Significant data on major disasters worldwide, 1900 to present.</u> Washington, DC: Author.

Weisaeth, L. (1989). The stressors and the post-traumatic stress syndrome after an industrial disaster. <u>Acta Psychiatrica Scandinavica Supplementum, 355</u>, 25-37.

ENDURANCE AND LIVING: LONG-TERM EFFECTS OF THE HOLOCAUST

Jacob Lomranz
The Herczeg Institute on Aging
Tel-Aviv University

"I feel very normal and well, but after the Holocaust either I or the world are completely insane" (A Holocaust survivor)

Introduction

50 years after, perhaps the most devastating man-inflicted trauma in human history, the Holocaust; obscurity, perplexity, and equivocality still characterize the scientific state of its investigations. The present chapter addresses itself to the disagreements, research problems and approach to the long-term effects of severe trauma, specifically the Holocaust. How can we explain our limited knowledge? Are our theories and methodologies perhaps inappropriate? How can we explain that extreme torment does not necessarily result in disorder, study trauma-experienced persons who seemingly are well adjusted and comprehend the human strength that copes constructively even with the severest trauma? Does trumatic stress interfere with normal adjustment, personality structure, aging, and life-span development? If so how? What impact does culture have on coping with trauma? What is the impact of mass trauma on the general culture?

This chapter deals with these questions and issues by first reveiwing the literature and its resulting problematic implications to which appropriate revisions are offered, both theoretical and methodological. This then serves as a bridge to the presentation of a multidimensional, integrative framework that includes the relationship between developmental stages, the traumatic sequelae and historical contexts on the one hand, and the various personal, interpersonal and cultural dimensions of coping with trauma on the other. The framework serves as the basis to an ongoing biographical research project with Holocaust, death camp, survivors, utilized here to illustrate some of the basic concepts characterizing coping and existence after trauma.

The chapter concludes with a discussion of certain cogent conceptual issues concerning personality, developmental aging and culture in posttraumatic perspective as well as methodological implications.

How Do we Comprehend The Long-Term Effects of Trauma?

Recent years have seen the development of the scientific discipline of Traumatology (Wilson & Raphael, 1993). Investigations of traumatic effects focus mainly on posttraumatic stress disorders (PTSD) as recognized and codified in the DSM-III (American Psychiatric Association, 1980). Human-inflicted trauma encompasses a variety of disastrous events or situations, including wartime casualities, battle fatigue, terrorism, victims of nuclear weapons and the Holocaust (Bergman & Jucovy, 1982; Davidson & Foa, 1993; Milgram, 1986, 1993). The Holocaust inflicted intense, prolonged, repeated, cumulative and unimaginably inhuman traumatic conditions. Its colossal impact created a tremendous challenge on its victims' ability to make lifelong adjustments. The nature and effects of the trauma, as well as coping modes have been reviewed elsewhere (e.g., Kahana, Kahana, Harel & Rosener, 1988; Krystal, 1987). Not surprisingly, the overall effect of the Holocaust on survivors has generally been considered physically and mentally damaging. But how do the majority of survivors function? How have such a wide array of traumatic conditions, differences in victims, and coping responses been investigated? Can we understand coping and long-term effects through a differentiating approach? What characterizes scientific investigations and findings up to this point?

A Review On Long-Term Traumatic Effects Of The Holocaust

I have attempted to review the research literature in terms of content, methodology, and findings, and to then draw upon the implications of this review. It is based on 108 articles regarding first generation Holocaust survivors that have appeared in Psychological Abstracts from 1974, the year such information began to be computerized, until 1990. Important research was also produced between the years 1946 and 1974. However, most of it was based on the Concentration Camp Survivor Syndrome Questionnaire (e.g., Eitinger, 1980), and is pathologically oriented. Several major studies which did not appear in the computarized search will also be referred to. Due to lack of space, the table below presents a condensed version, providing the information needed for the purposes of the present chapter.

Table 1 indicates that most studies have the following limitations. They are: 1) anchored in a psychoanalytic or psychodynamic theoretical orientation; 2) are limited mainly to intrapsychic dimensions; 3) are seldom empirical; 4) use extremely small samples and clinical case studies; 5) disregard the importance of sample selection procedures; 6) have patients as their subjects; 7) overinclude and do not specify the exact nature of the trauma (whether concentration camps, in hiding, etc.); 8) lack

Table No. 1. Research on the Holocaust: 1974-1990

Yrs. and No. of Pub.	Theoretical Orientation	Dimension or Variable	Method
1974 until 1990	Psychoanal.(35)	Psychopathology (38)	Theoretical(42)
	Psychodyn. (38)	Intrapsychic. (23)	Clinical & Case Studies (37)
	Med.Psy. (13)	Family (8)	
	Pers. & Psycho-soc. (8)	Psychotherapy (6)	Empirical (29)
108 Studies			
	Cognitive (6)	Personal-Dev. (6)	
	Fam. Appro (4)	Interps.-Soc. (6)	
	Eclectic (2)	Communication (5)	
	Rehab (1)	Well-Being (4)	
	Coping (1)	Miscellaneous (12)	

Trauma Specif.	Sample Pop. (Studies)	Contr. Gr.	Major Focus of Investigation (No. of Studies)
(33)	Not Specified (42)	(29)	Clinical, Intrapsychic defense mechanisms and pathology (21)
			Psychoanalytic, psychotherapeutic technique (17)
	Patients (38)		Family and parenting (8)
			Severity of traumatization (6)
			Treatment effects (6)
	Community (26)		Communication; documentation (5)
			Psychopathology & Development (5)
			Differentiation in pathology (5)
			Attitudes: Religion, politics (3)
			Memories (3)
	Representative (2)		Sleep & dreams (3)
			Well-being (3)
			Health & illness (3)
			Rehab. projects (2)
			Vulnerability (2)
			Time perspective (2)
			Role of support
			Fear of death
			Impact of previous Trauma on present one.

control groups and 9) have as their major focus of investigation, themes which are deficiency, symptomatological, or psychopathological in nature.

On the whole, research on the Holocaust displays several major trends. Nadler (1994) detects three of them. First, in the fifties and early sixties, studies focused directly on the survivor and the atrocities they underwent. In the late sixties and seventies, the focus shifted to long-term, generalized, psychopathological effects. Finally, since the eighties, we have seen a broader focus, relating the Holocaust to the general PTSD framework as well as to social variables and, producing somewhat more empirical research.

To a certain extent the more empirical studies based on broader theoretical perspectives, samples and validated instruments (e.g., MMPI; Life Satisfaction; Morale Scales), have underscored the remarkable adaptive capacities of survivors, revealing minimal, if any, differences with nonsurvivor control groups. These show survivors experience well-being, satisfaction in their work, marriage, and family, and enjoy social interactions. In some aspects of adaptation and well-being, survivors sometimes score even higher than non-Holocaust populations (e.g., Harel, Kahana & Kahana, 1988a, 1993; Leon, Butcher, Kleiman, Goldenberg & Almagor, 1981). Such findings raise serious questions as to the validity of earlier generalizations. What is the significance of this? Does it mean that these phenomena have not been properly studied in terms of theory, questions asked, and methodology.

Implications For The Present State Of Holocaust Research

The general impression after reviewing the Holocaust studies, is that major modifications in terms of approach and methodology have to be made. Perhaps the horrors of the Holocaust have not yet been fully realized and integrated by the world at large (Danieli, 1981a) so that the magnitude of the trauma has also hindered its appropriate investigation. However, the lack of clarity in the field, the initial questions raised by me and the above review, clearly lead to one conclusion: We must be open to different approaches and explanations, proceed inductively as well as deductively, generate hypotheses and adhere to scientific scruples. Some of our basic theoretical and methodological approaches to this area would have to be reconsidered, and I infer that the study of the long-term effects of the Holocaust will necessitate the following modifications and changes.

Required Perspectives In Theory And Methodology

A shift in approach; normal functioning, PTSR and total lives. Scientists hold different images of mankind and a "scientific community" may share such images. These, together with cultural factors, determine the nature of the scientific product to a great extent (Lomranz, 1986; Polanyi, 1964). They may explain, in part, why the pathogenetic, rather than the salutogenic, orientation (Antonovsky, 1979), spearheaded by all editions of the DSM, has dominated posttraumatic research. The mere experience of even the most extreme traumatic event does not necessarily result in a disorder. Attempting to deal with the impact of stress and trauma on communities we should not neglect the majority of victims who experienced the trauma, but show no signs of pathology. If we wish to comprehend the effects on all those who experienced trauma, we should supplement the deficit-oriented PTSD approach with an approach which also highlights successful adjustment, physical and mental health, efficacy, perception of control, resourcefulness, ego strength and competence, wellness models and human strength, growth, self-actualization and creativity (Antonovsky, 1979; Breznitz, 1983; Lazarus & Folkman, 1984, Pearlmuter & Monty, 1977; Rosenbaum, 1990; White, 1985). The term posttraumatic stress reaction (PTSR) would thus seem more appropraite allowing for a more differentiated, including a positive, approach to posttrauma and the formulation of different research questions. This again would compliment and balance the attempt to enlarge the definition of "disorders of extreme stress," DES (van der Kolk, Roth, Pelecovitz & Mandel, 1994). Posttraumatic difficulties have to be researched not only in terms of psychopathology. We should strive to understand people as organisms and total lives in their environments.

Conceptualization of traumatic stress. Next, we should remember that specific and generic dimensions of a trauma are of the utmost importance, as is its specific identification at the individual level (Green, 1993). The above review indicates that most studies did not differentiate between the diverse traumatic experiences undergone by survivors. First, the term "survivor" with no further explanation, describes most samples. The experience of a child in a ghetto, in a concentraion camp, living with a false identity, with a Christian family or in a convent, may all have different impact on posttraumatic adjustment. Second, duration, variation, intensity of threat, and specific human environment, are all part of the traumatic experience (Lazarus & Folkman, 1984), and similarly have not been differentiated. Such an undifferentiated, overgeneralized, approach rests on the assumption of what I have termed a "bulldozer effect," i.e., that the extremely intense traumatic impact of the Holocaust actually obliterated diverse and individual effects (Lomranz, 1990). A more fruitful approach may be to examine the different aspects of the trauma, relating them to individual differences, and to follow such an interactional course as it unfolds in the survivor's life cycle. Novel categories are needed to comprehend diagnostically the impact of trauma (Herman, 1992). Only then may we be able to specify generic dimensions that might apply to the variance in the trauma (Green, 1993), as well as to that of coping.

A perspective on coping. Coping must be considered a multifaceted, mediating operation aimed at reestablishing homostasis in a disequilibrated organism. Coping modes, strategies and effects have been researched extensively (e.g., Hobfoll, 1988; Lazarus & Folkman, 1984; Lieberman & Tobin, 1983; McCann & Pearlman, 1990; Pearlin & Schooler, 1978; Wilson, Harel & Kahana, 1988). Our review indicates that Holocaust researchers did not provide a clear definition of coping. Nor do the types of coping processes or modes appear as the main specified target in most studies, but are only invoked indirectly in clinical studies. Addressing psycho-social questions of coping requires the elaboration of different coping styles and their use.

Furthermore, coping is always on a time dimension so that long-term effects are facets of coping. When investigating life-span effects, we have to clarify whether coping modes are consistent or a change in time (Peskin & Livson, 1981), consider the impact of changing culture, and how coping, in the same person, can be constructive on one level and fail on another level. The effect of prior stress, traumatically or developmentally-related, on a person's reaction to a new crisis should be more intensively studied. Such issues can be dealt with only after further differentiation of the concept of coping, as related to the long-term effects of the Holocaust will be provided.

The centrality of the cultural dimension. The absence of sufficient psychological studies focusing on the cultural component of survivors is astonishing. Also the impact of cultural historical-normative events (Baltes, Reese & Lipsit, 1980), such as wars or economic crises have only recently been related to Holocaust survivors (Hantman, Soloman & Prager, 1994; Soloman, 1993). The notion of mass trauma deserves special attention in this context since it involves community stress and carries cultural implications. Research referred to what was the absorbing culture's responses to those victimized (Charny, 1992; Danieli, 1981). However, in mass trauma, where total communities have been traumatized, and partly reassembled, I believe we should also always ask the opposite question: What is the impact of the victims on the culture? All these issues will require much greater contributions on the part of social psychologists to Holocaust studies.

Methodology. Most Holocaust studies exhibit major faults in methodology. Pretrauma demographic variables, such as the personal familial, social and cultural background of the subjects, are almost uniformly missing. Current demographic variables are seldom reported. The age and sex components are ignored. The above-mentioned drawbacks in definitions of stress and coping, sample selection procedure, sample population research tools and questionnaires are often inappropriate for posttraumatic populations. Control groups are either absent or poorly described and the issues of what constitutes comparison or control groups are seldom addressed (Kulka & Schlenger, 1993). Faults in basic research designs further act to limit generalization of findings.

The improvement in methodology in some recent studies that use validated instruments and control groups should be encouraged, yet many pitfalls remain. To detect long-term posttraumatic adjustment requires highly sensitive instruments. We must ask what the levels of experience to be detected are and whether our research tools are sensitive enough. Some studies, yielding minimal differences between survivors and nonsurvivors have used brief questionnaires or limited self-report measures to examine mental health or well-being. Such tools cannot always appropriately tap sensitive and intricate aspects in adjusted survivors, aspects that could in fact indicate differences between them and controls. Similar criticism has been voiced regarding the methodology of "social indicator" research. Our conclusion must be twofold: (1) we should further elaborate our methodological approach, use more cross-sectional variables and groups, and develop instruments that are more sensitive and discriminatively appropriate to the posttraumatic populations and (2) different conceptualizations and methodology altogether should be employed.

Here I would like to point out that recent psychological studies have developed new methodologies that combine ideographic and nomothetic approaches. These have become the center of attention in the fields of assessment, personality and gerontology (Alexander, 1988; Kenrick & Stringfield, 1980; Zarit, Eiler & Hassinger, 1985) and have spurred renewed interest in the biographical method (Denzin 1989; Rosental, 1993). In psychology, "narratology" (Sarbin 1986) represents a renewed interest in "narratives of the self" (Gergen and Gergen 1988; McAdams & Ochberg, 1988; Shotter and Gergen 1989) and the narrative has increasingly become the focus of psycho-social discourse and research (e.g., Bruner, 1990; Kohli, 1986; Runyan, 1982; Schafer, 1992; Spence, 1982). The combined ideographic-nomethic approach seems to hold promise for a richer theoretical and methodological avenue for comprehending traumatizing effects of the general population. These considerations have led our research groups to undertake a research project applying such an approach. It seems to us the most appropriate manner by which to elicit the relevant questions and generate hypotheses. Furthermore, such approaches also carry major theoretical implications, they require a different conceptualization, and may result in novel models.

The theoretical component: Long-term effects along long-term living. Most of the studies reviewed are not theory derived, and have an exploratory descriptive nature, rather than a hypothetical structure. Indeed, except for the psychoanalytic orientation, a theoretical basis is rare and needs to be applied. The application of concepts from the behavioral and social sciences could contribute substantially to Holocaust research. Rich potential theories such as that of Baltes (1993) and Hobfoll (1988) both emphasizing conservation of resources and reserves could be applied to a posttraumatic elderly population and to narrative features of coping (Michenbaum & Fitzpatrick, 1992; Meichenbauam & Fong, 1992). I, however, propose to comprehend long-term effects of trauma at large, and especially in regard to Holocaust survivors in the light of life-span, adult developmental and aging theories.

Gerontology and long-term effects in traumatology. "Aging" and "long-term effects" are inseparable, both denoting human existence and behavior in temporality. Moreover, the normal "old-old" population of elderly are themselves "survivors" of age-related life stresses and losses. Fifty years after the Holocaust, all the survivors are virtually, if still alive, elderly people who have to cope with the double hazard of old age and posttraumatic effects (Kahana, Kahana, Harel & Rosner, 1988). Adult developmental theory (Nemiroff & Colaruso, 1990), Gerontology (Gutmann, 1987; Lieberman & Tobin, 1983; and Traumatology (Wilson & Raphael, 1993) all deal with the impact of life events and change across time. Thus, the ability to cope with developmental tasks in late adulthood can also be examined in light of the impact of long-term effects. Do Holocaust survivors, we ask, age differently than non-Holocaust survivors and, if so, how? These questions should be examined in light of the manner the survivor accomplishes developmental tasks reflected in behaviors and activities such as coping with milestones and transitions such as, for instance, the empty nest, retirement, the life-review processes or adapting to physical changes.

To summarize, the research reviewed indicates theoretical, methodological, and attitudinal problems, including contradictions in findings regarding adjustment of survivors. These must be compreheneded in a broader perspective allowing for diversity and variance on an intricate complex personal level. In case of the Holocaust survivor, adaptation includes a coping process that has incorporated 50 years of long-term traumatic effects. Such coping operates on various levels. It may have intrapsychic, interpersonal, social and cultural manifestations that, in various developmental stages and situations, may be either destructive to the organism or integrated into its personality structure and environment. Depending on multiple factors, long-term traumatic effects, may be adaptive or nonadaptive; they may vary in kind, intensity, delay of onset, duration and course. These considerations, along with the six issues and proposed strategies outlined above, and our biographical combined ideo-nomothetic investigation, have all led me to a specific conceptualization and derived methodology which I present below and which has been applied in our biographical research project of Holocaust survivors at the Tel-Aviv University. A full report on that research project will appear separately. However, data from the investigation is used here to illustrate and clarify the various components of the conceptualization (statements by survivors are referred to only when related by them to the Holocaust and not just the present).

A Multidimensional Integrative Framework Examining the Long-Term Effects of Trauma

The following conceptualization was initially introduced elsewhere (Lomranz, 1990), but the present scheme contains important modifications. Figure 1 incorporates stress, coping and integration occurring on multidimensional levels in a temporal, developmental, life-span perspective. The horizontal movement of the different sequale may be seen as depicting survivors coping in various interactive contexts throughout their lives, whereas the vertical movement indicates the between-dimensional interaction. Three separate time lines represent contextual courses and their resultant stressors that at any given moment in time all operate simultaneously on all levels. A stressor that originates in one context cuts across, and impacts all other contexts as well. These are coped with, as indicated in the lower part of Figure 1, by the Self and its different personality components as well as by other interpersonal and socio-cultural contexts, all related to specific resources (Hobfoll, 1989) and enabling the survivor to adjust and grow.

Trauma Time-Line

The trauma sequale will be mentioned here only briefly (see Lomranz, 1990). The principle here is to conceive the differential impact of trauma, its specific changing forcefulness across the life span, as it interacts with other contextual sequalae. The sequelae of stress in this framework has five temporal periods representing the sequale of trauma, which are interwoven with the processes in the developmental and historical dimensions, as well as with the coping personality structure and the environment.

The first entry indicates the onset of the trauma; the conditions under which a person was first bombarded by specific stressors. In our case, later in time, ongoing, "routinized traumatization" (Laufer, 1988) was part of the ongoing sequale of torment in the death camps. Reawakening, (Levi, 1987), refers to the conditions, shock and adjustment accompanying stepping out of the trauma. In the Laying Foundation stage, investments are in foundations established in various domains in life, e.g., work, family, etc., for future adaptation. Maintenance is often the survivors longest posttraumatic period, ending in old age. Resources are invested continuously in the central domains of life and the developmental tasks. We investigate the manner in which such energy is invested. Does it carry a forceful avoidance quality so that PTSR is prevented? Or does Maintenance, as opposed to Laying Foundations, require less total investment, so that perhaps in this period past memories and PTSR may re-emerge?

Finally, the last period, representing the traumatic sequale, is termed vulnerability (Solomon, 1993). Survivors may be caught here in the cross-pressures of posttrauma and the future threat (Breznitz, 1983) and losses of aging. The weakening of the body, as well as social prejudice and cultural discord may all interfere with aging processes and at the same time render the vulnerability of the aged to PTSR higher. In some cases this may lead to the reactivation of trauma, in others to the hardening of defenses and character, or depression, and still in others, to development, sublimation and creativity.

The Developmental Time-Line

The developmental time-line incorporates the above adult perspective, the principle being to comprehend the trauma in the developmental context. Long-term traumatic effects should be dealt with in light of the intersection between the trauma and the developmental stages and tasks, examining how the various tasks are achieved or complicated in posttraumatic existence.

We should consider developmental, life-long, consequences with survivors who claim they "had no childhood" or "never saw how elderly parents are treated." The Holocaust has prevented many from developing certain emotional maturities such as intimacy in the Eriksonian sense. Young adulthood and early middle age are crucial stages for the love and work-career lines that intersected with "Reawakening" and

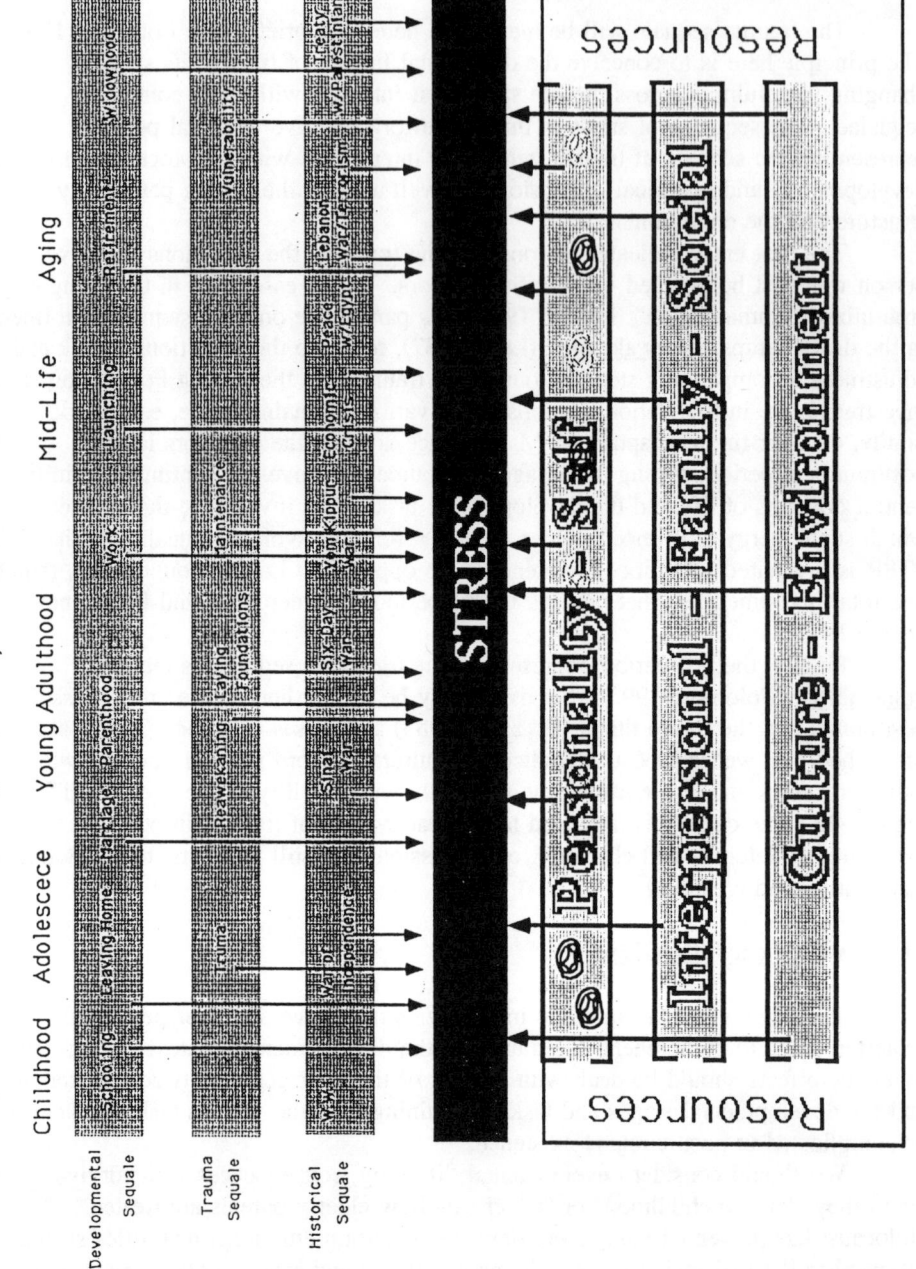

Figure 1. A Multidimensional Integrative Schema of Adaptation to Long Term Stress

"Laying Foundations" in the trauma sequale. In fact, our research shows the centrality of the issues of family, work and aging processes.

Family and parenting. While most survivors express pride and satisfaction in their families, they also emphasize complexities. Generally, children and grandchildren, not the spouse, were addressed. Marriages were often referred to as "marriages of despair" or "marriages of convenience" (Danieli, 1981). In light of traumatic memories and fears, e.g., many women commented that they were "afraid that the child would not be normal," the postponement and limitation of pregnancies became apparent. Although survivors seem to live in a different time dimension altogether (Lomranz, Shomotkin, Zochovoi, 1985), being "off-time" (Neugarten, 1977) on the lifespan carries a potential for stress and maladjustment. While the birth of a first healthy child often caused the survivor to feel "re-born," complexities were related to childrens' upbringing, education ("what you have learned cannot be taken away even by torture"), spoiling, fears of death and relationships with children and grandchildren ("I can love him, his presence proves that Hitler failed"). Many survivors reflected on their inability to convey their Holocaust experiences, thinking that their children accused them of subscribing to helplessness and being led as "lambs to the slaughter." Communicative networks of survivors' families similarly related to the inability of family members to listen to the horrors "If I begin to talk, he immediately shuts me up." These phenomena provide us with the basis to the transmission of trauma and the presence of "the second and third generations of the Holocaust" phenomena (Bar-On, 1994). In sum, parenting and the creation of new families was central to the adjustment of many survivors and enabled many to work through some of their past losses. However, while the family is perhaps the absorber of PTSR and the major vehicle for adaption, at the same time it is a major arena of trauma-related conflict. Aged survivors may be more prone to trauma-derived familial difficulties, especially in the later-life family.

Work and career. Work and career lifelines are basic to adult existence. The Holocaust as an event rapturing every existential cycle is also pronounced in the work cycle. We must examine how career choice comes about in a person who could not go through the earlier stages of the work cycle and what happens to people who are in the midst of building a self-concept based on work as that foundation is eliminated (Super, 1957).

Many survivors drew a line between their post-Holocaust occupation and the work they did during the Holocaust or before. For some, the concentration camp provided work experiences that they later turned into a profession in Israel (e.g., carpentery, shoemaking). Others tried to reconnect and reestablish pre-Holocaust occupations, thus creating continuity in their lives. For some, the theme of work became a "life theme" and they felt fortunate that they had actualized their real potential and invested most of their energies in work, living a constructive life, mainly in the "Maintenance" stage of the trauma sequale. However, these people may also be those who are most prone to retirement difficulties. Many respondents suggested their intensive career and workacholism as a possible means of coping. In terms of

Conservation of Resources (COR) theory (Hobfoll, 1988), this may be understood as an investment of resources in order to preserve other resources and offset further loss. It is generally in this area of work that social institutions may play a crucial role in supporting work, choice and guidance for the posttraumatic person, especially in the "Reawaking" period.

Aging in light of the Holocaust. In this last stage on the developmental line, some basic issues will be emphasized. While the midlife years may be conducive to the "Maintenance" levels of trauma, with energies invested in gains and power in the outside world (B.Green, here), aging may be unfavorable to those who have experienced severe trauma in childhood.

Old age brings with it various physical and mental processes and losses. It has repeatedly been confirmed that survivors suffer more in terms of lower health and medical problems (Dasberg, 1992). Many of them require geropsychological treatment (Gatz, Popkin, Pino & Vander Boss, 1985), but most of them cope adequately with adult developmental processes. Investment of personality energies are shifted; the aged emphasize mental qualities and change from an out-world to inner-world orientation, described as "interiority" (Neugarten, 1977), passive styles of coping are preferred (Gutman, 1987), the elderly turn toward closer circles of family and friends, and take an increased interest in the spiritual and philosophical (Jung, 1960). The elderly's pre-occupation with the Self, "life review," (Butler, 1963), "meaning" (Erikson, 1963), and "religion" as modes of adjustment (Moberg and Taves, 1965), and the predominance of stress, coping, and survival (Liberman & Tobin, 1983), are all integral parts of the aging process and the research agenda of aging studies and as such, the manner they are dealt with by survivors is of major interest.

Life review and survival. The life-review is considered, although debated, as a basic, developmental, universal, coping process occurring in the second half of life and especially in the shadow of death (Butler, 1963). While considered a prerequisite for successful aging, it may also constitute a source of significant stress. The bleaching away of childhood memories, the effort to bridge continuity including the painful years of the Holocaust, the inability to mourn, the availability of guilt and shame, the intensive appearance of traumatic memories, and trauma-related fears (Horowitz, 1986) and the need to confirm one's past life (Erikson, 1963), all render the life-review a complicated process and perhaps impossible task for the elderly survivor (Lomranz, 1990).

Biographical coping in the life-review of survivors. A biography presents an attempt at integrating one's life. This seems an almost impossible task for survivors. In the case of Holocaust survivors it would seem too simple to assume the classic notion that traumatic memories have become a nucleus of later psychopatholoy. The narratives of survivors may be characterized more as "traumatic memory" rather than "narrative memory" (van der Kolk & van der Hart, 1991). However, within the context of a dual mentality, we also find the attempt to integrate the Holocaust in autobiography.

Most survivors in our study considered the Holocaust as having had a pivotal role in shaping their lives. The variance of such attributions are, however, significant. There is a self-feeling that they have endured hell "there is no such thing as a Holocaust survivor; no-one survived the Holocaust, we are merely remnants of it." One called himself the "phoenix from Auschwitz." Many stated that the Holocaust had left them crippled and with scars for ever, but, as another said, "successfully coping cripples." The Holocaust was conceived of as a turning point that had split the narrator's life into two. Several respondents distincly referred to the passage from the Holocaust to their "new" life as a kind of "re-birth." Some respondents referred to the Holocaust as "a whole university," while others felt that "it helped me through life." As one stated "you see, I am successful and rich, and the Holocaust played a crucial role in making me the way I am today. Who knows, without it I may have been just an ordinary simple poor follow." Some argued that it made them stronger and self-sufficient, even in old age, while others claimed that the Holocaust had made them more sensitive to human suffering. Others insisted that they "were not changed by it," or said that "the Holocaust only accentuated what was in me previously." A significant related developmental issue is the fact that most of the respondents claimed that as they grow older it becomes more and more difficult for them to deal with the Holocaust memories or to watch films or observe ceremonies. This may be related to the vulnerability in the traumatic sequale.

Many biographies convey the survivor's considerable difficulty in finding words to describe their still unutterable experiences, even after fifty years. Language reflects survivors ongoing attempts to grieve and mourn (Charny, 1992; Moses, 1993). Indeed, the choice of language can be seen as part of the attempt to restore self-assumptions that have been shattered by severe trauma (Janoff-Bulman, 1992). For many, the losses were never worked through, but the life-review process may also provide the opportunity for some corrective experience. We have recently witnessed more and more survivors coming forward to "give account" of their experiences, and many discuss them more freely in family and in public. The Holocaust is also dealt with more directly on the cultural level. It seems no coincidence that an Oscar-winning film on the subject, such as Schindler's List, could only be produced fifty years after the traumatic event.

Religion may be conceived as one aspect of interiority and is a theme raised by many survivors. Many survivors became religious after the Holocaust and found religion helpful in stress resistance (McIntosh, Silver & Wortman, 1993; Wardak, 1992). However, traumatic stress entails an assult on basic values (Antonovsky, 1979). All in all, a variety of (inconsistent) approaches towards God emerge, ranging from total denial, to disbelief, to belief in some divine power. For many, it was impossible to reconcile a just God with the Holocaust. "What kind of God would kill children?" was a frequently voiced phrase. Men presented the most extreme atheistic attitudes, some defining themselves as "anti-religious." Women were, in general, less extreme. It is, however, remarkable that many between those "disappointed" in religion, exhibited religious feelings and even practices and rituals. A survivor's position on the issue of religion may have implications for affects and experiences such as guilt, morality, continuity and immortality, often cogent issues for posttraumatic people.

Meaning is a concept relevant to the adult person's struggle with personal history, old age and trauma. Among the meaning-giving concepts we find mainly: the mission to bear witness ("the meaning of my life is to tell the future generations what really happened"), ideology and Zionism ("our existence depends upon having a state for all the Jewish people") and generativity ("I now have great-grandchildren which shows that Hitler failed"). In part, these were also cognitive solutions to the dissonance of how a person who believes (as most survivors do) that it was through fate or luck that he or she survived, can endow his or her life with meaning. However, many survivors confronting this search for meaning concluded: "There is no meaning." For many, the quest for meaning led to paradoxes as they felt that although the Holocaust was a turning point it still left them unchanged, that it was both a place of burial and a re-birth. Survivors pondered whether the trauma can be meaningful and purposeless at the same time, or can the Holocaust, as a transhistorical event, be conceived as part of one's biography. Daily life, many thought, is meaningful but life as a whole, after the Holocaust, is not. These processes of meaning may be related to the community level where it has been shown that when disasters, such as wars, include loss of meaning, as was the case for Americans in the Vietnam War and for Israelis in the Yom Kippur War, vulnerability may be increased (Milgram & Hobfoll, 1986).

These responses reflect cognitive endeavors by which traumatized persons may cope with long-term effects of trauma. Zionism can be seen as an answer to helplessness and dependency. Generativity reinstitutes continuity and bearing witness, like a life-review, serves as an avenue to relate and grieve the lost loved ones, and at the same time fulfills the function of enabling one to feel part of history (Moses, 1993) and reconcile a paradoxical sense of being. All these provide opportunities for working through, as well as for the catharsis of inarticulate experiences and agonizing associative feelings. The interesting process to be observed is the relationships between the public and the private; how, in the case of community stress, meaning-giving endeavors directed towards the historical and the general are integrated with the personal meanings sought by the survivor.

The Historical Line

The Historical Line in Figure 1 consists of historical and cultural stressful and traumatic events inflicted upon survivors. These include 1) the political situation, ideology, values, and stress provoking attitudes of the absorbing culture and 2) the historical-normative-cultural events that impinge on the survivor's posttraumatic existence. In Israel they include primarily, wars, continuous tension and the loss of lives from acts of terrorism, economic upheavals, and social and ethnic tensions.

The impact of such factors on the course of readjustment is crucial. Ideology can determine well-being, as we can also learn from the Vietnam experience (the survivor who claims "they made me feel ashamed"), economics may provide opportunities for recovery ("the best thing that happened to me after I stepped off the boat was that I immediately found a job") and confrontation with wars and death raises the question as to how does present stress and trauma relate to the previous ones (Solomon, 1993). ("After I have lived with death, funerals do not really sadden me"). These issues will be addressed next.

Stress

Stress, in Figure 1, is in various degrees and intensity, the resultant of the three interactive dimensions and time lines. This has to be confronted by the living organism who must cope with it to achieve adjustment and possible growth. We shall now focus on such coping and adaptive aspects, represented in the lower part of Figure 1. These include resources that people have, value and use (Hobfoll, 1989, 1991), but the focus here will be on specific personal, interpersonal and cultural dimensions and properties.

Multidimensional Coping

The research on effects of the Holocaust, and, to a certain extent, that of stress and coping in general, has not been sensitive enough to the multidimensional interactive structures of coping. This has often led to a more undimensional focus in terms of the psycho-social issues examined (e.g., health, psychopathology, control, support groups, coping styles, resources) rather than to an interactive approach, including personality, idiosyncratic self and cultural mechanisms that are, in fact, responsible for certain aspects of PTSR.

The Cultural Dimension

Our mentality and humaneness is a product of our constant creation of evolvement from, and interaction with culture. Involved here is an ongoing formative mutual process between personal dynamics, development, history and culture. The attempt to comprehend how governments, societies and cultures react in psychological terms, to community stress and trauma (Giel, 1990; Hobfoll, Lomranz, Eyal, Bridges & Tzemach, 1989; Lomranz, Hobfoll, Johnson, Eyal & Zemach, 1994) and promote or hinder adjustment, is both intriguing and challenging. Its importance has recently been expressed in the metaphor that "societies function like therapists for the potential and real stress reactions and disorders of their members" (Milgram, 1993, p.819). In perspective, the Israeli culture has related problematically to its Holocaust survivors until more recently, it incorporated the Holocaust as a collective memory, visible on various socio-cultural levels.

It is important, especially as we are dealing with mass trauma - a collective experience - not just to consider the impact of cultural events on survivors' coping processes, but to also examine the opposite effect, the impact of the mass trauma on the absorbing culture and its reciprocal impact on the coping process. Here we ask how such impact occurs, on what levels, through what aspects: beliefs, values, ideology, the zeitgiest, cultural institutions and customs, national identity?

<u>Culture and the recovery from trauma</u>. The cultural climate in which posttraumatic persons are absorbed is crucial. A passitve, enthusiastic, or negative welcome may determine adjustment. The adjustment of severely wounded Israeli army veterans is clearly aided by the positive support they obtain from, not only authorities, but the total culture (Milgram & Hobfoll, 1986). The Holocaust carries specific cultural sensitivities since victimization was socially based on genocide. Several basic themes emerge: 1) the destruction and disappearance of the survivors' home culture; 2) the kind of reception extended by the absorbing culture; and 3) the opportunities for rebirth provided by the absorbing culture (Lomranz, 1990). Our biographies yielded three meaningful categories relating to culture:

(1) <u>Reception in Israel</u>. Survivors frequently mentioned the disbelief with which their stories were met, and their feelings of inferiority in relation to native Israelis. Thus, communal pride and a psychological sense of the greater community basic to readjustment (Sarason, 1974), was prevented from the survivor. The past local attitude reflected avoidence and often criticism. "You were slaughtered without resisting" was the charge hurled by a newly established, fighting for its independence, state and people. Basically, we note here a clash of world views (Jackson & Sears, 1992) and a threat to basic values (Hobfoll, et al., 1989) create stress, and interpersonal mistrust (van de Kolk, 1987) and render posttraumatic, personal and communal, adjustment more difficult.

(2) <u>National identity</u>. Survivors of mass trauma have the need for their national identity to be a source of pride, freedom and support. "Only here the Holocaust cannot happen again." The appropriation of a new national identity was also revealed through accounts of how it was the Holocaust survivors "who built this country after the first pioneers." Of interest here are double-bind feelings since it was Israeli society that freed survivors of their "yellow badges," which also labelled them as `lambs being led to the slaughter' and `soap.' One respondent expressed this double jeapordy in a nutshell: "there I was, the filthy Jew, different from everyone....Here I was also different - rejected. Think about it." Many survivors involved the present Jewish-Arab conflict and argued that "it is not us who should suffer, we were already the victims." The concept of vulnerability reappeared repeatedly in this context through use of the Hebrew word "korban" meaning "sacrifice," which may symbolically be connected to the cultural idiom of "lamb to the slaughter."

(3) <u>A culture of survivors</u>. I relate here to the survivors' impact on the total culture that has remedial adjustive implications. It seems that a dialectical process in which the negative receptive features of the absorbing culture, as well as survivors yearning for the culture and the identification with it, results in the modification of the culture altogether. Many survivors expressed the feeling that since their arrival, the culture had become much more understanding of their traumatic experiences and the Holocaust. This was revealed in comments such as: "Israel is the heir to the Holocaust." "As the years go by, people have come to understand that we were not led like lambs to the slaughter;" "this state has a Diaspora mentality, and believe me its a good thing that it does."

The almost unification of the victimized and the local culture can be recognized on the individual, community, as well as at the national levels. The extent to which the Holocaust is absorbed in daily communal living would be much beyond the scope of this chapter. Its presence is felt constantly in daily life, on the streets, in the press, language, including trigger words such as "soap," "gas," "trains," etc., in art, symbols and in official ceremonies. The fact that Israel exists under a constant threat to its existence evokes in many people political attitudes, positions and feelings that are associated with the Holocaust. During the Gulf War, for instance, a stream of Holocaust related expressions appeared, and the memory of the Holocaust was invoked. Bumper stickers identified Sadam Hussein with Hitler, chemical weapons were reminiscent of Nazi warfare, gas masks generated fearful associations, as did sealed and sheltered rooms, and the press contained extensive daily references to the Holocaust (Zukerman, 1993).

While the view that Israel was "built out of the ashes of the Holocaust" is a rather prevailing point of view with many Israelies, Israel, as a state, views itself, to a certain extent, as the representative of the survivors. Visitors to the country are taken to Yad Vashem Remembrance Authority as an essential part of their visit to view the history and horrors of the Holocaust, transmitting the message that relating to the Holocaust is a requirement to the comprehension of Israel as a state (Moses, 1983). History provided the occasion for two kinds of "rebirth," state and survivor, to occur simultaneously, powering and fertilizing one another. This accentuated the crucial role of the culture in the process of adjustment after a severe trauma. Like the victim, culture is a continuously changing process: from a stance of rejecting important aspects of the victims, to providing them with time to pause and divert energies towards other objectives, presenting them with opportunities to identify, be active and achieve goals, up to the incorporation of the victims' past into the receiving culture, thus changing it in a manner which fully integrates, or reintegrates the victims who, in a sense, were outcasts. To conclude, it is inconceivable to attempt to comprehend the long-term effects of mass trauma without taking into serious consideration the mutual survivor-culture impact. We should learn from this to prepare cultures absorbing survivors, to develop active coping mechanisms for survivors and to also consider the impact of values and ideology on survival, coping and growth.

The Interpersonal Dimension

The interpersonal-social dimension cuts across the total developmental line. The issues of family stresses and support, communication characteristics and the relation to children and interpersonal losses, have all elicited research and have been reviewed (e.g., Lomranz, 1990). Contradictory findings of problematic (Danieli, 1981) versus constructive (Harel & Kahana, 1993) families of survivors and social pictures result from differing attitudinal, theoretical and, especially methodological approaches. Certain issues emerged from our study, indicating unique posttraumatic coping in this area and should therefore be mentioned.

Social relations. Survivors reflected a certain quality of social restriction and mistrust along with tendencies toward isolation. Most of them comment that their best social relations are kept with other survivors. A prevailing feeling was that "only those who went through hell, like me, can understand." Related here is the issue of Cohort Identity (Rosow, 1978). Several respondents refer to survivors as a reference group, having a collective character, "we are immune to hardships, we can survive anything, no matter how bad." Many survivors also adhere to a "survivor identity" based on their social reference group, but at the same time, they yearn to be incorporated in the larger local Israeli social group. Many respondents also expressed a feeling of basic interpersonal distance. They claimed that they expect nothing from others, and that everyone is "on his own." This did not, however, prevent them, as they admitted, from being very sensitive and easily hurt. Some of such "asocial survivors" reflect, simultaneously, a tremendous need for warmth and supportive relationships.

The Personal Dimension

I refer here to personality and the self levels of organization, spheres of experience, cognitions and effect that are conducive in explaining how to cope with PTSR. It appears that concepts regarding a multiple-boundaries-balanced self may be the most appropriate. I perceive such a conceptualization as being based on a conjecture of stress theory, developmental life-span perspective, personality theories, and especially Lewinian structural personality and field theory (Lewin, 1935). For lack of space, I can only note that Lewin defines a person as a differentiated region in the life space. His basic concepts of "life space," "permeability," "valences," "vectors," "psychological ecology," and his emphasis on levels of reality, the degree of connectedness, firmness-weakness, fluidity-rigidity, interdependence and differentiation of "regions" and "boundaries," all allow for a flow of experiences in which inconsistencies can be endured, encapsulated, properties can change positions, be focal, or reside in the background. Thus, the most terrible, stressful memory can turn from figure to ground, be invaded or shut off completely. Survivors, as other traumatized persons (van de Kolk & van der Hart, 1991), can exist on the realm of trauma as well as that of normal ordinary life. Constructive behavior can be conceived despite psychological problems or the coexistence of contrasting thoughts, all depending on the state of the field and the qualities of the regions and boundaries and their position in the total life space. Other important features of such a personality configuration include a self that strives for balance, copes with demands and stress and has a measure of elasticity by which it incorporates them, and yet is competent and able to continuously change, develop and grow (White, 1985).

Theoretical And Methodological Implications

The lack of a comprehensive theory makes it difficult to understand and predict long-term adaptation to trauma. Research still awaits the clarification of the distinction between "clinical defense mechanism" and "coping patterns" (e.g., Lazarus & Folkman, 1984). We are still unclear as to whether to hold to a "wear or tear" or an "immune" conception of the effect of stress. We have yet to explain why and how people react differently to severe trauma. How to comprehend continuity between "pathology" with "normality" so that a well-functioning person can be understood despite PTSR or even PTSD. How may PTSR be expressed on different levels of experience. Whether delayed reactions to trauma have a time limit, when are they are liable to reappear and how are traumatic effects and coping mutually related to victim and total culture.

The aim of this chapter was to develop a framework for studying the long-term effects of the Holocaust. An attempt has been made as to how to approach the general traumatic-experienced population without labelling it pathological, but rather conceive of humans as coping and developing despite mass trauma. To do so, I first reviewed the research in the area and the implications for future research and theory. With that background in mind, I then presented a multidimensional conceptualization for studying long-term traumatic effects. This conceptualization is based on the sequale of the trauma and life-span development and history, all resulting in traumatic stress, handled by the survivor in reference to cultural, interpersonal, and personal dimensions. I have attempted here to relate specific points of references between various concepts and methodologies so that new theoretical propositions can be developed and different questions asked. On the basis of that conception I wish to emphasize the following theoretical and methodological implications:

The Multi-Dimensional Self

Holocaust survivors astonishingly express numerous inconsistencies and paradoxes, some of which are ingrained in daily life. They seem most prominent to us in areas such as basic values, assumptions, ideologies, approach to religion, temporality, or personal, social and national identity. They appear in self perceptions as related to continuity, feelings of strength despite vulnerability, and in attempts to comprehend the meaning of the Holocaust and integrate the past traumatic experience in the existential present.

Living with such daily inconsistencies and sometimes even deleterious effects, should be considered a result of trauma and part of its long-term effects (Lomranz, 1990). This has been recognized and eloquently dealt with through the focus on memory processes (Langer, 1990; van der Kolk & van der Hart, 1991). We have to conceive of a personality configuration equipped to handle posttraumatic impact and allowing for seemingly dual, contradictory, yet coexisting, modes of experience. I have suggested that coping with these can be comprehended in the framework of a multidimensional personality structure or "paradoxical self." The mentioned inconsistencies are lived with unresolved. They exist within a boundary-balanced self able to absorb contradictions, whose normalcy is embodied in its ability to reconcile such antitheticals and preserve the boundaries between the various, sometimes conflicting, life domains. This approach does not disregard situational determinants or idiosyncrasies. Thus, the personality study of the life of Holocaust survivors can become a test case for psychological personality coping modelling in general and the acquisition of the paradoxical self as a posttraumatic phenomena specifically. Future formulations of hypotheses in the study of the Holocaust will have to be based on the mentioned dual aspects.

A Developmental Perspective: Posttrauma in Light of Aging

This is another perspective wherein I propose to generate hypotheses and comprehend the extended long-term effects of trauma. The accomplishment of certain developmental tasks can promote constructive posttraumatic coping while others may forward vulnerability. Basically, trauma does not promote successful aging and the posttraumatic elderly are indeed characterized by vulnerability. However, this vulnerability may also be conceived metaphorically in terms of the ancient Greek figure of Achilles who may always have appealed to us because of his combination of power and weakness. Like many survivors, of old age, as well as of trauma, he is powerful, and yet he has an irreparable frailty, breaking point, in his heel. Depending on his or her resources and reserves (Baltes, 1993; Hobfoll, 1988), the elderly survivor may similarly possess ego strength amidst vulnerability and cope constructively with the combined losses of trauma and old age.

Mass Trauma, Its Impact on Culture and Coping

This is the third cogent issue I wish to emphasize, especially the impact of survivors on culture. The interaction of survivor and culture plays a major role in coping in general and in long-term effects in particular. Israel presented its survivor-immigrants with an opportunity to reestablish their lives, but at the same time received them with great ambivalence and complexity. However, an intriguing, still uninvestigated, process occurred. Survivors, in time, altered the community so that

Israel today is, in many ways, a culture landmarked and characterized by its Holocaust survivors. This process greatly contributed, and still does, to the adjustive functions the culture provides to its posttraumatic Holocaust victims.

The process by which survivors change the culture can be understood, in addition to political factors and processes, through the work of Durkheim (1953): The Holocaust has become a collective and "national memory" and as such, it constitutes a "collective representation" the system of which, in a given society, presents its "collective conscience." Such collective representations maintains Durkheim have both intellectual and emotional components. They are reflected in "social solidarity," in "anomies," in language, in professional practices, in group emotions, in systems of written laws and in works of art and literature. In fact, in all these domains, the Holocaust is distinctly visible in Israeli culture.

Another way to explain the dialectics between survivors and culture may be found in the concept of "secondary victims" of stress and trauma, i.e., those who are family, friends, bystanders and audiences of mass media depicting horrors of trauma and war (Milgram, 1986). Such secondary victims, indeed almost the entire Israeli public, were at first closed to the information about the Holocaust, but have, in time, become exposed, to the degree of identifying with it. This may also explain the fact that even those Israelies who are culturally removed from European immigrants now feel an emotional investment and identification with the memory of the Holocaust.

Theoretical and Methodological Perspectives.

PTSD as presented in the DSM III, seems to carry a blessing as well as an obstacle. It reinforces research and helps to integrate and generalize posttraumatic experiences. In fact, it has brought rapid progress to the field of traumatic stress studies and interventions. However, the comprehension of posttrauma solely as a disorder is an obstacle, especially where mass trauma and community stress are concerned. It does not deal with the majority of victims, biases the researcher to illness oriented concepts, and neglects positive and growth developments not imbedded in psychiatric frameworks. The spectrum of investigation has to be expanded and the nonclinical position should be strengthened, so that not only delibitating or disturbing behaviors come under investigation, but also those that reflect the normal, individual processing of the most traumatic events in a manner enabling life to proceed constructively. We would also do well to broaden our interdisciplinary framework to include the behavioral and social sciences such as personality and social psychology, learning theories, anthropology, sociology, medicine and others.

Research on the effects of the Holocaust has to improve and adhere to more strict methodology. We may, however, now be approaching a period in which studies of survivors will seem appropriately sound in methodologically, and reveal the better adjustment of Holocaust survivors with fewer delibitating long-term traumatic effects. I believe that such a swing of the pendulum, as has often happened in the history of science, is an artifact of the Zeitgeist (Boring, 1950). I therefore propose a multidimensional framework, open to different approaches in terms of theory and methodology. Our research review has reinforced the need to focus on a longitudinal course, emphasizing the multidimensional factors. I believe at this stage we should activate a network that allows for sound but different kinds of methodological applications. Our own biographical and combined ideo-nomothetic approach demonstrates the rich potential for tapping various levels of experience and making it possible to generate hypotheses.

References

Alexander, I. (1988). Personality, psychological assessment and psychobiography. In D. McAdams & R. Ochberg (Eds.). Psychobiography and life narratives. Durham: Duke University Press, 265-294.

American Psychiatric Association (1980). Diagnostic and statistical manual of mental disorders (3rd ed.) Washington, D.C. Author.

Antonovsky, A. (1979). Health, stress and coping. San Francisco: Jossey-Bass.

Baltes, P. (1993). The aging mind: Potential and limits. The Gerontologist, 33 (5) 580-594.

Baltes, P., Reese, H. & Lipsitt, L., (1980). Life-span developmental psychology. Annual Review of Psychology, 31, 65-110.

Bar-On, D. (1994). Fear and hope. Tel-Aviv: Getto Fighters' House Publishers.

Bergmann, M. & Jucovy, M., (1982). Generations of the holocaust. New York: Basic Books.

Breznitz, S. H. (1983). Anticipatory stress and denial. In: S. H. Breznitz (Ed.). The denial of stress. International Universities Press Inc., 225-255.

Bruner, J. (1990). Acts of meaning. Cambridge: Harvard University Press. Butler, R. (1963). The life review: An interpretation of Reminiscence in the Aged. Psychiatry, 26, 65-75.

Charny, I. (1992). Holding on to humanity: The Shamai Davidson Papers. New York: New York University Press.

Danieli, Y. (1981). Families of survivors of the Nazi Holocaust: Short and long- term effects. In: C. Spielberger, N. Sarason & N. Milgram (Eds.), Stress and anxiety. Vol. 8, 405-421. Washington, D.C.: Hemisphere.

Danieli, Y. (1981a). On the achievement of integration in aging survivors of the Nazi Holocaust. Journal of Geriatric Psychiatry, 14(2), 191-210.

Dasberg, H. (1987). Psychological distress of Holocaust survivors and their off-spring in Israel. Forty years later: A review. Israel Journal of Psychiatryand Related Sciences, 24, 243-256.

Davidson, J. T. and Foa, E. B., (1993). Posttraumatic stress disorder: DSM-IV-and beyond. Washington, DC: American Psychiatric Press Inc.

Denzin, N.K. (1989). Interpretive Biograph. Sage.

Durkhiem, E. (1953). Sociology and Philosophy. London & Glencoe, Ill.

Eitinger, L. (1980). The concentration camp syndrome and its late sequelae. In: J.Dimsdale Surivors, victims and perpertrators: Essays on the Nazi Holocaust. New York: Hemisphere, 67-89.

Erikson, E. (1963). Childhood and society. New York: W. W. Norton.

Gatz, M., S. J. Popkin, C. D. Pino & Vanden Boss, G. R., (1985). Psychological Interventions with Older Adults. In: J. Birren & K. W. Schaie (Eds.). Handbook of the Psychology of Aging. Ch. 28, 755-788, New York: van Nostrand.

Gergen, K. & Gergen, M., (1988). Narrative and self as relationship. In: L. Berkowitz (Ed.) Advances in Experimental Social Psychology, 17-56 New York: Academic Press.

Giel, R. (1990). The psychological aftermath of two major disasters in the Soviet Union. Journal of Traumatic Stress, 4, 381-392.

Green, B. (1993). Identifying survivors at risk. In: P. Wilson & B. Raphael (Eds.) International handbook of traumatic stress syndromes. New York: Plenum Press. 135-144.

Green, B. L. (this volume). Long-term consequences of disasters. In S. E. Hobfoll & M. W. deVries (Eds.), Extreme stress and communities: Impact and intervention. Dordrecht, the Netherlands: Kluwer.

Gutmann, D. (1987). Reclaimed powers. New York: Basic Books.

Hantman, S., Solomon, Z. & Prager, E., (1994). How the gulf war affected aged Holocaust survivors. In: T. Brink (Ed.). Holocaust survivors' mental health. New York: The Haworth Press, 27-37.

Harel, Z., Kahana, B. & Kahana, E., (1988). Predictors of psychologicall well-being among Holocaust survivors and immigrants in Israel. Journal of Traumatic Stress Studies, 1, 413-429.

Harel, Z.,Kahana, B. & Kahana, E., (1993). Social resources and the mental health of aging Nazi Holocaust survivors and immigrants. In: P. Wilson & B. Raphael (Eds.). International handbook of traumatic stress syndromes. New York: Plenum Press, 241-252.

Hazan, H. (1992). Managing change in old Age: The control of meaning in an institutional setting. New York: Suny Press.

Herman, J. (1992). Trauma and recovery. New York: Basic Books.

Hobfoll, S. E. (1988). The Ecology of stress. Washington, DC: Hemisphere.

Hobfoll, S. E. (1989). Conservation of resources: A new attempt at concept-ualizing stress. American Psychologist. 44(3), 513-524.

Hobfoll, S. E. (1991). Traumatic stress: A theory based on rapid loss of resources. Anxiety Research, 4, 187-197.

Hobfoll, S., Lomranz, J., Eyal, N., Bridges, A. & Tzemach, M., (1989). Pulse of a nation: Depressive mood reactions of Israelis to the Israel-Lebanon War. Journal of Personality and Social Psychology, 56, 1002-1012.

Horowitz, M. (1986). Stress response syndromes. New York: Yason Aronson.

Jackson, A. & Sears, S., (1992). Implications of an Africentric worldview in reducing stress for African American women. Journal of Conseling and Development, 71, 184-190.

Janoff-Bulman, R. (1992). Shattered assumptions. New York: Free Press.

Jung, C. (1960). Collected works. Princeton. New York: Princeton University Press.

Kahana, E., Kahana, B., Harel, Z., & Rosner, T., (1988). Coping with extreme stress. In: J. Wilson, Z. Harel and B. Kahana (Eds.). Human adaptation to extreme stress: From The Holocaust to Vietnam, 55-78.

Kahana, B., Harel, Z. &.Kahana, E., (1988a). Predictors of psychological well-being among survivors of the Holocaust. In: J. Wilson, Z. Harel and B. Kahana (Eds.). Human adaptation to extreme stress: From the Holocaust to Vietnam, 171-218.

Kenrick, D. & Stringfield, D., (1980). Personality traits and the eye of the beholder. Psychological Review, 87, 88-104.

Kohli, M. (1986). Social organization and subjective construction of the life course. In: A. Sorensen, F. Weiner & L. Sherrod (Eds.). Human development and the life course, 271-292. Hillsdale, New Jersey: Lawrence Erlbaum.

Kulka, R. & Schlenger, W. (1993). Survey research and field designs for the study of posttraumatic stress disorders. In: P. Wilson & B. Raphael (Eds.). International handbook of traumatic stress syndromes. New York: Plenum Press. 145-155.

Krystal, H. (1987). The impact of massive trauma and the capacity to grieve effectively: Later life sequelae. In: J. Sadavoy & M. Leszez (Eds.). Treating the elderly with psychotherapy. Madison, WI: International University Press, 95-156.

Langer, L. (1990). Holocaust testimonies: The ruins of memory. New Haven: Yale University Press.

Laufer, R. (1988). The serial self: War trauma, identity and adult development. In: J. Wilson, Z. Harel & B. Kahana. Human adaptation to extreme stress. New York: Plenum, 33-54.

Lazarus, R. & Folkman, S., (1984). Stress appraisal and coping. New York: Springer.

Leon, G., Butcher, J., Klienman, M., Goldenberg, A. & Almagor, M., (1981). Survivors of the Holocaust and their children: Current status and adjustment. Journal of Personality and Social Psychology, 41, 503-506.

Lewin, K. (1935). A dynamic theory of personality. New York: McGraw-Hill.

Leiberman, M. A. & Tobin, S., (1983). The Experience of old age: Stress, coping and survival. New York: Basic Books.

Levi, P. (1987). The reawakening. New York: Collier Books.

Lomranz, J., Shmotkin, D., Zechovoy, A. & Rosenberg, E., (1985). Time orientation in Nazi concentration camp survivors: Forty years after. American Journal of Orthopsychiatry, 55, 230-233.

Lomranz, J. (1986). Personality theory: A position and derived teaching implications in clinical psychology. Professional Psychology: Research and Practice, 17 (6), 551-559.

Lomranz, J. (1990). Long-term adaptation to traumatic stress in light of adult development and aging perspectives. In: M. P. Stephens, J. Crowther, S. Hobfoll & Tennbaum, D. (Eds.). Stress and coping in later-life families, New York: Hemisphere, 99-121.

Lomranz, J., Hobfoll, S., Johnson, R., Eyal, N. & Zemach, M., (1994). A nation's response to attack: Israelis' depressive reactions to the Gulf war. Journal of Traumatic Stress, 7, 55-69.

McAdams, D. & Ochberg, R. (1988). Psychobiography and life narratives. Durham: Duke University Press.
McCann, L. & Pearlman, L., (1990). Psychological trauma and the adult survivor. New York: Brunner/Mazel.
McIntosh, D., Silver, R. & Wortman, C., (1993). Religion's role in adjustment to a negative life event: Coping with the loss of a child. Journal of Personality and Social Psychology, 65, 812-821.
Meichenbaum, D. & Fitzpatrick, D., (1992). A constructivist narrative perspective on stress and coping: Stress inocoulation applications. In: L. Goldberg & S. Breznitz (Eds.). Handbook of stress. New York: Free Press.
Meichenbaum, D. & Fong, G., (in press). How individuals control their minds: A constructive narrative perspective. In: D. Wegner & J. Pennebaker (Eds.). Handbook of mental control. New York: Prentice-Hall.
Milgram, N.A. (Ed.) (1986). Stress and coping in time of war: Generalizations from the Israeli experience. New York: Brunner/Mazel.
Milgram, N.A. (1993). War-related trauma and victimization: Principles of traumatic stress prevention in Israel. In: P. Wilson & B. Raphael (Eds.). International handbook of traumatic stress syndromes. New York: Plenum Press, 811-821.
Milgram, N. (1993). Stress and coping in Israel during the Persian Gulf War. Journal of Social Issues, 49(4), 103-123.
Milgram, N.A. & Hobfoll, S., (1986). Generalizations from theory and practice in war-related stress. In: N. A. Milgram (Ed.). Stress and coping in time of war: Generalizations from the Israeli experience. New York: Brunner/Mazel, 316-352.
Moses, R. (Ed.) (1993). Persistent shadows of the Holocaust. Madison: International Universities Press.
Nadler, A. (1994). A perspective on the research on the Holocaust. Paper presented at the Conference on Aging and the Holocaust, The Herczeg Institute on Aging, Tel-Aviv University.
Nemiroff, R. & Colarusso, C., (Eds.) (1990). New dimensions in adult development. New York: Basic Books Inc.
Neugarten, B. (1976). Adaptation and the life cycle. Counseling Psychologist, 6, 16-20. Neugarten, B. (1977). Personality and aging. In: J. Birren & W. Schaie (Eds.). Handbook of the psychology of aging. 626-649.
Pearlin, L. (1980). Life stains and psychological distress among the adults. In: N. Smelser & E. Erikson (Eds.). Themes of work and love in adulthood. London: Grant McIntyre, 174-192.
Pearlin, L. & Schooler, C., (1978). The structure of coping. Journal of Health and Social Behavior, 19, 2-21.
Pearlmutter, L. C. & Monty, R. A., (1977). The importance of perceived control: Fact or fantasy? American Scientist, 65, 759-765.

Peskin, H. & Livson, N., (1981). Uses of the past in adult psychological health. In: B. Eichorn et al. (Eds.). Present and past in middle life. New York: Academic Press, 148-164.

Polanyi, M. (1958). Personal knowledge. Chicago: University of Chicago Press.

Recker, G. & Wong, T., (1985). Personal optimism, physical and mental health. In: J. Birren & J. Livingston (Eds.). Cognition, stress and aging. New York: Prentice-Hall, 134-173.

Rosenbaum, M. (1990). Learned resourcefulness: On coping skills, self control and adaptive behavior. New York: Springer.

Rosenthal, G. (1993). Reconstruction of life stories. In: R. Josselson & A. Lieblich (Eds.). The narrative study of lives. New York: Sage, 59-91.

Rosow, I. (1978). What is a cohort and why. Human Development, 21, 65-75.

Runyan, W. (1982). Life histories and psychobiography. New York: Oxford University Press.

Sarason, S. B. (1974). The psychological sense of community: Prospects for a community psychology. San Francisco: Jossey-Bass.

Sarbin, T.R. (1986). Narrative psychology: The storied nature of human conduct. New York: Praeger.

Schafer, R. (1992). Retelling a life. New York: Basic Books.

Shotter, J. & Gergen, K. (Eds.) (1989). Texts of identity. Sage Publications.

Solomon, Z. (1993). Combat stress reaction: The enduring toll of war. New York: Plenum Press.

Spence, D. (1982). Narrative truth and historical truth. New York: Norton.

Super, D. (1957). The psychology of careers. New York: Harper.

van der Kolk, B. (1987). Psychological trauma. Washington, D.C.: American Psychiatric Press Inc.

van der Kolk, B. & van der Hart, O., (1991). The intrusive past: The flexibility of memory and engraving of trauma. American Imago, 48 (4), 425-454.

van der Kolk, B., Roth, S., Pelcovitz, D. & Mandel, F., (1994). Complex post traumatic stress disorder: Results from the DSM IV field trail for PTSD. (unpublished manuscript).

Wardak, A. (1992). The psychiatric effects of war stress on Afghanistan society. P. Wilson & B. Raphael (Eds.) (1993). International handbook of traumatic stress syndromes. New York: Plenum Press, 349-364.

White, R. (1985). Strategies of adaptation: An attempt at systematic description. In: A. Monat & R. Lazarus (Eds.). Stress and coping. New York: Columbia University Press, 121-143.

Wilson, J., Harel, Z. & Kahana, B., (1988). Human adaptation to extreme stress. New York: Plenum Press.

Wilson, P. & Raphael, B., (Eds.) (1993). International handbook of traumatic stress Syndromes. New York: Plenum Press.

Zarit, S., Eiler, J. & Hassinger, M., (1985). Clinical assessment. In: J. Birren & W.Schaie (Eds.). Handbook of the psychology of aging. New York: van Norstrand Reinhold, 725-789.
Zukerman, M. (1993). Holocaust in a sealed room. Tel-Aviv: Zukerman Publications.

Acknowledgement
The author is grateful to the Naftali Frankel Research Project on Holocaust Survivors, for the support in the preparation of this chapter.

REVERBERATION THEORY: STRESS AND RACISM IN HIERARCHICALLY STRUCTURED COMMUNITIES

James S. Jackson & Marita R. Inglehart
Institute for Social Research
University of Michigan
Ann Arbor, Michigan, USA

In the 21st century, historians of the social sciences and particularly psychology might look back and conclude that two research topics, stress and racism, received an exorbitant amount of attention in the 20th century. They might argue that this scientific interest reflected the fact that these two issues -- stress and ethnic and racially based conflicts -- were of central personal, social and political significance in this era. While researchers engage in specific, relatively isolated analyses of these issues, however, a person living in the 20th century will not experience these two problems in the neatly compartmentalized way that researchers treat them. Quite the contrary, on a personal as well as on a community level, stress and racism are uniquely intertwined. In this chapter we propose that it is time for social scientists to recognize the intimate intermingling among community stress, racial and ethnic conflict, and racism and to bring together these concepts in one theoretical framework.

The purpose of this chapter is to investigate and explore the role of community stressors and perceived economic stress on dominant group prejudice, subordinate group economic stress and well-being outcomes. The Reverberation Theory of Stress and Racism conceptualizes stress and racism as mutually inter-related phenomena (see figure 1) and points to their combined reciprocal relationship with (social, psychological and physical) health outcomes.

Furthermore, we argue that it is crucial to explore the relationships among stress, racism and health within racially and ethnically hierarchically structured societies (see figure 2). The theory states that: (a) personal as well as community level stressors influence members of dominant as well as subordinate groups in a society, (b) this stress contributes directly to increased intergroup conflict/racism in these groups, which in turn will increase the stress level experienced by these different groups, and (c) this stress will influence social, psychological, and physical health outcomes of group members at all hierarchial positions.

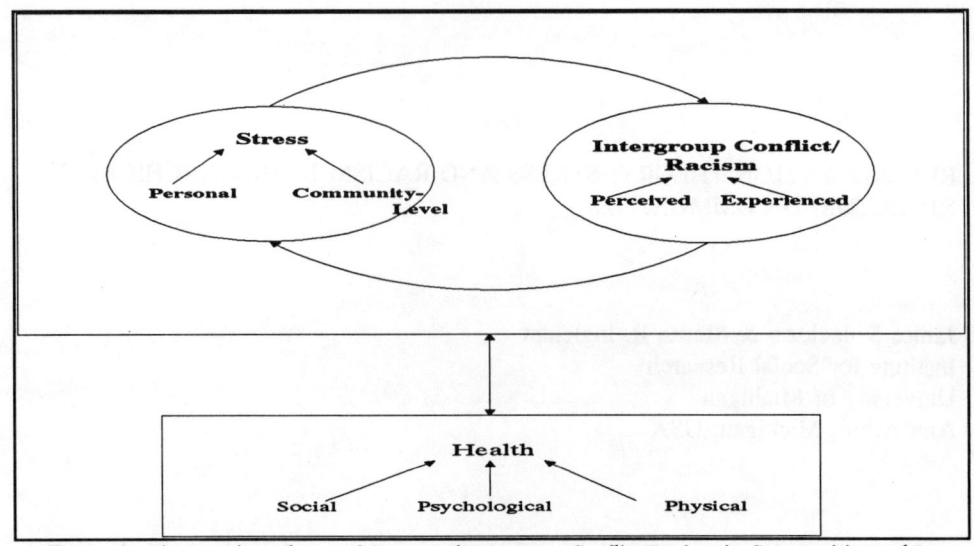

Figure 1. The Interdependence of Stress and Intergroup Conflict/Racism in Communities and Its Significance for Health Outcomes

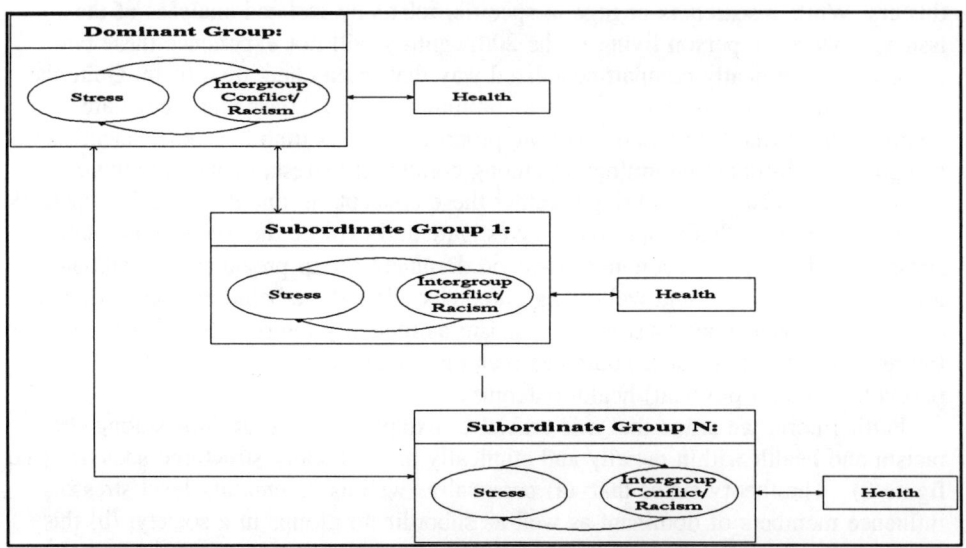

Figure 2. The Interdependence of Stress and Intergroup Conflict/Racism in Hierarchically Structured Communites

Data from two cross-national studies conducted in the United States and several Western European countries will be used in a preliminary test of the Reverberation Theory of Stress and Racism.

Racism in the United States and Western Europe

Recent studies in the United States have found a decrease in prejudice or racial intolerance over the years but no concomitant increase in support for policies oriented toward assistance for these same groups (e.g. Schuman, Steeth & Bobo, 1985). Some researchers have argued that this is due to the fact that racism has taken a new form today and that it has become subtler and intertwined with conservative orientations (Sears, 1988). Others have taken striking exception (e.g. Sniderman & Tetlock, 1986) arguing that conservative ideology is not necessarily related to racism nor discrimination. Other researchers have argued that real and perceived group conflict exerts significant influence on support for government policies designed to assist outgroups and on specific government actions designed to overcome discrimination (e.g. Bobo, 1983). None of these studies, to our knowledge, have investigated these issues outside of the United States, and few outside the confines of white-black superordinate and subordinate relationships.

The collapse of Eastern European communism has revealed that ethnic group antipathies lie just below the surface and can be easily aroused. A striking example is the ongoing armed conflict in former Yugoslavia. Additionally, it has become apparent that the social, political and economic status of immigrant and refugee groups who have less rightful claims (in the eyes of many) to the resources of European nations will be sorely tested over the coming years. Countries such as Great Britain and Germany have already provided unfortunate showcases of what may happen. Ongoing ethnic wars in the former Soviet Republics and Yugoslavia and anti-Semitic tensions in Poland and other Eastern European countries demonstrate the power of ethnic group boundaries in contributing to armed conflict, bloodshed and human atrocities. The enduring and virulent religious conflicts in the Middle-East and Northern Ireland reinforce the fact that neither simple nor short-term solutions are readily available.

Increased immigration and swelling numbers of economic and political refugees will continue, especially in Western Europe. These changes in demographic composition may portend many "hot summers" as experienced in the United States in the late 1960's and 70's, as well as more recently in the 1980's in Great Britain. Many European countries have closed their borders to general immigration. This is an option that may not be politically feasible in the European Union (EU) countries. Many of these nations have colonial ties and political arrangements with immigrant sending countries, e.g. Great Britain and Hong Kong; relationships that place domestic immigration and minority rights policies in a larger international diplomatic context. This is a problem that the United States avoided in its conflicts and legal struggles with Americans of African descent, but will itself increasingly face as immigration accelerates from Asia, Mexico and Central and South America; one vivid example is the international furor over recent changes in national and state immigration legislation.

The causes of current ethnic conflicts are deeply rooted in histories of prior conflict and bloodshed. The potential danger of these conflicts are much greater today than earlier in this century. The wide distribution and availability of historically unparalleled weapons of mass destruction demand the undivided attention of all nations to address the root causes of racism and intergroup conflict. Intergroup conflict is a problem that may threaten the peace and security of future generations. Indeed, finding workable solutions for reducing ethnic and racial conflict may be the major problem facing the world community today (Jackson, Kirby, Barnes & Shepard, 1993).

Prejudice and Racism: Theoretical Considerations

Theories of individual prejudice and racism range from intra-personal and psychodynamic models to economic conflict theories (e.g. Allport, 1954; Adorno, Frankel-Brunswik, Levvinson & Sanford, 1950). During the lengthy period of research on ethnicity, race and intergroup relations, no one theoretical position has emerged as an accepted, encompassing explanatory system. The scientific controversy over the role of personality, position in the social structure (e.g. educational level) and situational factors (e.g. national and group norms) as proximal causes of racism and anti-Semitism has existed since the beginnings of this century. The rise of fascism in Europe during the 1920's and 1930's and the prevailing Freudian psychoanalytical viewpoint enticed many scholars to examine the individual psychological determinants of fascist ideology. The writings of Reich, Fromm and Maslow were prominent during this period. It was, however, the emergence of the Third Reich, culminating in the shocking events during the Second World War, that fully brought the issue to a head. Faced with the inexplicable horror of Nazi death camps, serious scholars pondered the possibility of whether individual personality factors, including psychopathology, could account for such deviant and widely shared behaviors.

Because individual psychopathology explanations seemed dubious in accounting for the extensive and mass adherence to fascism and the repugnant actions of the Third Reich during the Second World War (as well as state supported racism in the United States and South Africa), most scholars turned to some type of general personality factors that might account for these behaviors. Research has focused on various aspects of personality, such as susceptibility to frustration, low self-esteem, political and religious conservative beliefs, and cognitive rigidity as correlates of prejudice, discrimination and anti-Semitism. Adorno's research became the most persuasive of these scientific efforts, though by no means the only serious scholarly work.

No one explanation produced the outpouring of research and criticism as the work of Adorno and his associates on the Authoritarian Personality and the Fascism Scale (Adorno et al, 1950). Their research attempted to operationalize the Authoritarian Personality as a response to a set of questionnaire items labelled the F (Fascism) Scale (and to a lesser extent the Ethnocentrism and Anti-Semitism scales as well). The problems which Adorno's work addressed have not dissipated over the decades and questions regarding the role of national character and individual personality factors in ethnocentric beliefs and behaviors remain unanswered.

It is as true today as it was forty years ago when Allport (1954) completed his famous monograph on *"The Nature of Prejudice"* that the field lacks an ordered system of underlying theory to guide research, especially in a cross-national and cross-cultural context. Even definitions differ greatly. Prejudice is generally considered as an attitude or set of attitudes held toward a group, encompassing a set of negative feelings (affect), beliefs (stereotypes) and intentions (behavioral dispositions) to act unfavorably toward groups or members of groups (Duckitt, 1992). These attitudes are considered to have been formed as part of a person's early social development and socialization and normally are thought to arise from direct parental tuition as well as indirect social learning from other family members, peers and increasingly the mass media (Duckitt, 1992). Ethnocentrism refers to both generally held positive attitudes about ones own group as well as negative views of a wide variety of other groups, groups that differ ethnically and racially from ones own group (Yinger, 1985)

Discrimination refers to intentional acts which draw unfair or injurious distinctions, that are based solely on ethnic or racial bases, and which have effects favorable to ingroups and negative to outgroups. Normally, discrimination is the set of observable behaviors that might ensue from ethnocentrism, prejudice or racism.

Racism usually refers to negative beliefs and behaviors towards racially categorized groups or members of groups involving elements of power differentials between dominant and subordinate groups, including strongly held beliefs about the racial or ethnic superiority of one's own group (Jones, 1983). At least three different forms of racism, all including strong beliefs about ethnic or racial inferiority, have been identified (Jones, 1983). Individual racism is most directly linked to the concept of prejudice and refers to individually held outgroup hatred, combined with ethnocentric views and beliefs of racial inferiority of the target groups. Cultural racism, linked to the concept of ethnocentrism, refers to the beliefs in the inferiority or non-existence of cultural traditions, implements and values of the target group. And Institutional racism refers to the system of laws, policies and political, economic and institutional arrangements that perpetuate and maintain subordinate and dominant group positions in a society.

In addition to issues of definition, some of the general problems with existing theories of prejudice and racism are: a) the confusion among etiology, process, and outcome; b) the lack of inter-disciplinary perspectives; and, c) a disproportionate focus on either the perpetrators of prejudice, or their victims, and not enough attention to the nature of inter-group interaction.

Racism, Stress and Health

Subordinate Group Perspectives

In this chapter we will use African Americans as an exemplar of subordinate groups. We recognize that other groups in all parts of the world share similar subordinate statuses. A substantial portion of the African American population lives in urban environments where they are likely to be exposed to a relatively high number of stressors (Jackson, Brown, Williams, Torres & Brown, 1994). Low socioeconomic status affects the options that an individual has in terms of the type and location of housing, as well as in the quality of life. Intertwined with low SES is a stressful lifestyle that may include poor nutrition, poor education, crime, traffic hazards, substandard and overcrowded housing, low-paying jobs, unemployment and underemployment, and a lack of health insurance and access to basic health services. It is frequently suggested that these factors contribute to the development of a wide range of problems in the black community, but empirical evidence in support of these notions is sparse. A study by Lipscomb and Trochi (1981), for example, suggested an important role for stress in affecting black drinking patterns. This survey of black adults ages 18-59 in two San Francisco neighborhoods found that marital problems, drug problems, family problems, being the victim of a crime, and police problems, were predictive of higher levels of alcohol consumption.

It is significant that current measures of stress are biased towards the stressors experienced by the middle class and do not adequately characterize the stressful conditions faced by the poor in general, and the black poor in particular. In addition to these middle-class biases, qualitative differences among ethnic and racial groups in the experience of stress may exist (Hobfoll & Jackson, 1991). For example, Wilson (1987) indicates that blacks have been increasingly concentrated in depressed inner-city neighborhoods, while the white urban poor is more evenly dispersed throughout the city with many residing in relatively safe and comfortable neighborhoods. There are important suggestions in the literature that the stress of urban residential areas may significantly impact health status. Some data suggest that perceptions of crime in the neighborhood has adverse effects on psychological well-being (White, Kasl, Zahner & Will, 1987). The classic ecological studies of Harburg and his colleagues (Harburg, Erfurt, Chape, Hauenstein, Schull and Shork 1973) found that residence in stressful urban areas (characterized by such factors as low median income and few years of formal education, residential instability, marital instability and crime) was adversely related to health.

Garbarino, Dubrow, Kostelny & Pardo, (1992) focused on the impact of community violence as a neglected variable in stress research. Their research indicates that individuals who live in inner-city housing projects are twice as likely to witness violence as other persons. The repetitive nature of witnessing these traumatic events may have an additive effect. Their research suggests that the increased likelihood of addiction is one of the consequences of chronic exposure to family and community violence. In addition, each homicide reflects the loss of an individual with social ties to others in the community, and thus a decline in available social support.

In addition, physical and sexual abuse are prevalent stressors in the lives of the urban poor that ordinary stress measures do not include (Bell, Taylor-Crawford, Jenkins & Chalmers, 1988). Non-lethal violence is a frequent antecedent to homicide, and there is growing evidence that the experience of violence impacts mental health status, including substance use as well as treatment outcome (Bell et al., 1988). Victimization screening in an urban African-American outpatient population revealed high rates of both sexual and physical assault (Bell et al., 1988). The literature indicates that sexual and physical assault is a risk factor for nervous breakdowns, drug abuse, alcohol dependence, depression, and other problems (Bell et al., 1988). It is well known that male alcohol use is related to the physical abuse of women and children. In addition, a recent study documented a significant association between alcohol use and being a victim of physical abuse among black and non-Hispanic white women (Berenson, Stiglich, Wilkinson & Anderson, 1991). It is not known whether these women were using drugs to escape the abuse in their lives, or whether drug use itself made them more prone to battering through the effects of drugs on their behavior.

It has been suggested that racism adversely affects the health status of African Americans. However, there have been few attempts to empirically assess racism and racial discrimination and to explore the consequences, if any, for the psychological well-being of African American children, adolescents, and adults (Jackson et al, 1994).

The concept of racial discrimination is frequently invoked in studies of race and health. Researchers uniformly note that it is an important factor in understanding African American health status and sometimes suggest that it may account for particular patterns of association. Little attention, however, has been given to the conceptualization and measurement of these constructs and their proposed relationships (Harvey, 1985; Franklin, 1988). The result is that racial discrimination is frequently inferred, but seldom measured, and its consequences for health status not directly assessed. Fernando (1984) indicates that racial discrimination is not just an added stress experienced by minority group members, but a pathogen that affects health. One recent study of black and white women by Krieger (1990) explored the relationship between rates of hypertension and the experience of racial and gender discrimination. She found that among black women who experience unfair treatment, those who kept quiet and accepted it were four times as likely to have high blood pressure as those who talked to others or took other action in response to the unfair treatment. Gender discrimination was unrelated to hypertension for white women. Instructively, black women were six times more likely than whites to respond passively to unfair treatment, suggesting that they, probably accurately, perceived themselves as having little control in these encounters. Krieger (1990) also found that black women who reported that they had experienced no incident of racial or gender discrimination were two to three times as likely to have high blood pressure as those who reported having experienced unfair treatment. An internalized denial of racial bias may also lead to adverse changes in health status. These findings suggest that racial discrimination may interact with personality characteristics and particular coping styles.

Dominant Group Perspectives

It is quite obvious that individual, cultural and institutional racism can be and are interpreted as stressors for the targets of this discrimination and can thus negatively affect health outcomes. However, the significance of understanding the effects of racism and intergroup conflict on the dominant groups' stress level and health status has been neglected topic. The Reverberation Theory of Stress and Racism points to this as a significant issue.

The relationship between (psychological) health and racism in the dominant group was traditionally seen as unidirectional: Psychologically unhealthy conditions (such as an authoritarian personality (Adorno et al. 1960), frustration (Dollard, Doob, Miller, Mowrer & Sears, 1939) or low self esteem (Crocker, Thompson, McGraw & Ingerman, 1987) were seen as causes of prejudiced reactions. And prejudiced reactions were sometimes even interpreted as serving a positive function for the racist: For example, one might have argued that by scapegoating a certain outgroup member, inner peace might have been reestablished (Duckitt, 1992).

It is significant to understand that by neglecting the fact that being a bigot can be "dangerous to one's health," a wide range of considerations have been excluded from empirical investigation and an important area for initiating changes in social policies has been overlooked. By placing intergroup conflict/racism and health together with stress hypotheses, a completely new perspective and research area has emerged.

The Reverberation Theory of Stress and Racism place the spot light on the fact that reducing intergroup conflict and racist behavior will be beneficial for all groups and individuals in a hierarchial racially ordered society. For the racist dominant group members several detrimental psychological effects accompany bigoted behavior. First of all, if one agrees that hostility is one crucial component of racism, then it is significant to recognize the research that shows a strong negative relationship between a person's degree of hostility and such health outcomes as ulcers, migraine headaches and asthma (Friedman & Booth-Kewley, 1987). Hostility and anger are often invoked in stressful situations pointing again to the interdependence of racism, stress and health outcomes.

Second, laboratory research on stress also shows that it may influences information processing. Under stress persons shift from a controlled mode of information processing to an automatic mode of information processing. In this situation, stereotypes of outgroup members might become more salient and more likely to determine reactions. Again this can have a clear impact on the degree of racism shown which in turn will influence stress and health outcomes.

Third, any form of discrimination can be interpreted as being based or resulting in an increased social distance from the targets of discrimination. Research on the role of social support as a mediator of stress effects (Inglehart, 1991) shows that this increased social distance and consequently the lack of social support may be a second mechanism that explains how racism, stress, and health are interrelated. For example, using a school class that is racially divided, the intergroup tension and the resulting lack of social support will lead to a more stressful class situation which in turn might lead to a lower subjective well-being of all students, to an impaired social functioning of the class as a whole, and eventually to keeping all students from living up to their full potentials. We believe that this same pattern of individual and group effects may occur in larger institutional and national settings as well.

In summary, the Reverberation Theory of Stress and Racism suggests the need to explore the ways in which everyone in a racially stratified society suffers from racism, how stress will affect racism and be affected by it, and how health outcomes relate to stress and racism among both dominant and subordinate group members.

Reverberation Theory of Stress, Racism and Health

Figures 3 and 4 provide concrete, graphic depictions of the proposed model. Figure 3 represents a hypothetical local situation involving one dominant group and several subordinate groups (e.g. former South Africa or the United States). In this case we argue that community stressors, such as unemployment and related macro social and economic conditions have affects on all hierarchically organized racial and ethnic groups. In addition, we suggest that this increased stress leads the dominant group to act in ways (discrimination, etc) that "cause" further stress in subordinate groups. We propose that the original stressful conditions and the racism displayed toward each successively hierarchically placed subordinate groups will lead to increased stress. Thus, in subordinate group three, there are four sources of stress in this model; the original community stressor (unemployment, poor economic conditions, etc) and the racism directed toward group three by the dominant group, and subordinate groups one and two. Stress and racism then reverberate in the community, lowering well-being and possibly increasing subsequent stress levels.

We propose that community level stressors, e.g. unemployment and downturns in macro-economic conditions, will influence the perceptions of both dominant and subordinate groups members. Among dominant group members we suggest that stress will directly lower psychological well-being and lead to increased racist sentiments toward subordinate groups. Among subordinate groups we argue that these same negative macro-economic conditions will contribute to the experiences of stress which in turn will lower well-being. In addition, we suggest that the racism directed toward subordinate groups by dominant groups will also be experienced as stressful and will contribute independently to lowering well-being even further. Thus, community level stressors contribute to individual level stress among both dominant and subordinate group members. This stress contributes to dominant groups acting in racist ways toward subordinate groups, which contributes even more stress to the lives of subordinate group members.

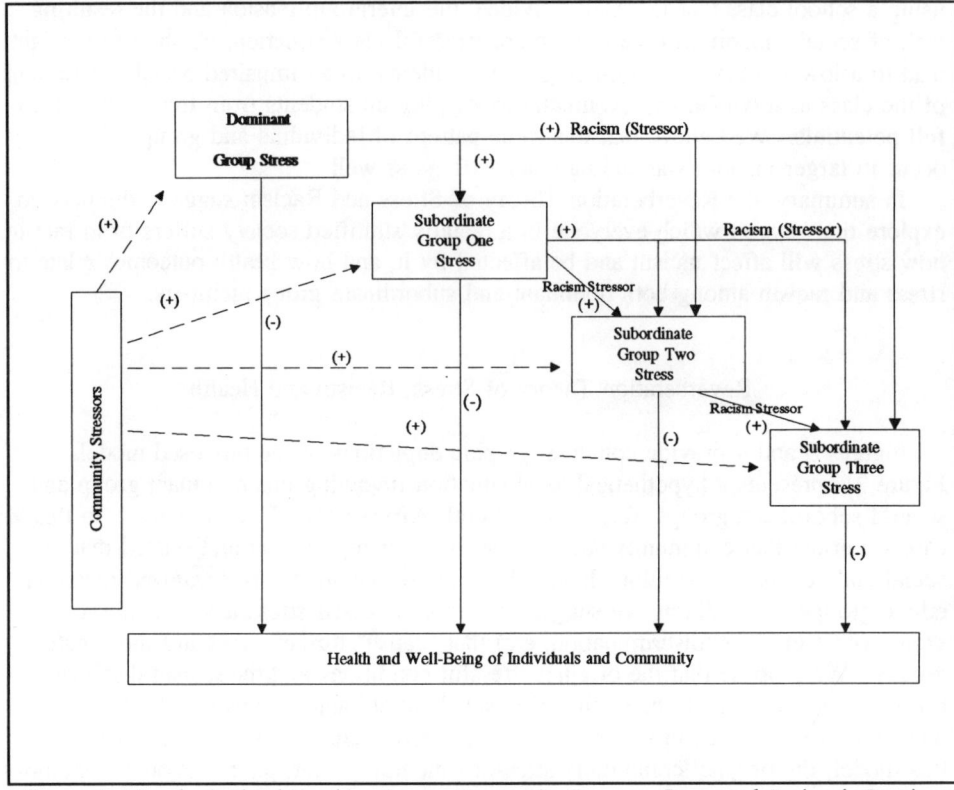

Figure 3. Hypothesized Relationships Among Community Stressors, Stress, and Racism in Dominant and Subordinate Groups

As shown in Figure 3, we hypothesize that: 1) community level stressors influence individuals in all dominant and subordinate groups; 2) stress contributes directly to increased racism in a hierarchial manner among relatively well and poorly situated dominant and subordinate groups; 3) racism is stressful to both dominant and subordinate groups; and, 4) the lower the subordinate group the higher the stress and associated experienced group conflict and group and individual mental health related disorders.

Figure 4 shows a set of hypothesized empirical relationships among stress, racism and well-being among dominant groups and stress, perceived/experienced racism and well-being among subordinate groups. Among dominant groups (shown at the bottom of Figure 4) we predict that economic stress will lead to increased racism and simultaneously lower well-being. Similarly, we predict that racism will lead to lowered well-being as well. Thus, there is a cost of being a racist and that cost is a lowering of ones own well-being. Although not immediately testable, we also predict that the racism of the dominant group will be reflected in increased perceptions and experiences of racism among the subordinate groups. This is reflected in the dashed arrow from racism among dominant groups members to perceived/experienced racism of the subordinate group. Similarly, we predict that racism will also contribute, over and above beyond that of community stressors, to the economic stress as perceived by the subordinate group.

Among the subordinate groups (shown at the top of Figure 4) we hypothesize that economic stress and perceived and experienced racism will both lower well-being. We also suggest that perceived and experienced racism will raise economic stress, but simultaneously economic stress may lead to an increase in perceived and experienced racism. In this chapter we test these relationships among dominant (White) and subordinate (African Americans) in the United States and among dominant groups (Europeans) in Western Europe. We lack the data to test these predictions among subordinate groups in Western Europe. Data are used from the National Panel Survey of Black Americans (1979-80 and 1987-88), the 1984 General Social Science Survey (GAS), and the 1988 Eurobarometer Survey using the selected countries of France, Great Britain, Germany and the Netherlands.

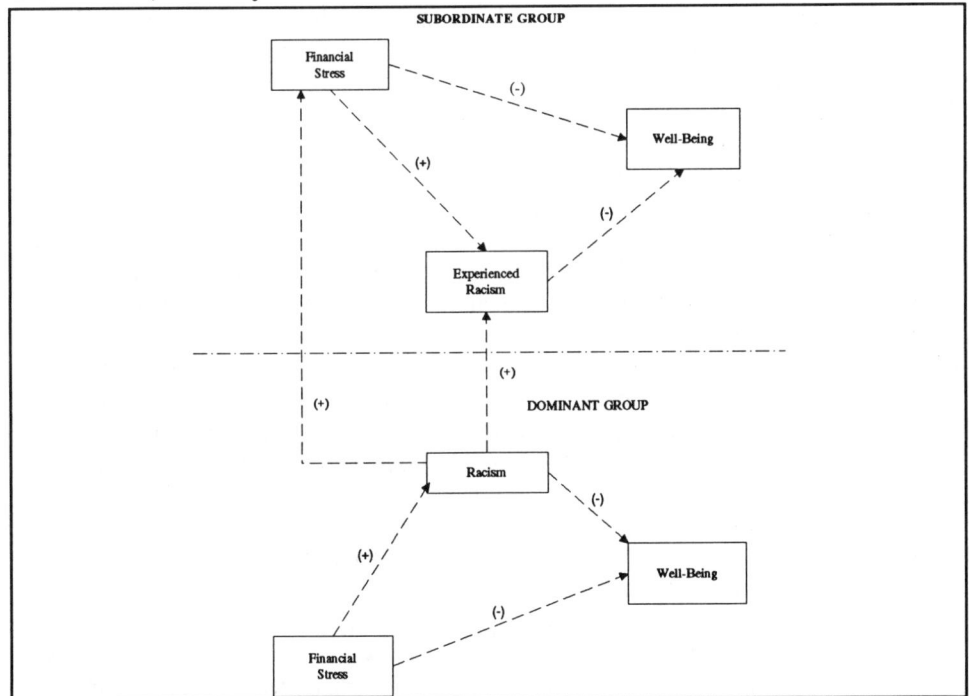

Figure 4. Hypothesized Relationships Among Economic Stress, Racism and Individual Poor Health and Well-Being

Data and Analytic Approach

Datasets

Eurobarometer. The Eurobarometer Surveys of the European Union (EU) are a long running set of opinion polls that are conducted twice yearly in the Spring and Fall on nationally representative samples of the EU. These surveys in varied form have been conducted since 1970. Although the themes of the surveys have changed on each occasion, a central concern has been with the attitudes of the EU publics toward the common market, attitudes toward other European countries, and the priority of goals and values within each country. Since 1973 the twice yearly polls have assumed a more traditional survey cast, with the addition of a continuing series of items related to subjective satisfaction and perceived quality of life as major aspects of the survey.

In 1974 the Commission of the European Communities initiated the Eurobarometer series. This is a supplemental survey within the European Omnibus Survey that is designed to provide a regular monitoring of social and political attitudes of the publics within the EU. The actual sampling and field work was conducted by the Gallup affiliates in each EU country. Representative samples were drawn of the adult populations 15 years of age and older. The sampling designs were a mixture of multi-stage national probability and national stratified quota procedures, similar to the Gallup polls conducted within the United States. Appropriate weights for the samples in each country, and the weights for a European sample are available.

Because of our interest in having salient populations of immigrants and ethnic outgroups for the study, and cost considerations, we limited our intensive research to only four of the 12 EEC countries: France (1,001), Great Britain (1,017), Netherlands (1,006), and West Germany (1,051). Data from these countries permit cross-national comparisons on the same and different groups. In keeping with the argument that more comparisons among different groups and cultural contexts are needed to study the nature of outgroup rejection, we used a split ballot questionnaire technique within each country (except Germany). This procedure had the advantage of providing two randomly drawn samples within each nation that reacts, respectively, to one of two preselected groups. For many purposes, such as the present paper, the data for each target group within and across countries may be combined to provide larger sample sizes.

National Survey of Black Americans (NSBA). The National Survey of Black Americans (NSBA) data were collected across four Waves beginning in 1979-80. The 1979-80 survey used face-to-face interviewing methods in a national multistage household probability sample of 2,107 self-identified black Americans living in the continental United States. The overall response rate was approximately 67%. This rate is quite good since 79% of the sample resided in urban areas, geographical locations that tend to be the most difficult locations for face-to-face interviewing. The 1979-80 NSBA data collection was followed by three more waves of smaller, yet comprehensive, telephone data collections in 1987-88, 1988-89 and 1992. The relatively large number of black Americans in the initial cross-sectional sample, its wide age range (18 to 101 years of age), and the thirteen year time span, provide a broad base from which our analyses were conducted. The 1987-88 NSBA Wave 2 was used in the analyses for this chapter.

General Social Science Surveys (GSS). The General Social Surveys are a set of yearly interviews on a sample of the American public conducted by the National Opinion Research Center (NORC) at the University of Chicago. The initial survey was conducted in 1972. Items that appear on the surveys are of three types, permanent questions that appear each year, questions that appear on two out of every three surveys, and occasional questions that appear mainly as the result of particular investigator interests. Approximately 1,500 interviews are taken yearly, though the numbers have fluctuated over the years (1,372 to 1,613). Each survey is an independently drawn sample of English-speaking persons eighteen years of age or older living in non-institutionalized housing arrangements within the continental United States. Both block quota and full probability sampling methods have been used in the twenty-one years of the GSS. The median length of the interview has been approximately ninety minutes. A total of 1,251 European background respondents from the 1984 GSS were used in the analyses for this paper.

Eurobarometer Measures

Traditional Racism. In the Eurobarometer this variable was operationalized as a three item index: 1) willingness to have sexual relations with a member of the targeted outgroup; 2) agreement with the statement that "outgroups take jobs that majority should have"; and 3) the extent of belief with the statement that the "majority can never really be comfortable with members of the outgroup". Overall, this four point index had a Coefficient Alpha of .68.

Financial Stress A three item index included unemployment status, financial changes on a four point response scale that asked, " in the past year has the financial situation of you and your family gotten worse", and income in quartiles. This five point index had a relatively low Coefficient Alpha of .32.

Subjective Well-Being This index included two items that asked, "in general, how satisfied are you with your life these days", and "how satisfied will you be with your life in five years". Individuals responded to each item on a ten point scale of very satisfied to very dissatisfied. The Coefficient Alpha for this ten point index was .79.

NSBA Measures

Experienced Racism. We used a dichotomous measure of experienced racism that asked respondents to indicate, "whether they or their family had been treated badly or not because of their race in the past month?".

Financial Stress. A four item index included unemployment status, financial changes over eight years on a four point response scale that asked, " in the past eight year has the financial situation of you and your family gotten worse", income in quartiles and whether the respondent worried about bills. This five point index had a Coefficient Alpha of .52

Subjective Well-Being. This six item index included, "in general, how satisfied are you with your life these days" and how satisfied are you with your friends, health, family, and family relationships, all measured on a four point scale of very satisfied to very dissatisfied. The final item in the index asked respondents on a three point scale, " taking all things together, how would you say things are these days, would you say you are very happy, pretty happy or not too happy these days". This five point index had a Coefficient Alpha of .66.

General Social Science Survey Measures

Traditional Racism. No really comparable measures of traditional racism measure was available in the GAS and an approximation was used. This is a slightly different operationalization of this racism construct but as shown later the same relationships observed among dominant group in the Eurobarometer Survey for traditional racism also holds in the GAS for this variable. A four item index was constructed form the following questions: 1. do you think that there should be laws against marriages between blacks and whites?; 2. how strongly would you object if a member of your family wanted to bring a black friend home to dinner? 3. white people have a right to keep blacks out of their neighborhoods if they want and blacks should respect that right. 4. do you think white students and black students should go to the same schools or to separate schools? This five point index had a Coefficient Alpha of .71.

Financial Stress. A four item index that included unemployment status, perceptions of financial changes over the last few years, income in quartiles and the opinion's of respondents about their family income was developed. This five point index had a Coefficient Alpha of .52

Subjective Well-Being This index included four satisfaction items and one happiness measure. The satisfaction items asked, "for each area of life I am going to name, tell me the number that shows how much satisfaction you get from that area" -- 1) city or place you live, 2) your family life, 3) your friendships, 4) your health and physical conditions, and individuals responded on a seven point scale of a very great deal to none. The second asked respondents on a three point scale, " taking all together, how would you say things are these days -- would you say that you are very happy, pretty happy, or not too happy ?". This seven point index had a Coefficient Alpha of .66.

Analysis Strategy

The analyses presented in this chapter provide a preliminary assessment of how racist feelings on the part of dominant group members, and the experiences of racism on the part of subordinate group members, may be related to economic stress and psychological well-being in each group, respectively. Correlations, Ordinary Least Squares and logistic regressions were the major analytical techniques employed. These analyses were summarized in a series of three path analysis models.

Our Findings and Conclusions

The path model in Figure 5 summarizes the interrelationships among perceived financial stress, racism and well-being in the Western European countries. As predicted, the path coefficient for financial stress is significantly related (.118, $p < .01$) to increased feelings of racism toward subordinate groups in Western Europe. Independently, financial stress is also related to lowered levels of well-being (-.609, $p < .01$). Also as predicted, increased feelings of racism are related to lowered levels of well-being as well (-.148 $p < .01$). These significant paths provide strong support for the independent influence of financial stress to simultaneously increase racist feelings and to lower well being among dominant group members. Simultaneously, increased levels of racism independently lower well-being. Thus, as hypothesized, perceived stress has both external (racism) and internal (lowered well-being) affects.

Figure 6 summarizes the path analyses for the United States. Among European Americans, as in Western Europe, increased perceptions of financial stress is related to higher levels of racism (.216, $p < .01$). Similarly to the European analyses, higher levels of financial stress are related to lower levels of the well-being index (-.359, $p < .01$). Racism, as in the European sample, is positively associated with lower levels of well-being, but it is not a reliable effect. Thus, in both Western Europe and in the United States, economic stress is highly associated with holding racist feelings about subordinate groups. These pattern of relationships are remarkably similar and provide strong support for our hypotheses and indirectly for the theory.

The upper half of Figure 6 presents the path coefficients among financial stress, experienced racism, and well-being. As found in the dominant groups, increased stress is directly associated with poor well-being (-.171, $p < .01$). Similarly, experienced racism is independently associated with lower levels of well-being (-.282, $p < .01$). Finally, financial stress is a significant independent predictor of experienced racism (.294, $p < .05$).

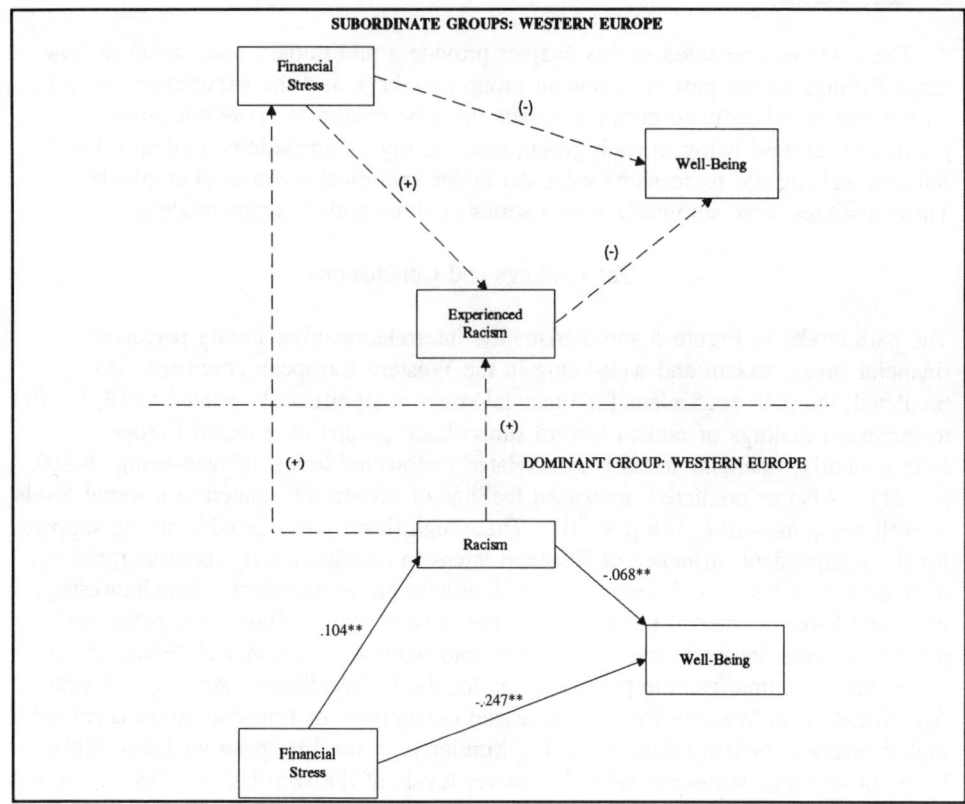

Figure 5. Observed Relationships Among Economic Stress, Racism, and Individual Health and Well-Being in Western Europe

Overall, these results provide strong preliminary evidence for the Reverberation Theory of Stress and Racism that we have hypothesized. Increased stress, represented in this paper by perceived financial strain, is associated with increased negative antipathy toward the outgroup(s). These relationships were found in national samples from the United States among Whites and also in combined national samples of Europeans across four major Western countries. It is also clear that while perceived economic stress directly reduces well-being, racism also has direct effects. Thus, there are costs associated with holding racist beliefs. While lower levels of well-being might lead to increased racism, the pattern of relationships and the direction of the stress effects argue against this interpretation.

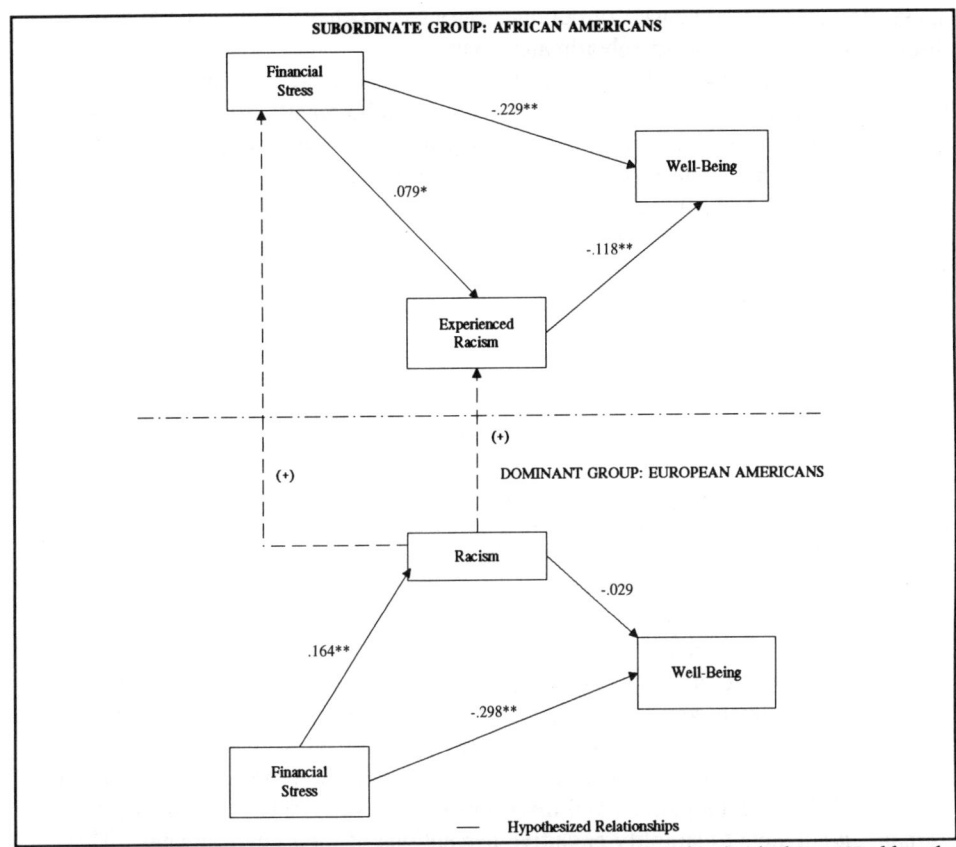

Figure 6. Observed Relationships Among Economic Stress, Racism, and Individual Poor Health and Well-Being in the United States

Finally, though not directly testable, racism among the dominant groups might be related to the nature of perceived racism, experienced stress, and well being among subordinate groups. A partial test of this hypothesis among African Americans (in both 1979-80 and in 1987-88) showed that reports of the experiences of racism and stress are both directly related to reducing well-being; and that economic stress may be more strongly related to experience of racism than experiences of racism are related to economic stress.

These findings support our Reverberation Theory of Stress and Racism in hierarchically organized mixed ethnic and racial communities. The results of our path models suggest that stressors like unemployment and poor economic conditions directly influence the extent of discriminatory responses and experienced stress among the major dominant and subordinate groups. Our results support recent theorizing that stress increases the propensity of dominant groups to behave in prejudicial and discriminatory ways toward subordinate groups.

The results of these analyses support our hypothesis that: 1) community level stressors influence individuals in all dominant and subordinate groups; 2) stress contributes directly to increased racism among relatively well and poorly situated dominant and subordinate groups; 3) racism (and the experience of racism) is stressful to both dominant and subordinate groups. The proposed Reverberation Theory appears to be a viable framework for assessing the role of community stress and racism in exacerbating divisions among ethnic and racial groups. And it points to the benefits that can be achieved for both subordinate and superordinate groups when racism is reduced.

Conclusions

In this chapter we have addressed the influence of macro level stressors on accumulated stress in dominant and subordinate groups. A Reverberation Theory of Stress and Racism was proposed to account for the interrelationships among community level stressors, dominant and subordinate groups status, and racism. Conceptually, it was suggested that stressors like unemployment and financial difficulties directly influence the extent of discriminatory responses and experienced stress among both dominant and subordinate groups. It is assumed that the dominant group and subordinate groups are hierarchically arranged, such that dominant status is relative to the group or groups positioned above and below at all points in this status ordering. Recent theorizing argues that stress increases the propensity of dominant groups to behave in prejudicial and discriminatory ways toward subordinate groups, perhaps in attempts to simplify cognitive perceptions of their environments. These stress effects are not limited to the major dominant group but appear among all hierarchically arranged subordinate social and political groups.

Thus, we hypothesized that: 1) community level stressors influence individuals in all dominant and subordinate groups; 2) stress contributes directly to increased racism in a hierarchial manner among relatively well and poorly situated dominant and subordinate groups; 3) racism is stressful to both dominant and subordinate groups; and, 4) the lower the subordinate group the higher the stress and associated experienced group conflict and group and individual mental health related disorders. Empirical support for the hypotheses derived from the proposed Reverberation Theory of Racism and Stress in ethnic and hierarchial racially organized communities was found in analyses of data from a national panel study of African Americans, the 1988 European Union Eurobarometer Survey, and the 1984 United States General Social Science Survey.

It is critical that we consider racism as a community stressor of a chronic and pervasive nature. The predicted relationships are modest compared to disasters, but given the hundreds of millions of people involved worldwide the impact is enormous both socially and financially. Racism creates a chronic health risk for the victim and perpetrator and deserves our intervention and research attention on a community level.

References

Adorno, T., Frenkel-Brunswik, E., Levinson, D., Sanford, R.N. (1950). The authoritarian personality. New York: Harper.

Allport, G.W. (1954). The nature of prejudice. Reading, MA:Addison-Wesley.

Bell, C.C., Taylor-Crawford, K., Jenkins, E.J., & Chalmers, D. (1988). Need for victimization screening in a black psychiatric population. Journal of the National Medical Association, 80, 41-48.

Berenson, A.B., Stiglich, N.J., Wilkinson, G.S., & Anderson, G.D. (1991). Drug abuse and other risk factors for physical abuse in pregnancy among white non-Hispanic, black, and Hispanic women. American Journal of Obsteric Gynecology, 164, 1491-1499.

Bobo, L. (1983). Whites' opposition to busing: Symbolic racism or realistic group conflict? Journal of Personality and Social Psychology, 45,1196-1210.

Crocker, J., Thompson, L.L., McGraw, K.M., and Ingerman, C. (1987). Downward comparison, prejudice,and evaluations of others: Effects of self esteem and threat. Journal of Personality and Social Psychology. 52, 907-916.

Dollard, J., Doob, L., Miller, N., Mowrer, O.H., and Sears, R.R. (1939). Frustration and aggression. New Haven, Ct: Yale University Press.

Duckitt, J. (1992). The social psychology of prejudice. New York: Praeger.

Fernando, S. (1984). Racism as a cause of depression. International Journal of Social Psychology, 30, 41-49.

Franklin, A.J. (1989). Dimensions of psychological well-being among blacks. In R.L. Jones (Ed.), Handbook of tests and measurements for black populations. Richmond, CA: Cobb & Henry Publishers.

Friedman, H.S., Booth-Kewley, S. (1987). The disease-prone personality: A meta analytic view of the construct. American Psychologist, 42(6), 539-555.

Garbarino, J., Dubrow, N., Kostelney, K. & Pardo, C. (1992). Children in danger: coping with the consequences of community violence. San Francisco: Jossey-Bass.

Harburg, E., Erfurt, J.C. Hauenstein, L.S., Chape, C., Schull, W.J. & Schork, M.A. (1973). Socio-ecological stress, suppressed hostility, skin-color and black-white male blood pressure: Detroit. Psychosomatic Medicine, 35, 276-296.

Harvey, W.B. (1985). Alcohol abuse and the black community: A contemporary analysis. Journal of Drug Issues, Winter, 81-91.

Hobfoll, S.E. & Jackson, A.P. Conservation of resources in community intervention. American Journal of Community Psychology, 19 (1), 111-121.

Ingelhart, M. (1991). Reactions to critical life events: A social psychological analysis. New York: Praeger Publishing.

Jackson, J.S., Brown, T.N., Williams, D.R., Torres, M., Sellers, S.L., & Brown, K. (in press, 1994). Perceptions and experiences of racism and the physical and mental health status of african americans. Ethnicity & Disease.

Jackson, J.S., Kirby, D., Barnes, L. & Shepard, L. (1993). Racisme institutionnel et ignorance pluraliste: une comparison transnationale. In (Ed.) M. Wievorka. Racisme et modernite. (pp. 246-264). Paris: Editions La Decouverte.

Jones, J.M. (1983). The concept of race in social psychology: From color to culture. In L. Wheeler and P. Shaver (Eds.), Review of Personality and Social Psychology, Vol. 4. Beverly Hills, CA: Sage Publications.

Krieger, N. (1990). Racial and gender discrimination: Risk factors for high blood pressure? Social Science and Medicine, 7, 1273-1281.

Lipscomb, W.R., & Tronchi, K. Black drinking practices study report to the Department of Alcohol and Drug Programs. Berkley, CA: Research Triangle Institute.

Sears, D.D. (1988). Symbolic racismm. In P.A. Katz & D.A. Taylor (Eds.), Eliminating racism: Profiles in controversy (pp. 53-84). New York, NY USA: Plenum.

Schuman, H., Steeh, C. and Bobo, L. (1985). Racial attitudes in America: Trends and interpretations. Cambridge, MA: Harvard University Press.

Sniderman, P.M. & Tetlock, P.E. (1986). Symbolic racism: Problems of motive attribution in political debate. Journal of Social Issues, 42, 173-188.

White, M., Kasl, S.V., Zahner, G.E.P., & Will, J.C. (1987). Perceived crime in the neighborhood and mental health of women and children. Envirment and Behavior, 19, 588-613.

Wilson, W.J. (1978). The declining significance of race: Blacks and changing American institutions. Chicago, IL: University of Chicago Press.

Yinger, J.M. (1985). Ethnicity. Annual Review of Sociology, 11, 151-180.

Author's Note

We would like to acknowledge with appreciation the work of Myriam Torres, Tony Brown and Sherril Sellers in assisting in the analyses and preparing the tables for this chapter. We would like to extend a very special thanks and acknowledgement to Ain P. Boone who provided incredible support in the analyses, production of the tables and preparing this manuscript. Our thanks also are extended to Eva Bates, Liza Chase, Dale Jerome, and Sally Oswald for their assistance in preparing the figures and typing the manuscript. Our appreciation to Kendra R. Jackson for reminding us of the contagion effects of stress and racism.

CULTURE, COMMUNITY AND CATASTROPHE: ISSUES IN UNDERSTANDING
COMMUNITIES UNDER DIFFICULT CONDITIONS

Marten W. deVries
University of Limburg, Department of Psychiatry and Neuropsychology, Section of
Social Psychiatry and Psychiatric Epidemiology, and the International Institute for
Psycho-Social and Socio-Ecological Research (IPSER), Maastricht, the Netherlands

At the end of this century, changes in the world's geopolitical landscape and its traumatic impact on individuals and their communities have taken center stage. Global communication and a growing universal awareness of the ecological interdependence of the earth's inhabitants have rendered personal suffering in one place of concern in another. Research over the last fifty years on stress, trauma and health in psychology (Lindeman, 1944; Brown and Harris, 1978; Caplan, 1981), physiology (Mason, 1968; Seyle, 1976), and sociology (House et al., 1983; Sarason et al., 1990), have further demonstrated the interrelatedness of human problems. Stress and trauma are not only universal, they are at once biological, psychological and social.

Stress in Individuals

Recent research has also alerted us to the fact that it is not only massive disruption in personal and social life (Holmes and Rahe, 1967) that affect individuals, but minor daily events, hassles and family problems do so as well. These studies represent a shift in research, design and methods, away from the clarification of a single event to an attempt at understanding the ongoing social and personal context of the individual as he or she adapts to environmental circumstances (deVries, 1987). Such studies record daily life events, activities and neuroendocrine responses and have shown that daily experience effects immunological (Stone et al., 1993) and neuroendocrine function (Nicolson, 1992) and thereby health outcomes (Meyer and Haggerty, 1962; Roghmann and Haggerty, 1973). Another body of data demonstrates that optimal, positive and supportive daily experiences (Csikszentmihalyi, 1991; Kanner et al., 1981; DeLongis et al., 1982), in particular, positively evaluated social contexts (deVries and Delespaul, 1988) and support (Sarason et al., 1990; Caplan, 1981), may improve or correct the negative effects of stressful events, both psychologically and physically. Daily life experience in actual community contexts is thus a key element in understanding human responses to stress, trauma and disaster.

There is an impressive history that attempts to link physiological response and behavior in traumatic and stressful situations. In 1871, Da Costa observed changes in gastric motility through a soldiers' abdominal wound in relation to emotional events. The relationship of emotions, circumstances and physiologic response, was in the 1950's systematically investigated by George Engel and his group (1962). The intensive case study of Monica, who like the soldier, had an abdominal fistula, provided a window through which to view physiological responses. Observations made as she interacted with her social environment as a baby girl and later as a young woman, made it clear that the vicissitudes of daily life and its socio-cultural structure had a direct, continual and often lasting impact on bodily functions. These studies led to the hallmark modeling of the bio-psycho-social adaptive process (Engel, 1977) that brought the study of behavioral and social complexity to attention in medicine.

Today studies in major and minor events that comprise stress and trauma create a complex physiological, psychodynamic and social picture. Both the environment, the community and the individual play key roles in whether or not a person can cope with or succumbs to disruptive events. The complexity is demonstrated by the influential work on life stress of Brown and his colleagues (1990). He and his associates examined the impact of loss and life events on depression, illustrating the embeddedness of individual risk and vulnerability in social contexts. For example, he found that loss and life events, only when accompanied by humiliation, loss of self esteem, and changes in social status, support, or role resulted with statistical significance in the occurrence of depression in women. This complex nexus of the individual, community and culture needs to be analyzed in detail to get a better understanding of traumatic reactions (Trickett, this volume).

Stress in Communities

To the question of what happens to a normal person's life under stress, trauma or disruptive events, this volume also asks what happens to his community. An unfortunate aspect of disasters and trauma is that they do occur with regularity, and this has resulted in cultures building up "social security systems" at least against some calamities, to protect its members and capital. Studies into individual reactions to extreme conditions have not paid sufficient attention to the complexity of the social environment and the cultural organization that could worsen or alleviate stress.

Historically, studies that included social factors clearly in research design began appearing following Eric Lindeman's landmark study of the Coconut Grove Fire in 1944 and World War II. Beginning in the 1950's, emotional and social reactions to catastrophic events were described (Tyhurst, 1957; Spiegel, 1954) and a National Academy of Science study highlighted the social consequences of disaster (Wolfenstein, 1957). Since then, other volumes have reviewed information on social responses to disaster (Baker and Chapman, 1962), specifically Hiroshima (Hersey, 1980), cyclones and tornados (Spiegel, 1957; Crawshaw, 1963), mine disasters (Lucas, 1969), and nuclear accidents (Bromet, 1980). High risk groups have also received attention such as the elderly (Friedsam, 1961) and children (Newman, 1976; Bloch et al., 1956).

Over the last ten years, studies on community reactions when disaster strikes have gained in momentum, expertise, and methodological sophistication. The work of Bromet at Three Mile Island (1980), the Chernobyl disaster (Bromet, this volume), the Holocaust survivors (Lomranz, this volume) the Buffalo Creek Disaster (Green, this volume), are good examples. These studies point to both the community as well as the individual's reactions under difficult conditions. Within this perspective, this chapter examines the complexity of community response in terms of the available cultural mechanisms that induce, facilitate or maintain community resources (Hobfoll, 1988). Third world and western examples of the adaptive possibilities offered by social contexts, cultural rules and community life will be discussed. Mechanisms of community response vary from culture to culture and community to community and as such are not always detectable by modern research strategies. Methods for detecting cultural strategies and variation must be included within more standard epidemiologic designs. In the last section of the chapter, strategies for including methods for the detection of cultural goals and social adaption will be presented.

This paper takes a social, ethnographic perspective on community stress. In understanding what cultures do, it is useful to borrow a process concept from embryology: induction, facilitation and maintenance. These stages of development provide a frame of reference for what cultures actually do to respond to problems, develop solutions and survive. The three stages globally describe the processes that are encoded in community responses to stress. By means of examples, these three areas of relevance to understanding trauma in communities will be described.

1. <u>Inducing</u>, legitimizing the individual communication of distress and mobilizing resources: taxonomic incorporation.
2. <u>Facilitating</u> resource mobilization embedded in community life: indigenous social security systems.
3. <u>Maintaining</u> resources and support after the immediate trauma has ended: self help healing alternatives.

Indigenous Possibilities: Mechanisms of Cultural and Community Response

Although disaster does not recognize cultural boundaries, traditional and third world settings have been overwhelmingly affected. Here, the often partial and incomplete shift to modernized society has left many communities poorly adjusted to new social, political as well as geographic conditions. Although often half forgotten, indigenous social aid resources and organization may still provide useful contributions. They should be investigated and used.

Traditional cultural responses are integrated within a frame of belief that holds that problems and illness, as well as their causes do not disappear with time or treatment. Traumatic events and their consequences are real and do not go away. They are inevitable and unavoidable. Trauma, grief and illness must therefore be continually managed and accommodated at both the personal and group level. Culture in part is adapted to help the community and individuals with this process. After trauma, problematic emotional and psychological reactions are generally responded to by the indigenous social security or filial (kin) system that orders an individuals' emotional reaction to life events. Society provides the rules for emotional expression and behavior, ultimately facilitating, understanding and inviting the help and participation of others. Society organizes the process of suffering, rendering it meaningful within a larger social framework. A response to stress or danger operationalizes society's essential capacity to support its members. Illness and suffering are, in this model, at once communications to the group as well as profound personal experiences.

Culture is in the business of assuring its own survival and that of its members. The community, as such, if still intact when threatened by disruption in the lives of its members, will make attempts to correct these unwanted processes in line with traditional strategies or in developing tolerance for new ones. Traditional medical practitioners (healers) are a key element in such a response in that they induce or activate cultural concepts of dependency, family roles, care seeking behavior and life cycle expectations. Materialistically, culture is a maintenance system assuring adequate physical and social resources for maintaining social structure and relationships, the distribution of goods, the organization of the human life cycle, and the securing of human reproduction (Whiting and Whiting, 1975). Culture provides a complex and flexible set of rules and values, as well as both practical and symbolic means to carry them out. Within the culturally prescribed social and community structure, life cycle roles and the emotional management of transitions from birth to death, marriage to divorce and the fusion and fission of family, kin and human relationships, are facilitated and ordered (LeVine, 1973). It is in this context that personal life events, trauma and illness will be mastered or not.

In traditional cultural settings, the body can not, even remotely, be isolated from the mind, nor the mind removed from its social context. Ethnographically, it is axiomatic that individuals grow up within a particular social context where cultural values and the meaning of health and disease are communicated from birth to death. Individuals in turn, experience their physical and mental functioning in the context of a larger social-cultural frame of reference (Schweder and LeVine, 1984). All cultures have their own medical system, that embodies ideas of illness and health as well as hope and the expectation for solutions. Medical systems are delicately interwoven with the group's ideas and feelings about the entire range of physical and social events possible or tolerable within a group. The medical system then plays a crucial role in shaping individuals' social world and experience (deVries et al., 1982). Cultures differ in their religious systems and social organization, and therefore each provides its own particular signature to the cause and the experience of illness; variations as to whether illness can be cured, must be endured or is a means of communicating (Kleinman, 1988), are the rule. Given this embeddedness, cultural differences in illness and health care seeking strategies need to be investigated and understood in order to streamline interventions.

Traditional cultures are largely animistic systems. This implies that the idiom of causation is either assigned to God, others (witchcraft), or ancestors (breaking of rituals or taboos). Animistic concepts of external causation have the social function of linking the individual's experience of illness and trauma directly to larger society. In these settings, filial responsibility and dependency are triggered by illness communication. Health is considered an intricate part of daily life function of the social person in most societies, while illness is then often viewed as a breach of social rules. This is in contrast to the West where the individual's "duty to be healthy" is the central concept and has become a key force in the self-help movement and responsibility for health. This individualized idiom for cause and cure is a major underpinning of Western medical intervention. In contrast, more "fatalistic," animistic cultures believe that problematic and traumatic events are externally caused and must be continually faced during life. Causes and consequences do not disappear, so ritual and symbolic places are necessary to reify and support group members during times of inevitable difficulty, and rituals support the individual, repair rents in the social fabric, and re-establish the group (Geertz, 1973). Individuals in traditional and to a lesser extent modern societies do not only lose their kin support network during social disruption but may also lose access to their rituals and symbolic places, thus limiting their ability to mobilize healing resources. Accordingly, rituals and the symbolic places required to carry them out should whenever possible be incorporated into medical treatments and rehabilitative programs for a community. Following major social disruption, the re-establishment of symbolic places, i.e. churches, mosques, trees for gathering, school yards, places for women to talk, and safe evening meeting places, should be a primary goal. Symbolic places make visible the normal demographic age distribution of a community, the range from young to old. This will help re-establish previously learned cultural rules and reinstate members of the community in appropriate life cycle role functions. Symbolic places and their prescribed behavior help reinstitute natural age hierarchies. These go a long way to facilitating mature defenses and the potential for altruistic action during times of disorganization and stress where regressive, primitive defenses such as projection, denial and narcissistic survival strategies tend to prevail.

Three aspects of the cultural and community responses to stress and illness will be examined highlighting the formal induction and legitimization of a problem for social attention, facilitating community responses, and the creation of self-help maintenance groups that secure resources over a longer period:

1. taxonomic incorporation: the traditional medical systems', or response;
2. indigenous social security systems: filial responsibility and social support;
3. self help healing alternatives.

1. Taxonomic Incorporation: The Traditional Medical Systems' Response

One formal social response is the expansion of the medical system itself, inducing and legitimizing the allocation of community resources. Digo medicine, for example, provides a case in which the scope of the medical taxonomy is increased to accommodate individual and community stress. The Digo of the East African coast, where I worked in 1974 (deVries and deVries, 1977), have lived at the edge of the Arab, Portuguese, Bantu and Nomadic worlds for some 600 years. They inhabited the coastal strip ranging from the deserts of Somalia into the fertile coastal plain of Kenya and Tanzania. The Bantu Digo, who also speak Swahili, have integrated many aspects of neighboring cultures in their social system. They have a flexible matriarchal social organization and a strong traditional medical system capable of responding to many internal and external threats to community cohesion (Gerlach and Hine, 1973).

The western Digo border overlaps with the eastern extension of Masai grazing land. The two cultures previously did not have much contact since they are separated by an irregular mountain range running North to South along the African coast. During the late 1960's, however, the Masai, largely due to drought and increased pressure on grazing land, began raiding peripheral Digo homesteads for cattle and supplies, creating panic and generalized anxiety throughout Digo land. The stress experienced by individuals and the group was often expressed in ad hoc trance dances. In these dissociated states, individuals could experience and relive their anxiety and fear by abreacting and behaving like the aggressor during the dance. Eventually, the traditional healers gave this specific stress response of anxiety, fear and behaving like a Masai warrior, a label and incorporated it within the traditional healing rituals. The dances were then formalized and used to alleviate stress as well as to accumulate resources for the protection of border communities from the Masai threat. Thus, personal fear and anxiety in reaction to community stress was labeled and transformed into an illness and social communication thereby securing attention and resources. Medicalizing the problem enabled both the group to protect itself against the Masai as well as to provide social support for individuals unable for both personal and social reasons to cope with this threat in their daily lives.

A similar expansion of taxonomy allowed stressful war reactions in the U.S. to be normalized. Following the war in Vietnam, veterans were able, through medical labeling and legal activity centered on the 'Agent Orange' controversy, to redress the social problems experienced upon their return to American society. The labeling of the post-traumatic stress syndrome in DSM III by the American Psychiatric Association, provided a formal place in the taxonomy of Western medicine for their experience and legitimized the suffering of these warriors as they demobilized back to normal life. In both Digo and U.S. society, stress experiences, while manifested at the individual level, are intricately tied to larger social problems. Society is constantly challenged and threatened, and individuals respond to such group stress. Their experiences and emotions need to be rendered meaningful and legitimized. Medicalization or labeling (deVries et al., 1982), achieves this by expanding the medical taxonomy. A medical label justifies and operationalizes social interventions and resource allocation. Culture then, by means of its medical system, may cast a net across disruptive human experience. Human experience thus remains understandable and under control. For the individual, it legitimizes suffering. The two examples demonstrate how a flexible medical taxonomy may accommodate the stress that individuals experience. This is a positive medicalization. The flip side of this problem is that while such labeling facilitates social support, it may impede self-help by medicalizing a problem and placing responsibility on experts rather than on friends, family and kin. We will return to self-help groups that arise to support the sufferers identity and maintain resources after the threat has subsided in section 3.

2. Social Security System: Filial Responsibility and Social Support

Indigenous social security systems are the mainstay of the community response. They are complex and must at least be partially understood before carrying out interventions. They facilitate in complex ways the provisions of help to dependents. The social security systems are based on filial piety and kin responsibility, since the family and kin group is chiefly responsibly for its members. Loss of social and kin structure in filially dependent societies, such as happens in times of disaster in the third world, compounds an already difficult personal situation. The complex workings of social security systems are in no instance clearer than in the ensuring of reproduction and the survival of young children. The bottom line of culture is whether or not it is able to reproduce both information and human capital. Assuring survival of infants by supporting families and mothers is therefore a key cultural responsibility. A case description of a Digo woman living in her homeland demonstrates how cultures stack up the social security system to assure survival by multiple levels of support.

> Fatuma, who did not expect or want twins, nor the caesarian section required to birth them, sat listless, almost mute, staring into the distance on the fourth day after delivery.
> One of the twins was considerably smaller than the other and scored poorly on neurological and behavioral tests. During the early postpartum period, Fatuma shunned both infants but eventually, on the 8th day, she began caring for the larger active infant while ignoring the smaller one. On the 10th day, time to leave the hospital, Fatuma still was not tending to the smaller infant in spite of the best efforts of the hospital staff and the other mothers. The smaller infant was thus at extreme risk given the negative maternal attitude, poor neonatal competence, harsh perinatal

experience and the stress that the twins would create in this economically marginal family.

At a two to three month follow-up visit, Fatuma still was negative toward the smaller infant and the grandmother and sister had assumed most of the caretaking. At the time, both infants were ill and the smaller one seemed extremely irritable. A traditional doctor had shrewdly diagnosed a complex of social and witchcraft causes that amounted to a rationale for maternal "neglect." He based his diagnoses on the Digo belief that infants have increased social needs at two to three months of age. He prescribed that Fatuma should attend more personally and directly to her infant's communications and that Fatuma's mother should teach her how to do this. It was determined that her depression was caused by the surgical intervention that had left her vulnerable to possession by spirits and witchcraft. These circumstances could be corrected by a ritual healing dance. Such healing rituals are also a means of activating ad hoc aid groups. All these prescriptions were carried out.

At the 4-6 month follow-up, tests showed that the now only slightly smaller infant, performed better on both social and coordination items of a developmental scale. The infant temperament profile showed a once difficult, withdrawn infant now was less distractable and rhythmic. The mother still reported not liking the infant and carried out only minimal caretaking, but the child's demanding style was a strong solicitor of care from the grandmother and other female kin. At four months, the "at risk" infant, with a "difficult" temperament and numerous predisposing risk factors had matched or surpassed her more able twin (deVries, 1994).

Here, we observe the impact of a correction by the traditional social security system. For example, Fatuma's form of marriage. She paid a low bride price which provided maximal freedom of choice and economic power. This gave her the freedom to elicit care from distant kin and to move her homestead closer to a supportive maternal uncle. Her well-to-do uncle (mother's brother) was capable of financing the healing ritual and providing subsequent support. Digo ideas about "what a baby is" and the expected sequence of infant development with rapidly increasing motoric and social competence during the first year, guided specific training interventions of both the grandmother and the traditional healer. The Digo notion of causality in pediatric illness, holding that the child's problems resulted from maternal resource depletion (Chirwa), created in this case by postoperative vulnerability to spirit possession, was correctly identified. The problem could thus be defined as a social one, spirit possession, enabling society to intervene directly by means of healing rituals to limit the threat to the infant. A second factor was the availability of competent female kin, who because of their own early child rearing experience as young girls had been trained in specific Digo infant care practices that facilitated the transfer of maternal care (deVries and deVries, 1977). These factors embedded the care of the twins (twins are also valued by the Digo in contrast to many other societies) in society at large supplementing maternal infant care deficits. This influx of support from society and maternal kin allowed the at-risk twin to pull up and surpass her sibling. Whether the smaller twin's better performance is based on her release from maternal depression, the superior rearing skills of other women, or better supplementary feeding cannot be completely ascertained, but the response of the social group certainly played a key role in this developmental effect.

The twin's story also points out the vulnerability of babies and other dependents in changing and uprooted social systems when new strategies for survival are inadequately available and old ones no longer viable. In contrast, in disrupted Digo society the traditional healer may not have been sufficiently active. The wife and husband might have moved away from kin. Both of these would have tended to maintain the risk. Moreover, if the idea of "what a baby is" had been Westernized, the child would not have been expected to act socially at two to three months. This more passive approach to the smaller infant could have resulted in mortality. Since even minor changes of modernization could have resulted in mortality, this highlights the greater vulnerability that occurs during times of upheaval stress and disaster. As others in this volume also point out, interventions must target and empower local support systems (see Sarason, Sarason, & Pierce, this volume) and on building collaborative resources (see Hobfoll, Briggs, & Wells, this volume).

3. Self-Help Healing Alternatives

The complex way society induces, facilitates and ensures the survival and well being of its members and how these may be helpful during interventions, has been explored above. These may, however, be insufficient for maintaining support and resources after the problem has abated. Individual or group self help strategies may then be required. For example, the anthropologist J. Janzen (1982a) describes how:

> "...on a cross-cultural basis, sufferers of modes of affliction have been brought from the isolation of their sickness together with others of the same affliction and have given each other mutual support to reenter society, indeed, even to become specialized healers of their affliction."

Cross culturally, Janzen uses the African term for these societies and refers to them as "drums ... anonymous," with common characteristics so striking that it is worthwhile to explore them as representatives of a much larger class of therapeutic activities particularly for chronic afflictions, and to analyze their common characteristics. For example, Janzen (1982a), citing from an ethnography by De Sousberghe (1958), describes the Pende of the Kasai region of Zaire who in 1930 before the advent of Western surgery, developed the "chiefship of the scrotal hernia."

The Pende were active hunters and traders for whom a scrotal hernia is a severe stress and handicap. The sufferers of this affliction began asserting themselves as leaders in their society, and gradually coalesced into a chiefly order. These individuals who were physically incapacitated, but otherwise perfectly intelligent, were transformed into an order of chiefs involved in judicial affairs. They became, in effect, sitting judges of the "chiefship of the scrotal hernia," an important, powerful, political and positive institution.

The gourd dance of southern Plains Indian societies is another example. It dates back to before the creation of reservations, when it was a warrior society. When the warriors put down their arms in the late nineteenth century and were placed on reservations, the gourd dance served as a means to work out their frustrations. At the end of the Vietnam war when the veterans came home, there were again warriors who had turned in their weapons. They were sitting around in cities and towns not knowing what to do, drinking, often getting into trouble, and lacking a sense of orientation. The gourd dance with its unique pulsating circular rhythm and the social activities surrounding it, re-emerged as one such orientation. Today, in the cities of the southern Plains states and on the reservations, one finds active gourd dance chapters. In local chapters veterans counsel each other on alcohol and other problems and dance together (Howard, 1976; Gephardt, 1977).

A common feature making one eligible for belonging to a self help group is that the affliction comes on the individual rather suddenly and in an overwhelming way, as in a disaster. Despite this initial helplessness, in the group process the "sufferer" gradually is transformed into a healer. In a striking contrast to orthodox professional medical models, the ill, or the evil is somehow converted into a virtue in these self help groups (Janzen, 1982b). For example, in the chiefship of the scrotal hernia, the "therapy" consists of re-creating the individual into a judge, thus providing a meaningful alternative role in society. It is apparent that these self help groups emerge when permanent maintenance of help and resources are required and, not one-time solutions. As in traditional settings in general, the sufferer never fully loses the illness. The affliction is seen as a permanent characteristic inherent in them that they cannot eliminate.

This maintenance of therapy or self help is a widespread, if not universal, mode of healing. The examples from the Euroamerican tradition (e.g., Alcoholics Anonymous, Parents Anonymous, cardiac rehabilitation units) (Janzen, 1982a), demonstrate that it is a viable specific form of therapy for chronic afflictions of particular use when the scientific system fails or is irrelevant. It is a model of care that stands midway, organizationally, between high-cost specialist's care of the dependent single patient and the non-professional practice of folk medicine. It is a unique and useful indigenous mechanism that may arise and be facilitated in traumatized communities with minimal cost and maximum impact.

Guidelines: Studying Persons in Disrupted Community Contexts

Although most of the data described above on community adaptation was gathered in participant observation studies, more systematic approaches are needed during times of crisis and when we need to evaluate interventions. We must, however, continue to rely on descriptions given by participants from the actual experiences in their daily lives. The need to know more about how traumatic stress is experienced by individuals as well as the risk and protective characteristics of the environment and community in which stress takes place, challenges the ready-made research questions of psychosocial research. To meet these new challenges, research under traumatic conditions cannot remain aloof to the specific personal and local variations and conditions that contribute to such events. We must transform often hidden, abstract cultural categories into data that may guide interventions.

Suitable multi-level methodologies need to be used to bring order to the confusing mix of qualitative and quantitative data that confront the clinician, researcher and help provider. Methods such as intensive time sampling of individuals (deVries, 1992), systematic ethnographic and participant observation techniques (Grund et al., 1991; Kaplan et al., 1987), targeted risk population sampling and focus groups (Krueger, 1988; Romme and Escher, 1989), have been developed and employed in multimethod, multistage designs in European cities, refugee camps, schools and in studies of mental disorders (deVries, 1987; de Jong and Clark, 1992; Kellam and Rebok, 1992; Kaplan et al., 1987). These epidemiological and ethnographic techniques target the actual places and times in which stress, psychopathology and health are experienced.

A dynamic metaphor characterizes the methodology advocated to bring about naturalistic assessment under difficult circumstances. The 'cascade approach' denotes such stepwise movement to gather information about aspects of illness and health at the multiple levels that exist between the population, community and the person. Sampling for us has become a case by case methodological preoccupation, and indeed, we draw the image of "cascade" from a site sampling technique that links natural places for problem areas where cases exist in enough density that they can be relatively easily detected, to the examination of individual experience from day to day in those settings. In choosing for a concept of "cascading" we are formulating a specific way of moving systematically from place to place in a search to detect cases and episodes of illness and relate these to the contexts in which we find them. Six stages are proposed, including two new intermediate stages between epidemiological techniques, experiments and standard care evaluation studies (see below).

MULTI-LEVEL MULTI-STAGE APPROACH
CASCADE APPROACH

STAGE 0   Clinical attention and field impression (ethnography and interview)
STAGE I   Identification of risks and problems in specific populations (<u>epidemiological surveys</u>).
STAGE II Target group selection through <u>Social Networks and Snowball Sampling,</u> followed by problem clarification with <u>focus groups</u>.
STAGE III Intensive small-size field sampling using <u>Experience Sampling Methodology</u> and systematic ethnographic observations.
STAGE IV <u>Laboratory testing</u> of hypotheses related to specific variables derived in stages II and III.
STAGE V   Conducting <u>clinical and field trials</u> with robust variables and outcome measures derived in stages I-IV (incl. brain and cultural structures.)

Although conceptually not entirely new (see Trickett, this volume), the development of methods, procedures and models that are sensitive to measuring change over time within the natural environment and under difficult conditions are new. These provide data with a level of detail that matches the precision of experimental psychology and the biological laboratory. Classic epidemiological approaches that seek central tendencies in large samples are too rough and global for the task of describing problems in context. The aggregation of intensively studied individuals nested in particular places is superior over methods that use a large number of subjects with few variables for solving the clinical and research problems under difficult conditions.

In this model, stage O, II and III are emphasized for describing communities. The goals of stage II are to clarify problems and locate the cases identified by stage "O" clinical impression or in the statistics of stage "I", population samples. Since much clinical and sub-population information may be hidden from stage I samples, i.e. disrupted or uprooted individuals, drug scenes, neighborhoods, etc., new methods are required to find them. <u>Snowball sampling</u>, a variant of social network analysis (Baars et al., 1988), is such a technique. Snowball sampling is essentially a method for detecting cases with similar characteristics by means of one key informant selecting others like himself (Kaplan et al., 1987). The underlying logic of techniques such as snowball sampling is to <u>focus</u> and <u>intensify</u> research attention and selection in a manner that increases the ethnographic reliability and validity of psychiatric research. A valuable "by product" of this case finding effort is to approach, by multiple snowball samples, a better estimation of the size of the "hidden populations" as well as a better level of generalizability (external validity) of given populations' parameters. Such "ethnographic samples" provide a way of bridging localized characteristics with more regional and even global patterns that are extremely efficient in evaluating the traits of such a population (Watters and Biernacki, 1989; Frank and Snijders, 1993).

This permits an economical and effective way of obtaining epidemiological and cultural profiles in disrupted communities where neighborhood and other sample techniques prove impossible.

In stage II, problems are located in actual social domains, neighborhoods, scenes, families, etc., and also clarified at the level of actual experience described by a group of subjects in focus groups. One of the key additions of Stage II is the creation of such focus groups. Focus groups are an improvement on key informant research strategies used in traditional anthropology. Not only do they allow distressed individuals to come together and discuss their problems in detail, and thereby garner social support and begin to take pro-active steps toward solution, the focus group is also a research tool. This tool is useful for clarifying the research problem, gaining new information and pre-testing research instruments for (member) validity (Mehan and Wood, 1975; Ericsson and Simon, 1985). The researcher is thus better able to match goals, aims and plans to target groups' actual experience and needs. Focus groups may moreover be used at different stages of an intervention to evaluate impact. Multiple focus groups therefore provide useful means of determining what is initially going on and later in checking what the results of interventions have been. Because of the group format and increased numbers of informants, a more efficient, powerful and systematic tool is created to gather detailed information about the social group and its structure. Focus groups also facilitate the creation of ongoing therapy maintenance groups, similar to the gourd dance or "drums" in Africa (Janzen, 1982b). Such groups are supportive and create a base for political solutions and action toward solving ongoing problems. Focus groups and snowball sampling may thus be used to stimulated self-help groups for problems that require longer term solutions or are not amenable to easy treatment.

In order to probe the information in stage II further, prospective intensive time sampling is needed. Such methods capture the unfolding emotions and reactions to severe stress in context; a step toward ecological validity (Bronfenbrenner, 1979). The Experience Sampling Method (ESM) (deVries, 1987, 1992) does this by providing a representative sample of moments in a person's daily life. It uses an electronic signaling device, often a wrist terminal, to alert subjects 4-20 (most usually 10) times a day to fill out self-reports at preselected but randomized time-points, thus providing detailed information about an individual's mental states or symptoms within the physical and social context and the flow of experience and emotion. Through the use of ESM we have been able to avoid bias (Wheeler and Reis, 1991) and add precision as well as physiological measures to the ecological validity of qualitative ethnographic approaches such as participant observation. This portable self report measurement technique accompanies the person on his daily routine in social settings. It thereby opens up areas for investigation that have remained hidden from other techniques. They thus may provide important personal and cultural information crucial for refining intervention.

Conclusion

Trauma in communities is today visible worldwide. Research into the individual experience of stress both on large catastrophic and a smaller daily life scale has demonstrated the complex relationship between social life and personal psychological and physiological responses. Community life may either buffer or worsen the impact of events. Examining social structure and its potential to help alleviate trauma thus becomes important for understanding and intervening in communities. The cross-cultural cases described above highlight a number of key issues: the important contribution of idiom, ritual and symbolic places that are needed to re-establish community life during crisis and afterwards, the legitimization of individual problems by the medical system that introduces the problem into social life, the role that filial-kin responsibility and the indigenous social security system play in facilitating community responses, and lastly, the stimulating of self help, therapy maintenance groups for problem solving after the disaster has ended. These processes go beyond the reach of current medical interventions and require new information provided by the subjects or group of subjects themselves so that the success of interventions may be improved and evaluated. These data further suggest that interventions need to find a balance between traditional Western medical strategies, the existing social system and cultural rules. Defining and negotiating indigenous community responses are important elements in finding such a balance. A particularly helpful contribution from research is the technique of snowball sampling which allows us to find key informants (even in disrupted situations) who share similar problems. When followed by focus groups, key informant interviews provide reliable new ethnographic information. Such data may be checked and used again to evaluate the impact of interventions later. The intervention team may thus gain insight and incorporate current observations of problems within the ongoing cultural system. This attempt to integrate traumatic reactions within the social system stands central to the ethnographically informed interventions proposed here. During subsequent stages of intervention, focus groups may stimulate self help therapy maintenance groups that will be necessary to maintain and allocate resources to those still in need after a crisis.

Although most of the data presented in the beginning of this paper is conceptual or has been gathered using participant observation techniques, the last half of the paper demonstrates a more empirical design and method. These designs may be used by researchers with relatively little ethnographic sophistication in a variety of different cultural and political settings. Although they do not provide the richness of more qualitative data, these methods are better at securing data that are both ecologically valid, less biased and more reliable. While this empirical research design is of great use in evaluating interventions and ongoing research, it in no way eliminates the need for "Stage 0" approaches that utilize key informants and participant observation techniques. The cascade approach, however, does move beyond another set of assumptions where information used for intervention is often based on vague population statistics and clinical impressions that are rarely checked for validity in the lives of individuals or the community.

The cascade then incorporates detailed information about two missing levels of research data necessary for intervention, the <u>small representative group</u> within community settings and the <u>person</u>. The design creates a pathway from which to move from population data to the person through representative samples, gaining in member and ecological validity as we go. In so doing, new profiles are created that include the illness experience as well as cultural, social, personal, and biological reactions. Herewith, rather than providing an abstract model of causality, a greater level of detailed description, as well as a better goodness of fit between the stress experience of the individual and medical intervention are achieved. Such data allow us to reason better with individuals and groups about their reactions to trauma, paving the way for tailored interventions. Moreover, it localizes the problem in actual social places and groups. It therefore may empower the victim toward self help and the provider to more specific interventions. Thus, the cascade approach is not only a generalized model for undertaking complex multilevel field trials and analyses; it is much more a protocol for a new science of prevention and intervention: a science that enables the voice of the sufferer and his group to be heard, extending the range of responsibility and practical clinical decision-making beyond the boundaries encountered today. Such optimism should be checked by the enormity of today's problems. Often, the community's social life may be so damaged that it is unable to take responsibility. Since we do not know how debilitating these problems may be at any point in time, the cascade, with its ethnographic and quantitative approach offers important information in this regard. Our optimism is not based on the fact the cascade approach will provide solutions. It is based on the fact that the approach may more systematically clarify the problem and empower both sufferers and helpers, while not ignoring the complexity of the human dimensions involved. By organizing research so that we gain insight into indigenous solutions, we may create a partnership with individuals in crisis, enabling us to take a step together out of this world of trauma.

References

Baars, H.M.J., Uffing, J.T.F. & Honnée, J.V. (1988). Use of social networks in mental health care. In Romme, M.A.J. & Escher, A.D.M.A.C. (Eds.) Research to practice in community psychiatry. Maastricht/Assen: van Gorcum.

Baker, G.W. & Chapman, D.W. (1962). Man and society in disaster. New York: Basic Books.

Bieleman, B., Diaz, A., Merlo, G. & Kaplan, C.D. (Eds.) (1993). Lines across Europe: Nature and extent of cocaine use in Barcelona, Rotterdam and Turin. Amsterdam/Lisse: Swets & Zeitlinger.

Bloch, D.A., Silber, E. & Perry, S.E. (1956). Some factors in the emotional reaction of children to disaster. American Journal of Psychiatry, 113, 416-422.

Bromet, E. (1980) Three mile island: Mental health findings. Final Report, National Institute of Mental Health.

Bronfenbrenner, U. (1979). The ecology of human development. Cambridge, USA: Harvard University Press.

Brown, G.W. & Harris, T.O. (1978). Social origins of depression: a study of psychiatric disorder in women. Tavistock, London, Free Press, New York.

Brown, G.W., Andrews, B., Bifulco, A. & Veiel, H. (1990). Self-esteem and depression. Social Psychiatry and Psychiatric Epidemiology, 25, 200-209.

Caplan, G. (1981). Mastery of stress: Psychosocial aspects. American Journal of Psychiatry, 138, 4, 413-420.

Crawshaw, R. (1963). Reaction to a disaster. Archives of General Psychiatry, 9, (2), 157-162.

Csikszentmihalyi, M. (1991). Flow. The psychology of optimal experience. Steps towards optimizing Quality of Life. Harper: New York.

Da Costa, J.M. (1871). On irritable heart: A clinical form of functional cardiac disorder and its consequences. American Journal of Medical Science, 61, 17-52.

De Sousberghe, L. (1958). L'Art Pende. Brussels: L'Académie Royale desSciences Coloniales (Tome IX, fasc. 2 Beaux-Arts).

DeLongis, A., Coyne, J.C., Dakof, G., Folkman, S. & Lazarus, R.S. (1982). Relationship of daily hassles, uplifts, and major life events to health status. Health Psychology, 1, 119-136.

deVries, M.W., Lipken, M. & Berg, R. (1982). The use and abuse of medicine. Praeger Scientific, NY, NY, pp. 296-.

deVries, M.W. (1987). Investigating mental disorders in their natural settings. Journal of Nervous and Mental Disease, 1275, pp. 509-513.

deVries, M.W. (Ed.) (1992). The Experience of Psychopathology: Investigating mental disorders in their natural settings. Cambridge. Cambridge University Press.

deVries, M.W. (1994). Kids in context: Temperament in cross-cultural perspectives. In W.D. Carey, & S.C. McDevitt, (Eds). Prevention and early intervention. Brunner Mazel, NY, pp. 127-139.

deVries, M.W. & deVries, M.R. (1977). Cultural relativity of toilet training readiness. Pediatrics, (60,) pp. 170-179.

deVries, M.W. & Delespaul, P.A.E.G. (1989). Social context and subjective experience in schizophrenia Schizophrenia Bulletin, vol. 15 (2), pp. 233-244.

Engel, G. (1977). The need for a new medical model: A challenge for biomedicine. Science, 196, 129.

Engel, G.L. (1962). Psychological development in Health and Disease. W.B. Saunders Company.

Ericsson, A.K. & Simon, H.A. (1985). Protocol analysis: Verbal reports and data. Cambridge, MA, MIT Press.

Frank, O. & Snijders, T. (1993). Estimating the size of hidden populations using snowball sampling. Paper presented at the third European conference on social network analysis. München, June 10-13.

Friedsam, H.J. (1961). reactions of older persons to disaster-caused losses:An hypothesis of relative deprivations. The Gerontologist, 1, (1), 34-37.

Geertz, C. (1973). The interpretation of cultures. New York: Basic Books.

Gephardt, L. (1977). The Affective Structure of the Gourd Dance, Anthropology M.A. thesis. Lawrence: University of Kansas.

Gerlach, L.P. & Hine, V.H. (1973). Lifeway leap: dynamics of change inAmerica, University of Minnesota Press, Minn. U.S.A.

Grund, J.-P., Kaplan, C.D. & Adriaans, N.F.P. (1991). Needle sharing in theNetherlands: An ethnographic analyses. American Journal of Public Health, 81, pp. 1602-1607.

Hersey, J. (1980). Hiroshima. New York: Knopf.

Hobfoll, S. E. (1988). The ecology of stress. New York, Hemisphere.

Hobfoll, S. E., Briggs, S., & Wells J. (this volume). Community stress and resources: Actions and reactions. In S. E. Hobfoll & M. W. deVries (Eds.), Extreme stress and communities: Impact and intervention. Dordrecht, the Netherlands: Kluwer.

Holmes, T.H. & Rahe, R.H. (1967). the social readjustment rating scale. Journal ofPsychosomatic Research, 11, 213-218.

House, J., Landis, K. & Umbessen, D. (1983). Social relationships and health.Science, 241, pp. 540-545.

Howard, J.H. (1976). The Plains Gourd Dance as a Revitalization Movement.Am. Ethnologist, 2, 243-59.

Janzen, J. (1982a). Drums Anonymous. In deVries, M.W., Lipken, M.,& Berg, R. The use and abuse of medicine. Praeger Scientific, NY, NY., pp. 154-166.

Janzen, J. (1982b). Lemba 1650-1930: A Drum of Affliction in Africa andthe New World. New York: Garland.

Jong, J.T.V.M. de & Clark, L. (Eds.) (1992). WHO/UNHCR Mental healthtraining manual. WHO, Geneva.

Kanner, A.D., Coyne, J.C., Schaefer, C. & Lazarus, R.S. (1981). Comparison oftwo modes of stress measurement: Daily hassles and uplifts versus major life events. Journal of Behavioral Medicine, 4, 1-39.

Kaplan, C.D. (1992). Drug craving and drug use in the daily life of heroinaddicts. In: deVries, M.W. (Ed.) (1992). <u>The experience of psychopathology: Investigating mental disorders in their natural settings</u>. Cambridge: Cambridge University Press, 193-218.

Kaplan, C.D., Korf, D. & Sterk, C. (1987). Temporal and social contexts ofheroin-using populations. An illustration of the snowball sampling technique. <u>Journal of Nervous and Mental Disease, 175</u>, pp. 566-574.

Kellam, S.G. & Rebok, G.W. (1992). Building developmental etiologicaltheory through epidemiologically based preventive intervention trials. In: McCord, J. & Tremblay, R.E. (Eds.) <u>Preventing deviant behavior: Experimental approaches from birth to adolescence</u>. New York: Guilford Press.

Kleinman, A. (1988). The illness narrative. New York: Basic Books.

Krueger, R.A. (Ed.) (1988). <u>Focus groups. A practical guide for applied research</u>. Newburry Park, California Sage Publications, Inc.

LeVine, R.A. (1973). <u>Culture, behavior and personality</u>. Chicage: Aldine.

Lindeman, E. (1944). Symptomatology and management of acute grief. <u>American Journal of Psychiatry</u>, vol. 101, pp. 141-148.

Lucas, R.A. (1969). <u>Men in crisis: A study of a mine disaster</u>. New York: Basic Books.

Mason, J. (1968). Organization of psychoendocrine mechanisms, <u>Psychosomatic Medicine</u>, vol. 30, pp. 365-608.

Mehan, H. & Wood, H. (1975). <u>The Reality of Ethnomethodology</u>. New York:John Wiley.

Meyer, R.J. & Haggerty, R.J. (1962). Streptococcal infections in families: Factorsaltering individual susceptibility. <u>Pediatrics, 29</u>, 539-549.

Newman, C.J. (1976). Children of disaster: Clinical observations at Buffalo Creek. <u>American Journal of Psychiatry, 133</u>, (3), 306-312.

Nicolson, N.A. (1992). Stress, coping and cortisol dynamics in daily life. In: deVries, M.W. (Ed.) (1992). <u>The experience of psychopathology: Investigating mental disorders in their natural settings</u>. Cambridge: Cambridge University Press, 219-232.

Roghmann, K. & Haggerty, R.J. (1973). Daily stress and the use of health servicesin young families. <u>Pediatrics Research, 7</u>, 520-526.

Romme, M.A.J. & Escher, A.D.M.A.C. (1989). Hearing Voices. <u>Schizophrenia Bulletin, 15</u>, pp. 209-217.

Sarason, I.G., Pierce, G.R. & Sarason, B.R. (1990). Social support and interactional process: A dyadic hypotheses. <u>Journal of social and personal relationships, 7</u>, pp. 495-506.

Seyle, M. (1976). <u>The stress of life</u> (rev. ed.). New York, McGrawhill.

Shweder, R.A. & LeVine, R.A. (1984). <u>Culture theory: Essays on mind, self,and emotion</u>. Cambridge University Press: Cambridge NY.

Spiegel, J.P. (1957). The English flood of 1953. <u>Human Organization, 16</u>, (2), 3-5.

Stone, A.A., Neale, J.M. & Shiffman, S. (1993). Daily assessments of stress andcoping and their association with mood. <u>Annals of Behavioral Medicine</u>, 15, (1), 8-16.

Trickett, E. J. (this volume). The community context of disaster and traumatic stress: An ecological perspective from community psychology. In S. E. Hobfoll & M. W. deVries (Eds.), <u>Extreme stress and communities: Impact and intervention</u>. Dordrecht, the Netherlands: Kluwer.

Tyhurst, J.S. (1957). Psychological and social aspects of civilian disaster. <u>Canadian Medical Association Journal</u>, 76, 385-393.

Watters, J.K. & Biernacki, P. (1989). Targeted sampling: Options for thestudy of hidden populations. <u>Social Problems</u>, 36, pp. 416-430.

Wheeler, L. & Reis, H.T. (1991). Self-recording of everyday life events:Origins, types and uses. <u>Journal of Personality</u>, 59, pp. 339-354.

Whiting, B. & Whiting, J. (1975). <u>Children of six cultures</u>. Cambridge,Mass.: Harvard University Press.

Wolfenstein, M. (1957). <u>Disaster</u>. Glencoe, Ill.: Free Press.

SECTION VI: PREVENTION AND INTERVENTION (OVERVIEW)

Stevan E. Hobfoll, Kent State University, Kent, Ohio, USA
Rebecca P. Cameron, Kent State University, Kent, Ohio, USA
Marten W. deVries, University of Limburg, Maastricht, the Netherlands

Section Six offers a wide variety of approaches to intervention into community stress processes. These range from traditional clinical interventions to community interventions, with targets of intervention ranging from schoolchildren to emergency response groups. Chapters challenge conventional wisdoms, such as the use of critical events debriefing as an intervention strategy. This section does a thorough job of setting the stage for the crucial next step of empirical investigation of community stress interventions.

Weiæsth (Chapter Eighteen) begins this section with a reminder that prevention efforts should include efforts to strengthen individuals and communities and promote resilience, as well as seek to limit risk factors. To that end, he presents several features of disasters and disaster responses that can affect outcomes.

One is the relationship of certain features of trauma to eventual outcome. These dimensions include physical stressors, threat to life, witnessing destruction and suffering multiple losses, and experiencing a conflict between self-preservation and offering assistance to others. Weisæth indicates that the experience of any one or more of these stressors predicts psychopathological outcome. A protective factor is the presence of others, which tends to mobilize and encourage supportive actions.

Additional features of disaster response that more directly relate to prevention efforts are emergency personnel selection, specific training efforts, and preventive interventions. Weisæth compares these three approaches to the three legs of a chair, with each being part of a coherent prevention effort. He goes on to outline several protective and vulnerability factors, including individual-level and group-level variables that predict disaster responses, and to provide evidence from his previous research indicating that high levels of training predict optimal coping with disaster. Personality factors and the ability of disaster-stricken individuals to find meaning are additional factors influencing coping. A major limitation of disaster training as a general community resource is that, in practice, training is usually conducted for specific occupations of workers learning to deal with job-related hazards. The potential for the positive effects of training to generalize beyond stressors encountered in particular work settings has not been tapped.

Weisæth next describes several features of early prevention efforts in the aftermath of disaster, drawing on his experiences following the capsizing of an oil rig. He characterizes that particular disaster as containing all of "the three c's": the social contexts of disaster involving the community, a company, and communication. By communication, Weisæth is referring to disasters in which the site of the occurrence is removed from the location of family members, necessitating efforts to bring families closer in order to communicate more effectively with them.

In instances where communication is an issue, it becomes necessary to establish an information and support center in order to keep family members apprised of developments related to their loved ones. In addition, this gives survivors a chance to provide the bereaved with meaning-enhancing details of the disaster. Through the center, several objectives can be met. Examples of these objectives include the rapid and humane provision of authoritative information, the facilitation of mutual support groups' development, and the efficient collection of legal and investigative data. Mobilization of support at levels ranging from self-help to highly skilled professionals' services is another important feature of prevention in the aftermath of disaster. In addition, attention must be paid to the need for early identification and screening of high-risk situations, persons, or reactions, to the extent that such screening is feasible and useful. Each of these responses constitutes a potentially important part of prevention efforts implemented in the aftermath of disaster.

Van der Kolk, van der Hart, and Burbridge (Chapter Nineteen) provide a thorough review of current thinking about post-traumatic stress disorder (PTSD). They characterize PTSD as a reaction to an experience of intense terror associated with the loss of normal feelings of predictability, controllability, and invulnerability. It is a very frequently-occurring disorder, and can result from a variety of traumatic stresses. These authors feel that physiological hyperarousal is the key to the development of PTSD. This hyperarousal is associated with dissociation, and with the failure to integrate the traumatic experience into a meaningful autobiographical set of memories. Thus, PTSD is a biologically based disorder related to longterm changes in neurochemical functioning that affect cognitive processing.

Van der Kolk et al. characterize current conceptualizations of the symptomatology of PTSD, which includes intrusive re-experiencing; autonomic hyperarousal; numbing of responsiveness; intense emotional reactions and sleep problems; learning difficulties; memory disturbances and dissociation; aggression against self and others; and psychosomatic reactions, all of which are processes that are affected by the individual's developmental level.

Next, Van der Kolk et al. outline principles of treatment. The primary tasks of treatment are the processing of the original overwhelming experience, controlling and mastering physiological stress reactions, and re-establishing the security of social relationships and interpersonal efficacy. Management of acute trauma requires special attention to the re-establishment of a sense of security, primarily through utilization of pre-existing support networks, ensuring predictability, and promoting active engagement in coping efforts. Treatment should be geared to phases of the affected individual's life and to stages of the disorder. Psychotherapeutic interventions that facilitate the process of integrating the unacceptable and overwhelming traumatic experience are: stabilization, identification of feelings by verbalizing somatic states, deconditioning traumatic memories and responses, restructuring trauma-related schemes of internal and external reality, and exposure to restitutive experiences. He argues that group psychotherapy and psychopharmacological treatments that block serotonin reuptake can also facilitate recovery.

Van der Kolk et al. conclude by saying that traumatic stress leaves indelible imprints on survivors. However, as introduced in previous sections of this book, interventions that facilitate the construction of integrated narratives, that increase the perception of available social support, and that enhance self-efficacy in the wake of trauma can do much to facilitate healing.

Pynoos, Goenjian, and Steinberg (Chapter Twenty) present a comprehensive and systematic strategy for disaster intervention with children and adolescents. They argue that not enough research has been focused on these age groups, despite the large frequency with which they are affected by traumatic stress.

An essential component of the effective provision of disaster-related services for children and adolescents is the recognition of the multiple levels at which services need to be coordinated: the government, the school, and the intervention team. Clarity about the appropriate roles of each of these institutions and of priorities for intervention is crucial to avoid resistance responses from individuals and organizations that are unsure how to respond to traumatized children. In addition, each member of the school staff and the intervention team needs to have her or his emotional reactions acknowledged and dealt with, so that she or he can function effectively. Staff people should be aware of the importance of their respective roles, and should be monitored for continued functioning under stressful intervention conditions.

A public mental health approach facilitates and coordinates the implementation of services. Features of a public mental health approach are the assessment of relative risk, the stratification of interventions, and monitoring of the course of recovery. Information that is obtained through these procedures can be provided to governmental agencies, relief organizations, schools, and intervention teams as needed to facilitate the optimal coordination of efforts. Pynoos et al. advocate a developmental model of traumatic stress that takes into account objective and subjective disaster experiences, exposure to traumatic reminders, and the presence of secondary stressors. Additionally, this model focuses attention on potential developmental disturbances that may emerge, and suggests appropriate early intervention.

The developmental model accounts for distress using a tripartite model, but also calls for consideration of contextual issues and the child's coping abilities. Treatments must attend to the complexities of child and adolescent experiences, including bereavement, guilt and shame, depression, and disturbances in attachment or autonomy. Length of separation from loved ones during the trauma and the inability of loved ones to protect the child are two important contextual issues of special relevance to children. Interventions should include efforts to increase the child's ability to cope with traumatic reminders and secondary stresses.

Stages of intervention include psychological first-aid, specialized initial interviews, brief therapy, pulsed interventions, and long-term psychotherapy. Goals of intervention include improving coping, normalizing responses, reworking the trauma in terms of meaning and in terms of developmental issues, such as the need for safety, and preventing or limiting developmental disturbance. Prevention strategies and preparedness are helpful in that they minimize the child's initial exposure to disturbing features of the traumatic stress experience. Specialized treatment approaches are implemented for the most severely disturbed children, many of whom have pre-existing or comorbid psychological difficulties.

Milgram, Sarason, Schönpflug, Jackson, and Schwarzer (Chapter Twenty-one) offer suggestions on how to effectively catalyze community support following extreme stress. They relate their discussion to stressors that can be considered to be community-wide disasters affecting largely intact communities in which support provision can be accomplished through resources internal to the community, rather than by relying on international aid. In presenting their discussion, they attend first to the definition of terms, then build on those definitions in making their suggestions. Support takes multiple forms, including the provision of information, encouragement, material assistance, empathy, and validation of worth. Support can be provided to people along a continuum of severity of need. Milgram et al. suggest that high-risk groups should be identified and targeted for prompt interventions. Some high-risk groups include the elderly, minors, and those who are relatively isolated. Assessment of what support is needed, when, and by whom is essential to maximize effectiveness, and can be accomplished with the aid of key informants. It is important to consider who may be able to provide needed support efficaciously, and to deal with issues related to support recipients' capacity to utilize support effectively.

Milgram et al. next address the issue of community, which they define as a group of people sharing common interests related to the nature of the stressor event. A proper understanding of community support interventions should include assessment of pre-disaster resources in the community, and mobilization of these resources as appropriate. Community leadership can be helpful in eliciting support by publicly endorsing the call for support mobilization. Community values may significantly affect the likelihood of successful support mobilization. The ability of support providers to empathize with support recipients' needs and values will facilitate support provision.

Finally, Milgram et al. consider the concept of catalyzing. They define this as an interpersonal process in which certain people change the viewpoints and actions of certain other people. The media can be a powerful means to catalyze support, and can be influenced through the various people who control the dissemination of information through that particular medium as well as by the activities of those coordinating volunteer supportive efforts. The intended audience of any particular message may influence its nature (i.e., different messages may be appropriate for the intended recipient of support, the provider of support, or the general public). One important form of communication that should not be overlooked is the messages that community leaders provide about the meaning of traumatic events. Leaders can develop helpful perspectives in conjunction with professionals in the field of traumatic stress, and then can develop and implement public healing rituals. The simple dissemination of information can be empowering if it is presented clearly and contains concrete suggestions of ways to be helpful. Milgram et al.'s analysis of the components of the process of catalyzing community support can be of significant value in conceptualizing strategies to enhance a community's self-efficacious response to stress.

Figley, Giel, Borgo, Briggs, and Haritos-Fatouros (Chapter Twenty-two) provide a concise summary of the key elements to consider when planning a course of action to implement within a disaster-stricken community. First, they categorize disasters according to two dimensions: sudden versus long-term and natural versus man-made. These distinctions provide initial insights into the character of the disaster impact and the types of interventions that are likely to be helpful. Next, they outline key types of information that need to be gathered.

An assessment should be conducted that attends to the following issues: demographic features of the stricken population; the nature of the disaster; customary community channels of communication; the formal and informal authority structure; available national resources; the availability of social support at the community and family level; attitudes towards and institutions dealing with loss and mourning; the full range of primary and secondary victims of the disaster; and the nature and extent of post-traumatic stress responses being experienced in the community. Disaster phase should guide the interventionist in understanding the attitudes and response of the community, since there is often an initial sense of community cohesion that dissipates over time, leaving individuals relatively isolated during the long process of rebuilding.

Figley et al. provide some recommendations to community interventionists. First, working within existing social values and structures, mobilize and organize existing or new self help groups to serve as the backbone of social support. Second, energize self help groups, providing appropriate guidance and direction as needed. Third, begin the process of organizing and planning for the future, again bearing in mind specific characteristics of the local community. Fourth, work with government officials by supporting them in handling the disaster constructively and quickly. And, fifth, educate and utilize the public information media to provide helpful messages and avoid unhelpful communications. A final suggestion is that interventionists should be on the lookout for signs of compassion fatigue among disaster workers. These guidelines have been provided so that mental health specialists can contribute to solving disaster-related problems, rather than create more problems for an affected community.

Ørner, in Chapter Twenty-three, discusses intervention strategies for emergency response groups, noting their special role in responding to modern disasters. In general, communities have a group of people specially sanctioned to respond to emergency situations. There are important rituals and conventions that facilitate these groups' handling of the burden of trauma that their role requires them to carry. These include special training, hierarchically defined roles, and the wearing of uniforms. The role of emergency workers is to shield the general public from direct exposure to extreme stress, and in return the host community finances and supports the emergency team. Nowadays, however, emergency teams are often deployed to communities far from home, where they are to respond to the needs of communities that may not be able to support them. This can serve to undermine the ritualized coping mechanisms the team is accustomed to using, and may heighten emergency workers' vulnerability to stress reactions.

It is important to note that emergency workers are not psychologically exempt from reactions to the traumatic situations they face. Instead, they face a host of psychological responses, including the use of rigid defense mechanisms and the experience of a full range of anxiety or depressive symptoms. They may also experience positive reactions, such as invigorated self-confidence and enhanced self-efficacy. Nor do emergency workers' emotional responses occur exclusively following their exposure to trauma. Instead, they often experience symptoms of distress in the midst of coping with the disaster.

A variety of interventions have been implemented with emergency responder groups, including critical incident stress management services (CISMS), which encompass a wide range of interventions implemented before, during, and after stress exposure. Interventions can include education, peer counseling, demobilization meetings, and professional counseling. Psychological debriefing is another seven-stage strategy developed specifically for emergency response teams. It should be noted, however, that these interventions have not been adequately evaluated to know if they are effective. Instead of repeating the call for outcome studies, Ørner offers a new conceptual framework to guide interventionists, and to hopefully inspire researchers. They key element of this conceptualization is the view of intervention strategies as transitional rituals. This approach gives a theoretical underpinning to outcome research and capitalizes on what we know about stress resistance among emergency workers.

Throughout this section, specific guidelines for disaster intervention are presented, along with their theoretical underpinnings. The need for empirical validation of interventions is clearly established. We are reminded of the scope and dimensions of disaster, the contextual factors that alter the nature of particular disasters, and the multiple players in any disaster context: interventionists, victims, bereaved families, school and government officials, the media, etc. Thorough and ongoing assessments must be conducted and attention must be paid to relationships between the different elements and players in the particular context in order to provide help, rather than hindrances to communities and individuals coping with issues of survival.

PREVENTIVE PSYCHOSOCIAL INTERVENTION AFTER DISASTER

Lars Weisæth
Division of Disaster Psychiatry, Dep. of Psychiatry, University of Oslo.
Oslo, Norway.

Prevention, Preparedness, and Mitigation

During the last 25 years 1 billion persons have been affected by natural disasters. The 1990's have been designated as a decade for natural disaster reduction (WHO, 1988). The smallest and poorest countries are affected most severely by natural disasters, and the poorest and most disadvantaged members of a disaster-affected community are likely to experience the most serious consequences. Therefore, in the majority of developing countries, disasters, because of their severity and frequency, represent a real public health priority (WHO, 1992a).

Disaster preparedness is a significant part of the overall strategy for achieving Health for All by the year 2000. One of WHO's strategies for emergency preparedness and response is strengthening the national capacity to cope with disaster. By 1995, the WHO's target for the Eight General Programme of Work is that 70% of all countries will have developed master plans to deal with the health aspects of emergency and disaster situations. These master plans should include a mental health component. A long range plan including a full scale mental health intervention strategy should be developed at national and international level. Models for a three step development, from international reliance through national to local reliance have been described by the World Health Organization (WHO, 1992a).

The key concepts and activities for coping with disaster risks and disaster are prevention, which includes all measures designed to prevent phenomena from causing or resulting in disasters; preparedness, which involves all actions designed to minimize loss of life and damage, and to prepare for timely and effective rescue, relief and rehabilitation should disaster strike; and mitigation, which means reducing the effects of an extreme hazard on man and his environment once it has occurred.

Psychological aspects need to be considered in each of these activities. Because psychosocial aspects play a part in forming the responses both before, during and after a disaster strikes, psychological knowledge and techniques can contribute to prevention at several points in each of the time phases of a disaster.

In the past there has been a general tendency to consider that the basic needs of a disaster-stricken population were to be met essentially in terms of providing shelter, food, sanitation, and immunization against epidemics. Psychosocial needs were seen as something too secondary to attract the attention of relief agencies or health services. In this paper some research findings and practical experiences our institute has made over a twenty year period with relevance for prevention of traumatic stress effects will be reviewed and applied in the context of disaster mainly as they are occurring in the technologically developed countries. Two issues will be our focus: The preventive effects upon post-traumatic stress problems by (1) a high level of disaster preparedness among potential disaster victims and professional disaster workers, and (2) establishing an Information-Support Center in the disaster aftermath, particularly for bereaved families. We will begin, however, by pointing out some problems in preventive psychiatry and some challenges in prevention in the field of traumatic stress.

Prevention in Psychiatry and in Traumatic Stress

Traditionally, it is stated that prevention of illness demands that the risk factors are known, can be identified, and modified. Studies of the psychopathogenic process can help us achieve this. For primary prevention the distress or illness risk factors are of greatest importance, for secondary and tertiary prevention, we need to gain insight into the nature of the prognostic factors.

An alternative approach, namely to strengthen the individual or the group, is even less used in psychiatry. But it was always there, we are just becoming aware of it: Increasing the resilience of a person is being understood to have a touch of health promotion to it. And it cannot be learned from studying patients.

In general, prevention in psychiatry is difficult because the etiology of nearly all psychiatric disorders is multifactorial and often over-determined, there are more than the necessary number of risk factors present. At the same time, as in most fields of medicine, the risk for developing the illness is low. Most high risk individuals are likely to remain well. The weakness of the high-risk strategy reflects our poor ability to predict which individual will become sick. Whereas risk factors may identify a group with a much increased relative risk, most clinical cases occur in those who were not a conspicuous risk: "A large number of people exposed to a small risk commonly generate many more cases than a small number exposed to high risk" (Rose 1992).

Progress in traumatic stress research during the last two decades may represent a serious challenge to prevention in psychiatry. In recent years strong links have, not surprisingly, been demonstrated between abuse in childhood and later adult psychiatric illnesses (Bryer et al 1987, Swett et al 1990). Certain diagnostic groups are apparently very strongly related to previous traumatization of a specific kind. For example, 95% of the patients in a study of multiple personality disturbance had been exposed to sexual abuse or physical violence as children (Ross et al 1990). In any dissociative disorder, the doctor should be alerted to traumas in the history of the illness (Spiegel 1991). Similarly, findings have been reported for borderline conditions by Herman et al (1989): They recently reported that 80% of children with diagnosis of borderline disorder had been exposed to traumas, most often violence, sexual abuse, or having frequently witnessed such traumas. In addition, one third of these children satisfied the diagnostic criteria of PTSD (Famularo et al 1991). That the psychic trauma is so often a main etiological factor in causing psychiatric illness represents a great challenge to mental health professionals. The problems in preventive work are well known, for example the fact that the children's network are so often responsible for the traumas, that traumas are not often reported when they occur.

Health Effects and Long Term Psychiatric Morbidity After Exposure to Disaster Stress

Mortality has been shown to increase after disasters (Adams and Adams 1984, Bennet 1970). With regard to the study of general morbidity, the methodological problems are difficult to overcome. Holen (1990, 1993) who studied survivors of an oil rig disaster found an increase in psychosomatic diagnoses during the first eight years after. A series of studies have established psychiatric morbidity levels from about 20% to 50% one year after disaster (Tierney and Baisden, 1979, Gleser et al, 1981, Powell and Penick, 1983, Green et al, 1983, Weisæth, 1985, Shore et al, 1986). In spite of the brief duration of the exposure, the man-made disasters with high shock show persisting levels of over 30% morbidity, with PTSD as the most frequent disorder, followed by depressions. Considering that some of the populations studied are positive samples in terms of prior health compared to the general population, and even trained to cope with disaster, such as industrial shift-workers (Weisæth 1985) or off-shore oil rig employees (Holen 1990), these morbidity rates are impressive, and a challenge to prevention. Survivors of such collective severe events should be very well suited as research subjects for the study of preventive interventions.

Research on Preventive Intervention

From a research view point it should be less difficult to demonstrate the effect of preventive efforts in the field of traumatic stress than in other branches of psychiatry. Compare, for example, the task of trying to demonstrate the success of attempts to reduce new cases of schizophrenia in a part of an urban area with that of studying the effects of preventive measures in a population of trauma exposed persons. In the latter case, such as a large accident, (1) the population is well defined,(2) the illness risk is high, depending, amongst other things, on the severity of the trauma, (3) the observation period can be relatively brief - a few years at the most, but much of the reactional pattern will be observable during the first year, (4) the illnesses in question, such as PTSD, can be reliably diagnosed, and (5) the interventions can be reasonably well described. In addition, (6) if the ideal level and type of interventions are compared with the average interventions practiced, the ethical objection involved of having untreated control groups can be handled and a controlled intervention design achieved (Schüffel et al, 1990). Internationally acknowledged standard research instruments are now available in the traumatic stress field, such as self-report scales, clinical rating instruments, and structured diagnostic interviews (Raphael et al, 1989).

From a preventive mental health view point, traumatic stress offers another advantage compared to other branches of psychiatry and medicine. Case definitions in the field of traumatic stress recognize the continuous distribution in the exposed population, it is "How much of it do they have?", rather than "Has this person got it?". Although evaluation for therapy may still need to be dichotomous, treat or not treat, rational early prevention may utilize a more graded risk case definition and interventions graded accordingly.

A most promising post-disaster result of a preventive intervention, was reported by Herlofsen (1994). There were no cases of PTSD at follow-up in his prospective, interventive study of survivors of a snow avalanche which killed 55% of a military unit. He points out that the social networks in the platoon consisted of the same elements as in civilian life, in addition to family, there were friends, colleagues and neighbors. In the military these are the friends in the platoon, squad members and roommates. The difference from a non-military situation is that fellow servicemen were present and available at all times. In the military system the chain of care from which one can mobilize support is more obvious than in the non-military context: Informal self-help, and formal support from comrades, commanders, military chaplains, medical corps personnel, and military psychiatry. Consistent with this, Holen (1990) has reported that support from colleagues was valued more highly than other support during the first year after a disaster by the survivors. In another study, getting back to work soon and being with work mates, were most highly valued by employees exposed to an industrial disaster (Weisæth 1984).

Traumatic Stress: Prepare or Repair?

Theoretically, primary prevention by a reduction of new cases can be achieved through (1) lowering the number of traumas, (2) increasing the stress tolerance of exposed subjects, i.e. by way of improved selection of personnel or of better preparedness and training, leadership, and support team building, and (3) early screening, identification of risk cases and implementation of interventions so that the pathological processes are aborted. The first two strategies aim at safety and preparedness, whereas the third approach tries to prevent a breakdown in coping attempts by repairing, or relieving individuals of their post-traumatic stress reaction. In one way, however, early intervention is also a preparatory approach, since so much of the effort is anticipatory guidance that aims to reduce uncertainty and helplessness.

Before returning to the question of prevention after disasters, it is necessary to describe some aspects of the destructive events and the settings in which prevention is to be implemented, before and after, for example for surviving disaster victims and disaster rescue workers. These are two of the groups likely to be among the most affected by of a disaster of some magnitude, the others are the next-of-kin, onlookers, body handlers, health personnel, persons holding responsibility, and evacuees. All these groups experience more or less of the three dominating dimensions of disaster trauma, danger, loss and exposure to the grotesque.

Taxonomy of Disaster, Psychological Aspects

Natural disasters include flood, tidal wave, storm, cyclone, hurricane, tornado, tsunami, earthquake, volcanic eruption, landslide, avalanche, drought, and wildfire. Natural disasters are often familiar to the victims, and the affected communities may have developed a lot of experience with these particular hazards. Traditionally these disasters are seen as unavoidable. Although early warning systems are being developed, the impact is extremely powerful and causes substantial destructions, social disruptions and many secondary stressors, such as loss of both home and income (total disaster).

Man-made disasters include fire in large buildings and cities, collapse of man-made structures (bridges, mines, dams, buildings, roads), transport system accidents (ship, railway, airplane, motor transport), and technological disasters (explosions, toxic, chemical, nuclear).

Because man-made disasters are rarely preceded by warnings they often have a sudden onset, producing shock traumas. While the impact is extremely powerful, the destructions are often concentrated and cause less social disintegration. These disasters result from a loss of control, for which someone or some agency may be seen as responsible.

Man-made disasters seem to be more traumatic to mental health (Weisæth, 1993,1994). Their higher unpredictability, uncontrolability and culpability may partly account for this. Another stressful aspect of some technological disasters such as nuclear accidents, is the lack of a clearly defined "low point", i.e. the worst day (Baum, 1986), in other words, when is the worst over?

The risk of exposure to disaster has increased in many populations, particularly in the developing countries, because of increase of population size, greater population density in vulnerable areas and the strong tendency of large populations toward urbanization. Because of the increase in communication, the concentration of industrial complexes and dependence on technological products, the possibility of man-made disasters may also have increased in the industrial countries, and magnified their potential destructions.

Accidents are a major cause of death in technologically developed countries. Technology is often able to prevent natural disasters or their destructive consequences, while failing technology is an increasing risk to human life.

In our experience there are on average 10-20 persons close enough to every person killed in a major accident to suffer a major loss. The circle of less affected people may be very wide: As many as 25% of the Estonian population of one million, and 10% of the eight million Swedes reported that they were close to or knew well one of the nearly thousand persons who perished when the ferry Estonia sunk in September 1994 or to some of the bereaved.

Because man's actions are upsetting ecological balance, a partly human causation may be thought of in what was earlier a typical natural disaster. In addition, there is a strong relationship between low socio-economic level and increased risk of exposure and number of deaths. Both these realizations may reduce the acceptance of disasters and somewhat resigned attitudes in the third world countries. If this happens, the psychological suffering is likely to increase until the matters are changed.

Definition of Disaster

Korver (1987) found more than 40 different scientific definitions of disaster in the literature. Common to most definitions and those of medicine, psychology and sociology which are of most relevance for our purpose, is that they stress that a disaster is a severe destruction which greatly exceeds the coping capacity of the affected community. Thus, the coping capacity and the psychosocial resources of a community are essential in defining when a destructive event is to be seen as a disaster. A disaster has no upward limit, and the limit downwards is not clear. A high frequency of catastrophic events may raise the threshold for consideration of an event as a disaster. To declare an event a disaster often has political, economic and emotional consequences.

The high expectations of rescue, support and care in the technologically developed countries may make it reasonable to have a lower threshold for when a disaster is declared. In the main, however, in these countries the lack of resources will be felt only during the first hours after the impact.

When it is necessary to reduce the standard of medical care because of the great number of injuries, a mass injury situation is said to exist.

The medical definition with its focus on victims who are so numerous that the treatment needs far outweigh the immediately available resources is operational, and serves to define when a hospital's disaster plan needs to be put into action. Until recently, however, the only criterion taken into consideration was the number of somatically injured or acutely ill individuals. The life-threatening conditions naturally have been given first priority. This narrow view of disaster has delayed the organization of psychosocial interventions in accidents or disasters in which everyone perished or none had been physically harmed. The hospitals, with their 24 hour preparedness serve as the basis for the disaster medical organization, would not mobilize. Thus, there was nothing to secure that psychosocial resources would be set in to deal with the psychosocial problems of bereaved families, rescue workers, body search and recovery teams or other disaster workers.

The medical definition of disaster also fails to identify the mass destructive event which destroys a large social system such as a major work place or a local community, in contrast to destructive events that mainly strike a great number of people who are not socially related to each other. Many transport accidents, for example, constitute mass scale injuries, but not disasters in the social sense.

Both for the disaster victim, rescuer, and health worker the sheer magnitude of the event makes the disaster different from other critical situations, such as accidents. When the needs far outrun the resources, the situation is easily felt to be overwhelming, especially for the individual who necessarily has to recognize his insufficiency. For the victim, in particular, the sense of powerlessness that is created by the magnitude of the event is added to the helplessness induced by the disaster impact.

Priorities in Disaster Medicine

In contrast to the everyday emergency decision making, in which the most severe injuries are given highest priorities, the prioritizing in disaster situations may seem paradoxical. Situations may occur in which injuries that are life-threatening and where lives can be saved by small expenditure of resources may be given first priority. Extremely severe injuries with small chances of survival and demanding a great deal of resources may be given low priority, so-called expectant or comfort treatment.

The Collective Perspective: Dimensions of Disaster Trauma.

Both for planning and practice it would be desirable for research to compare the effect of exposure to small versus exposure to large magnitude events. Studies of severe, but limited everyday highly stressful events, such as accidents, tend to yield lower incidences of psychiatric morbidity than the findings from the large scale events (Weisæth 1985, Raphael 1986, Malt 1988). In a country like Norway where approximately 5% of all deaths are violent deaths, only 5% of these deaths occur in events that cost 5 or more lives.

During the disaster impact of an accident or disaster, the victim is 1) likely to experience severe physical stressors, the worst of which is the serious physical injury. 2) Every degree of threat to life may be experienced, and of various duration. Most everyday accidents have very brief duration so that the death threat may not be so intensely experienced as in a disaster. This may account for the low PTSD rates after most traffic accidents (Malt 1988). In addition 3) the disaster victim is likely to witness enormous destructions, suffer multiple losses, and witness mass injuries and deaths. Finally, 4) collective situations often create a responsibility trauma, which is the experience of conflict between incompatible choices of action, for example between ensuring one's own survival versus rescuing others. In two studies of disaster impacts, about 25% of the survivors were found to have had experienced such significant intrapsychic conflicts (Weisæth 1984, Holen 1990). The presence of one or more of the four stressors of disaster trauma seem to predict psychopathological outcome (Weisæth, 1984).

The presence of others, however, increases the possibility of receiving help, of being recruited by spontaneous leaders who organize rescue activities, and in fact help to turn victims into rescuers. This has been shown to have a significant preventive effect (Weisæth 1984).

On the whole, the disaster victim is likely to be exposed to more extreme stressors, to experience more overwhelming powerless and helplessness than the accident victim. In the immediate aftermath, the disaster victim is more at risk of suffering from the lack of rescue - and treatment resources and a longer exposure than the accident victim who benefit from an intact framework.

In the post-disaster phases, when victims of disaster have been kept together and offered information and support services, observations indicate that collective situations may synchronize post-traumatic stress reactions, reinforce individual reactions and shorten the shock phase (Berle et al 1991). Among children Terr (1985) has reported symptom contagion.

Selection, Training and Preventive Intervention: The 3-Legged Chair.

Military experiences during war have been a virtual laboratory for testing out the preventive effects of selection to screen out susceptible individuals, training and other factors believed to increase resilience, and preventive interventions on soldiers with combat stress reactions (Gal and Mangelsdorff, 1991). Each of these approaches have had their successes and their backlashes, all three are needed; after all: Which leg is most important on a three-legged chair? The preventive effects upon psychiatric morbidity by selection of suitable personnel will not be discussed at length. Selection is usually practiced as a part of an employment process for jobs that may expose the person to severe stress. Often, however, these jobs (military personnel, pilots, sailors, oil workers. high risk industry workers, fire fighters, police officers, engine drivers, and others) also provide other circumstances that are likely to increase a person's stress tolerance. For example, team building, competence and training, motivation, leadership, psychological and medical support and so on. It seems to be a general finding that stringent selection, except in the form of screening out the definitely unfit, becomes less important the more the above factors are made present (Belenky, 1987).

There is yet a scarcity of studies on coping with major traumatic events (Vaillant 1979, Antonovsky 1987), but nevertheless the extensive literature provide us with a lot of interesting and, not the least, fruitful material.

Rachman (1978) noted that academic psychology had drawn little learning from the stress studies and experiences of World War II. He also states that there has been a shortage of useful terms in our professional literature to describe elements that are extremely important in our adaptive psychological handling of stressful life events. When I tried to characterize people who managed to maintain their health after exposure to a severe psychic trauma, an industrial explosion that happened in 1976, I was struck by the lack of theory, of concepts, and measuring instruments that could be used in describing their coping process (Weisæth 1984).

In the study mentioned, I measured their previous education, training and personal experience in coping with physical dangers. This crude variable, "level of disaster training," correlated strongly with the immediate functional capacity during the exposure to trauma ("disaster behavior") (Weisæth, 1989a). This was no surprise, industry and the military have always believed it would. What was more surprising were the low rates of subsequent PTSD in those who had coped well during the exposure. This was surprising because PTSD apparently was just as much the result of a failure to cope during the initial trauma, as a failure in recovering from the post-traumatic stress reactions caused by the traumatic exposure.

Some of the relationships between trauma, disaster behavior and the post-disaster course of the post-traumatic stress syndrome that came out of that study, can be seen from Figure 1.

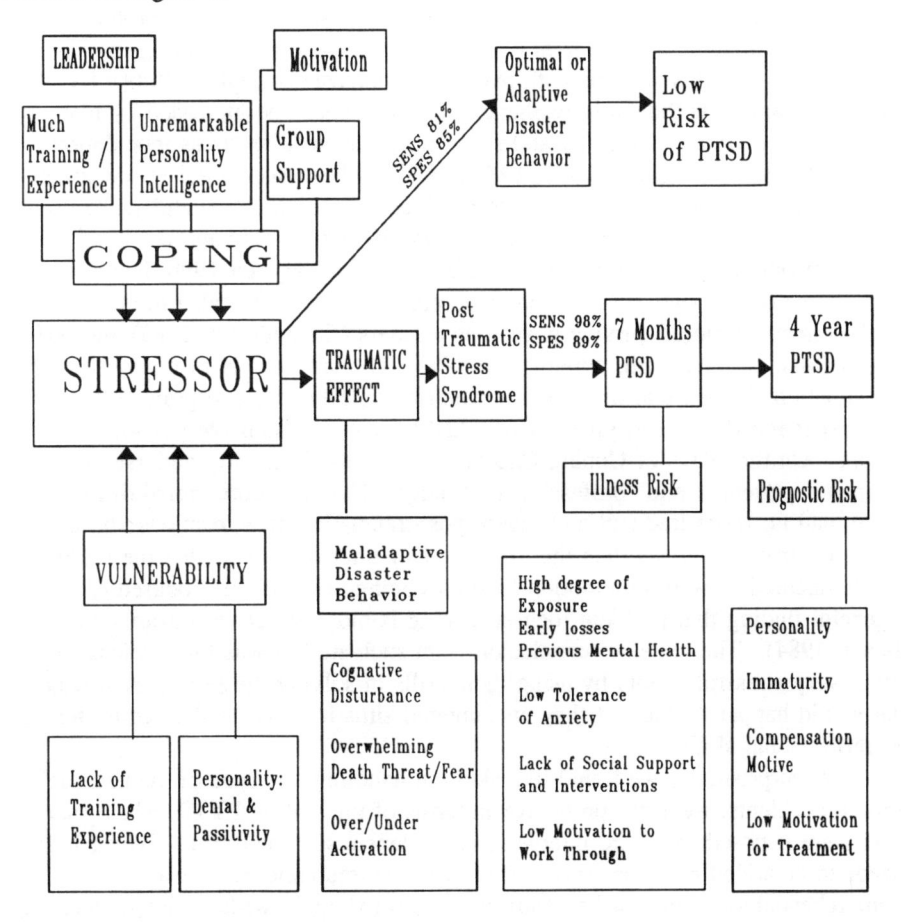

Figure 1: Risk- and protective factors for disaster behavior, and acute and long-term post-traumatic stress reactions in 125 survivors of an industrial explosion in 1976 (Weisæth, 1984).

The left side of the figure shows the protective and vulnerability factors that were found to affect the responses during disaster impact. Shown is the high sensitivity (81%) and specificity (86%) of a high level of training in predicting an optimal disaster behavior. The latter correlated with a low risk of later development of PTSD.

Lack of training, and denial and passivity as personality traits, correlated with maladaptive disaster behavior. This mainly behavioral measure correlated very strongly with a traumatic experience of particularly severe death threat, emotional storm or mental and motoric paralysis.

To the right in Figure 1 can be seen the strong predictive validity (sensitivity 96%, specificity 89%) of the one week post-traumatic stress syndrome for the diagnosis of PTSD seven months post-disaster, which again correlated strongly with the four-year outcome.

Since training for danger situations seemed to be an important protective factor, studies were conducted to shed light on what mechanisms in the training process were important for the ability to cope with real trauma exposures (Hytten 1989, Hytten and Hasle, 1989) and how the stress resilience of people could be increased by new methods derived from psychology and stress medicine such as stress inoculation training (SIT) (Meichenbaum, 1977, 1985). SIT has been successful in preparing individuals for combat training (Novaco, Cook and Sarason, 1983) and scuba diving (Deikis, 1983) and other stressful situations. Promising results were achieved in preparing people for occupational traumas by using SIT (Hytten 1990, Hytten et al 1990). Some of our later studies have supported these findings, also in other groups than the directly exposed survivors, such as rescuers (Ersland et al 1989) and body handlers (Malt and Weisæth, unpublished data). The latter study of coping in a mass death situation showed that the professionals (forensic experts and police officers) highly experienced in identifying corpses, had hardly any intensive post-traumatic stress reactions. On the Ways of Coping Checklist they most frequently endorsed the items "previous experience" and "professional attitude." The non-professional disaster workers had far more frequent and severe post-traumatic stress reactions and used more emotion control techniques than the experts. Our impression was that the findings fit with the distinction between emotion-focused coping and problem focused coping and the general finding that problem focused coping is more effective (Lazarus and Folkman 1984). The tentative conclusion from such studies was that professionals manage very stressful events by using their skills in solving the problems at hand. What would happen to them if they encountered situations where they could not use their professional skills?

Not surprisingly, we found that skills in handling one type of danger, such as maritime accidents, were not protective in terms of preventing PTSD, when seasoned sailors were exposed to severe interpersonal violence, such as torture (Weisæth 1989b). It needs to be added however, that in this case, the traumatic event was uncomprehendable, could not be controlled and was largely without deeper meaning. Thus, according to Antonovsky (1987), some of the basic conditions, comprehensibility, manageability and meaningfulness, needed in order to cope with stress, were absent.

Another study (Weisæth, unpublished data) of well-trained sailors who were unable to rescue passengers during a ship's fire, resulting in 159 deaths, also supported the hypothesis; about 50% of the crew suffered from PTSD and other stress-related disorders two years after the fire. It would seem that the event here produced a sense of failure to perform the very tasks for which the personnel were trained.

Summing up, studies like those mentioned, indicate that disaster training appears to be a very effective preventive measure for post-traumatic stress, for victims and disaster workers. The limitation of the approach is that so much of the preparedness work is limited to job related hazards. The protective role of training may generalize to other traumatic situations than the job-related, but the general situation in society is still unsatisfactory. Women, for example, have been found to have far less competence in how to handle accidents (Weisæth, 1989a).

Prevention in the Aftermath: Where We've Been and Where We Might Go

Clinical psychologists and psychiatrists have a strong identity as therapists, but a weak and unclear role and identity when it comes to preventive work. Prevention often implies working through others, mobilizing human resources at various levels in the community, and utilizing mass strategies. Mental health professionals may feel particularly out of place when prevention is to be practiced after traumatization of large numbers of people, or when working in technologically underdeveloped countries with poorly developed health services (WHO, 1992). Our own experiences have been made largely in such collective stress situations, and military settings, and our strategy and approach have been colored by this.

In the following section, some of the background, principles and organization of the so called Information and Support Center are described.

It began with a personal observation. In 1980, on the day after the capsizing of an oil rig in the North Sea (which eventually turned out to have killed 123 oil workers), I experienced the strong need among the many who had family members missing, of meeting survivors and enquire what they might know about the fate of their close ones. By that time our disaster rescue and medical organization had developed a psychosocial intervention program for survivors, disaster workers and bereaved families. It turned out that we had seen these groups as too separate. They had more of shared interests and needs than we had realized. Until 1980, our experiences with psychosocial intervention programs had mainly been local community and company accidents and disasters. We had no comprehensive plan for a combination of a community, company and communication disaster, which the oil rig disaster turned out to be. By communication disaster we mean transport disasters and others where the disaster victims are removed from their social networks, such as hotel fires, military accidents and many others.

The Three C's

Because of the different social context of the community, company and communication disaster, there has been a need to design specific models for psychiatric interventions. The agencies with which one should establish a working relationship in order to be an effective catalyst of support services will vary in each case.

In communication disasters the uncertainty of who has been killed may be particularly high when there are no definite passenger lists, which is the case for ferries, trains and public transport. On one occasion in Norway 64,000 telephone calls were registered during a few hours when thousands of families tried to find out whether their family member were among the victims of a military accident which had been reported in the media without delay, and without identifying who were the victims. Even rapid and effective announcements through the media of telephone numbers to which inquiries can be directed for information cannot meet such a convergence.

In the communication category of traumatic stress, people die or are severely injured often far away from home. Their social network is not there. We started to bring in the families.

Establishing an Information/Support Center

The psychosocial organization can be located either at a hospital or at a convenient place not too far from the disaster area, (hotel, school, etc.) or both. If the identity of the dead is uncertain (which is frequent), or the number of dead is unknown for a time, a great number of families are affected until they ascertain that their missing family member is safe. The existence of such a center and its telephone numbers should be distributed by radio and television. The Center is run by the Police who has the coordinating responsibility for the disaster rescue organization. Health personnel, chaplains, police officers and employees of the transport company or other hit by the disaster, will staff the Center (Weisæth, 1991). Families with suspected missing members should be invited to come to the center and survivors may also be asked to gather there, later also rescuers and personnel who has a function in relation to the disaster that make them important for those affected by the disaster. The Center gives the bereaved a chance to meet survivors to get a first hand report about what happened to their loved ones, how they died, perhaps even what they uttered before they perished, where, why, - and what efforts were made to rescue them. The survivors and possibly also onlookers and rescuers have information that often cannot be given by others. Such information will often be crucial in helping the bereaved to understand, and finally to accept, the new reality. For the survivors, it is often an important experience to be of help to the bereaved.

The main functions of such an Information/Support Center are:
(1) To provide rapid, authoritative information about tragic news that can be conveyed in a humane, direct way in a setting sheltered from public and media attention.

(2) To provide support and a holding environment for the affected persons (health personnel, clergy, police and others).
(3) To serve as a forum or meeting place where affected individuals and families can support each other. Self-help groups/organizations may develop from this forum.
(4) To be a place where the police can collect identification data about missing/dead persons from their close ones.
(5) If necessary the police should be able to use the center to interrogate survivors about the disastrous chain of events as a part of their investigation.
(6) The information/support center may also help to reduce the convergence of people on the disaster site that may create congestion and therefore mobility problems for rescuers.
(7) To provide linkage to local helpers when the initial assessment indicates that some kind of help or service would be needed over a longer period of time than the existence of the center.

A meeting may be organized for everyone affected (this may be possible for up to one thousand people) or at least one or two representatives from each affected family can attend and be given information about rescue, identification, investigation of causes, insurance, psychosocial support services and religious services.

Mobilizing Support at Different Levels

Other questions that need to be asked are Who should help? When? In what way? The chain of care from which one can mobilize support at different levels may run like this:

(1) Self-help (advice to victims about intrapsychic, interpersonal, and activity-related coping techniques).
(2) Social network (mobilizing support from family, friends, workmates, and neighbors).
(3) Helpers outside the health care and social services: Leaders, clergy, police, rescuers, firemen, volunteer organizations.
(4) General and specialized somatic health care services.
(5) Mental health professionals.
(6) Traumatic stress teams.

Early Screening

For mental health personnel working in an Information Support Center, another question is: Who ought to be helped? Assessment of traumatization in victim groups can, in principle, be carried out in three ways, by identifying:

(1) *High-risk situations*, the presence of particularly severe trauma dimensions in the individual's or the family's exposure.
(2) *High-risk persons*, the presence of high-risk factors (vulnerability) in exposed persons (for example, lack of training in survivors, a history of psychiatric problems) in survivor or family.
(3) *High-risk reactions*, the presence of early response variables that predict later illness.

In medicine there is an enthusiasm for screening. Frequently, however, screening is a pursuit of early diagnosis and should not be confused with prevention. The ability to identify individuals at high risk of developing an illness is traditionally characterized by the method's sensitivity and specificity. Sensitivity yields the proportion of the real risk cases that the method is able to identify. For example, in the mentioned study we found a sensitivity of 0.96 1-week post-disaster when screening was based upon a Traumatic Anxiety Index made up of the State Anxiety Inventory Score, degree of traumatic sleep disturbance, startle reaction, and fear/phobia of the scene of the accident and degree of social withdrawal (Weisæth 1985). Thus, 96% of those who developed a PTSD 7 months post-disaster could be identified at an early stage by this method (Fig. 1).

The specificity of a screening method depends on its ability to identify those who are not at risk of developing the disorder. In the mentioned study, 89% of the healthy group seven months post-disaster had been identified as such one week post disaster. If it is important not to overlook any risk cases, one will choose a lower cut-off point on the screening instrument, yielding higher sensitivity and fewer false negatives. If the interventive resources are limited, the effect of preventive intervention modest, or there is a risk of being stigmatized by early identification, one must tolerate that a proportion of the risk cases will not be detected. Improved accuracy, theoretically at least, may be obtained by choosing a higher cut-off point that gives a maximal specificity and the lowest number of false positives.

Findings as the above, of a high predictive validity of the acute stress reactions and the post-traumatic stress syndrome support a practice of early diagnosis. The introduction of the diagnoses Acute Stress Reaction in the ICD-10 (WHO, 1992b) and the Acute Stress Disorder in the DSM IV (APA, 1994) will be helpful in this respect. But then we may no longer be talking of primary prevention in the strict sense, but of screening for early diagnosis.

The resistance or avoidance of the traumatized person in seeking help is also a major problem in preventive work. In the study of the effects of the industrial explosion we found that approximately 42% of the post-traumatic psychopathology (PTSD) had been lost, and as many as 64% of the severe cases, if only 82% had been reached of those exposed, namely those who joined the preventive program upon the first call (Weisæth 1989c). The non-response was highest in those with most severe exposure. If predictions had been made solely based on those who willingly registered, and not based on the final follow-up response rate of a 100%, the predictor value of severe exposure would have become far too low. The initial resistance in many who later developed PTSD was found to relate to the psychological defenses such as avoidance against the re-experience in the acute post-traumatic stress syndrome. For primary and secondary prevention, the implication may be that early outreach must be very active. Thus, a paradox in trying to implement preventive measures after psychic trauma appears to be that those with the highest risk may be least likely to seek help or accept out-reach programs.

It is also important to improve our early identification tools. We developed the Post Traumatic Symptom Scale (PTSS-10), in 1980 (Holen, 1990). The PTSS-10 seems to have promising predictive validity; it correlates strongly with instruments like HSCL-90 and the Impact of Event Scale in describing clinical cases of PTSD (Stæhr et al 1993).

How consistent a finding is the high predictive validity of early risk reactions? It needs to be asked to what extent a high predictability depends upon certain characteristics of the psychic trauma, of the persons exposed, and of other factors that would be expected to influence the pathogenetic process, such as experiencing additional stressful life events or receiving social support.

In her study of rape victims, Dahl (1993) found that the severity of the post-traumatic stress syndrome during the first weeks and months after the traumatic event did not particularly well predict PTSD 1 year after the exposure. The normal, average reaction pattern was so strong, it did not reflect adaptation or maladaptation (What Lomranz calls the bulldozer effect of trauma, this volume). However, combining risk factors relating to the stressful event, the exposed person and the social network, yielded a high predictive validity of the screening process, for certain groups of the victims. For example, the triad (1) use of weapon by the rapist (2), a history of previous psychological instability in the victim and (3) blaming of the victim from her close social network, defined a risk of 90% of developing a PTSD within the first year after the rape. Thus, after certain types of traumas it seems to be necessary to base predictions upon a combination of data about high-risk exposure, high-risk persons, and high-risk reactions.

References

Adams, P. R., Adams, G. R. (1984). Mount St. Helens' ashfall: Evidence for a disaster stress reaction. American Psychologists, 39, 252-260.

American Psychiatric Association (1994). Diagnostic and Statistical Manual of Mental Disorder. Fourth Edition. Washington, DC: American Psychiatric Association.

Antonovsky, A. (1987). Unraveling the Mystery of Health. Jossey-Bass.

Baum, A. (1986). Toxins, Technology, Disasters. In Van Der Bos, G. R., Bryant, B. K. (Eds). Cataclysms, Crisis, and Catastrophes: Psychology in Action (pp: 9-53). Washington, DC: The American Psychological Association.

Belenky, G. (1987). Contemporary Studies in Combat Psychiatry. New York: Greenwood Press.

Bennet, G. (1970) Bristol floods 1968: Controlled survey of effects on health of local community disaster. Br Med J, 3, 454-458.

Berle. J.Ø., Haver, B., Karterud, S. (1991). Group reactions as observed in crisis intervention programs in hospitals. Nord Psykiatr Tidsskr, 45, 329-335.

Bryer J. B., Nelson, B. A., Miller, J. B, Krol, P. A. (1987). Childhood sexual and physical abuse as factors in adult psychiatric illness. Am J Psychiatry, 144, 1426-1430.

Dahl, S. (1993). Rape - A Hazard to Health. Oslo: Scandinavian University Press.

Deikis, J. G. (1983). Stress Inoculation Training: Effects on Anxiety, Self Efficacy, and Performance in Divers. Doctorial thesis, Temple University.

Ersland, S., Weisæth, L., Sund, A. (1989). The stess upon rescuers involved in an oil rig disaster. "Alexander L. Kielland 1980". Acta Psychiatr Scand Suppl, 335, 38-49.

Famularo, R., Kinscherff, R., Fenton, T. (1991). Posttraumatic stress disorder among children clinically diagnosed as borderline personality disorder. J Nerv Ment Dis, 179, 428-431.

Gal, R., Mangelsdorff, A. D. (1991). Handbook of Military Psychology. Chichester. John Wiley & Sons.

Gleser, G. C., Green, B. L., Winget, C. N. (1981). Prolonged psychosocial effects of disaster: A study of Buffalo Creek. New York: Academic Press.

Green, B. L., Grace, M. C., Lindy, J.D., Titchener, J. L., Lindy, J. G. (1983). Levels of functional impairment following a civilian disaster: The Beverly Hills Supper Club fire. J Consult Clin Psychol, 51, 573-80.

Herlofsen, P. (1994). Reactions to trauma: an avalanche accident. In Ursano, R.J., Mc Caughey, C. S., Fullerton, C. (eds). Trauma and Disaster. The Structure of Human Chaos (pp. 248-266). Cambridge: Cambridge University Press.

Herman, J.L., Perry, J.C., van der Kolk, B.A. (1989). Childhood trauma in borderline personality disorder. Am J Psychiatry, 146, 490-495.

Holen, A. (1990). A Long Term Outcome Study of Survivors from a Disaster. Oslo: University of Oslo.

Holen, A. (1993). The North Sea Oil Rig Disaster. In Wilson, J. P., Raphael, B. (eds). International Handbook og Traumatic Stress Syndromes (pp: 471-478). New York: Plenum Press.
Hytten, K. (1989). Helicopter crash in water: Effects on simulator escape training. Acta Psychiatr Scand Suppl, 355, 73-78.
Hytten, K. (1990). Studies on stress and coping: Psychosocial and physical dangers. Establishment and manifestations of negative and positive outcome expectancies. Oslo: Medical Faculty, University of Oslo.
Hytten, K., Hasle, A. (1989), Fire Fighters: A Study of Stress and Coping. Acta Psychiatr Scand Suppl, 355, 50-55.
Hytten, K., Jensen, A., Skauli, G. (1990). Stress inoculation training for smoke divers and free fall lifeboat passengers. Aviat Space Environ Med, 983-988.
Korver, A. J. H. (1987). What is a disaster? Prehospital and Disaster Medicine, 2, 152-153.
Lazarus, R.S., Folkman. S. (1984). Stress, Appraisal and Coping. New York: Springer Publishing.
Malt, U. F. (1988). The Long-Term Psychiatric Consequences of Accidental Injury. Br J Psychiatry, 153, 810-818.
Meichenbaum, D. (1977). Cognitive Behavior Modification. New York: Plenum Press.
Meichenbaum, D. (1985). Stress Inoculation Training. New York: Plenum Press.
Novaco, R. W., Cook, T. M., Sarason, I. G. (1983). Military Recruit Training. An Arena for Stress-Coping Skills. In Meichenbaum, D., Jaremco, M. E. (Eds). Reduction and Prevention (pp: 377-418). New York: Plenum Press.
Powell, B. J., Penick, E. C. (1983). Psychological distress following a natural disaster: A one-year follow-up of 98 flood victims. J Community Psychology II, 269-276.
Raphael, B. (1986). When Disaster Strikes. How Individuals and Communities Cope with Catastrophe. New York: Basic Books.
Raphael, B., Lundin, T., Weisæth, L. (1989). A research method for the study of psychological and psychiatric aspects of disaster. Acta Psychiatr Scand, Suppl, 353.
Rose, G. (1992). The Strategy of Preventive Medicine, Oxford: Oxford University Press.
Ross, C. A., Miller, S. D., Reagor, P. (1990). Structured interview data on 102 cases of multiple personality disorder from four centers. Am J Psychiatry, 147, 96-601.
Schüffel, W., Lopez-Ibor, J. J., Rosser, R., Weisæth ,L. (1990). A concerted European action for coping with disaster. Brussels: E.C. Research and Development Coordination Programme.
Shore, J. H, Tatum, E., Vollmer, W. M. (1986). Evaluation of mental health effects of disaster. Am J of Public HEalth, 76, 76-83.

Spiegel, D. (1991). Dissociation and Trauma. In: Tasman, A., Goldfinger, S. M. (eds). American Psychiatric Review of Psychiatry, Volume 10, (pp. 261-276). Washington, DC: American Psychiatric Press.

Stæhr, A., Stæhr, M., Behbehani, J., Bøjholm, S. (1993). Treatment of war victims in the Middle East. Copenhagen: International Rehabilitation Council for Torture Victims.

Swett, C., Surrey, J., Cohen, C. (1990). Sexual and physical abuse histories and psychiatric symptoms among male psychiatric patients. Am J Psychiatry 147, 632-636.

Terr, L. C. (1985). Children traumatized in small groups. In: Eth. S., Pynoos, R. (eds). Post-Traumatic Stress Disorder in Children. (pp: 47-70). Washington, DC: American Psychiatric Press.

Tierney, K., J., Baisden, B. (1979). Crisis intervention programs for disaster victims: A source book and manual for smaller communities. Rockville: National Institute of Mental Health, 203. (DHEW publication).

Vaillant, G. E. (1979). Health consequences of adaptation to life. American Journal of Medicine, 67, 732-734.

Weisæth, L. (1984). Stress Reactions to an Industrial Disaster. An Investigation of disaster behaviour and acute post-traumatic stress reactions, and a prospective, controlled, clinical and interventive study of sub-acute and long-term post-traumatic stress reactions. Oslo: University of Oslo.

Weisæth, L. (1985). Post-traumatic stress disorder after an industrial disaster. In Pichot, P., Berner, P., Wolf, R., Than, K. (eds). Psychiatry - The State of the Art (pp.299-306). New York: Plenum Press.

Weisæth, L. (1989a). A study of behavioural responses to an industrial disaster. Acta Psychiatr Scand Suppl. 355, 13-24.

Weisæth, L. (1989b). Torture of a Norwegian ship's crew. Acta Psychiatr Scand. Suppl. 355, 63-72.

Weisæth, L. (1989c). Importance of high response rates in traumatic stress research. Acta Psychiatr Scand Suppl, 355, 63-72.

Weisæth, L. (1991). The information and support centre. Preventing the after-effects of disaster trauma. In Sørensen, T., Abrahamsen, P., Torgersen, S. (eds). Psychiatric Disorders in the Social Domain (pp: 50-58).Oslo: Norwegian University Press.

Weisæth, L. (1993). Disaster: Psychological and Psychiatric Aspects. In Goldberger, L., Breznitz, S. (Eds). Handbook of Stress (pp. 591-616). New York: The Free Press.

Weisæth, L. (1994). Technological disaster: Psychological and psychiatric effects. In Ursano, R. J., McCaughey, C. S., Fullerton, C. (Eds). Individual and Community Response to Trauma and Disaster. The Structure of Human Chaos (pp72-102). Cambridge: Cambridge University Press.

World Health Organization. (1988). Resolution on the International Decade for Natural Disaster Reduction. Geneva: WHO, A/44/832/Add. 1.

World Health Organization. (1992). <u>Psychosocial consequences of disasters. Prevention and management</u>. Geneva: WHO, MNH/PSF/91.3, 1992.
World Health Organization. (1992). <u>International Classification of Disease ICD-10.</u> Geneva: WHO.

THE TREATMENT OF POST TRAUMATIC STRESS DISORDER

Bessel A. van der Kolk
Onno van der Hart
Jennifer Burbridge
Harvard Medical School
Brookline, MA

Terrifying experiences that rupture people's sense of predictability and invulnerability can profoundly alter the ways that they subsequently deal with their emotions and with their environment. The syndrome of Post Traumatic Stress Disorder (PTSD) can follow such widely different stressors as war trauma, physical and sexual assaults, accidents, and other natural and man-made disasters. Mirroring the confusion and disbelief of people whose basic assumptions are shattered by traumatic experiences, the psychiatric profession periodically has been fascinated by trauma, followed by sudden disbelief in the importance of trauma in the genesis of psychopathology. Over the past decade our profession has experienced the third intense wave of efforts to grasp the reality of trauma on body and soul, after the first at the Salpetriere during the closing decades of the 19th century, and the second, spearheaded by Abram Kardiner (1941), in the 1940s. The findings about the consequences of trauma and what constitutes effective treatment have been extraordinarily consistent over these 120 years.

    Several studies in recent years have shown that Post Traumatic Stress Disorder (PTSD) is among the most common of psychiatric disorders. The National Vietnam Veterans Readjustment Study (Kulka et al, 1990) found that approximately twenty years after the end of the Vietnam war 15.2% of Vietnam theater veterans continued to suffer from PTSD. However, PTSD is not confined to combat soldiers, but is quite common in the general population, particularly among psychiatric patients. Various studies have demonstrated a life time prevalence of between 1.3% (Helzer et al, 1987) and 9% (Breslau & Davis, 1991) in the general population and at least 15% in psychiatric inpatients (Saxe et al., 1993). Although PTSD is associated with high levels of chronicity, co-morbidity and functional impairment, the general level of functioning varies a great deal between affected individuals.

    Lack of predictability and controllability are the central issues for the development and maintenance of PTSD. The combination of intrusive and numbing symptoms has been consistently noted over the past century (e.g. Janet, 1904; Kardiner, 1941), and forms the basis of our understanding of the nature of PTSD. What distinguishes people who develop posttraumatic stress disorder (PTSD) from people who are merely temporarily overwhelmed is that people who develop PTSD become "stuck" on the trauma, keep re-living it in thoughts, feelings, or images. Evidence during the past decade supports the notion it is the intrusive re-living, rather than the traumatic event itself that is responsible for the complex biobehavioral change that we call PTSD (McFarlane, 1988). Once they become dominated by intrusions of the trauma, traumatized individuals begin organizing their lives around avoiding having them (van der Kolk & Ducey, 1984). Avoidance may take many different forms: keeping away from reminders, ingesting drugs or alcohol that numb awareness of distressing emotional states, or utilizing dissociating to keep unpleasant experiences from conscious awareness. The helplessness, conditioned hyperarousal, and other trauma-related changes may permanently change how a person deals with stress, alter his/her self-concept and interfere with the view of the world as a basically safe and predictable place.

A relative sense of safety and predictability are preconditions for effective planning and personal action. Freud (1911/1959) described how, in order to function properly, people need to be able to define their needs, anticipate how to meet them and plan for appropriate action. In order to do this, people need to be able to mentally entertain a range of options, without resorting to action. He called this capacity: "thought as experimental action". Traumatized people seem to lose this essential capacity and have difficulty turning inwards to utilize their emotions as guides for action (van der Kolk & Ducey, 1984). Instead, their internal world becomes a danger zone and they seem to spend their energies on NOT thinking and planning.

The therapeutic relationship with these patients tends to be extraordinarily complex. It confronts all participants with intense emotional experiences, forcing them to explore the darkest corners of the mind, and to face the entire spectrum of human glory and degradation. The devastating effects of trauma on affect modulation, attention, perception, and the giving and taking of pleasure bring us face to face with the full destructive impact of traumatic stress to dominate, use and control others.

The Role of Memory and Dissociation

Pierre Janet (1889) first described how the central issue in trauma is dissociation: memories of what has happened cannot be integrated into one's general experiential schemes and are split off from the rest of personal experience. Physiological hyperarousal seems to be a central precondition for dissociation to occur (Rauch et al, 1995). Lack of integration on a schematic level causes the experience to be stored as affect states or as somatosensory elements of the trauma (van der Kolk & Fisler, in press 1995), which return into consciousness when reminders activate customary response patterns: physical sensations (such as panic attacks), visual images (such as flashbacks and nightmares), obsessive ruminations, or behavioral re-enactments of elements of the trauma.

Most studies of people who develop PTSD find significant dissociative symptomatology (Bremner, 1993; Marmar, 1994) The most extreme form of post-traumatic dissociation is seen in patients who suffer from Dissociative Identity Disorder. Janet (1889) first described how traumatized people become "attached" (Freud would later use the term "fixated") to the trauma: "unable to integrate traumatic memories, they seem to have lost their capacity to assimilate new experiences as well. It is .. as if their personality definitely stopped at a certain point and cannot enlarge any more by the addition or assimilation of new elements (p.532)." This suggests that traumatized people are prone to revert to earlier modes of cognitive processing of information when faced with new stresses.

Since the core problem in PTSD consists of a failure to integrate an upsetting experience into autobiographical memory, the goal of treatment is find a way in which people can acknowledge the reality of what has happened without having to re-experience the trauma all over again. For this to occur merely uncovering memories is not enough: they need to be modified and transformed, i.e. placed in their proper context and reconstructed into neutral or meaningful narratives. Thus, in therapy, memory paradoxically becomes an act of creation, rather than the static recording of events which is characteristic of trauma-based memories.

PTSD as a Biologically Based Disorder.

Abram Kardiner (1941) introduced the notion that "traumatic neuroses" are "physioneuroses" and that patients with PTSD remain on constant alert for environmental threat.: "(t)he subject acts as if the original traumatic situation were still in existence and engages in protective devices which failed on the original occasion..." (p. 82). In PTSD, the physiological state of chronic overarousal is accompanied by difficulties in attention and concentration, as well as distortions in information processing, including narrowing of attention onto sources of potential challenge or threat. It appears that for traumatized people *all* emotions become angerous. While the function of their hyperarousal is to prepare them for some form of action in the face of threat, it does not build up specific skills and feelings of mastery and control, because the anticipated action is not specific.

Over the past few years it has become increasingly evident that the intensity of the initial somatic response to a potentially traumatic experience is the most significant predictor of long term outcome. If the stress is sufficiently overwhelming, the resulting trauma sets up a conditional emotional response in which the body continues to go into a fight, flight, or freeze responses at the least provocation: traumatized people keep experiencing life as a continuation of the trauma, and remain in a state of constant alert for its return. Many traumatized people who have consciously put the trauma behind them continue to experience anxiety and increased physical arousal when exposed to situations that remind them of the trauma, or even to unexpected events such as loud noises, and go into fight/flight reactions, without necessarily being aware of the origin of these extreme behaviors.

Though the biological underpinnings of response to trauma are extremely complex, forty years of research on humans and other mammals have demonstrated that trauma (particularly trauma early in the life cycle) has long term effects on the neurochemical response to stress, including the magnitude of the catecholamine response, the duration and extent of the cortisol response, as well as a number of other biological systems, such as the serotonin and endogenous opioid system. (For an extensive review on the psychobiology of trauma, see van der Kolk, 1994).

The Symptomatology of PTSD

While post traumatic stress has been recognized in the poetry of Homer, Shakespeare and Goethe, psychiatry has consistently recognized its existence only since 1980 when PTSD was introduced into the DSM III. Table I shows the diagnostic criteria for simple PTSD. Since that time, there has been a growing literature documenting the posttraumatic symptoms of hyperarousal, hyper-reactivity to stimuli reminiscent of the trauma, avoidance and emotional numbing in a large variety of traumatized populations, including war veterans, children who have experienced physical or sexual assaults, women who have been battered and raped, people exposed to natural disasters, refugees and political prisoners. Regardless of the origin of the terror, the Central Nervous System (CNS) reacts consistently to overwhelming, threatening, and uncontrollable experiences with conditioned emotional responses. For example, rape victims may respond to conditioned stimuli, such as the approach by an unknown man, as if they were about to be raped again, and experience panic.

Intrusive Re-experiencing

Remembrance and intrusion of the trauma is expressed on many different levels, ranging from flashbacks, affective states, somatic sensations, nightmares, interpersonal re-enactments, including transference repetitions, character styles, and pervasive life themes. Laub and Auerhahn (1993) organized the different forms of knowing along a continuum according to the distance from the traumatic experience, each form also progressively represents a consciously deeper and more integrated 'level of knowing.' The different forms of remembering trauma range from 1)not knowing; 2) fugue states (in which events are relived in an altered state of consciousness); 3) retention of the experience as compartmentalized, undigested fragments of perceptions that break into consciousness (with no conscious meaning or relation to oneself); 4) transference phenomena (wherein the traumatic legacy is lived out as one's inevitable fate); 5) its partial, hesitant expression as an overpowering narrative; 6) the experience of compelling, identity-defining and pervasive life themes (both conscious and unconscious); 7) its organization as a witnessed narrative. These various forms of knowing are not mutually exclusive.

TABLE I
SIMPLE PTSD (DSM IV)

A. 1) Exposure to life threatening experience
    2) Intense subjective distress upon exposure

B. Reexperiencing the trauma:
    1) recurrent intrusive recollections, or repetitive play,
    2) recurrent dreams
    3) suddenly acting or feeling as if the traumatic event were recurring
    4) intense distress upon re-exposure to events reminiscent of trauma
    5) physiological reactivity upon re-exposure

C. Persistent avoidance or numbing of general responsiveness.
    1) efforts to avoid thoughts or feelings associated with   trauma
    2) efforts to avoid activities
    3) psychogenic amnesia
    4) diminished interest in significant activities
    5) feelings of detachment of estrangement
    6) sense of foreshortened future

D. Persistent symptoms of increased arousal
    1) difficulty falling of staying asleep
    2) irritability or outbursts of anger
    3) difficulty concentrating
    4) hyper-vigilance
    5) exaggerated startle

Autonomic Hyperarousal

While people with PTSD tend to deal with their environment by emotional constriction, their bodies continue to react to certain physical and emotional stimuli as if there were a continuing threat of annihilation. Conditioned autonomic arousal to trauma-related stimuli has consistently been shown to occur in a variety of traumatized populations. Autonomic arousal, which serves the essential function of alerting the organism to potential danger seems to loose that function in traumatized people: the easy triggering of somatic stress reactions causes people with PTSD to be unable to rely on bodily sensations to warn them against impending threat. Instead, the persistent warning signals loose their functions of signals of impending danger, and cease to alert the organism to take appropriate action.

Numbing of Responsiveness

Aware of their difficulties in controlling their emotions, traumatized people seem to spend their energies on avoiding of distressing internal sensations, instead of attending to the demands of the environment. In addition, they loose satisfaction in matters that previously gave them a sense of satisfaction and may feel "dead to the world". This emotional numbing may be expressed as depression, as anhedonia and lack of motivation, as psychosomatic reactions, or as dissociative states. In contrast with the intrusive PTSD symptoms, which occur in response to outside stimuli, numbing is part of these patients' baseline functioning. In children, numbing has been observed among elementary school children attacked by a sniper, among witnesses to parental assault or murder, and among victims of physical or sexual abuse. They become less involved in playful social interactions, and often are withdrawn and isolated. After being traumatized, many people stop feeling pleasure from exploration and involvement in activities, and they feel that they just "go through the motions" of everyday living. Emotional numbness also gets in the way of resolving the trauma in psychotherapy: they give up on recovery and it keeps them from being able to imagine a future for themselves.

Intense Emotional Reactions and Sleep Problems

The loss of neuromodulation that is at the core of PTSD leads to loss of affect regulation. Traumatized people go immediately from stimulus to response without being able to first figure out what makes them so upset. They tend to experience intense fear, anxiety, anger and panic in response to even minor stimuli. This makes them either overreact and intimidate others, or to shut down and freeze. Both adults and children with such hyperarousal will experience sleep problems, both because they are unable to still themselves sufficiently to go to sleep, and because they are fearful of having traumatic nightmares. Many traumatized people report dream-interruption insomnia: they wake themselves up as soon as they start having a dream, for fear that this dream will turn into a trauma-related nightmare. They also are liable to exhibit hyper-vigilance, exaggerated startle response and restlessness.

Learning Difficulties

Physiological hyperarousal interferes with the capacity to concentrate and to learn from experience. Aside from amnesias about aspects of the trauma traumatized people often they have trouble remembering ordinary events, as well. Easily triggered into hyperarousal by trauma-related stimuli, and beset with difficulties paying attention, they may display symptoms of attention deficit disorder. After a traumatic experience, people often loose some maturational achievements and regress to earlier modes of coping with stress. In children, this may show up as an inability to take care of themselves in such areas as feeding and toilet training; in adults, it is expressed in excessive dependence and in a loss of capacity to make thoughtful, autonomous decisions.

Memory Disturbances and Dissociation

Increased autonomic arousal not only interferes with psychological comfort, anxiety itself also may trigger memories of previous traumatic experiences. The administration of lactate, which stimulates the physiological arousal system, elicits flashbacks and panic attacks in people with PTSD. Yohimbine injections (which stimulate NE release from the Locus Coeruleus) are able to induce flashbacks in Vietnam veterans with PTSD. Any arousing situation may trigger memories of long-ago traumatic experiences and precipitate reactions that are irrelevant to present demands (see van der Kolk & Fisler, 1994).

In addition to hypermnesia and intrusive memories, chronically traumatized people, particularly children may develop amnestic syndromes related to the traumatic event. During the stage of life that children, in a stage-appropriate way, try on different identities in their daily play activities, children who are exposed to prolonged and severe trauma may be capable of organizing whole personality fragments in order to cope with traumatic experiences. In the long term, this may give rise to the syndrome of Dissociative Identity Disorder, which may occurs in about 4% of psychiatric inpatients in the USA (Saxe et al, 1993).

Patients who have learned to dissociate in response to trauma are likely to continue to utilize dissociative defenses when exposed to new stresses. They develop amnesia for some experiences, and tend to react with fight or flight responses to feeling threatened, neither of which may be consciously remembered afterwards. People who suffer from dissociative disorders are a clinical challenge, including helping them acquire a sense of personal responsibility for both their actions and reactions, while forensically, they are a nightmare.

Aggression Against Self and Others

Numerous studies have demonstrated that both adults and children who have been traumatized are likely to turn their aggression against others or themselves. Being abused as a child sharply increases the risk for later delinquency and violent criminal behavior. In one study of 87 psychiatric outpatients (van der Kolk et al., 1991) we found that self-mutilators invariably had severe childhood histories of abuse and/or neglect. There is good evidence that self-mutilative behavior is related to endogenous opioid changes in the CNS secondary to early traumatization. Problems with aggression against others have been particularly well documented in war veterans, traumatized children and in prisoners with histories of early trauma.

Psychosomatic Reactions

Chronic anxiety and emotional numbing also get in the way of learning to identify and articulate internal states and wishes (Pennebaker, 1993). People traumatized as children frequently suffer from alexithymia - an inability to translate somatic sensations into basic feelings, such as anger, happiness or fear. This failure to translate somatic states into words and symbols causes them to experience emotions simply as physical problems. This naturally plays havoc with intimate and trusting interpersonal communications. These people have somatization disorders and relate to the world through their bodies. They experience distress in terms of physical organs, rather than as psychological states (Saxe et al., 1994).

Developmental Level Affects the Behavioral and Biological Concomitants of Trauma

Over the past thirty years people have slowly started to unravel the differential effects of trauma at various age levels. Modern psychiatry has begun to reconsider the ways in which failure of attachment and traumatic separation affect the developing organism. Bowlby (1969) has emphasized that attachment behavior is first of all a vital biological function, indispensable for both reproduction and survival. A rapidly expanding body of research has shown that disturbances of childhood attachment bonds can have long term neurobiological consequences. In addition to the disturbances in affect regulation, a large variety of studies, both in animals and in humans, have shown that childhood abuse, neglect, and separation have far-reaching biopsycho-social effects, including lasting biological changes which affect the capacity to modulate emotions, difficulty in learning new coping skills, alterations in immune competency, and impairment in capacity the to engage in meaningful social affiliation. Aided by work on other animal species, a voluminous research literature on the effects of childhood physical and sexual abuse, and the Field Trials for the DSM IV, it has become understood that there are critical stages in the development of the CNS that make children particularly vulnerable to develop lasting disturbances secondary to abuse, neglect and separation. Aware of the fact that trauma at an early age has profound effects on affect regulation, levels of consciousness, tendency to organize experience on a somatic level, and to make characterological adaptations to chronic exposure to danger and fear, the DSM IV PTSD committee recommended an expanded definition of PTSD for inclusion in the DSM IV. The DSM IV classification system now recognizes the pervasive effects of trauma on the totality of a person's personality functioning in its new section on "associated features". Table 2 shows the features of the associated features of PTSD in the DSM IV.

TABLE 2
COMPLICATED PTSD.

I. Alteration in Regulation of Affect and Impulses

   A. Affect Regulation   D. Suicidal Preoccupation
   B. Modulation of Anger   E. Difficulty Modulating Sexual involvement
   C. Self-Destructive   F. Excessive Risk taking

II. Alterations in Attention or Consciousness

   A. Amnesia
   B. Transient Dissociative Episodes and Depersonalization

III. Somatization

   A. Digestive System   D. Conversion Symptoms
   B. Chronic Pain   E. Sexual Symptoms
   C. Cardiopulmonary Symptoms

IV. Alterations in Self-Perception

   A. Ineffectiveness   D. Shame
   B. Permanent Damage   E. Nobody Can Understand
   C. Guilt and Responsibility   F. Minimizing

V. Alterations in Perception of the Perpetrator

   A. Adopting Distorted Beliefs
   B. Idealization of the Perpetrator
   C. Preoccupation with Hurting Perpetrator

VI. Alterations in Relations with Others

   A. Inability to Trust
   B. Re-victimization
   C. Victimizing Others

VII. Alterations in Systems of Meaning

   A. Despair and Hopelessness
   B. Loss of Previously Sustaining Beliefs

Principles of Treatment

The treatment of PTSD has three principal components: 1) processing and coming to terms with the horrifying, overwhelming experience, 2) controlling and mastering physiological and biological stress reactions, 3) re-establishing secure social connections and interpersonal efficacy.

The aim of these therapies is to help the traumatized individual to move from being dominated and haunted by the past to being present in the here and now, capable of responding to current exigencies with his or her fullest potential. Thus, the trauma needs to be placed in the larger perspective of a person's life, as a relatively isolated historical event, or series of events, that occurred at a particular time, and in a particular place, and that can be expected to not recur if the traumatized individual takes charge of his or her life. Tragically, many traumatized people are involved in situations of ongoing trauma, in which they have little or no personal control over what happens to them. However, even under those circumstances, learning how to properly assess what is going on and planning one's responses, possibly in collaboration with other people, still can be expected to have significant psychological benefits.

Acute trauma

Immediately after the trauma, the emphasis needs to be on self-regulation and on rebuilding. This means the re-establishment of a sense of security and predictability, and active engagement in adaptive action. Only a limited proportion of people who are traumatized develop PTSD. Most traumatized people seem to be able to successfully negotiate these initial adaptive phases without succumbing to the long term progression of their acute stress reaction into PTSD. For them, the trauma becomes merely a terrible experience that happened to them some time in their past. It is quite unclear whether talking about what has happened is always useful in preventing the development of PTSD. Some surprising findings have come out of careful Critical Incidence Stress Debriefing research: the few controlled studies that have examined the preventative effect of debriefing immediately following exposure to a traumatic event have suggested a poorer outcome following debriefing as compared with no intervention (McFarlane, 1994). Give the paucity of controlled studies, we are left with the clinical impression that the initial response to trauma consists of reconnecting with ordinary supportive networks, and of engaging activities that re-establish a sense of mastery. It is obvious that the role of mental health professionals in these initial recuperative efforts is quite limited.

The Need for Phase Oriented Treatment

Trauma needs to be treated differently at different phases of people's lives following the trauma, and at the different stages of the disorder PTSD. Treatments that may be effective at some stages of treatment might not be effective at others. For example, on a pharmacological level, initial management with drugs that decrease autonomic arousal will decrease nightmares and flashback, promote sleep, and are likely to prevent the kindling effects that are thought to underlie the long-term establishment of PTSD symptomatology. These same drugs, once the Disorder has been established have, at best, a palliative function, and serotonin re-uptake blockers, which seem to have little immediate benefit, can be immensely helpful in allowing people to attend to current asks, and not to dwell on past fears, interpretations, and fixations. In this context, it is interesting to note that Foa et al. (1991) found that in the initial stages of treatment of rape victims Stress Inoculation Training turned out to be as effective a treatment of PTSD as was Prolonged Imaginal Exposure. However, on follow-up, imaginal flooding had superior results to stress inoculation. If there are differential effects of therapeutic modalities within a four month time frame, it is likely that there would be differential effects over longer time spans. It is likely that some forms of therapy might be effective at some stages, but have negative outcomes at other phases of the illness. Another instance is abreaction. It appears that abreaction as a treatment is most effective early in the course of the illness, and that its effectiveness decreases over time. For example, exposure therapy using "flooding" techniques have been found to worsen the symptoms of some patients, particularly in those in whom the focal trauma was decades earlier (Pitman et al., 1991). When intrusions of fragments of the trauma are the predominant symptom, exposure and desensitization may be what is most required. At a later stage of the progression of the disorder, when people have organized their entire lives around avoidance of triggers of the trauma, and approach other people as potential triggers of traumatic intrusions, helplessness, suspicion, anger, and interpersonal problems may dominate the symptom picture. When that is the case, primary attention needs to be paid to stabilization in the social realm.

Psychotherapeutic Interventions

The key element of the psychotherapy of people with PTSD—as perhaps for all psychotherapy—is the integration of the alien, the unacceptable, the terrifying, the incomprehensible. Life events initially experienced as alien, as if imposed from outside upon passive victims, must come to be "personalized" affectively as integrated aspects of one's history and life experiences (van der Kolk & Ducey, 1989). The massive defenses, initially established as emergency protective measures, must gradually relax their grip upon the psyche, so that dissociated aspects of experience do not continue to intrude into one's life experience and thereby threaten to re-traumatize an already traumatized victim.

Psychotherapy must address two fundamental aspects of PTSD: the deconditioning of anxiety, and the pervasive effects that trauma has on the way victims views themselves and the world. In only the simplest cases will it be sufficient to decondition the anxiety associated with the trauma. In the vast majority of patients, both aspects will have to be treated, which means the use of a combination of procedures for deconditioning anxiety, for changing beliefs, and for developing a cognitive system that somehow allows a person to continue to cope effectively in a world that now is known to be capable of great destructiveness (Epstein, 1991).

1) Stabilization. In the treatment of simple cases of PTSD, it is perhaps possible to move quickly, to activating the traumatic memory. In more complex cases, it should be part of a more encompassing treatment model, which must include careful preparation, with an eye on providing the patient with a capacity to feel safe while accessing traumatic material (e.g. Brown & Fromm, 1986). For the past century, psychotherapeutic clinicians have basically adopted a phase-oriented model that consists of (1) reintegration and rehabilitation (cf. van der Hart, Brown & van der Kolk, 1989; Herman, 1992). In the first phase the foundation is laid that enables patient to deal with the challenge of confronting the trauma. The patient is helped with establishing more stability and safety in daily life, including social support, stress inoculation, ways of controlling symptoms and ways of containing intrusive memories (e.g. van der Hart et al., 1993). Psychopharmacological management often is an integral part of stabilization.

2) The identification of feelings by verbalizing somatic states. The function of emotions is to alert people to the occurrence, significance, and nature of subjectively significant events (Krystal, 1978) Ordinarily, emotions are de-activated when schemes and situations have been realigned (e.g., by taking action that conforms situations to schemes, or by amending schemes to better fit situations) (Horowitz, 1986). Thus, emotions function as signals to readjust one's expectations of the world and to take adaptive action. Krystal (1978) first noted that in people with PTSD emotions seem to loose much of their alerting function: a dissociation is set up between emotional arousal and goal directed action. Traumatized people loose their capacity to interpret the meaning of their emotional arousal, which thus becomes irrelevant is a current signal. Unable to interpret the meaning of their emotional arousal, feelings themselves become endowed with a negative valence: because no release can be found in adaptive action, emotions merely become reminders of one's inability to affect the outcome of one's life. Hence, aside from the concrete, usually visual, reminders of the trauma, feelings in general come to be experienced as traumatic reminders, and are to be avoided (van der Kolk & Ducey, 1989).

Unable to neutralize affects with adaptive action, traumatized people tend to experience their affects as somatic states: either through their smooth, or striated musculature. Thus, people with PTSD tend to somatize (Saxe et al, 1994,) or to discharge their emotions with actions that are irrelevant to the stimulus that precipitated the emotion: with aggressive actions against self or others (van der Kolk et al ,1991). When the disorganizing intrusions can be understood as failures of integration of traumatic experiences into the totality of one's life, the psychotherapist is in a position to recognize seemingly overwhelming affective experiences as actual reliving of past terror. One's natural proclivity in psychotherapy is to help the patient avoid experiencing undue pain; yet the patient's affective experiences are part and parcel of healing and integration. The psychotherapist who understands the nature of trauma can aid the process of integration by staying with the patient through his suffering, by providing a perspective that the suffering is meaningful and bearable, and by helping in the mastery of trauma through putting the experience into symbolic, communicable form, such as words, thoughts, and feelings. The patient's "repeating" the trauma in action is the forerunner to his "remembering" and symbolizing it in words, which in turn is the precursor accompaniment to his "working it through" in emotional experience

3) Deconditioning of traumatic memories and responses. This consists of: (a) controlled activation of the traumatic memories, and (b) corrections of faulty traumatic beliefs. The critical issue is to introduce the capacity to flexibly remember the trauma. In order for this to occur, some new information that is incompatible to the traumatic memory must be introduced (Foa et al., 1989). The most important new information is probably the fact that the patient is able to confront the traumatic memory by a trusted therapist in a safe environment (van der Hart & Spiegel, 1993). In order to help the patient regulate emotional arousal, secure attachment may be even more important than evoking the traumatic memories. Therefore, it is important for the patient to establish and maintain an emotional connection with the therapist. While behavioral therapists speak about exposure-procedures, which are either systematic desensitization procedures or implosive therapy or flooding procedures, they neglect to write about the intensely personal element in all psychotherapeutic procedures, which is a critical element in the success of effective treatment. So, while these clinicians and researchers almost exclusively present their data about decreases of fear or anxiety through controlled exposure to (a) the stimulus components (environmental cues), (b) the response components (e.g. motoric actions, heart pounding), and the meaning elements (e.g. cues regarding morality and guilt) of the traumatic memory (Foa & Kozack, 1986; Foa et al., 1989; Lidz & Keane, 1986), their results are most likely heavily affected by their personal investment in the well-being of their patients, which is communicated and translated into a subjective sense of safety.

According to Foa & Kozak (1985) two conditions are required for anxiety reduction in the treatment of PTSD: 1) a person must attend to fear-relevant information in a manner that will activate his/her own fear memory. As long as the fear is not experienced, the fear structure cannot be modified. 2) in order to form a new, non-fear structure, some of the information that evoked the fear must be absent in the new context in which the fear is being provoked. Exposure to information consistent with a fear memory would be expected to strengthen the fear (i.e., sensitize and thereby increase the likelihood of developing PTSD). Hence the critical issue in treatment is to expose the patient to an experience that contains elements that are sufficiently similar to an existing traumatic memory in order to activate it, and at the same time for it to be an experience that contains aspects that are incompatible enough to change it (for example experiencing a traumatic memory in a safe and controllable environment, being able to evoke a traumatic image, without feeling overwhelmed by the associated emotions).

There are at least two significant problems with this exposure technique: 1) Because excessive arousal interferes with the acquisition of new information, excessive arousal impedes habituation (Strian & Klicpera, 1978). When that occurs, the fear structure will not be corrected, but instead, will be confirmed: instead of promoting habituation, it accidentally fosters sensitization. 2) An additional serious obstacle to effective treatment is that the strong response elements in the PTSD structure may promote avoidance: strong fear and discomfort motivates people who suffer from PTSD to avoid or escape confrontation with situations that remind him/her of the trauma, in order to overcome the intrusive, sensorimotor elements of the trauma, a person must transform the traumatic (non-verbal) memory into a personal narrative, in which the trauma is experienced as a historical event that is part of a person's autobiography. This entails being able to tell the story of the shocking event without reexperiencing it. It is generally assumed that once all relevant elements of the total traumatic experience have been identified and thoroughly and deeply examined and experienced in the therapy, successful synthesis will take place. The work by Resick & Schnicke (1992) supports the notion that exposure of all elements of the trauma, and their associated shifts in perception of self and others does lead to successful resolution of trauma-related symptomatology.

4) Restructuring of trauma-related schemes of internal and external reality. Apart from treatment needing to address specific trauma-related memories, and fostering de-conditioning, treatment needs to address the effects of the trauma on people's perceptions of themselves, and the world around them. People are meaning-making creatures. As we develop we organize our world according to a personal theory of reality, some of which may be conscious, but much of which is an unconscious integration of accumulated experience. These mental schemes organize psychological experience via the process of assimilation and accommodation and assure continuity of one's identity (Horowitz, 1991). Although most people cannot clearly articulate the content of their mental schemes, they nonetheless determine what sensory input is selected for further coding and categorization. Adaptive resolution to a stressful experience consists of the modification, or accommodation one's view

of self and others that permits adaptive action and continued attention to the exigencies of daily life. In order to successfully deal with a distressing experience, it is necessary to not generalize from that experience to the totality of existence, but to view it merely one terrible event that has taken place at a particular place at a particular time (Epstein , 1991).

Traumatic experiences, i.e. experiences that do not fit into people's personal schemes, may be assimilated (directly taken in) ("That never happened." "I caused it to happen."), or people may accommodate to the experience by altering their conceptions of the world ("There is no safe place." "This happened because people are out to hurt me.")(Resick & Schnicke,1992, Hollon and Garber,1988).

Traumatic experiences are not only processed by means of currently existing mental schemes, but they may also activate latent self-concepts and views of relationships that were formed earlier in life. This activation of latent schemes is particularly relevant for people with prior histories of trauma, even in those who subsequently have been able to make a successful adaptation. When trauma activates these earlier self-schemes, these will compete and co-exist with more mature schemes in explaining cause and effect relationships in regards to the trauma. These different, and often competing mental schemes then will determine the psychological organization of the traumatic experience.

Psychotherapy needs to specifically address how the trauma has affected people's sense of self-efficacy, their capacity for trust and intimacy, their ability to negotiate their personal needs, and their ability to feel empathy for other people (McCann & Pearlman, 1990).

5) Exposure to restitutive experiences. Considering the fact that the central psychological preoccupation of traumatized people is either the reliving or the warding off of the memory of the trauma, there is little room for new, gratifying experiences which might allow for reparation of past injuries to the self. Patients need to actively expose themselves to experiences that provide them with feelings of mastery and pleasure. Engagement in physical activities, such as sports or wilderness ventures, gratifying physical experiences, such as massages, or artistic accomplishments may be experiences that patients build up that are not contaminated by the trauma, and which may serve as a core of new gratifying experiences.

Group Psychotherapy

Emotional attachment is the primary protection against being traumatized: people have always gathered in communities and organizations to help them deal with outside challenges: we seek close emotional relationships with others in order to help us anticipate, meet and integrate difficult experiences. Contemporary research (e.g. Quanterelli, 1985; Holen, 1990) has shown that as long as the social support network remains intact, people are relatively well protected against even catastrophic stresses. For young children, the family usually is a very effective source of protection against traumatization, and most children are amazingly resilient as long as they have a care giver who is emotionally and physically available (Wender, 1989; van der Kolk, Perry & Herman, 1991, McFarlane, 1988). Mature people also rely on their families, colleagues and friends to provide such a trauma membrane. In recognition of this need for affiliation as a protection against trauma, it has become widely accepted that the central issue in acute crisis intervention is the provision and restoration of social support (Lystad, 1988; Raphael, 1986; Mitchell ,1983). However, curiously, research has not supported the efficacy of standardized Stress Debriefing interventions following trauma.

The task of group therapy and community interventions is to help victims regain a sense of safety and of mastery. After an acute trauma, fellow victims often provide the most effective short-term bond because the shared history of trauma can form the nucleus of retrieving a sense of communality.

Regardless of the nature of the trauma, or the structure of the group, the aim of group therapy is to help people actively attend to the requirements of the moment, without undue intrusions from past perceptions and experiences. Group therapy is widely regarded as a treatment of choice for patients with trauma histories. It has been used for victims of interpersonal violence (Mitchell, 1983) natural disasters (Lystad, 1988; Raphael, 1986), childhood sexual abuse (Herman & Shatzow ,1987, Ganzarian & Buchele, 1987; Schacht et al, 1990), rape (Yassen & Glass, 1984), spouse battering (Rounsaville et al, 1979), concentration camps (Danielli, 1985) and war trauma (Parson, 1985). In a group of people who have gone through similar experiences, most traumatized people eventually are able to find the appropriate words to express what has happened to them. As was observed almost fifty years ago: "by working out their problems in a small group they should be able to face the larger group, i.e., their world, in an easier manner" (Grinker & Spiegel, 1946).

There are many levels of trauma-related group psychotherapies, with different degrees of emphasis on stabilization, memory retrieval, bonding, negotiation of interpersonal differences, and support. However, to varying degrees, the purpose of all trauma related groups is to 1) stabilize psychological and physiological reactions to the trauma, 2) to explore and validate perceptions and emotions, 3) to retrieve memories, 4) to understand the effects of past experience on current affects and behaviors and 5) to learn new ways of coping with interpersonal stress (see van der Kolk, 1992) .

Psychopharmacological Treatment

While it is widely recognized that PTSD is a "physioneurosis", i.e. that it is based on psychological manifestations of biological changes, systematic psycho-pharmacological studies of PTSD are scarce and almost entirely limited to tricyclic antidepressants and MAO inhibitors. As of July, 1994, a total of only 134 patients with PTSD had been studied in double-blind placebo controlled studies. The treatment effects of the psychotropic agents examined in these systematic studies have been quite modest (Davidson, 1992). In addition, in open studies and clinical reports, usefulness has been claimed for benzodiazepines, lithium carbonate, carbamazepine, clonidine and beta adrenergic blockers (van der Kolk, 1987; Davidson, 1988; Friedman, 1988), but their efficacy has not been confirmed in double-blind, placebo controlled studies.

Three double-blind trials of tricyclic antidepressants have been published (Frank et al., 1988; Kosten et al., 1991; Davisdon et al., 1990; Reist et al., 1989), two of which demonstrated some improvement in PTSD symptoms (Frank et al., 1988; Kosten et al., 1991; Davidson et al., 1990). Davidson et al (1990), studying in-patient and out-patient veterans of World War II and Vietnam, showed that amitriptyline caused a decrease in overall PTSD, primarily by decreasing avoidant symptoms. In two reports of essentially the same sample, Frank et al. (1988), Kosten et al. (1991) and their collaborators found that imipramine was more effective than placebo in out-patient Vietnam veterans, particularly decreasing intrusive symptoms. On the other hand, Reist et al (1989) found no significant difference between desipramine and placebo in a four week crossover trial. All three studies report a lack of placebo response in war veterans with chronic PTSD.

Phenelzine sulfate has been used in two double-blind trials, with a total of 40 subjects. One study was positive (Frank et al., 1988; Kosten et al., 1991) showing improvement in intrusive symptoms of PTSD, without significant effect on avoidant symptoms. The other failed to demonstrate a positive effect of phenelzine on PTSD symptoms in a mixed civilian/combat veteran population (Shetatsky, 1988).

During the past few years evidence has accumulated that the serotonin reuptake blockers are likely to be the most effective drugs in the treatment of *chronic* PTSD (e.g. Davidson et al., 1991; March, 1992; Nagy et al., 1993). In our own studies (van der Kolk et al 1994) we were able to show that fluoxetine can have profound effects on numbing arousal, and, to a lesser degree, on intrusions. Fluoxetine had a significant positive effect on the dimensions of affect dysregulation, distorted relationships with others and loss of sustaining beliefs. Positive effects became evident after five weeks on active drug was sufficient to demonstrate significant improvement Fluoxetine was not only effective in alleviating the core symptoms of PTSD, but also the associated features: affect dysregulation, distorted relationships with others and loss of sustaining beliefs. Our study showed that the beneficial effect of fluoxetine on PTSD is not a function of its antidepressant effects, but, instead, by making people with PTSD feel less numb and more in tune with their surroundings, fluoxetine is likely to make them feel better equipped to deal with residual trauma-related fears, recollections and intrusions.

The efficacy of this serotonin reuptake blocker on PTSD symptomatology raises intriguing questions about the possible role of serotonin in the psychopathology of PTSD. The increased availability of serotonin in the hippocampus may activate inhibitory pathways in the limbic system that prevent the initiation of habitual emergency responses (van der Kolk, 1994). Animal research has shown that serotonin receptor blockers reverse the suppression of fear-induced behavior, probably because an increase in available serotonin in the limbic system amplifies the signals necessary to distinguish punishment from reward (Gray, 1988)

Concluding Remarks

After a trauma which fully confronts people with their existential helplessness and vulnerability, life can never be exactly the same: the traumatic experience will somehow become part of a person's life. Sorting out exactly what happened and sharing one's reactions with others can make a great deal of difference in one's eventual adaptation. Putting the feelings and cognitions related to the trauma into words is essential in the treatment of post traumatic reactions. After intense efforts to ward off reliving the trauma, therapists cannot expect that the resistances to remember will suddenly melt away under their empathic efforts. The trauma can only be worked through when a secure bond is established with another person; this then can be utilized to hold the psyche together when the threat of physical disintegration is re-experienced.

Failure to approach trauma related material gradually is likely to lead to intensification of posttraumatic symptomatology, leading to increased somatic, visual or behavioral reexperiences. Once the traumatic experiences have been located in time and place, a person can start making distinctions between current life stresses and past trauma, and decrease the impact of the trauma on present experience. Talking about the trauma is not enough: trauma survivors need to take some action that symbolizes triumph over helplessness and despair. The Holocaust Memorial Yad Vashem in Jerusalem and the Vietnam Memorial in Washington, DC, are good examples of symbols for survivors to mourn the dead and establish the historical and cultural meaning of the traumatic events. Most of all, they serve to remind survivors of the ongoing potential for communality and sharing. This also applies to other survivors who may have to build less visible memorials and common symbols around which they can gather to mourn and express their shame about their own vulnerability. This may take the form of writing a book, taking political action, helping other victims, or any of the myriad of creative solutions that human beings can find to defy even the most desperate plight.

References

Bowlby, J. (1969). Attachment and loss: Vol. 1. Attachment. New York: Basic Books.
Bremner, J.D., Steinberg, M., Southwick, S.M., et al. (1993). Use of the structured clinical interview for DSM-IV dissociative disorders for systematic assessment of dissociative symptoms in posttraumatic stress disorder. American Journal of Psychiatry, 150, 1011-1014.
Breslau, N., Davis, G.C., & Andreski, P. (1991). Traumatic events and post traumatic stress disorder in an urban population of young adults. Archives of General Psychiatry, 48, 216-222.
Brown & Fromm. (1986). Hypnoanalysis and hypnotherapy. Hillsdale, NY: Lawrence Erlbaum Associates.
Danielli, Y. (1985). The treatment and prevention of long-term effects and intergenerational transmission of victimization: A lesson from holocaust survivors and their children. In C.R. Figley (Ed.), Trauma and Its Wake (Vol. 1). New York: Brunner/Mazel.
Davidson, J.R.T. (1992). Drug therapy of post traumatic stress disorder. British Journal of Psychiatry, 160, 309-314.
Davidson, J.R.T., Nemeroff, C.B. (1989). Pharmacotherapy in PTSD: Historical and clinical considerations and future directions. Psychopharmacology Bulletin, 25, 422-425.
Davidson, J.R.T., Kudler, H., Smith, R., Mahorney, S., Lipper, S., Hammett, E., Saunders, W., & Cavenar, J.O. (1990). Treatment of post-traumatic stress disorder with amitryptilene and placebo. Archives of General Psychiatry, 47, 259-266.
Davidson, J.R.T., Roth, S., & Newman, E. (1991). Treatment of post-traumatic stress disorder with fluoxetine. Journal of Traumatic Stress, 4, 419-423.
Epstein, S. (1991). The self-concept, the traumatic neurosis, and the structure of personality. In D. Ozer, J.M. Healy, Jr., & A.J. Stewart (Eds.), Perspectives in personality (Vol. 3, Part A, pp. 63-98). London: Jessica Kingsley.
Foa, E.B. & Kozak, M.J. (1985). Treatment of anxiety disorders: Implications for psychopathology. In A.H. Tuma & J.D. Maser (Eds.), Anxiety and Anxiety Disorders. Hillsdale, NY: Lawrence Erlbaum Associates.
Foa, E.B., & Kozak, M.J. (1986). Emotional processing of fear: Exposure to corrective information. Psychological Bulletin, 99, 20-35.
Foa, E.B., Steketee, G. & Olasov, B.R. (1989). Behavioral/cognitive conceptualizations of post-traumatic stress disorder. Behavior Therapy, 20, 155-176.

Foa, F., Rothbaum, B. O., Riggs, D. S., & Murdock, G. B. (1991). Treatment of post traumatic stress disorder in rape victims: Comparison between cognitive behavioral procedures and counseling. <u>Journal of Consulting and Clinical Psychology, 59</u>, 715-725.

Frank, J.B., Kosten, T.R., Giller, E.L., & Dan, E. (1988). A preliminary study of phenelzine and imipramine for post-traumatic stress disorder. <u>American Journal of Psychiatry, 145</u>, 1289-1291

Freud, S. (1959). Formulations on the two principles of mental functioning. In J. Strachey (Ed. and Trans.), <u>Complete psychological works, standard edition</u> (Vol. 12). London: Hogarth Press. (Original work published 1911)

Friedman, M. (1988). Toward rational pharmacotherapy of post traumatic stress disorder. <u>American Journal of Psychiatry, 145</u>, 281-285.

Ganzarain, R. & Buchele, B. (1987). Acting out during group psychotherapy for incest. <u>International Journal of Group Psychotherapy, 37</u>, 185-200.

Gray, J. (1988). <u>The psychology of fear and stress</u> (2nd ed.). Cambridge: Cambridge University Press.

Grinker, R., & Spiegel, H. (1946). <u>Men under Stress</u>. New York: Basic Books.

Heltzer, J.E., Robins, L.N., & McEvoy, L. (1987). Post-traumatic stress disorder in the general population. <u>New England Journal of Medicine, 317</u>(26), 1630-1634.

Herman, J.L. (1992). <u>Truama and recovery</u>. New York: Basic Books.

Herman, J.L. & Schatzow, E. (1987). Recovery and verification of memories of childrehood sexual trauma. <u>Psychoanalytic Psychology, 4</u>(1), 1-14.

Holen, A. (1990). <u>A long term study of survivors from a disaster</u>. Oslo: University of Oslo Press.

Hollon, S.D., & Garber, J. (1988). Cognitive therapy. In L.Y. Abrahamson (Ed.), <u>Social cognition and clinical psychology: A synthesis</u> (pp. 204-253). New York: Guilford Press.

Horowitz, M.J. (1991). <u>Person schemas and maladaptive interpersonal patterns</u>. Chicago: University of Chicago Press.

Horowitz, M.J. (1986). <u>Stress response syndromes</u> (2nd ed.). Northvale, NJ: Aronson.

Janet, P. (1889). <u>L'Automatisme psychologique</u>. Paris: Alcan.

Janet, P. (1904). L'amnesie at la dissociation des souvenirs par l'emotion. <u>Journal de Psychologie</u>, 1, 417-453.

Kardiner, A. (1941). <u>The traumatic neuroses of war</u>. New York: Hoeber.

Kosten, T.R., Frank, J.B., Dan, E., McDougle, C.J., & Giller, E.L. (1991). Pharmacotherapy for post traumatic stress disorder using penelzine and imipramine. <u>Journal of Nervous and Mental Disorders, 179</u>, 366-370.

Krystal, H. (1978). Trauma and Affects. <u>Psychoanalytic Study of Children, 33</u>, 81-116.

Kulka, R.A., Schlenger, W., & Fairbank, J. (1990). Trauma and the Vietnam war generation. New York: Brunner/Mazel.

Laub, D., & Auerhahn, N.C. (1993). Knowing and not knowing massive psychic trauma: Forms of traumatic memory. International Journal of Psychoanalysis, 74, 287-301.

Lidz, B.T., & Keane, T.M. (1989). Information processing in anxiety disorders: Application to the understanding of post-traumatic stress disorder. Clinical Psychology Review, 9, 243-257.

Lystad, M. (1988). Mental health response to mass emergencies. New York: Brunner/Mazel.

March, J. (1992). Fluoxetine and flovoxamine in PTSD [Letter to the editor]. American Journal of Psychiatry, 149, 413.

Marmar, C.R., Weiss, D.S., Schlenger, W.E., et al. (1994). Peritraumtic dissociation and post-traumatic stress in male Vietnam theater veterans. American Journal of Psychiatry, 151, 902-907.

McCann, I.L., & Pearlman, L.A. (1990). Psychological trauma and the adult survivor: Theory, therapy, and transformation. New York: Brunner/Mazel.

McFarlane, A.C. (1988). Recent life events and psychiatric disorder in children: The interaction with preceding extreme adversity. Journal of Clinical Psychiatry, 29(5), 677-690.

McFarlane, A.C. (1994). Individual psychotherapy for post-traumatic stress disorder. Psychiatric Clinics of North America, 17(2), 393-408.

Mitchell, J. (1983). The critical incident stress debriefing. Journal of Emergency Medical Services, 8, 36-39.

Nagy, L.M., Morgan, C.A., Southwick, S.M., & Charney, D.S. (1993). Open prospective trial of fluoxetine for post traumatic stress disorder. Journal of Clinical Psychopharmacology, 13, 107-114.

Parson, E.R. (1988). Post traumatic accelerated cohesion: Its recognition and management in group treatment of vietnam veterans, Group, 9(4), 10-23.

Pennebaker, J.W. (1993). Putting stress into words: Health, linguistic, and therapeutic implications. Behav. Res. Therapy, 31(6), 539-548.

Pitman, R.K., Altman, B., Greenwald, E., Longpre, R.E., Macklin, M.L., Poire, R.E., & Steketee, G.S. (1991). Psychiatric complications during flooding therapy for posttraumatic stress disorder. Journal of Clinical Psychiatry, 52(1), 17-20.

Quarantelli, E.L. (1985). An assessment of conflicting views on mental health: The consequences of traumatic events. In C.R. Figley (Ed.), Trauma and Its Wake (Vol. 1). New York: Brunner/Mazel.

Raphael, B. (1986). When disaster strikes: How individuals and communities cope with catastrophe. New York: Basic Books.

Rauch, S., van der Kolk, B.A., Fisler, R., Alpert, N., Orr, S., Savage, C., Jenike, M., & Pitman, R. (in press). A symptom provocation study using Positron Emission Tomography and Script Driven Imagery. Archives of General Psychiatry.

Reist, C., Kaufman, C.D., & Haier, R.J. (1989). A controlled trial of desipramine in 18 men with PTSD. American Journal of Psychiatty, 146, 513-516.

Resick, P.A., & Schnicke, M.K. (1992). Cognitive processing therapy for sexual assault victims. Journal of Consulting and Clinical Psychology, 60(5), 748-756.

Rounsaville, B., Lifton, N., & Bieber, M. (1979). The natural history of a psychotherapy group for battered women. Psychiatry, 42, 63-78.

Saxe, G., van der Kolk, B.A., Hall, K., Schwartz, J., Chinman, G., Hall, M.D., Lieberg, G., & Berkowitz, R. (1993). Dissociative disorders in psychiatric inpatients. American Journal of Psychiaty, 150(7), 1037-1042.

Saxe, G.N., Chinman, G., Berkowitz, R., Hall, K., Lieberg, G., Shcwartz, J., & van der Kolk, B.A. (1994). Somatization in patients with dissociative disorders. American Journal of Psychiatry, 151, 1329-1335.

Schacht, A., Kerlinsky, D., Carldon, C. (1990). Group therapy with sexually abused boys: Leadership, projective identification, and countertransference issues. International Journal of Group Psychotherapy, 40(4), 401-417.

Shetatsky, M., Greenberg, D., & Lerer, B. (1988). A controlled trial of phenelzine in post-traumatic stress disorder. Psychiatry Research, 24, 149-155.

Strian, F., Klicpera C. (1978). Die bedeuting psychoautotonomische reaktionen im entstehung und persistenz von angstzustanden. Nervenartzt, 49, 576-583.

van der Hart, O., Brown, P., & van der Kolk, B.A. (1989). Pierre Janet's treatment of posttraumatic stress. Journal of Traumatic Stress, 2,(4).

van der Hart, O., & Spiegel, D. (1993). Hypnotic assessment and treatment of trauma-induced psychoses: The early psychotherapy of H. Breukink and modern views. International Journal of Clinical and Experimental Hypnosis, 41, 191-209.

van der Hart, O., Steele, K., Boon, S., & Brown, P. (1993). The treatment of traumatic memories: Synthesis, realization, and integration. Dissociation, 6, 162-180.

van der Kolk, B.A. (1987). The drug treatment of post-traumatic stress disorder. Journal of Affective Disorders, 13, 203-213.

van der Kolk, B.A. (1992). Group psychotherapy with post traumatic stress disorders. In H. Kaplan & B. Sadock (Eds.), Comprehensive Group Psychotherapy (pp. 550-560). Williams & Wilkins.

van der Kolk, B.A. (1994). The body keeps the score: Memory and the evolving psychobiology of post traumatic stress. Harvard Review of Psychiatry, 1, 253-65.

van der Kolk, B.A., Dreyfuss, D., Berkowitz, R., Saxe, G., & Michaels, M. (1994, December). Fluoxetine in post traumatic stress. Journal of Clinical Psychiatry.

van der Kolk, B.A., & Ducey, C. (1984). Clinical implications of the Rorschoch in post-traumatic stress disorder. In B.A. van der Kolk (Ed.), Post-traumatic stress disorder: Psychological and biological sequelae (pp. 30-42). Washington, D.C: American Psychiatric Press

van der Kolk, B.A., & Ducey, C.P. (1989). The psychological processing of traumatic experience: Rorschach patterns in PTSD. Journal of Traumatic Stress, 2, 259-274.

van der Kolk, B.A., & Fisler, R. (1994). Childhood abuse & neglect and loss of self-regulation. Bulletin of Menninger Clinic 58:145-168.

van der Kolk, B.A., & Fisler, R. (1995, in press). Dissociation and the fragmentary nature of traumatic memories: Background and experiemental evidence. Journal of Traumatic Stress.

van der Kolk, B.A., Perry, J.C., & Herman, J.L. (1991). Childhood origins of self-destructie behavior. American Journal of Psychiatry , 148, 1665-1671.

Yassen, J., & Glass, L. (1984). Sexual assault survivor groups. Social Work, 37, 252-257.

STRATEGIES OF DISASTER INTERVENTION FOR CHILDREN AND ADOLESCENTS

Robert S. Pynoos, Armen Goenjian, Alan M. Steinberg
Trauma Psychiatry Service, Department of Psychiatry and Biobehavioral Sciences
University of California at Los Angeles, U.S.A.

Children are frequently victims of disasters and, until recently, little attention has been paid to their plight. This chapter presents recommendations for the design and implementation of school-based disaster-related mental health interventions for children and adolescents, their families, schools and communities. It proposes that three levels of organization are required for the implementation of such a public mental health disaster program, and recommends the use of a developmental model of traumatic stress to guide intervention strategies in addressing risks of psychological, interpersonal and developmental disturbances. Recommendations are made regarding strategies for the evaluation of primary and secondary preventive interventions and clinical mental health services. Public policy should make provision for the allocation of resources for disaster safety at schools and post-disaster services for children and adolescents.

Prevalence of Disasters and Childhood Exposures

Over the past two decades, natural disasters have taken the lives of 3 million people worldwide and adversely affected the lives of over 800 million more (Weisaeth, 1993). No epidemiological data exist on death or morbidity of children exposed to major disasters. However, in the United States, early access to affected children and their families after disaster is mandated as a public health measure by the Disaster Relief Act to "help preclude possible damaging physical or psychological effects" (U.S. Government, 1976).

Whereas the morbidity and mortality rates associated with natural disasters are decreasing in the more industrialized countries, in developing countries there is often widespread death, injury and destruction, with large numbers of affected child survivors (Pynoos, Goenjian, Tashjian et al., 1993; International Federation of Red Cross and Red Crescent Societies, 1993). Berz (1989) reported that, of 109 disasters occurring between 1960 and 1987, the 41 disasters that occurred in developing countries killed 758,000 people compared to 11,441 killed by 68 disasters that occurred in developed countries.

The rates and severity of children's exposures to specific traumatic experiences during natural or technological disasters are strongly influenced by socioeconomic factors (Breslau, Davis, Andreski & Peterson, 1991). For example, housing conditions, school building standards, advanced warning and evacuation plans, and disaster relief capabilities affect the rate at which children are injured or trapped, or witness injury or death to others. The UCLA Trauma Psychiatry Program has had extensive experience in implementing child mental health services, ranging from circumscribed disasters affecting school communities to major catastrophic disasters severely affecting an entire child population of a large region (Nader & Pynoos, 1993; Pynoos, Goenjian et al., 1993).

Disaster-Related Services for Children and Adolescents

A public health approach to disaster intervention requires an efficient means to access children and their families within an affected community or region. Whereas in the past in the United States, disaster services have been traditionally administered through county and city mental health agencies, there is a growing trend to centralize efforts at information gathering, screening, outreach, and intervention within the school setting (Bucker, Trickett & Corse, 1985). The UCLA Program has complimented the use of public schools with added intervention modules at private and religious schools. The school offers a familiar, non-stigmatizing setting for provision of disaster-related mental health services, increasing child, parent and teacher involvement, and facilitating the coordination of mental health and educational responses.

Figure 1

THREE LEVELS OF ORGANIZATION
1. Governmental and Social Institutions ▸ Educational, Health and Mental Health ▸ Public, Private and Volunteer 2. School Community 3. Intervention Teams

There are three levels of organization that are typically necessary as a prerequisite to implementing a post-disaster population-based intervention for children and adolescents (see Figure 1). Such interventions require a well-organized governmental response to mobilize educational, health, and mental health resources, including public, private, and volunteer. In the mental health care of children and adolescents, the most common conflicts to be resolved are those between educational, health and political institutions over their appropriate roles and authority, the allocation of resources including man-power, and the relative priorities of mental health and educational goals. Initiating a disaster response for children and adolescents often elicits intense protective responses over what is considered in their best interest. These responses need to be understood within the particular culture and bureaucratic structure of the affected area and pre-existing inter-agency and institutional conflicts. Proper attention to these issues both acutely and over time, is necessary to prevent individual or organizational resistance that would otherwise significantly obstruct or prematurely terminate even demonstrably successful intervention programs.

The second level of organization involves the school community. This includes administrators, teachers, school health personnel, support staff, parents and children, all of whom may have been affected in differing degrees by the disaster itself and by differing responsibilities and adversities in its aftermath. Assistance to school personnel and administrative staff is essential to restore the school community, an important component of children's recovery environment. For the first time, following the recent Northridge earthquake in California, the Los Angeles Unified School District implemented a program for debriefing and assistance for all school personnel concurrent with the implementation of a mental health program addressing the specific needs of students.

Special attention should be given to the disaster-related emotional needs of principals, whose cooperation is necessary to insure the participation of teachers and parents. For example, one of the first actions of the Armenian Earthquake Relief Society after the 1988 earthquake in Armenia, was to provide special services to principals in the earthquake zone, all of whom were severely traumatized by their earthquake experiences and the overwhelming losses in their schools (Goenjian, 1993). In situations where principals were bypassed, we have observed traumatic avoidance leading to abrupt post-trauma decisions that impede early efforts to assist teachers and students, and the creation within the school of an intolerant atmosphere of unrealistic expectations about recovery. Strategies for assisting principals include debriefing sessions and ongoing assistance with problem-solving. These sessions can be conducted among all principals within an affected area, among the principal and administrative staff within a given school, and with an individual principal.

Work with teachers begins with addressing their own disaster experiences and those of their families, especially children and elderly parents. Special attention must be given to teachers whose students were killed or badly injured during a disaster, or have suffered family losses, residential damage and dislocation and financial loss. Teachers must be assisted with the emotional demands created by a disrupted school environment, loss of their personal teaching materials, sometimes accumulated for years, changes in students' classroom behavior and academic performance and parent's intense interactions with school personnel and urgent requests for advice on managing children's post-disaster emotional and behavioral problems. At the same time, special outreach programs to provide educational and therapeutic interventions to parents are necessary to assist their recovery and to assure their continued cooperation in the care of their children.

The third level is the organization of intervention teams that will be responsible for sub-populations of children. Because intervention teams will include professionals and para-professionals with varying training and experience, there is a need to establish a training program that provides an overview of the importance of their individual contributions. For example, a para-professional who is responsible for outreach to students who are absent from school due to their or their family's traumatic reactions, is as critical to the overall success of the intervention program as expert clinicians who help children resolve intense intrusive images. In addition to providing expert training in issues of childhood trauma, all members of the intervention teams must be prepared for the realities of working in the disaster area as well as their own emotional reactions. For example, in Armenia, prior to engaging in field work, intervention teams were shown a videotape depicting the physical hardships of working in the earthquake zone and the condition of the victims.

The selection and monitoring of intervention team members should take into consideration their emotional capacity to work with severely traumatized children and their capacity to withstand post-disaster adversities. The monitoring of field workers in Armenia revealed a spectrum of problems. One clinician could not tolerate the distress exhibited by children, and systematically under-identified overt posttraumatic stress symptomatology. Another, an extremely sensitive clinician, overidentified with the survivors, and eventually chose to work outside the earthquake zone, characterizing it as a "massive graveyard." A third clinician exhibited continued morning nausea and vomiting prior to going to work with child survivors. Special monitoring, assistance, and, at times, substitution, are needed for members of the intervention team who are direct victims of the disaster, who face ongoing post-disaster adversities, and whose children have been badly affected.

A Public Mental Health Approach

Over the past decade, advances in our understanding of children's post-disaster reactions, the psychometric assessment of children, and strategies of intervention have paved the way for taking a public mental health approach to child populations affected by disaster (see Figure 2). The first step of such an approach is an assessment of the extent and nature of exposures and the degree of morbidity in the target population. This effort should be conducted in conjunction with provision of acute psychological assistance provided directly to children in their classrooms or alternative group settings. Rigorous, systematic and periodic screenings also permit identification of affected individual children or groups at risk, and monitoring of course of recovery. Sampling strategies should include schools from a spectrum of exposures, including degree of life-threatening experience, injury and mortality, and extent of damage to school, home and community. If possible, a comparison sample should be drawn from a similar child population outside the disaster zone.

Figure 2

A PUBLIC MENTAL HEALTH APPROACH

1. Risk Assessment
   Stratification of Interventions
   Monitoring Course of Recovery
   • Initial and Periodic Screening
     ▸ Exposure
     ▸ Psychological Distress
     ▸ Adversities
2. Provision of Information
   • Governmental Agencies
   • Relief Organizations
   • School
   • Intervention Teams

The initial screening should include basic exposure information about where they were and what happened to them and those around them. A general inquiry should be followed by specific questions about high risk experiences, for example, experiencing direct life-threat, being trapped or injured, witnessing injury, hearing screams of distress and seeing mutilated bodies, being separated from family members or caretakers, or injury or loss among family members. Additional exposure screening questions should address the child's subjective appraisal and associated emotional responses during the disaster. These exposure questions should be complemented with a brief evaluation of posttraumatic stress and grief reactions.

Such a procedure can be carried out with school-age children and adolescents with good reliability and validity. The screening of pre-school children remains more problematic, although methods to improve assessment procedures for this age group are under investigation. Children's self-reports should be supplemented with information from teachers and parents (Nader, Stuber & Pynoos, 1991). Such procedures have been implemented in areas of major disasters under extremely difficult circumstances, as in Armenia, where screenings were conducted in tents and make-shift schools, and in situations of ongoing warfare, as in the UNICEF program in the former Yugoslavia region. In addition to providing useful screening and triage information, the screening interview within the framework of psychological first-aid, can a serve a psycho-educational function with measurable benefit. Direct screening of children should be supplemented by information gathered through other public health efforts assessing disaster-related damage, ongoing health risks and disruption of community services.

A public health approach requires periodic screening to assess the course of recovery among children with different exposures. These later screenings should include additional assessments of the nature and frequency of traumatic reminders and secondary stresses and adversities faced by children and their families. Several disaster studies have suggested that longitudinal monitoring of children include additional self-report of depressive symptoms (Yule & Udwin, 1991; Goenjian, 1993). The use of continuous scales for evaluating posttraumatic stress and depressive reactions rather than categorical diagnostic classifications, may provide better information for risk assessment, stratification of interventions and monitoring course of recovery (Pynoos et al. 1993).

Sharing of information derived from screening interviews with governmental agencies can serve to promote judicious allocation of resources and support for appropriate intervention efforts. For example, in Armenia, the screening data was used by the government to assign resources to the most needy areas, and by philanthropic organizations to provide immediate housing to reunite families rather than to rebuild public buildings. In Croatia, additional screenings demonstrated the mental health advantage to war-traumatized children of their families living with a host family rather in multifamily resettlement camps or hotels (Hobfoll, 1991).

Sharing of information at the school level will contribute to an appreciation of the extent of psychological distress and adversities among the student body, the admixture of services that may be required, and the length of time to be expected for recovery of the students and the school community. Additional monitoring and renewed interventions may be prompted by school-related adversities such as school reconstruction, the occurrence of physical reminders such as aftershocks, high winds or heavy rains, and commemorative activities or anniversaries. This additional information can assist teachers and administrators to modify educational methods and goals to accommodate to these circumstances, and to provide appropriate supportive interventions.

The clinical intervention team can use the screening information to better define the most acutely at risk populations. This information can then be used to guide immediate case finding and outreach efforts. It also provides a basis for estimating the amount of classroom, family, group and individual work that may be required, including personnel requirements, planning the timing of interventions with different at risk groups, and selecting appropriate treatment techniques. Lastly, the intervention team can use these estimates to decide on the team's requirements for supervision and ongoing debriefing and group support. Ongoing monitoring contributes to the evaluation of the efficacy of interventions and permits prompt recognition of exacerbation due to unanticipated occurrences or intercurrent traumas or adversities. In addition, sharing of clinical information among the intervention team regarding the evolution of clinical themes, for example, towards grief-related themes, and in clinical profiles, for example, the intensification of intrusive images or depressive reactions, can alert team members to needed modifications in treatment approaches.

Finally, information regarding a child's disaster-related exposure, reminders and losses should included as a part of a permanent health or school record. Such a record can help prevent mislabelling later behavioral or emotional responses to future reminders or disaster-related adversities, and permit timely identification and intervention for renewed symptoms or subsequent academic, interpersonal or developmental disturbances.

The Developmental Model of Traumatic Stress: An Overview

The developmental model of traumatic stress (Pynoos, Steinberg, Wraith, in press) indicates how the interaction over time of many critical factors plays a role in the progression from traumatic exposure(s) to subsequent pathology. It attributes a tripartite etiology to traumatic distress that includes the child's objective and subjective disaster experience, the nature and frequency of traumatic reminders and the type and severity of secondary stresses. It emphasizes that outcome measures must extend beyond those of traditional physical health and psychiatric morbidity to include proximal and distal developmental disturbances, impact on emerging personality, changes in life trajectory and vulnerability to future life stresses. The ecology of the child's environment is conceptualized as pervasively interacting with the course and outcome of traumatic stress. The key concepts represent potential foci for primary and secondary prevention, intervention and treatment. The model also suggests the importance of early intervention to minimize traumatic distress, reduce the risk of psychiatric co-morbidity and chronicity, and promote normal developmental progression (see Figure 3).

Treatment Implications of the Developmental Model

The developmental model assigns a tripartite etiology to posttraumatic distress. An accurate characterization of the disaster experience includes the context in the child's life, objective features of the experience, the child's subjective appraisal of external and internal threats, coping strategies during the disaster to address the situation and to manage their own reaction and associated concerns. Such concerns can include worry about the safety of a significant other who may or may not be with the child, the experience of loss of a loved one, even as the life-threat continues, and reminders during the course of the event(s) of a prior trauma (Pynoos & Nader, 1988).

The nature of disaster experiences varies considerably across disasters and among children, even within the same disaster zone. An accurate characterization of the disaster-related experiences of the target child populations will contribute to the selection of intervention strategies and appropriate treatment modalities. Certain disasters may be associated with extreme levels of life-threat and witnessing of grotesque injury and death, and pervasive traumatic loss. For example, a ten year old

Figure 3
DEVELOPMENTAL PSYCHOPATHOLOGY AND PTSD

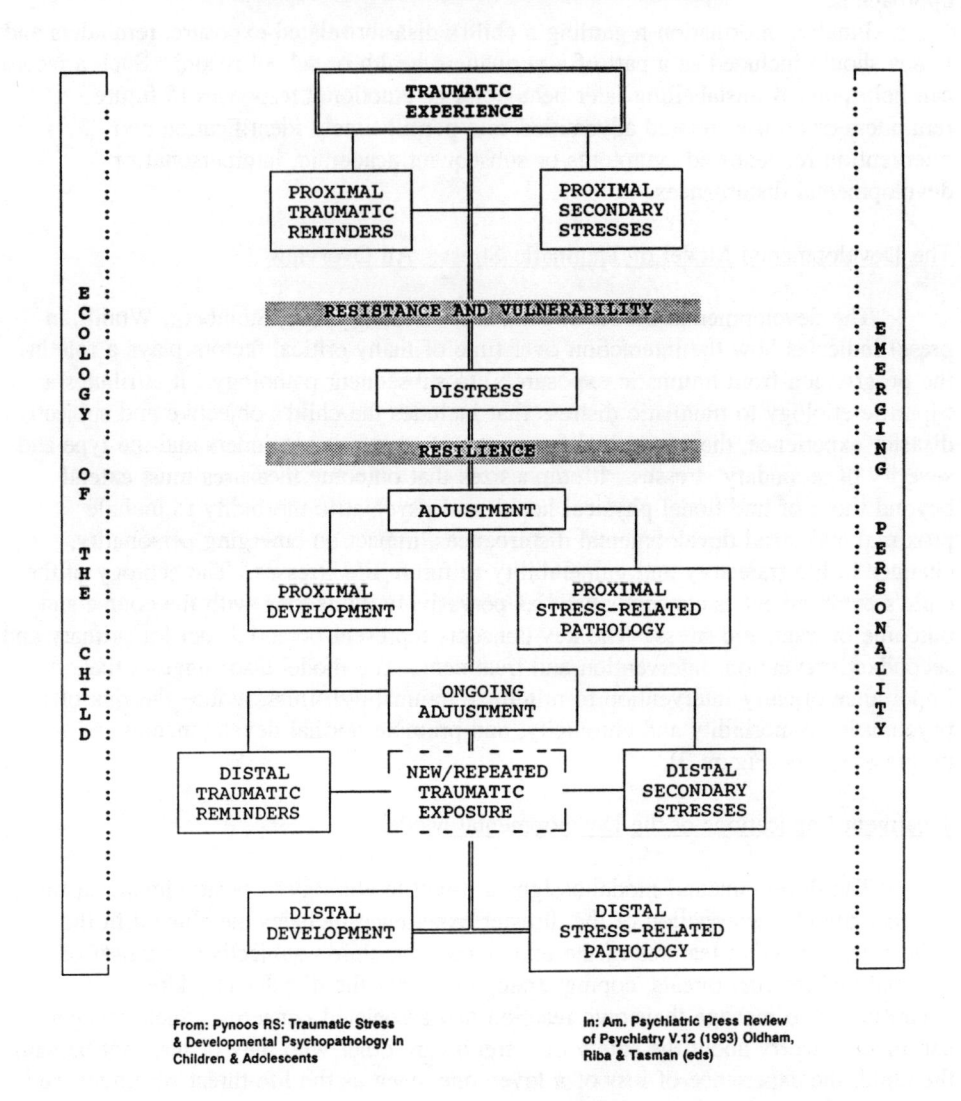

```
                          ┌──────────────┐
                          │  TRAUMATIC   │
                          │  EXPERIENCE  │
                          └──────┬───────┘
                    ┌────────────┴────────────┐
            ┌───────┴────────┐        ┌───────┴────────┐
            │   PROXIMAL     │        │   PROXIMAL     │
            │   TRAUMATIC    │────────│   SECONDARY    │
            │   REMINDERS    │        │   STRESSES     │
            └───────┬────────┘        └───────┬────────┘
                    └────────────┬────────────┘
             ▓▓▓▓▓▓▓▓ RESISTANCE AND VULNERABILITY ▓▓▓▓▓▓▓▓
                            ┌────┴─────┐
                            │ DISTRESS │
                            └────┬─────┘
             ▓▓▓▓▓▓▓▓▓▓▓▓▓▓▓▓ RESILIENCE ▓▓▓▓▓▓▓▓▓▓▓▓▓▓▓▓
                          ┌──────┴───────┐
                          │  ADJUSTMENT  │
                          └──────┬───────┘
                    ┌────────────┴────────────┐
            ┌───────┴────────┐        ┌───────┴────────┐
            │   PROXIMAL     │        │   PROXIMAL     │
            │  DEVELOPMENT   │        │ STRESS-RELATED │
            │                │        │   PATHOLOGY    │
            └───────┬────────┘        └───────┬────────┘
                    └────────────┬────────────┘
                          ┌──────┴───────┐
                          │   ONGOING    │
                          │  ADJUSTMENT  │
                          └──────┬───────┘
                    ┌────────────┼────────────┐
            ┌───────┴────────┐ ┌─┴──────────┐ ┌┴───────────────┐
            │    DISTAL      │ │NEW/REPEATED│ │    DISTAL      │
            │   TRAUMATIC    │ │ TRAUMATIC  │ │   SECONDARY    │
            │   REMINDERS    │ │  EXPOSURE  │ │   STRESSES     │
            └───────┬────────┘ └─┬──────────┘ └┬───────────────┘
                    └────────────┼─────────────┘
                    ┌────────────┴────────────┐
            ┌───────┴────────┐        ┌───────┴────────┐
            │    DISTAL      │        │    DISTAL      │
            │  DEVELOPMENT   │        │ STRESS-RELATED │
            │                │        │   PATHOLOGY    │
            └────────────────┘        └────────────────┘
```

Left vertical label: ECOLOGY OF THE CHILD

Right vertical label: EMERGING PERSONALITY

From: Pynoos RS: Traumatic Stress & Developmental Psychopathology in Children & Adolescents

In: Am. Psychiatric Press Review of Psychiatry V.12 (1993) Oldham, Riba & Tasman (eds)

boy drew a picture of his earthquake experience in Armenia, depicting his partially collapsed apartment building that had caught on fire, his escape after he burned his hand, and his viewing of someone falling from the building while another person shouted for help. He depicts himself as standing by waiting to "rescue" whoever he could assist, expressing feelings about his ineffectualness. He then sadly told of his father's death and of the loss of a close friend. When describing the worst moment of the earthquake, he told of seeing a dead child "right in front of me."

Where these types of experiences are wide-spread, child mental health programs need to be designed to treat severe posttraumatic stress reactions and their exacerbation by extreme feelings of guilt or shame. Empirical studies of acutely traumatized children and adolescents have increased clinical awareness of the complexity of traumatic experiences and the mental activity during and in the immediate aftermath (Pynoos, 1993). All forms of treatment involve varying degrees of assessment and therapeutic attention to these complex factors. Therapeutic attention includes both assisting the child in reprocessing the experience, increasing tolerance for traumatic anxiety and addressing traumatic helplessness through engagement of constructive fantasy and action. The social-environmental interventions are directed at increasing the understanding and responsiveness of caretakers to the child.

At the same time, the treatment programs must address the significant interplay of trauma and grief over an extended period of time, and the potential risks of pathological bereavement, depression and developmental disturbances, especially in the areas of attachment behavior and autonomous strivings. In circumstances like the collapse of the Niemetz highway during the 1989 Loma Prieta earthquake, where most of the victims were on their way home from work, there may be a high frequency of traumatic bereavement among a large number of children and their families, and, a comparatively lower frequency of traumatic stress reactions. Outreach programs such as those provided by Cruse in the United Kingdom (Hendriks, Black, & Kaplan, 1993) and grief counselling and treatment services, for example, those described by Raphael (1986), are especially indicated in these situations.

Different magnitude disasters are associated with alternative symptomatic, behavioral or developmental outcomes. In comparison with Armenia, the 1994 Northridge earthquake in Los Angeles was associated with less widespread destruction, injury and loss of life. Because the earthquake occurred in the early morning hours, the disaster experiences of most children and their parents included extreme fear during the tremor, and difficulty in parents being able to quickly get to their children. As a consequence, children and parents experienced a dramatic lapse in the expected "protective shield" to be provided by parents in the face of danger. These types of experiences can be associated with pervasive and persistent disturbances in sleeping arrangements as both parents and children out of fear of recurrence seek to assure physical proximity to one another. Treatment approaches include attention to the child and parents experience of this failure of a developmental expectation, and, the use of flexible, jointly constructed plans to restore more normal family functioning and sleeping arrangements. In the 1989 Loma Prieta earthquake, which occurred in late afternoon, many children were in afterschool activities while their parents were either at work or at home. As a consequence, many parents were concerned for the safety of their children, and, many children experienced prolonged worry about the welfare of a parent who did not arrive home for many hours afterwards (Bourque, Aneshensel & Goltz, 1991). Such an experience can result in anxieties and symptoms unrelated to PTSD and require a specific therapeutic program to address separation issues regarding continued preoccupations with the safety of a significant other.

Traumatic reminders are embedded in the external and internal cues specific to the child's traumatic experience. The frequency of traumatic reminders is dependent, both on the nature of the traumatic experience and the post-disaster environment circumstances. These contribute to both the phasic nature of posttraumatic stress reactions and their persistence, the appearance of behavioral changes, and, over time, the increased risk of heightened neurophysiological reactivity and slower neurophysiological recovery after arousal. Unanticipated reminders can reevoke a sense of unpreparedness that exacerbates fears of recurrence. The treatment of reactivity to traumatic reminders requires identification of the reminders, increasing the child's understanding of the traumatic reference, assistance with cognitive discriminations, increasing internal tolerance for expectable reactivity, and utilizing strategies to promote the child's ability to recovery after reminders (see Figure 4).

Figure 4

TREATMENT OF REACTIVITY TO TRAUMATIC REMINDERS
1. Identification of Traumatic Reminders
2. Increase Child's Understanding of the Traumatic Reference
3. Assistance with Cognitive Discrimination
4. Increase Tolerance for Expectable Reactivity
5. Address Missed Developmental Opportunities Due to Traumatic Avoidance

The social environmental interventions are three-fold. One addresses reducing the impact of traumatic reminders by enhancing parent, teacher or care-taker appreciation of the role of traumatic reminders, promoting appropriate communication over their anticipation or occurrence and provision of extra assistance to reduce both the intensity and duration of reactivity. The second is to institute appropriate environmental interventions to reduce the frequency of traumatic reminders through repair or rebuilding, to reduce unnecessary exposures from physical reminders and to graphic disaster depictions in the mass media. A third is to provide assistance and support to parents and teachers in order to similarly to reduce reactivity and unnecessary exposures. Their reactive behavior to reminders may accentuate children's anxieties and interfere with parent or teacher skills.

Disasters are frequently associated with acute and long-term adversities and secondary stresses. These include medical, surgical and rehabilitative treatment for acute injuries and subsequent disabilities, relocation, resettlement, immigration, secondary health and nutritional problems, change in family finances, alterations in role performance or school performance due to posttraumatic stress reactions, and demands on new social skills to respond to social questioning and stigmatization. Secondary stresses increase the risk of comorbidity, complicate efforts at adjustment, initiate maladaptive coping, interfere with the availability of social support, family functioning and reintegration with peers. They challenge the child's social skills to respond to social questioning, stigmatization and altered role performance. Therapeutic attention includes assisting the child in identifying the sources of secondary stresses, addressing the resulting internal emotional conflicts, and enhancing coping skills. Socio-environmental interventions to minimize adversities and secondary stresses often require a child-advocate role on the part of the intervention team (See Figure 5).

Figure 5

INTERVENTION STRATEGIES TO ADDRESS SECONDARY STRESSES
1. Monitor Secondary Stresses for the Child and Family
2. Assist Child in Identifying Sources of Secondary Stresses
3. Address Emotional Responses
4. Address Interference with Developmental Opportunities
5. Enhance Coping Skills

Intervention strategies needed to address proximal developmental disturbances vary and differ from those employed in the clinical assessment and treatment of posttraumatic stress related psychopathology. For example, redressing an interruption in learning to read subsequent to the witnessing of violence may require remedial educational assistance along with therapeutic attention to the disturbance in visual information processing. Prevention of the secondary repercussion of academic failure with attendant loss of self-esteem and disturbances in peer relations may reduce the risk of other subsequent development disturbances and psychopathology. In disaster where a significant portion of the children within a school have had severe levels of exposure, there may be a measurable decline in academic achievement (Yule, 1991) that may necessitate developing a graduated curriculum to assist the most affected children to retain their self-esteem while they recover adequately from their posttraumatic stress and grief reactions.

Stages of Intervention

This model can be applied at different temporal stages of post-disaster intervention. We have previously described five types of interventions that are typically applied at successive post-disaster stages: psychological first-aid, specialized initial interview, brief therapy, pulsed interventions and long-term psychotherapy (Pynoos & Nader, 1993). These progressive therapeutic modalities are typically employed in the temporal sequence given. However, it may be appropriate, depending on the need, to reintroduce (or introduce for the first time) interventions from earlier stages.

The common goals at each stage are to: 1) normalize and legitimize the disaster experience and assist children in gaining greater tolerance of their reactions; 2) assist children in reworking the meaning of the disaster experience in terms of developmental schematizations of safety, trust, risk, injury, loss, parental protection, dependency and autonomy; 3) increase children's recognition of, and adaptation to, traumatic reminders; 4) ameliorate disaster-related stress reactions and facilitate grief work in order to minimize the consolidation of symptoms into persistent stress-related psychopathology; 5) foster the continued adaptation of resilient children and promote competence in effective adaptation to the crisis situation, including secondary adversities; 6) prevent interferences with the achievement of progressive developmental competencies; 7) promptly address early signs of maladaptation that would otherwise lead to secondary developmental disturbances and psychopathology; and, 8) enhance the responsiveness of the child's social support network and the child's capacity to engage others in providing support. We have also identified five different sites for these interventions including: the individual, family, group, the school, and community (Pynoos & Nader, 1993).

Proper disaster preparedness plans not only contribute to reduced mortality and physical morbidity but, by including appropriate guidelines and training, can significantly enhance secondary prevention during and in the immediate aftermath of a disaster. One major goal is to minimize the exposure of children and adolescents to the most traumatogenic disaster experiences. Proper evacuation, if possible, reduces the risks of injury or death, minimizes such exposures, and reduces the realm of potential traumatic reminders. Family or school personnel disagreements over evacuation decisions, witnessed by children, can exacerbate children's disaster reactions. During an evacuation, efforts should be made to keep children with familiar primary caretakers and to minimize unnecessary separations or reduce the duration of separation from parents and siblings. It is important that parents be made aware of school disaster evacuation plans regarding where their children may be transported. It is especially important to have a system to record information about hospitalization of children to avoid unnecessary delays in parents locating them. During any prolonged separation of parents and children, it is important to provide adequate information and psychological support. Lastly, disaster preparedness plans need to include guidelines about reuniting children with their families (Nader & Pynoos, 1993).

Short of evacuation, children should be protected from unnecessary witnessing of injury and grotesque death, for example, having an injured or dead child brought into their classroom where they witness an unsuccessful effort at resuscitation. Caution should be observed in engaging adolescents in rescue work (as is routinely planned in many schools in the U.S.), especially without appropriate pre-disaster training and immediate debriefing (see Ersland, Weisaeth & Sund, 1989). Teachers and other school personnel assigned to participate in medical first aid and morgue duty need to be trained for the emotional risks of this work, in order to minimize the post-disaster impact on themselves, and, in turn, their students.

Psychological first-aid refers to the provision of emotional relief and assistance with problem solving in the immediate aftermath of a disaster and, at subsequent times when traumatic reminders, secondary stresses and new developmental challenges may renew or exacerbate disaster reactions. Pynoos and Nader (1988) have described developmentally-related variations in the type of acute reactions and recommended a range of caretaking (including parents and school personnel) responses and crisis affective and cognitive interventions. These age-related variations, for example, regressive behavior in younger children, have been explained on the basis of development-linked expectations regarding protective intervention in the face of external and internal dangers (Pynoos, Steinberg and Wraith, in press).

In disaster and war zones around the world, public, private and international relief organizations have come to recognize the need to reestablish the school environment as soon as possible, even under continued adverse circumstances and with more limited educational goals. Interruption of schooling and the peer milieu that it provides represents a significant developmental disruption. Schooling has been resumed in tents, in parks, in basements, and in trailers after disasters. The resumption of schooling reinforces expectations about the continuation of more normal predisaster roles and provides an important intervention site.

A major goal of an organized classroom or group interventions is to normalize and legitimize childrens' disaster-related experience and their acute reactions. A number of complimentary techniques have been used to achieve this psycho-educational goal. These include classroom or group discussions in which trained personnel (in conjunction with their teachers) assist children to participate in specialized disaster debriefing procedures. These can make use of drawing and story telling, play and books, pamphlets and cartoons (Frederick, 1985). The procedures depend, in part, on how diverse or uniform the disaster experiences are among the child group. Where there is a spectrum of exposures, it is preferable to have an introductory general discussion of the range of experiences and reactions without introducing unnecessary graphic details of any one child's extreme experience, coupled with individual child debriefing within the group setting, and followed by a second group discussion that includes more directive suggestions about immediate adjustment.

This second discussion provides an opportunity to enhance cohesion of the group or classroom by increasing understanding of the range of exposures among the children and what that may mean in terms of their expected reactions and course of recovery. This portion of the discussion includes explanations of typical posttraumatic stress and grief reactions in age-appropriate language (e.g., "if you see something terrible happen to someone, you may see pictures of it in your mind for longer than you think" or "its pretty hard to concentrate as well right after going through something as frightening as this"), of the distress of failed developmental expectations (e.g., "it's hard not to have your mommy or daddy be able to get to you right away when the earthquake started"), of the role of traumatic reminders (e.g., "it's hard to walk by that building that fell down without thinking about what happened during the earthquake" or "we are all likely to get more afraid the next time there is a high wind") and of the impact of adversities ("it's okay if things don't seem as much fun as they used to, for now; this is a lot to go through").

It also provides an opportunity to enhance helpful adjustment responses, especially help-seeking behavior. For example, "it helps to let someone know when something reminds you of what happened, because even your mommy or daddy taking your hand at that moment can make you feel better," or "if you are having bad dreams, it helps to let your parents know," or "if you are having pictures of what happened bother you at school which make it hard for you to learn, it will help to let your teacher know." It is also important to address age-related risks of reckless behavior, especially among adolescents, who may need specific instruction about the increased risk of abrupt changes in interpersonal relationships, substance abuse, radical decisions in regard to future plans, of aggressive and thrill seeking behavior.

This follow-up discussion also permits the intervention team to address fears of recurrence and their disruptive effects on the child, family, classroom and school community. It provides an opportunity to present factual information about the type of disaster which occurred, post-disaster safety status (e.g., the safety of school buildings), and possible recurrence (how to discriminate high winds from another hurricane or tornado or the expectable course of earthquake aftershocks). Such information can be used to correct confusions, distortions and misappraisals. For example, some school-age children in Armenia thought at first that they were under attack by bombs dropped by Azeris, and, even as they got free from the rubble, thought the uniformed rescue workers were enemy soldiers. Another group of children attributed the cause of the earthquake to nuclear explosions ordered by Gorbachev. Each of these misinterpretations were addressed within the classroom intervention. It is important with preschool and younger children to insure opportunities for repeated and ongoing clarification of misattributions, lack of understanding and misinformation obtained from rumors and other children.

In the individual debriefing with a child and in the classroom discussion, it is important to move beyond the immediate anxieties and disaster-related reactions toward a more active psychological engagement of constructive fantasy, play, thoughts and actions. It has become common practice to permit children to express their disaster experience in classroom exercises. However, the Galante and Foa (1986) study after the 1980 Italian earthquakes demonstrated no measurable reduction in anxiety or fear of recurrence until the children began to rebuild their villages in play with improved construction and earthquake safety. This constructive response is common in adult adaptive responses, but its importance is often overlooked in therapeutic work with children. With younger children, this work may primarily involve the use of constructive fantasy. For example, after the Northridge earthquake, a six year old child, asked to draw what happened to her during the earthquake, readily illustrated how her stuffed animals had fallen onto to her from above her bed. When asked, what would she like to see happen to make her feel safer about earthquakes, she thought for a moment and, in an animated voice, responded, "They should glue (e.g., super glue) the plates together and tape them so they cannot move", referring as she told the interviewer to the plates of the earth that she had learned about in school. She could then move to more active problem solving, including her thought that younger children should be on the first floor of the school building so they can evacuate more quickly. Adolescents can be encouraged to participate in constructive activities to achieve similar protective goals. For example, after the 1993 devastating residential fires in Laguna Beach, California, adolescents, on their own, started a community movement to replace the burned tress with more fire-resistant Pacific Oaks.

The individual debriefing within the group setting not only can be used for screening purposes but may also permit clinical intervention to address an acute problematic behavior. For example, two brothers witnessed the death of their mother in the 1988 Armenian earthquake while they watched from under a table during the collapse of their roof. Two days later, the seven year old brother began to exhibit serious aggressive outbursts. During the individual debriefing of the classroom intervention, he first avoided drawing his mother. When asked about his mother, he stabbed the paper. When the interviewer interpreted to the child that it is understandable to be angry about his mother dying as she did, the child's behavior calmed down. He then drew his mother in a coffin, expressed his anger over not attending her funeral, and began to cry over her loss.

The use of drawings can often facilitate an understanding of childrens' traumatic experiences and current emotional state, prior to more verbal expression. It can also assist a child who is emotionally overwhelmed, and facilitate their entrance into more individual or group clinical care. For example, one nine year old girl in Spitak had remained mute and withdrawn after witnessing her mother crushed to death. With the presence of an intervention team member, she was able to draw the mutilated body of her mother. Asked about the picture, she was able to nod, and then allowed herself to be comforted while she cried. She was then able to continue to see a mental health counsellor.

Care must be taken in recognizing the limitations of classroom and individual debriefing. One reason to conduct individual debriefings when there is a spectrum of exposures within the child group is to minimize the risk of secondary exposure of children to graphic details and fears beyond their own level of exposure. In addition, one cannot adequately treat the intrusive symptoms of children discussed above who witnessed the grotesque death of a parent, nor the associated guilt or grief. At the same time, the loss of a parent represents a major secondary adversity which clearly cannot be adequately addressed in this format. As has been demonstrated with combat veterans (Marmar, Foy, Kagan & Pynoos, 1993), an initial set of individual sessions may be a necessary prerequisite to subsequent group treatment among highly exposed children and adolescents.

Care must also be exercised in recommending certain treatment techniques in a non-specific fashion without adequate recognition of their risks for certain exposure groups. For example, relaxation exercises are often taught to children to use at home for post-disaster-related anxieties. However, these exercises may actually be accompanied by increased vividness of traumatic imagery (Rachman, 1980) and are most appropriately used among severely exposed children only within the context of ongoing cognitive-behavioral therapy. In addition, these techniques may be most suitably used to assist in a program to decrease reactivity in anticipation of, or response to, traumatic reminders.

The developmental model indicates that a child's efforts at post-disaster adjustment are strongly influenced by the family, school and community environment. There are educational and clinical interventions with parent's that can enhance the child's recovery. Referring to the tripartite model of distress, parenting functions can be compromised by reactions stemming from their own disaster experience, including posttraumatic and grief reactions, by their reactivity to traumatic reminders and fears of recurrence, and by demands and strains of post-disaster adversities.

Our experience has been that a prerequisite to providing parents with educational information, either in the form of printed material, through telephone hot-lines or during group meetings, about how to assist their children is to attend to the parents' disaster responses and adjustment efforts. In our attention to children's reactions, many opportunities are overlooked to provide early interventions to parents that may significantly improve parenting function. Identification of children at risk and monitoring their course of recovery includes targeting children whose parents are at risk for impaired functioning. Highly traumatized parents may compulsively describe their subjective intrusive images, exacerbating the child's distress. Their traumatic anxiety and fears of recurrence may markedly interfere with their ability to formulate a constructive plan to assist their own children's recovery, for example, a plan to gradually return to more normal sleeping arrangements. Their traumatic avoidant behavior may compromise their ability to be open to hear of the child's own experiences or distress. Their own reactivity to reminders may increase a child's anxious responses, and impede their ability to support a child with their own reactions to reminders. Dysregulation of aggression can lead to more domestic violence and child abuse within the family setting.

Secondary adversities, for example, unemployment or relocation, carry mental health risks for the parent, and, parental demoralization or depression can seriously increase the mental health risks for the child. The interaction of traumatic reactions and adversities can lead to impaired decision-making and maladaptive coping. Impaired decision making can lead to impulsive relocation or delayed efforts at repair, that can compromise mental health efforts on behalf of an individual child. Maladaptive coping in the form of alcohol or drug abuse can seriously erode parental functioning.

Parenting skills can be enhanced when parent's are educated regarding their own and their childrens' post-disaster stress reactions, realistic expectations about the course of recovery, differing psychological agendas among family members, and the importance of incurring open communication with their children on an ongoing basis. For example, after the 1994 Northridge earthquake, parental meetings helped parents to better understand how their own anxious attachment because of their difficulty in getting to their children quickly, was contributing to the delay in supporting children to return to sleeping in their own bedrooms.

Specialized Treatment Approaches

Treatment interventions beyond classroom interventions and psychological first aid should be designed to address prominent psychological, behavioral, social, and developmental consequences in the child population. Each disaster may result in a particular configuration of risks in these categories and require different treatment goals. For example, after the 1989 Hurricane Hugo where there was a successful evacuation effort, children and adolescents had few of the most traumatogenic experiences and exhibited mild to moderate posttraumatic stress reactions (Lonigan, Shannon, Finch, Daugherty, & Taylor, 1991; Belter, Dunn, & Jeney, 1991) In this range, child intrinsic and parental factors may play a significant role in mediating the development and persistence of disaster-related anxieties and other co-morbid conditions. Child and parent premorbid anxiety renders them more vulnerable both to fears of recurrence and to retarded recovery from reactivity to traumatic reminders. Lonigan et al. (1991), reported, that in addition to the level of exposure, children's trait anxiety was a significant predictor of the severity and chronicity of posttraumatic stress reactions. Similarly, after the Northridge earthquake, many of the children referred to the Federal Emergency Management Agency supported Los Angeles Unified School District mental health counsellors by teachers and parents for acute counselling had histories of prior anxiety and related behavioral disturbances. The treatment in these situations includes psycho-educational and pragmatic approaches to improve cognitive discrimination among potential reminders, supportive individual, group and family work to minimize exacerbation of anxious conditions and to contain or avert the contagion of anxiety within the family setting, and treatment of underlying conditions among children, where their reactivity, rather than receding, persists or increases over time.

In disaster circumstances where there has been a significant prevalence of traumatic death or an accumulation or persistence of severe post-disaster adversities, or both, it will be important to screen for comorbid conditions, especially depression. Interventions for traumatic bereavement extend from the immediate issues of death notification, to issues of participation in funeral and commemorative rituals, to the interplay of trauma and grief over an extended period of time. Especially for children, secondary issues surrounding loss of nuclear family members, including grief-related disturbances in a surviving parent's functioning, variations in the quality of substitute care-taking and the child's response, and developmental risks associated with the process of bereavement. Interventions to address secondary adversities include close monitoring of parental and child functioning with intercurrent stresses, by early treatment of serious depressive symptoms and by pro-active emergency efforts to prevent socio-environmental actions that might precipitate the acute onset of depression or demoralization. For example, Yule reports having been able to avert a serious depressive reaction in a school aged boy by getting his teacher to rescind her demand that he redo his school notebook lost in a ferry boat disaster (Yule, 1991). Conversely, after a devastating community fire, the adaptational resources of a school-age child were overwhelmed by a fourth relocation of residence in the span of one year, precipitating an acute depressive reaction with conduct disturbance. From a developmental perspective, preventive intervention may include ensuring opportunities to continue friendships disrupted by disaster-related relocations.

Specialized treatment techniques are required in circumstances where there is widespread traumatic exposure and the predominant symptom profile is severe posttraumatic stress reactions. We are beginning to accumulate evidence that such a specialized program can be efficacious in reducing posttraumatic symptomatology in children and adolescents. In Armenia, the use of classroom debriefings followed by individual and group sessions conducted 1 1/2 years after the earthquake significantly reduced the severity of posttraumatic stress reactions compared to untreated controls. At three years the treated group showed a significant reduction on the Child Posttraumatic Stress Disorder Reaction Index compared with controls who remained unchanged. Yule (1992) reported similar findings after treatment of adolescents in a more acute phase following a catastrophic transportation disaster.

Although the theoretical orientations may differ, the interventions include a core of common components. These components include: 1) recognition of the complexity of the child's disaster experience and its representation in memory; 2) that the meaning of the emotional and cognitive reactions are embedded in the details of the experience; 3) that children can be engaged in a safe and secure therapeutic setting to thoroughly reexplore their disaster experience, acutely and over time; 4) the importance of characterizing the hierarchy of traumatogenic aspects of the experience, including "the worst moment" and the attribution of meaning to each; 5) that, over time, differing traumatogenic aspects may emerge with more importance and differences in attribution or meaning, due to traumatic reminders, developmental challenges, resolution of extra and intrapsychic conflicts, and changes in socio-environmental circumstances; 6) the importance of working through the anxiety and developmental implications for each of the traumatogenic elements; and 7) that effectiveness is not only to be measured in the diminution of posttraumatic stress symptoms but in the restoration or acquisition of adaptive resources to address secondary changes in the child's life.

Specialized interview techniques have been described for the early in-depth exploration of traumatic experiences with children and adolescents (Pynoos & Eth, 1986). The initial interview(s) may provide some acute benefit to the child. They also serve two other important functions. First, the sharing of the child's experience, reactions, responses to reminders and current concerns with parents constitutes a critical intervention for enhancing parental responsiveness which is a major source of social support during the recovery period. Second, they facilitate children's acceptance of referral to further therapy, including individual, group or family modalities.

The following is a case example of brief individual and family therapy from Spitak, Armenia:

> A fourteen year old boy was seen in a relocation hotel in Yerevan, a city at the periphery of the earthquake zone. By self report, he was suffering from severe posttraumatic stress symptoms. He displayed restless, intrusive behavior, especially by his compulsive interference with others in an effort to help them. Having begun treatment by saying that he was not aware of having any difficulties, he eagerly engaged in a specialized interview to explore his disaster experience and its personal consequences. He described how, at the time of the earthquake, he was sitting at home with his father, sister and a friend when he heard, what he interpreted to be, an explosion. As his home was collapsing, his father pulled him and his sister out of the building. The boy then described his experience of the immediate aftershocks, the sight of burning buildings, the smell of smoke and "cracks in the ground." His first appraisal was that "the Turks were attacking them." He then spoke of hearing children crying and witnessing a neighbor's wife burning to death and hearing the husband's cries of anguish. He then described his fear over the safety of his mother, who was not at home at the time and his later relief at reunion. He then described seeing many dead bodies, including a friend of his father. Toward the end of the first session, he began spontaneously to discuss his distress over having been relocated twice and the difficulties he and his family had faced.

In the next session, he described many traumatic reminders, especially earthquake-related sounds, including hearing anyone cry, even on TV. As the treatment progressed, he began to describe feelings of terror and horror as he related even worse moments than any he had previously described. He had seen the corpse of a close friend whose leg had been severed and whose face had been "cracked". He then quickly retreated into describing witnessing people who he thought had become "crazy", as they "sung and danced" in frenzied behavior. He became afraid at the time that he would become like them. The therapist was able to address his fears of losing control and becoming crazy and his current hypomanic behavior as a form of denial in action, similar to the people he described, in response to the horrifying site of his friend.

The next phase of treatment included an exploration of his anger and guilt. First, he described how upset he was with himself over his unusual irritability and his yelling at people. His self-reproach lead to a discussion of his aunt who died. He had had a thought about going to rescue his aunt after his own escape from his collapsing house that he excluded from his mind as he, his father and sister "went the other direction" to seek safety. He had feelings, not only of guilt, but of cowardliness. In treatment, it was possible to relate his overly helpful behavior as an agitated reenactment in an effort to redress his bad feelings over not going to the aid of his aunt. As a consequence, he became more settled down, and began to discuss his grief over the loss of his aunt, who was one of his favorite relatives. He then related reunion dreams in which his aunt and his dead friend interacted with him, which helped him begin the difficult process of grieving.

In the termination phase of treatment, the boy spoke about how his parents had prohibited him from speaking of his experience and how beneficial it had been for him to be able to communicate his thoughts and feelings and to gain an understanding of his reactions and their meaning. He reflected on the developmental impact of relocation, exclaiming his longing to return to Spitak to be with his friends, "Even if it were for just one minute". By the end of his therapy, his posttraumatic stress symptoms had improved, and, his behavior was markedly less intrusive and agitated.

Concomitant with the treatment, the parents received brief counselling in regard to their traumatic experience and loss. With a reduction in their own traumatic avoidance and suppression, and psycho-education about their child's need for communication, they were able, in a subsequent session, to be made more aware of their child's subjective experience, continued concerns and need for support. The parents were able to be counselled to permit their son to make a short visit to Spitak in order to see his close friends and his demolished home.

In a five month follow-up consultation, the boy described how he was especially pleased by being able to make this visit, and expressed more hopeful feelings about his future, as well as more sadness over his acceptance of the losses and changes in his life. He had maintained the improvement in his posttraumatic stress condition.

Brief therapy permits contextual understanding of the traumatic experience(s) within the circumstances and culture of the individual, family and community. It facilitates ongoing emotional and cognitive reworking of the succession of traumatic moments, the developmental implications, and the influence of traumatic reminders and secondary stresses (Foy, Resnick, Carroll & Osato, 1991; Horowitz, 1986; Pynoos & Nader, 1993). As in the above example, children and adolescents require appropriate therapeutic work to lessen the psychological focus on the circumstances of disaster-related deaths, in order to promote a psychological shift toward exploring the meaning of losses and facilitating the mourning process.

Different clinical intervention strategies may complement one another, although each may have a different emphasis and role in an the over-all intervention program (Marmar et al, 1993). Clinical case reports and clinical research have begun to demonstrate the potential effectiveness of cognitive-behavioral treatment strategies with school-aged children and adolescents. This approach focuses on overt-behavioral avoidance and reenactment, stimulus and response components that have become part of the fear memory or signal of danger, and a detailed understanding of biological and psychological conditioning occurring during exposure. Behavioral observation, self-report of anxiety and physiological measurement have all been used with children to monitor the working through of a complicated hierarchy of fearful moments that emerge or evolve from traumatic events (Saigh, 1988). There is increasing interest to understand the developmental dimension of how to assist children in reworking the meaning of the event as dangerous and assisting children in constructing a coherent narrative (Foa & Kozak, 1986; Meichenbaum & Fitzpatrick, 1992).

Psychodynamic approaches add attention to a developmental hierarchy of internal dangers as well as external dangers, and to the complex affective states which characterize the child's experience and subsequent response (Pynoos, Steinberg & Wraith, in press). They recognize that meaningful associations are linked to each moment of the traumatic event and its aftermath and that these associations recruit unconscious conflict from current and earlier developmental periods and emerging self-regulatory mechanisms. They focus on the emerging mental schemas of danger, protection and intervention and concerns regarding safety, risk, injury, loss and parental protection or supervision, including transference and countertransference issues. Pynoos and Nader (1993) have proposed that special attention be given to intervention fantasies, including their evolution over time. These intervention fantasies provide indications of a child's conflicts over traumatic helplessness and the efficacy of self and other, which often involve viridical and non-viridical representations.

Pharmacotherapy targets psychobiological mechanisms underlying hyperarousal, cue specific hyperreactivity, sleep disturbances and co-morbid anxiety and depressive disorders. Amelioration of intense and persistent arousal symptoms, for example, those associated with non-REM sleep disturbances, may be essential to restore a child's sense of restfulness and daytime concentration and attention. The reduction of tonic and phasic physiological arousal may contribute to the therapeutic process by permitting fuller registration and tolerance of traumatic reminders and improved cognitive discrimination. There is preliminary evidence that specific pharmacologic agents that reduce fear-enhanced startle in animal models, including clonidine and propranolol, can be effective in treating arousal symptoms in children and adolescents (Ornitz & Pynoos, 1989; Famularo, Kinscherff & Fenton, 1988; Perry, 1994).

It has been our observation that the most common overlooked adverse influence on the child's recovery environment is the disturbed interpersonal matrix of the family due to variability in psychological agendas among family members as a result of differences in exposure and response to loss (Pynoos & Nader, 1993). A primary goal of family therapy, therefore, should be to help family members validate and legitimize each others disaster-related experiences and to enhance an understanding of the developmental impact on the family, thereby facilitating continued mutual support. The skills of family members can be enhanced through education regarding posttraumatic stress reactions, realistic expectations about the course of recovery, differing psychological agendas, the management of temporary behavioral alterations or regressions, and the importance of encouraging open communication. For example, after the 1994 Northridge earthquake, we found that one of the most common problems among families was the failure to develop a flexible plan to restore normal sleeping arrangements or to address episodes of renewed anxiety. Family interventions proved useful in assisting families in developing such plans, individualized to the level of exposure of family members, their developmental stage, and realistic expectations about the course of recovery.

The small group has proven to be an important therapeutic intervention during the immediate weeks or months after a disaster (Yule, 1989). Group therapy offers the opportunity to reinforce the normative nature of reactions and recovery, to share mutual concerns, to address common fears and traumatic reminders and avoidant behaviors, to increase tolerance for disturbing emotions, to provide early attention to depressive reactions, and to aid recovery through age-appropriate and situation-specific problem solving (Pynoos & Nader, 1993). Groups may become especially valuable in the treatment of adolescents by permitting the working-through of any potential serious disturbances in peer relationships. When there has been a peer death related to the disaster, group therapy can take on an added importance for those close acquaintances. It provides on ongoing setting to normalize grief responses, provides an additional emotional support and a reserved time for reworking the loss, permits professionally-assisted shared reminiscing, and reinforces efforts at recovery.

A developmental model of traumatic stress would suggest that a component of an optimal intervention strategy would include pulsed interventions, potentially at all levels, which include planned periods of consultation after an acute phase of treatment. After initial treatment, the child is seen at certain critical junctures, determined by anticipated or reported reminders, subsequent adversities, or important life-transitions or challenges that may be compromised by renewed symptoms (Pynoos & Nader, 1993). These interventions assist the child with future experiential and maturational reappraisals in an effort to maintain normal developmental progression (Budman & Gurman, 1988). At the school level, pulsed interventions may be planned for future occurrences, for example, renewed occupancy of repaired school buildings or graduation of a class from which their were many disaster deaths, where the focus of a circumscribed group discussion may include self-reflection on the developmental impact on their lives currently and in the future.

Conclusion

The model presented in this chapter suggests that the complex interaction over time of many critical factors plays a role in the outcome of traumatic exposure. Each of these factors can be seen as a potential focus for prevention and treatment. The model therefore implies that prevention and intervention must be multidimensional and that outcome measures must extend beyond those of traditional psychopathology. As Jensen and Shaw (1993) have commented, there is an urgent need to clarify the optimal level of intervention for children and their families, both acutely and over time. Because early intervention may prove most efficacious, there will be important public health and ethical issues regarding the conduct of biomedical research involving traumatized children and adolescents and the allocation of mental health resources.

Beyond the individual child, family or community, traumatic stress studies are beginning to consider how the repercussions of regional catastrophic disasters or violence may alter the social and political character of a nation. After massive trauma, a large segment of the child population may experience posttraumatic stress reactions. As evidenced by the rates of chronic psychiatric morbidity among Armenian children after the 1988 earthquake (Pynoos et al 1993), the existence of thousands of traumatized children in different stages of recovery places special burdens on society. These can include the consequence of widespread maladaptation in terms of schooling, disturbances in intrafamilial and peer interactions and diminished resistance or resilience to future stress. Changes in future orientation may not only affect the individual child, but, on a massive scale, permeate and transform cultural expectations, altering the social ecology of the next generation. Disasters and war can lead to radical shifts in fundamental beliefs and philosophical outlook. For example, Luke and Reeves (1978) reflected on how the famous Spanish earthquake of 1755 "not only shattered Lisbon but severely shook the optimistic theodocy of the Enlightenment (pp 16)." War and political violence can also radically alter expectations about the social contract, leading to upsurges in democratic convictions or more Machiavellian political ideologies (Pynoos, 1992). Recently, out of an awareness of the alarming extent to which children are exposed to massive violence and the grave psychological repercussions, the United Nations General Assembly adopted a Convention on the Rights of the Child which requires countries to file and publicize regular progress reports on compliance (UNICEF, 1991). There is also increased international interest in elevating the standard of care provided to children after disasters. Researchers and clinicians in the field of traumatic stress can help to make prevention more of a national and international concern by giving continued scientific voice to the legacy of trauma.

> The authors gratefully acknowledge support for the writing of this chapter from the Armenian Relief Society, the Robert Ellis Simon Foundation, the Bing Fund and the Foundation of the Milken Families.

References

Belter, R.W., Dunn, S.E., & Jeney, P. (1991). The psychological impact of Hurricane Hugo on children: A needs assessment. Advances in behavior research and therapy. 13, 1155-161.
Berz, G. (1989). Lists of major natural disasters, 1960-1987. Earthquakes and volcanoes 20, 226-228.
Bourque, L.B, Aneshensel, C.S., & Goltz, J.D. (1991). Injury and psychological distress following the Whittier Narrows and Loma Prieta earthquakes (abstract), in Proceedings of the UCLA International Conference on the Impact of Natural Disasters, Agenda for Future Action, Los Angeles, University of California, 1991.
Breslau, N., Davis, G.C., Andreski, P., Peterson, E. (1991). Traumatic events and posttraumatic stress disorder in an urban population of young adults. Archives of General Psychiatry, 48, 216-222.
Budman, S.H., & Gurman, A.S. (1988). Theory and practice of brief therapy. New York: Guilford Press.
Bucker, J., Trickett, E.J., & Corse, S.J. (1985). Primary prevention and mental health: An annotated bibliography DHHS Publication No. ADM 85-1405) Washington, D.C. Government Printing Office.
Ersland, S., Weisaeth, L., & Sund, A. (1989). The stress upon rescuers involved in an oil frigate disaster. "Alexander L. Kielland" 1980. Acta Psychiatrica Scandinavica Suppl. 335, 80, 38-49.
Famularo, R., Kinscherff, R., Fenton, T. (1988). Propranolol treatment for children with acute post-traumatic stress disorder. American Journal of Diseases of Children, 142, 1244-1247.
Foa, E.B., & Kozak, M.D. (1986) Emotional Processing of fear: Exposure to corrective information. Psychological Bulletin, 99, 20-35.
Foy, D.W., Resnick, H.S., Carroll, E.M., & Osato, S.S. (1991). Behavior therapy. In A.S. Bellack & M. Hersen (eds.), Handbook of comparative treatments for adult disorders. New York: Guilford Press.
Frederick, C, (1985). Children traumatized by catastrophic situations. In Eth S, Pynoos R (eds): Post-traumatic stress disorder in children, (pp 71-99). Washington DC, American Psychiatric Press.
Galante, M.A., & Foa, D. (1986). An epidemiological study of psychic trauma and treatment effectiveness for children after a natural disaster. Journal of the American Academy of Child and Adolescent Psychiatry, 25, 357-363.
Goenjian, A. (1993) A mental health relief program in Armenia After the 1988 earthquake: Implementation & clinical observations British Journal of Psychiatry, 163, 230-239.
Hendriks, J.H., Black, D., & Kaplan T (1993). When father kills mother: Guiding children through trauma & grief. New York, London; Routledge.

Hobfoll, S.E. (1991). Traumatic stress: A theory based on rapid loss of resources. Anxiety Research, 4, 187-197.

Horowitz, M. (1986). Stress response syndromes (2nd edition). North Vale, NJ: Aronson.

International Federation of Red Cross and Red Crescent Societies (1993). World disaster report, 1993 Dordrecht, The Netherlands: Martinus Jijoff.

Jensen, P.S., & Shaw, J. (1993). Children as victims of war: Current knowledge and future research needs. Journal of the American Academy of Child and Adolescent Psychiatry, 32, 697-708.

Lonigan, C.J., Shannon, M.P., Finch, A.J., Daugherty, T.K., & Taylor, C.M. (1991) Children's reactions to a natural disaster: Symptom severity and degree of exposure. Advances in Behavior Research and Therapy, 13, 135-154.

Marmar, C., Foy, D., Kagan, V., & Pynoos, R. (1993). An Integrated approach for treating posttraumatic Stress. In J. Oldham, M. Riba & A. Tasman (Eds.), American psychiatric press review of psychiatry Vol 12. (pp 238-272). Washington, DC: American Psychiatric Press.

Meichenbaum, D, & Fitzpatrick, D. (1992). A constructivist narrative perspective on stress and coping: stress inoculation applications. In, L. Goldberger & S. Breznitz (eds.), Handbook of stress: Theoretical & clinical aspects, 2nd edition (pp 706-723). New York: Free Press.

Nader, K., Stuber, M, & Pynoos, R. (1991). Posttraumatic stress reactions in preschool children with catastrophic illness: Assessment Needs. Comprehensive Mental Health Care , 1, 223-239.

Nader, K., & Pynoos, R. (1993). School disaster: Planning and initial interventions. Journal of Social Behavior and Personality, Handbook of Post-disaster Interventions, 8, 1-22.

Ornitz, E.M., Pynoos, R.S. (1989). Startle modulation in children with post-traumatic stress disorder. American Journal of Psychiatry, 147, 866-870.

Perry B.D. (1994). Neurobiological sequelae of childhood trauma. Post-traumatic stress disorders in children. In M. Murberg (ed.), Catecholamine function in post-traumatic stress disorder: Emerging concepts, (pp 233-255). Washington, DC: American Psychiatric Press, Inc.

Pynoos, R.S. (1992). Violence, personality and politics. In A. Kales, C.M. Pierce, M. Greenblatt (eds.), The mosaic of contemporary psychiatry in perspective, (pp 53-65). New York: Springer Verlag.

Pynoos, R.S. (1993). Traumatic stress and developmental psychopathology in children and adolescents. In J. Oldham, M. Riba & A. Tasman (Eds.), American psychiatric press review of psychiatry Vol 12, (pp 205-238). Washington, D.C.; American Psychiatric Press.

Pynoos R, & Eth, S. (1986). Witness to violence: The child interview. Journal of the American Academy of Child Psychiatry, 25, 306-319.

Pynoos, R. & Nader, K. (1988). Psychological first aid and treatment approach for children exposed to community violence: research implications, Journal of Traumatic Stress, 1, 445-473.
Pynoos, R.S., Nader, K. (1993). Issues in the treatment of post-traumatic stress in children and adolescents. In J.P. Wilson, & B. Raphael (eds.), The international handbook of traumatic stress syndromes (pp 535-549). New York: Plenum Press.
Pynoos, R., Goenjian, A., Tashjian, M., Karakashian, M., Manjikian, R., Manoukian, G., Steinberg, A.M., Fairbanks, L. (1993). Posttraumatic stress reactions in children after the 1988 Armenian earthquake. British Journal of Psychiatry, 163, 239-247.
Pynoos, R.S., Steinberg, A.M., & Wraith, R. (In press) A developmental model of childhood traumatic stress. In D. Cicchetti, D. & D.J. Cohen (eds.), Manual of developmental psychopathology New York: John Wiley & Sons.
Rachman, S. (1980) Emotional processing. Behavior research and therapy, 18, 51-60.
Raphael, B. (1986). When disaster strikes: How individuals and communities cope with catastrophe. New York: Basic Books, Inc.
Saigh, P.A. (1988). T he use of an in vitro flooding package in the treatment of traumatized adolescents. Journal of Developmental and Behavioral Pediatrics, 10, 17-21.
Yule, W. (1991) Working with children following disasters. In M. Herbert (ed.), Clinical child psychology: Social learning, development and behavior, (pp 349-363). Chichester: Wiley.
UNICEF (1991). The state of the world's children. Oxford University Press
U.S. Government (1976). Rules and regulations for the Disaster Relief Act, PL 93-288, Section 413. Federal Register, November 6.
Weisaeth, L. (1993). Disasters: Psychological and psychiatric aspects: In, L. Goldberger & S. Breznitz S (eds.), Handbook of stress: Theoretical and clinical aspects, 2nd edition, (pp 591-616). New York; Free Press.
Yule, W. (1991) Working with children following disasters. In M. Herbert (ed.), Clinical Child Psychology: Social Learning, Development and Behavior, (pp 349-363). Chichester: Wiley.
Yule, W., & Udwin, O. (1991). Screening child survivors for post-traumatic stress disorders: Experiences from the `Jupiter' sinking. British Journal of Clinical Psychology, 30, 131-138.
Yule, W., Bolton, D., & Udwin, O. (1992). Objective and subjective predictors of PTSD in adolescence. Presentation at the World Conference of the International Society for Traumatic Stress Studies Amsterdam, The Netherlands, June 1992.

CATALYZING COMMUNITY SUPPORT[1]

Noach Milgram, Tel-Aviv University, Ramat-Aviv, Israel
Barbara R. Sarason, University of Washington, Seattle, Washington USA
Ute Schönpflug, Freie Universitat, Berlin, Germany
Anita Jackson, Kent State University, Kent, Ohio USA
Christine Schwarzer, Heinrich Heine Universitat, Dusseldorf, Germany

There are many complex issues associated with catalyzing community support in behalf of members of a community adversely affected by major stressful events. Intervention planning must assess important features of the stressor (e.g., intensity, duration, foreseen versus unforeseen, rare versus common occurrence, etc.), the stress resistant resources of potential support providers, the strengths and vulnerabilities of potential support recipients, and the socio-economic, ethnic, religious and cultural context of the community in which providers and recipients reside. The first step in dealing with this topic is to identify the kinds of stressful life events that come within the scope of this paper.

Stressors

Community-Wide Disasters

This paper addresses stressors that affect many people at the same time (e.g., war or a massive flood) rather than events that affect many individuals at different times (e.g., rape, physical assault, life-threatening illness). Rape is a wide-spread societal problem that justifies mobilizing community support to deal with its legal, educational, social, and psychological implications. It requires, however, different

---

[1]This paper is based on the input of a working group at the NATO, Advanced Research Workshop on Stress in Communities held at Bonas, France in June, 1994. Group members were Jasem Al-Khawaf, Dina Berman, Joop de Jong, Anita Jackson, Noach Milgram (Co-Chair), Alexander McFarlane, Barbara Sarason (Co-Chair), Irwin Sarason, Ute Schönpflug, Christine Schwarzer, and Edison Trickett.

perspectives and interventions from those applied to people whose lives were disrupted by natural (e.g., wind, flood, or forest fire) or man-made disasters (e.g., war, plane crash, or atomic radiation leakage). These disasters evoke coordinated community support for affected community members, and call for potentially well-defined interventions.

One may make a legitimate case for including in our discussion other chronic and wide-spread community problems such as long-term unemployment and homelessness. These stressors do not traumatize people in the same way as a hurricane or a plane crash and do not elicit an urgent and unequivocal desire to help, but they do affect many people at one and the same time in a given community and elicit some perspectives and interventions comparable to those applied to natural and man-made disasters. By contrast, some community problems--for example, efforts to eliminate war or racism or to preserve the ozone layer against ecological depredation-- are not amenable to these analyses and interventions. These causes require concerted actions on many levels and go well beyond the professional expertise of mental health researchers and crisis interventionists.

Intact Communities

This paper is further restricted to largely intact communities that provide the support needed by distressed members. It does not deal with recruiting lay and professional people who reside in one country to travel to another and provide its citizens with support. Intervention at the community level is a complex, difficult task for well-intentioned and well-trained "insiders" trying to help people in their own community with whom they share language, culture, and values. Intervention is far more complex and difficult when well-intentioned and well-trained "outsiders" attempt to do the same (see de Jong, this volume). Hence, our decision to focus exclusively on the effort to mobilize intact or relatively intact members of a community to help members victimized by events beyond their control.

The next step in dealing with our topic is to define the key terms--support, community, and catalyzing, in that order. The order of defining major terms is not accidental. It appeared wiser to proceed from more familiar terms to less familiar ones.

Support

Definition

Support had typically been conceptualized in terms of what is provided: information, encouragement, material help, empathy, and reassurance of personal worth. Sarason (this volume) has stated that support for disaster victims consists of the same elements found in any helpful interpersonal relationship--attachment, social integration, opportunity for receiving nurturance, reassurance of worth, sense of reliable alliance, and guidance.

Support may also be conceptualized in terms of the severity of the distress of the groups requiring support and the professional training of the source of the support. In any disaster some groups are more vulnerable than others. These require immediate support to prevent symptom formation and exacerbation while others continue to function without breakdown. Weisath (this volume) has proposed the following pyramidal hierarchy:

(a) Helping oneself or accepting a little help from one's neighbors, friends, or relatives (the base of the pyramid).

(b) Spontaneous nonprofessional and professional activation of existing social networks in behalf of mildly distressed people (e.g., activating parents in behalf of children, adults in behalf of relatives, and close friends or neighbors in behalf of distressed peers).

(c) Encouraging volunteer lay strangers to meet with and help support-seeking distressed people.

(d) Mobilizing and training lay or semi-professional workers to provide brief professional support to moderately distressed people on a voluntary basis.

(e) Referring highly distressed people to professional mental health clinics and practitioners for treatment.

As may be noted, the sources of support correspond to symptom severity. The milder the symptoms, the more likely persons will draw upon their own resources or those of close friends and family; the more serious the symptoms, the more likely they will draw upon the resources of a professional worker.

A comprehensive literature has accumulated on the many theoretical and applied issues that relate to support. Some of these issues are cited and briefly discussed here.

<u>To Distinguish Between High- And Low-Risk Groups</u>

In any disaster some groups are more vulnerable than others and require immediate support to prevent symptom formation and symptom exacerbation. Others have less immediate, urgent needs for support and will continue to function without breakdown. Research has identified a number of high risk groups cited below. It is important to identify still others.

(a) Elderly people are especially vulnerable for many reasons. They are overlooked or less likely to receive assistance in disaster situations by silent agreement, cannot rely on the few surviving kin for support beyond a minimum level, and have lost many self-sustaining activities and supporting people (Giel, 1990a).

(b) Minors are highly vulnerable. On the one hand, children are more appealing than the elderly and more likely to receive support. On the other hand, their very helplessness exposes them to well-intentioned, misinformed adults or to adult predators.

(c) People living in rural areas are far away from service facilities, are less likely to receive support, and if they do, to receive it relatively late in the disaster cycle (Kaniasty, Norris, & Murrell, 1990).

(d) Working class people in general and economically disadvantaged and poorly educated people, in particular are less knowledgeable than well-educated, middle-class people about soliciting support in their own behalf, and when they do so, are less likely to receive it (Riley & Eckenrode, 1986). They are also less likely to have insurance coverage to provide financial support subsequent to the stressful event.

(e) People who lack kin support, a basic interpersonal resource, are likely to become depressed and less able to mobilize support in their own behalf or to utilize it well when it is offered (Kaniasty & Norris, 1993).

(f) People who have experienced distress in prior disasters but received little help come to expect even less the next time. Moreover, those who expect less support actually receive less (Kaniasty, et al., 1990).

To Provide What People Need When They Need It

It is not an easy task to determine what different groups of people need at different stages in the stress and coping time frame. MacFarlane (1994) has distinguished the following stages: Planning, threat, impact, inventory and rescue, remedy and recovery, and the aftermath of traumatization. If we use the example of a hurricane, planning refers to efforts undertaken to prepare people who live in an area where hurricanes often occur to cope with this hypothetical eventuality. Other efforts become necessary when a particular community is threatened by a hurricane (threat). Still other types of support are required when the hurricane strikes the community (impact), the hurricane passes on and people assess damage and strive to minimize it (inventory and rescue), and when they begin the process of rehabilitation and restoration of their community, their homes, and their lives (remedy and recovery).

On the face of it, the identification of who needs what kind of support and when it is needed is an extremely complex assessment task. The meeting of these needs is an even more demanding organizational task. At the practical level, however, these tasks are less overwhelming. Many conceptually distinguishable kinds of support are not empirically distinguishable, either at the giving or the receiving end. Support providers who provide information or material help are also demonstrating to recipients that they care about them (emotional support) and that they are persons of worth. Nevertheless, there is a clear distinction between accelerating financial loans and insurance payments to injured parties on the one hand and providing them with emotional support and reassurance, on the other. It is important to determine when we should provide each of these support services in a community-wide disaster. It is recommended that intervention workers maintain close contact with key informants in the community in order to be updated concerning service timing.

To Identify People Capable of Providing Needed Support

We will briefly comment on several key issues in this process.

First, do we actively recruit volunteers with specific criteria in mind or do we accept self-selected volunteers? We tend to assume that people who volunteer to provide support services for afflicted community members select those tasks with which they are comfortable and if they find themselves doing something upsetting or difficult, transfer to a more comfortable assignment or drop out altogether. On the other hand, some well-meaning, energetic support providers may be unaware of their lack of appropriate skills and do considerable damage before others become aware of it. Still other helpers may be accomplishing a great deal, but experience burnout due to stressful situations with which they are dealing. These possibilities require us to do light screening of volunteers and to provide an avenue for helpers to seek professional help and peer support when they, themselves, become distressed or begin to question the efficacy of what they are doing.

Second, do we encourage family members to help people cope with disasters and do we encourage strangers to provide the necessary support? Research on relationship-based social support (Sarason, Sarason, & Pierce, 1994) points to circumstances when support from family members may be highly beneficial. These circumstances arise when the recipient believes (a) the provider can be relied upon to give the needed assistance, (b) the provider values their relationship and is committed to it, and (c) their prior relationship has been relatively free of conflict or ambivalent feelings. When these circumstances are absent, the help provided by family members will not be helpful and may even be damaging. It is advisable to speak frankly with potential recipients of support from family members to ascertain whether they would welcome support from prospective family members, friends, or strangers.

Third, should we recruit people who experienced similar disasters in the past? We recommend doing so when these people have been able to rebuild their lives successfully. Such people have high credibility in the eyes of current disaster victims and are more likely to achieve effective rapport in a relatively brief period. They are also able to draw upon their experiences and provide effective support. We also recommend recruiting people caught up in the current disaster who possess unusual personal resources and are able to help themselves and at the same time to help others.

Fourth, when do we employ professional workers vs. natural or lay helpers? Recent research by Memmott (1993) provides some specific answers to this question with a rural community. According to his field study, lay helpers tend to attribute less responsibility for the disastrous situation to older and younger people as compared to professional social workers. Also, lay helpers expect less problem-solving initiatives from older and younger people as compared to professional social workers. In general, professionals will expect more self-reliance of people in need of support. So when there is a shortage of resources for support, professionals will probably be able to instigate more self-support on the part of those in need.

We like to think that interventions help or at least cause no harm, but, in fact, many interventions--medical, psychological or societal--have deleterious effects on the recipients. It is imperative to monitor the support-giving effort and its effects with heightened alertness to the possibility that it may be detrimental to some of those to whom help is provided. Helpers, either family members or strangers, need to be appraised of the risk of iatrogenic disorders. We assume that all volunteers receive initial briefing and ongoing review. During this briefing and review we should apprise helpers of the possibility that they may harm rather than help the very people they wish to help, notwithstanding their own good intentions, if they ignore subtle or obvious cues that the intervention is not going well.

Efficacy of Coping Behavior by Support Recipients

Some people obtain and use support better than others. Depressed, lonely people exposed to stressful situations receive less support because they are less likely to solicit support, more likely to discourage it, and less likely to use it because of their depleted energy resources (Jerusalem, Schwarzer, & Hahn, this volume). Follow-up studies of recipients are necessary to identify those people who are unable to utilize the conventional forms of support and to ascertain what special support efforts should be undertaken in their behalf.

Empirical investigation of these issues is demanding and difficult. Deciding what to do in the present, imperfect state of knowledge on these issues is even more difficult. Giel (1990a,b) has suggested that all disasters are unique and must be understood in terms of the prior crises and disasters that affected the community as well as their cultural interpretation of the present crisis. Practical decisions in the field are based on the accumulated empirical wisdom achieved thus far in the field and on the idiosyncratic features of a particular large-scale disaster affecting particular people within a particular community. By monitoring our own efforts, we may be able to minimize iatrogenic side-effects and correct for our mistakes.

Community

Definition of the Term

Is a community a particular geographic or political area? We assume that the affected parties who require support and the parties who provide this support reside in the same or a nearby community, but this may not be literally true. A town may have been wiped out wholly or in part by a mudslide, and remote urban centers may become involved in damage control, interpersonal intervention, and reconstruction and rehabilitation. The community from which support is forthcoming may be a small township, a large city, a sprawling district, an entire country, or it may consist of groups living in different parts of a country or of the world.

The term community may be defined as a group of people who share common interests. The community in question is defined by common interests. All of humankind share some common interests (e.g., having air to breathe) and would react as a global community to dangerous pollution of the air we breathe. By contrast, only a few people have a common interest in preventing an angry wife from divorcing her errant husband (e.g., the husband, children, friends and family). The common interests that define the community in the present context are determined by the location, intensity and scope of the threat or damage, and by geographic, legal-political, and socio-psychological considerations.

Pre-Disaster Resources in the Community

Many communities possess resources that are mobilized by pre-planning or by spontaneous response to need, so that deliberate efforts to recruit support at large may be unnecessary. On the other hand, planning and coordination of resources and efforts to provide support are always necessary (Baum, 1986). Prudent pre-planning may have produced a comprehensive survey of the various support-providing organizations that operate within the community--governmental organizations (local, state, federal) and volunteer organizations--and what each organization does. If the survey does not exist or is out of date, it should be undertaken and completed before efforts are made to recruit support at large. The urgency of the situation will determine the speed and thoroughness with which the survey is conducted.

When the survey of support demand and support supply is completed, the following recommendations are in order:

(a) Existing organizations should do what they know best, if (a big "if") what they know best is what is needed.

(b) Existing organizations should be encouraged to acquire new skills or modify their existing repertoire of skills so as to better serve affected people in the community. It is more efficacious for an existing organization to adapt to new circumstances than to establish a new organization from the ground up to provide the necessary services. It is recommended that we approach intact organizations such as the police, teachers, or the churches through their leaders. These groups already have a tradition of established support relationships within their ranks and may be able to recruit volunteers from their membership in large numbers. They may also have some of the necessary skills. For example, teachers already know a lot about children and working with groups. Police are trained to keep their cool under pressure. Experts can give these groups the additional skills and knowledge that they require.

(c) As a last resort, ad hoc organizations should be created to deal with the special support requirements of situations that would not otherwise be met.

Endorsement of Community Support Recruitment

Launching a community-wide effort to recruit support for targeted groups is an important step. The public support of many groups is essential, especially the respected leadership of the community--the elected officials, religious leaders, prominent people in the world of business, the arts, and the universities. The endorsement of these leaders is a necessary, but not a sufficient basis for a successful support recruitment campaign. Support will be more forthcoming from a given community when respected leaders in the community publicly endorse the support mobilization effort and when no respected leader opposes it.

Community Values

Do the members of the community share common values and attitudes toward the disaster and how to cope with it? We have spoken of a larger community of interest in defining the community from which support will be forthcoming for those who require it. There may be major ethnic, socio-economic, religious, and psychosocial differences within the community or between support providers and recipients. Consequently there will be differences of opinion about who should provide what to whom. These discrepancies may lead to differences between support providers and recipients in perceived trust, communication style, values placed on such relevant concepts as God, fate, and charity, and the actual versus the anticipated resource potential in providers and recipients.

Consider the implications of the following scenario: The neighborhood hit by a tornado consists wholly of socio-economically disadvantaged working class people. The majority of professional workers and volunteers who enter the neighborhood to provide needed services belong to the more affluent, better educated middle class. These differences may be serious barriers to effective support provision for several reasons:

(a) The support providers have been spared the destruction and dislocation that affects those who require their support. This difference may be a barrier to establishing rapport and good working relationships.

(b) The socio-economic and ethnic differences alluded to earlier may block optimal communication and support. The financial losses incurred by the less affluent group may be inconsequential to the more affluent. The necessity to move to a new neighborhood may mean different things for upper class people who make frequent desirable moves than for lower class people who may never have moved from their community before and had no intention of doing so until the disaster occurred.

(c) Different attitudes toward divine providence and tragic fate, and different interpretations of personal and social disaster serve to distance one group from another (Meichenbaum, 1994).

These points reinforce our earlier thesis that visible representatives from within the affected community must be partners in planning in order to provide key information and translate values subscribed to by the community into action. They also bear witness to the thesis that recovery is a partnership effort that transcends group differences and animosities.

If it is difficult to locate those in need of support or those able and willing to provide it, it is even more difficult to insure shared community interests and values held by support providers and recipients. The process of catalyzing is designed to do both: To utilize the available means of communication to locate support providers and support recipients, and to educate, persuade and motivate them to develop interpersonal relationships that will benefit the community in general and those adversely affected by the disaster, in particular.

Catalyzing

Definition

Catalyzing is a difficult term to define. In chemistry the term refers to a substance that modifies or increases a chemical reaction between two or more reactants without being decreased or affected by the process. In the humanities and social sciences the term has come to mean an idea, event, person or group that serves as a necessary cause for change. We regard the term as referring to an interpersonal process whereby some people change the perceptions, cognitions, motivations, and actual behaviors of other people.

(a) Perceptual: We wish to change how people--the general public, potential helpers and recipients of help--view the disaster.

(b) Cognitive: We wish to inform these groups of the dire straits in which some people find themselves and of their need for certain kinds of support, and how the others may help them.

(c) Motivational: We wish to enable or persuade people--helpers and recipients alike--to do something they would otherwise be unable or reluctant to do.

(d) Behavioral: We wish to provide manuals and models of behaviors that we would like helpers and recipients to emulate.

To insure that the message reach its intended audience, we must consider a number of issues.

Importance of the Media

People are more likely to provide support to others when they become aware of the human dimensions of the disaster. People become aware of these dimensions only when they learn about them. The existing electronic media are the most rapid and probably the most efficient means of informing the public of what is being done. Communication and response may be so automatic that it is unnecessary to "catalyze" support in a given community for a given disaster. It may arise spontaneously or follow smoothly and automatically from preplanned intervention programs. This spontaneous development should not absolve researchers and practitioners from assisting and monitoring the process so as to making recommendations for present and future crisis intervention efforts.

Groups Involved in Catalyzing Support by the Media

Many different groups play an essential role in this process. Their involvement may be initiated by and is influenced by the communication network selected. Starting from the top,

(a) Media communicators, invariably salaried professional workers, create or adapt the support recruitment message and place it before the public. They cannot operate without the cooperation of the groups cited below.

(b) Sponsors are prestigious people in the community, whose name lends credibility and value to the effort. They may be the same people identified earlier as community leaders or may include additional people from outside the community whose reputation enhances the catalyzing effort.

(c) Gate-keepers are members of the organizational and political structure of the community who either permit the support endeavor to take place or help it along. If gatekeepers choose not to cooperate, they may throw up political and legal roadblocks to thwart the support recruitment campaign or the subsequent provision of support to those who need it.

(d) Planners coordinate the efforts to bring support from those who have the resources to those who need them.

(e) Directors head the organizations that send people into the field to provide the support.

(f) Field leaders supervise and assess what is happening in the field.

(g) Field workers, typically volunteers, provide the actual support under the supervision of field leaders.

All of these groups must be enlightened by knowledgeable "insiders," people familiar with the community and its current crisis, in order to insure their cooperation and enlist their expertise in the communication and persuasion process.

Preferred Medium, Targets, and Messages

Which medium will deliver the message best? The message may be delivered by any of the media--television, radio, newspaper, handbill, or personal communication. All have the potential for providing support. It is necessary to consider the message and the intended audience in the context of the disaster in order to select the preferred medium.

The media are utilized to communicate relevant messages to three groups: Those who will provide support, those who will receive it, and the general public who may encourage or discourage the other two groups in the community endeavor. All groups need to become knowledgeable and willing to do their part. The distressed people themselves need information in order to appraise their personal situation and to identify what they need and where they can hope to find it. Potential support providers need information to know what they will be required to do, where, when, and for how long.

The messages directed to support providers may not be appropriate for recipients. For example, a communicator might elect to make a group more appealing to potential support providers by emphasizing its tragic plight. In so doing, one may gain many providers, but lose many more potential recipients. People in need of help may find the description of their plight so odious or humiliating that they are reluctant to come forward and accept help under those terms. In using a public medium to promote a community social support program, we must tailor our messages so that they achieve their purpose with some groups without offending others. Where this cannot be accomplished, the organizers may use a private medium, letters or meetings by invitation only, to convey a message that is intended for some, but not others.

Communicating the Meaning and Implications of the Disaster

It is necessary to identify and communicate widely an existential healing context by which we understand and interpret the disaster so as to mobilize effective community support for distressed members. This context will differ for one kind of disaster versus another, for one group within the community versus another, and from community to community.

Consider the differing contextual implications of a man-made versus a natural disaster. If the disaster is man-made, there is the temptation to become involved in recrimination, scapegoating, and litigation. People's energy, a valuable, but scarce resource in all disasters, may be squandered by engaging in counter-productive activities directed against (1) those perceived to be responsible for the disaster, or (2) those who might have prevented the disaster from happening to begin with, or (3) those who might have controlled the damage better, once the disaster occurred.

This anger of people directly affected by the disaster and the anger of other concerned groups, if properly expressed and channeled, can accelerate government cooperation in all stages of reaction to disaster and reconstruction. The same anger can be counterproductive by itself rather than a means to recovery and reconstruction. Anger should not determine the priorities of the individual or the group, rational analysis should. Accordingly, people struggling to cope with current pressing problems may postpone appeals to government or to the courts for compensation to a later date. Hence, the importance of the media in educating potential helpers and receivers about meanings, priorities, and appropriate behaviors is clear. The media should be used, for example, to educate the general public about the potential damage that unbridled anger can cause: The exaggeration of disaster-related damage, physical harm to targets of the anger, pointless destruction of property, and social divisiveness.

It is as important to use the media to discourage counter-productive acts as to encourage productive ones.

If a disaster is of natural origins, the psychological problems brought about by some attributions may be equally debilitating. We may blame the natural disaster on God or on ourselves, and either blame assignment is likely to be detrimental to our functioning. To blame God for the disaster is to confirm that cherished assumptions about God's grace and the natural order in the world have been shattered with detrimental consequences for our present and future value systems. To blame ourselves is to acknowledge that we have erred or sinned in some way and to engage in compulsive self-flagellation.

We recommend that the civic and religious leaders of the community develop a series of perspectives about the disaster in consultation with professional workers. These perspectives should provide some reassuring answers to why the disaster took place and should minimize damage to pre-existing belief systems.

We further recommend that these leaders select or create religious and civil ceremonies and rituals that pay proper respect to the afflicted who have lost valuable resources and that encourage all to participate in rebuilding the stricken community (Meichenbaum, 1994). Rituals are important because they make it easier for people in need of support to become available to those able and willing to provide it. Ørner (this volume) states that rituals are important for providers as well. Specialized emergency helping teams wear uniforms, pledge allegiance to the goals of their organization and obedience to its chain of command. These rituals (e.g., special costumes or badges, oaths, prayers) identify the members as public servants with a defined mission, and reinforce a cohesive group identity and associated esprit de corps.

Information is Catalytic and Empowering

This section discusses the kinds of information that will enhance support activity: What to do, why it is worth doing, and how to cope with losses and ongoing stresses.

People are more likely to volunteer if they are given clear and precise instructions. Receipt of information in terms of general principles or vague instructions may be dismaying to people when they require structure. Hence, it is important to phrase media communications to the public in a clear, practical manner.

People volunteer when they become aware of the genuine needs of distressed community members, and when they come to believe that the help they are being asked to provide will be appreciated and will actually be helpful. Negative stereotypes held by some members of the community about those in need of help are a barrier to this awareness and to constructive beliefs. If you believe that the help you are asked to provide will be rejected, or will not be appreciated or helpful, you are less likely to offer it. Appeals for volunteers may be strengthened when accompanied by community surveys showing that large numbers of potential recipients welcome the help they receive. Information of this kind is important when either the support providing group or the recipient group is an ethnic minority that elicits unfavorable stereotypes from some segments of the community.

The media is a proper avenue to educate people about the economics of investment. Investing our resources to help others to help themselves is a worthwhile investment, because it does not diminish the resources of the investors and it increases the resources of the recipients, thereby helping the community as a whole. People are likely to be receptive to an informed appeal that stresses the gains of investing community resources to control damage and to accelerate reconstruction versus the costs of inactivity (see Hobfoll, Briggs, & Wells, this volume).

The same notion applies to the psychosocial concept of empowerment. When we provide distressed people with the means to do things in their own behalf and to recover thereby from adverse circumstances, we are enhancing their sense of empowerment. We may also speak of empowerment for the helpers. When we approach the community with an appeal to their sense of social responsibility, we are creating conditions in which some people will voluntarily help others. Their involvement in behalf of others enhances their sense of control over their own lives and over what transpires in their community. In other words, they become more powerful from the experience of helping others regain power over their lives. This psychoeducational concept is worth communicating in the messages directed toward potential volunteer support groups.

Information about compensation for injury or damage should be introduced at a time when it facilitates rather than interferes with recovery. Depending on the kind of disaster, some may derive positive benefits from pursuing the issue forcefully shortly after the disaster, others may not. We are well aware that efforts to receive compensation may be detrimental to recovery and rehabilitation. This caveat applies to people who elect to emphasize their current disability so as to increase the size of the claim they are making, and to people who invest most of their energy in obtaining compensation and invest little in rehabilitation efforts. It is essential that those representing the media consult with mental health and forensic authorities when they provide information about this sensitive issue.

The media may be used as a therapeutic educator, informing the public about the kinds of cognitive mechanisms that may enhance positive, optimistic affect in otherwise depressed victims or support providers. These include: (a) Contrasting our situation with that of less fortunate groups elsewhere, (b) Imagining a potentially worse situation, (c) Manufacturing normative standards for affect, cognition, and behavior that makes our responses "normal," and (d) Identifying positive benefits that may accrue from this unfortunate disaster and from our efforts to cope with it (Taylor, Wood, & Lichtman, 1983).

We tend to approach the public with an optimistic, activist orientation toward disaster. Such a perspective is regarded as a major personal resource in stressful situations in many Western societies. On the other hand, many distressed people tend to adopt a fatalistic orientation to life in general and toward disaster in particular. Lay and professional workers who come in contact with people professing this fatalist orientation may become discouraged from helping such people to help themselves. We recommend that helpers not interpret this orientation in terms of their own Western stereotypes. Fatalism does not necessarily imply passivity on the one hand or pessimism on the other. Many religious people profess a constructive formulation of fatalism that mandates active efforts on one's behalf with a recognition that personal effort is a necessary, but not a sufficient condition for the desired outcome. We recommend that those who develop educational and inspirational communications directed to such audiences broaden their personal orientation and consider the subtle nuances of the orientations of others.

Group identity and group consciousness are community assets. They place the good of the group above that of the individual and encourage those less affected by the disaster to help those who are more affected. It is important to inculcate in all community members the awareness that the nature of these disasters is such that today's support providers may become tomorrow's support recipients. Media communications should emphasize this musketeer imperative (one for all and all for one).

Overview

There have been many revolutionary changes in the science and practice of psychology in its brief history. Three of these changes are implicit in this report: (1) The shift in focus from the individual to the group, (2) The shift from treating illness to promoting health, and (3) The shift of focus from internal to external determinants of disturbed behavior.

In the beginning the scientific and professional goals of psychology were directed toward the individual. Fields as diverse as psychophysiology and clinical psychology illustrate common focus. Theories were developed to describe and explain an individual's behavior, and professional services were provided on an individual basis. In recent years, organizational psychology, military psychology, and community psychology have come to emphasize theoretical understanding and professional intervention with large groups of people, if not entire communities.

This shift was accompanied by a shift from a pathogenic orientation--we treat sick people and cure their illnesses--to a salutogenic one--we try to make people healthy or to help them stay healthy (Antonovsky, 1979). The assumption that the absence of illness was health has been rejected, and in its place has come an effort to understand what makes and keeps people well-adjusted and well-functioning in the face of health-threatening forces.

The third revolutionary change has been the focus on external rather than internal determinants of abnormal behavior. Psychoanalysis and its offshoots assumed that people behaved in a disturbed manner in their day to day lives because of their aberrant perceptions, thoughts, motivations, and feelings. Major attention was given to the inner workings of the personality and scant attention was paid to the nuances of the environment. The shift came with the rise of interest in stress, stressful life events, traumatic events, and large-scale disasters in that order. We now assert that people behave inappropriately because they are currently exposed or were exposed in the past to unusual, aversive, threatening circumstances.

The two approaches are complementary rather than contradictory because each specializes in different life circumstances. When some people behave in a bizarre fashion in response to ostensibly normal events (e.g., driving through a tunnel, meeting unfriendly people)--while most do not--we focus upon inner world torment. When many, if not most, people exposed to an abnormal set of external circumstances (e.g., war, rape) behave in a bizarre fashion, we regard their behavior as "normal" and understandable, given these difficult circumstances. When some of these people continue to show disturbed behavior long after these tormenting circumstances have ceased, we continue to attribute their current behavior to the after-effects of this torment.

Unfortunately, many professional workers do not make these distinctions and only offer individual, inner-world oriented treatment to people suffering from various kinds of external world torment. This confusion is very evident in the planning and treating of large scale community disasters. Hence, the reason d'etre of this volume in general and our report on catalyzing community support in particular.

We have defined the relevant terms, identified the various phases in the process of providing the right kind of help to those in need of it, elaborated on some of the considerations in each phase, and focused in on the communicative processes that are essential. These phases, considerations and recommendations are consistent with a group-oriented, salutogenic, preventive approach toward highly stressful large-scale disasters.

Finally, we have a confession to make. We were not comfortable in preparing this report because of the competing demands of a research versus an intervention orientation. Research takes place in a relatively quiet working environment in which researchers investigate without time pressure human suffering before or long after the fact. Intervention--whether primary, secondary or tertiary--takes place in a tumultuous, time-driven world in which professional workers consult and cooperate with many other people in providing help to still larger numbers of people in a fluid, life threatening catastrophe unfolding in real time. These are very different working conditions, and in dealing with the one, we felt we were not doing justice to the other. We consoled ourselves with the thought that the information and insights from the one fertilize the work in the other, and decided to take a definite tack in our analysis of the topic. The decision was in favor of intervention and this decision is reflected in the practical recommendations offered throughout the paper.

References

Antonovsky, A. (1979). Health, stress, and coping. San Francisco: Jossey-Bass.

Baum, A. (1986). Toxins, technology, and natural disasters. In G.R. Vandenbos and B.K. Bryant (Eds.), Cataclysms, crises and catastrophes: Psychology in action (pp. 1-53). Washington DC: APA Master Lectures.

Giel, R. (1990a). Psychosocial processes in disasters. International Journal of Mental Health, 19, 7-20.

Giel, R. (1990b). The psychosocial aftermath of two major disasters in the Soviet Union. Journal of Traumatic Stress, 4, 381-392.

Kaniasty, K., Norris, F.H., & Murrell, S.A. (1990). Received and perceived social support following natural disaster. Journal of Applied Social Psychology, 20, 85-114.

Kaniasty, K., & Norris, F.H. (1993). A test of the social support deterioration model in the context of natural disaster. Journal of Personality and Social Psychology, 64, 394-408.

Memmott, J.L. (1993). Models of helping and coping: A field experiment with natural and professional helpers. Social Work Research and Abstract, 29, 11-21.

Riley, D., & Eckenrode, J. (1986). Social ties: Subgroup differences in costs and benefits. Journal of Personality and Social Psychology, 51, 770-778.

Sarason, I.G., Sarason, B.R., & Pierce, G.R. (1994). Social support: Global and relationship-based levels of analysis. Journal of Social and Personal Relationships, 11, 295-312.

Taylor, S., Wood, J., & Lichtman, R. (1983). It could be worse: Selective evaluation as a response to victimization. Journal of Social Issues, 39, 19-40.

PREVENTION AND TREATMENT OF COMMUNITY STRESS: HOW TO BE A MENTAL HEALTH EXPERT AT THE TIME OF DISASTER

Charles Figley, Florida State University, USA
Robert Giel, Academisch Ziekenhuis Groningen, The Netherlands
Stefania Borgo, Centro di Ricerca in Psicoterapia e Scienze del Comportamento, Italy
Sylvester Briggs, Ohio Dept. of Rehabilitation and Correction, USA
Mika Haritos-Fatouros, Aristotelian University, Greece

In an extraordinary document, Cater, Revel, Sapir, and Walker (1993) provided a four section report of community disasters. These sections include (1) why a report was needed, (2) a world picture of disasters, (3) the dynamics of disasters, and (4) disaster database. Among the more interesting revelations is found in this last section. Following is a topology of disaster types, in outline form:

1.	**Sudden, Natural**	1.12	Tsunami and Tidal Wave
1.1	Avalanche	1.13	Volcanic Eruption and Glowing Avalanches
1.2	Cold Wave		
1.3	Earthquake	**2.**	**Long-term Natural**
1.4	Aftershock	2.1	Epidemics
1.5	Floods	2.2	Drought
1.5.1	Flash Flood	2.3	Desertification
1.5.2	Dam Collapse	2.4	Famine
1.6	Heat wave	2.5	Food Shortage or Crop Failure
1.7	High wind cyclone		
1.7.1	Storm	**3.**	**Sudden Man-Made**
1.7.2	Hail	3.1	Structural Accident
1.7.3	Sand Storm	3.1.1	Structural Collapse
1.7.4	Storm surges	3.1.2	Building Collapse
1.7.5	Thunderstorm	3.1.3	Mine Collapse or a Mine Cave-in
1.7.6	Tropical Storm		
1.7.7	Tornado	3.2	Transport Accidents
1.8	Insect Infestation or Animal Infestation	3.2.1	Air Disasters
		3.2.2	Land Disasters
1.9	Landslide	3.2.3	Sea Disasters
1.10	Earth Flow	3.3	Industrial/Technological Accidents
1.11	Power Shortage		

3.4	Explosions	3.6	Fires
3.4.1	Chemical Explosions	3.6.1	Forest/grassland Fire
3.4.2	Nuclear Explosions or Thermonuclear Explosions	3.6.2	Urban
		4.	**Long-term Man-made**
3.4.3	Mine Explosions	4.1	National (civil strife, civil war)
3.5	Pollution		
3.5.1	Acid Rain	4.2	International
3.5.2	Chemical Pollution	4.3	Displaced Population
3.5.3	Atmosphere Pollution	4.3.1	Displaced Persons
3.5.4	Chlorofluoro-carbons (CFC)	4.3.2	Refugees(Cater, Revel, Sapir, and Walker (1993),
3.5.5	Oil Pollution		pp. 94-97).

In addition, the section provided a topology of the disaster effects. They noted, in addition to the population that was either dead or injured, those who were the primary affected population, the exposed population, the population at risk, the target population, the secondary affected population, and the homeless as a result of the disaster.

Scope of This Chapter

It is well beyond the scope of this chapter and, indeed, the volume in which it resides, to discuss the prevention and treatment tenets of each of these disaster contexts and the population affected. However, it is critical for disaster workers experienced in working with disasters in any part of the world to recognize that their experiences may not be applicable to any other types of disasters and in any other parts of the world (Lystad, 1988).

In this chapter we attempt to consolidate the views of a working group comprised of twelve internationally recognized experts[1] in the general area of community stress. An important theme throughout our discussions was the importance of the role of mental health experts at the scene of a community disaster.

Nowadays, a common feature of any disaster is the tidal wave of experts on the scene, trying to do good but often adding to the confusion. This is in itself a stressful experience. This chapter is aiming at helping the mental health expert in overcoming this embarrassment by developing a plan of action as quickly as possible.

The tenet of this disaster inventory is that the relationship between the disaster experience and the traumatic responses of the individual is not a direct one. It is mediated by the perception of the disaster as a risk and a threat to the community at the individual level. It is also mediated by culture which determines the coping styles in case of loss and the social networks and resources. These are all contextual features defining the impact of the disaster.

Information Gathering:
What We Need to Know First

Demographic Profile of the Stricken Population

Identifying the stricken population is a vital first step. If possible, attempt to identify those that fall into one of the categories noted above: primary affected population, the exposed population, the population at risk, the target population, the secondary affected population, and the homeless as a result of the disaster. Note the subgroups in each category: Children, elderly, internal or external migrants and refugees, institutionalized or otherwise dependent people, materially deprived subgroups requiring more than average protection and rehabilitation. Who is most effected by the disaster? Which groups who had been "marginalized" in the community prior to the disaster are most vulnerable to the negative impact of the disaster? (e.g. poor, unemployed, minorities, psychiatric population, young, untrained emergency workers such as adolescents, etc.) A close, inter-related community may be knocked out by an earthquake, for example. Another way to state this question is "What have I done to conduct a community diagnosis?" Always keep in mind long-term follow up.

Nature of the Disaster

Consistent with the World Disasters Report, it is important to be able to classify the disaster, especially with regard to it being either man-made or natural, because of the issues of culpability and compensation in the rehabilitation phase. The type and rapidity of impact (radiation, chemical, flood, fire, earthquake, etc.) is important to note because the lack of time to prepare has important indirect and long-term consequences for, among other things: (1) The magnitude of loss (deaths, number of injured, material losses); (2) the known or unknown hazard, in the latter case with more lasting anxiety; (3) recurring risk, and degree of warning and preparedness at the community and individual level; (4) the scope of impact is the central, intermediate or peripheral to community functioning; (5) the degree to which escape was or was not possible during or immediately following the disasaster. The above items apply to the community as a whole, in addition to this, the expert should have an idea of the full range of personal exposures and experiences to be expected under the conditions of the disaster.

Channels of Communication

The expert should be aware of the customary channels of the communication in the community, and of the habits of the authorities and the public in this aspect. Intactness of these channels; how open and public are they; and through whom is experience shared? Where will people go for information and explanation? Which source do they consider reliable?

Authority Structure

It is important to determine the formal and informal lines of authority, and their intactness and inherent strengths and weaknesses in an emergency. Did the political structures and agencies that survived the community disaster effectively represent and have the trust of its people? What is the degree of credibility of the authorities? Did a disaster preparedness plan and structure exist?

National Resources

This includes material resources available and transportable from elsewhere in the country; rescue and emergency health services (e.g. the military and Red Cross), likely to be involved; existing non-governmental and religious agencies and their roles in an emergency.

Social Support at the Community and Family Level

At the community level, what voluntary associations and mutual support systems are available and can be utilized by the victims of the disaster? What support within the (extended) family is customary? Who is the head of the family, and to whom is leadership delegated in case of a crisis? To what extent is the family free to act and move, independent of the authorities? What is characteristically the locus of control of the family? What are important differences between the social strata?

Attitudes Towards and Institutions Dealing With Loss and Mourning

Funeral rites and customs differ widely across cultures, and serve to pay homage to the victims and come to terms with their loss. This latter aspect is important to resolve whatever negative feelings (guilt) prevail in the survivors. This includes memorial services and monuments. At the personal level the survivors often wish to have an explanation and to know about the last moments of the victim. In other words, the expert should acquire knowledge about cultural coping behavior and defensive styles, as well as details regarding the disaster.

Victims

Nowadays, it is accepted that the category of the victims includes more people than those primarily affected by the disaster: e.g. relatives and friends whether or not present at the time and the site of the disaster; rescuers; accidental witnesses, those who should have been a victim but escaped by accident; onlookers drawn to the site of the disaster etc. The expert should be aware of the range of victims and on whom it is to focus.

Post-Traumatic Stress Responses

DSM-IV, with its clear description of PTSD, has somewhat obscured the fact that other morbid reactions can be more numerous and severe.
- Generally increased mortality, particularly in the underprivileged or socially deprived;
- more serious course (less responsive to treatment) of all kinds of diseases due to deficiencies in the immune system;
- more serious course of physical illness, due to co-morbidity of physical disease and depression, anxiety or PTSD;
- increases in illness behavior, i.e. increased awareness of any symptom, followed quickly by contact with the health services;
- and finally, changes in mental morbidity; depression, anxiety, suicide, psychosis and PTSD.

The expert should identify the needs and demands in this respect, avoiding modelling all suffering in one way more convenient to himself. The above points should serve to help the expert obtain a fuller picture of the emergency situation. In addition, he or she should explore in which post-impact phase the community is. During the recoil phase the community is more united, cohesive and optimistic than during the protracted rehabilitation phase, when people are on their own again, less hopeful and less certain of the future. During that phase, the need for individual psychosocial support may be greatest and more prolonged.

Some Recommendations

Armed with the above information, mental health specialists can serve a vital role to communities affected by catastrophe. Among those that immediately come to mind are the following:

A. Mobilize and Organize Existing and/or New Self Help Groups Which Will be the Back Bone of Social Support.

We believe that any outsider must be careful not to create an artificial and temporary program of intervention that can not be maintained by those who will remain long after the disaster clean up. It is vital to recognize and build upon the community's strengths and natural, social resources. Among the recommended actions are:

1. Recruit advisors and helpers and/or people from existing self help groups. Turn survivors into helpers.

2. Consider the importance of who is perceived to initiate and provide appropriate help.

3. When establishing new groups identify individuals involved in existing community provision.

4. To recruit people for self help groups consider using local rituals and ceremonies; neighborhood and existing patterns of social bonding.

B. Energize Self Help Groups

Similarly, self help groups are the single most important element to recover, beyond naturally existing systems such as family, neighborhood groups (both informal and formal) and other community institutions. Among our recommendations for mobilizing support groups are:

1. Use first self help groups (two at most; 15-30 people, one session) as focus groups to map out and pinpoint problems, to be discussed and faced in self help groups. Give priority to basic issues of security and stability.

2. Support general and existing values; families; respect of elderly; care of children. Consider that the threat to values are often more threatening than the actual threat (Hobfoll, Briggs, & Wells, this volume).

3. Support initiatives for those who are the "formal" providers of help (Ørner, this volume).

4. Consider that perceived support is more important than actual social support (Sarason & Sarason, this volume).

5. Be advised by past experiences of what has been helpful and what was not: e.g. family placements for children are better in some situations than others.

6. Bring in experts to work with specific groups.

7. Follow up and evaluate work of self help groups.

C. General Actions:

Other, more general interventions we would recommend include the following:

1. Foster reliance and trust in local services (for social support).

2. Recognize usefulness of local cultural patterns (de Vries, this volume).

3. Organize general umbrella supports using overall organizational facilities- national, political, etc.

4. Identify and plan for handling the ongoing and escalating adversities. Disasters change over time. To be prepared one must know how to monitor the impact of the disaster over time and how to use this information in formulating an intervention strategy.

5. Make plans to insure that the survivors have been permitted to do as much as they can for themselves. Those survivors who are empowered and enabled will be better prepared to carry on after outsiders depart (de Jong, this volume).

6. Determine which specific interventions can be provided both in acute, immediate past and long terms. For example, provide debriefing immediately following the disaster, support groups after that, and group treatment for disaster-related PTSD after that. Illustrative educational materials are useful throughout to prepare the population for recovery.

D. Working with Government Officials

Invariably, mental health specialists will be working with local, regional, and national government officials regarding all the issues noted above. It is wise to gain the confidence of these officials to insure that effective prevention and intervention programs are effectively developed and implemented. Following are some recommendations in terms of providing useful information to officials:

1. Urge them to provide consolation and condolence to the families of the disaster victims and to note that families will require time and assistance of the community to recover.

2. Recommend that they use experts to give information (e.g. Hurricane center)

3. Warn them not to promise something they can not provide, avoid false hope.

4. Train them in the immediate and long-term wanted and unwanted consequences of disasters and insure that this knowledge is provided to the officials who deal with the media.

5. Urge them to establish methods for controlling rumors.

6. Overall, be certain that your message to these officials are simple, clear, and do not overload them.

7. Suggest that burials should be completed within 72 hours and prevent reexposure.

8. Urge them to avoid unnecessary separation of those affected from friends and family.

9. Urge them to try to clear up and remove reminders of the disasters as quickly as possible.

E. Public Information Media

The media are, by definition, the primary resource for public education. Most media representatives are eager to help recovery efforts. Following are some recommendations for mental health experts in working with these professionals:

1. Spend sufficient time in educating them about their role in the recovery process; that the general public needs answers to vital questions. The answers will help them shift from fright and fear to rebuilding their lives and community. Among the questions are (1) What happened to us? (2) Why did this happen to us? (3) How did others react during the disaster and now? (4) How have people like us survived other, similar disasters elsewhere (the more similar the community the more useful the

information)? (5) What can we do now to make things better for ourselves, our loved ones, and our community?

2. Establish special disaster report teams that can be a resource to media about various aspects of the disaster and the recovery.

3. Be sensitive to signs of respect for both living and dead.

4. Critique the quality of public information reports in various media and communicate these evaluations to influential officials inside and outside the respective media.

5. Be cautions about the use of certain terms that would instill panic, and increase anxiety and uncertainty.

6. Urge media representatives to include stories of coping models and past history of successful coping efforts (available and representative.)

Compassion Fatigue

Mental health specialists can also be helpful in recognizing and carefully monitoring those whose work most with the suffering. These include, but are not limited to police, dispatchers, soldiers, fire fighters, medical personnel, and other emergency responders who are exposed directly to the injured, the dead, and those who mourn their death. However, others such as clean up crews, morgue workers, red cross workers, and, yes, even mental health workers are affected emotionally. The reactions are similar to those who suffer from traumatic stress and, in some cases, posttraumatic stress disorder: startle responses, flashbacks, social withdrawal, aggression, depression, sleeping problems, and general stress reactions. These reactions are a normal reaction to the extraordinary conditions of post-disaster work. At one time these reactions were known simply as "burnout." Now they are recognized as a special and more definitive form of burnout known as "compassion stress" and "compassion fatigue" (Figley, 1995). The most important point in either prevention or treating Compassion Fatigue is to treat it like a traumatic stress reactions and implement treatment procedures accordingly, even though persons exhibiting the symptoms were not directly in "harms way." We now know that working with those in harms way who suffer can be equally as stressful as direct exposure to the danger of the disaster.

Conclusion

Mental health specialists can be a part of the solution or part of the problem. Gathering vital information is the first step. Based on this information, the recommendations noted above should be useful in helping to develop a comprehensive, temporary plan for the emotional recovery. At the same time, mental health specialists should be cautious about their own mental health while attending to the suffering of others.

References

Cater, N., Revel, J., Sapir, D. and Walker, P. (1993). World Disasters Report 1993. Geneva: The International Federation of Red Cross (IFRC) and Red Crescent Societies (RCS).

de Jong, J.T.V.M. (this volume). Prevention of the consequences of man-made or natural disaster at the (inter)national, the community, the family, and the individual level. In S. E. Hobfoll & M. W. de Vries (Eds.), Extreme stress and Communities: Impact and Intervention. Dordrecht, The Netherlands: Kluwer.

deVries, M. W. (this volume). Culture, community and catastrophe: Issues in understanding communities under difficult conditions. In S. E. Hobfoll & M. W. de Vries (Eds.), Extreme stress and Communities: Impact and Intervention. Dordrecht, The Netherlands: Kluwer.

Figley, C. R. (Ed.) (1995). Compassion Fatigue: Secondary Traumatic Stress From Treating the Traumatized. New York: Brunner/Mazel.

Hobfoll, S. E., Briggs, S., & Wells, J. (this volume). Community stress and resources: Actions and reactions. In S. E. Hobfoll & M. W. de Vries (Eds.), Extreme stress and Communities: Impact and Intervention. Dordrecht, The Netherlands: Kluwer.

Ørner, R. J. (this volume). Intervention strategies for emergency response groups: A new conceptual framework. In S. E. Hobfoll & M. W. de Vries (Eds.), Extreme stress and Communities: Impact and Intervention. Dordrecht, The Netherlands: Kluwer.

Lystad, M. (Ed.) (1988). Mental Health Response to Mass Emergencies: Theory and Practice. New York: Brunner/Mazel.

Sarason, I. G., Sarason, B. R., & Pierce, G. R. (this volume). Stress and social support. In S. E. Hobfoll & M. W. de Vries (Eds.), Extreme stress and Communities: Impact and Intervention. Dordrecht, The Netherlands: Kluwer.

Notes:
1. In addition to the authors, they included James Jackson, Jacob Lomranz, Donald Meichenbaum, Roderick J. Ørner, Robert Pynoos, Bessel van der Kolk, Lars Weisæth

INTERVENTION STRATEGIES FOR EMERGENCY RESPONSE GROUPS: A NEW CONCEPTUAL FRAMEWORK

Roderick J Ørner
Department of Clinical Psychology, Baverstock House
Lincoln, England.

Emergency Responders, Their Host Communities And A New World Order

Emergency responder groups now encompass a broader variety of expert professionals and organizations than our local police, firebrigades, health care organizations, ambulance services or social services departments. This is an important development of relatively recent origin. A further change is that in many instances operational commitments may be geographically removed from their host communities. Historically, emergency services were established to respond to critical incidents and disasters affecting particular localities. In return for services that aim to minimize damage within a community, that same community supports and meets the costs of maintaining emergency response capabilities. This damage limitation and containment is affected at a physical and a psychological level. By largely confining exposure to extreme situations to specialist emergency services personnel the broader public is protected from traumatic events that, as predicted by Janoff-Bullman and Frieze (1983), might destabilize belief systems that underpin a given social order.

To promote the accomplishment of these socially stabilizing functions a range of rituals and ceremonies are practiced. This is most obviously observed in the case of staff selection, training, initiation, rituals centered on the wearing of uniforms, of subservience to hierarchical command structures and rituals reinforcing service loyalty. These rituals achieve the double feat of setting emergency responder groups apart from the general public they serve and protect, whilst simultaneously identifying these individuals as public servants of the community.

Crucially, this mutuality of interest is not so apparent when emergency responders are deployed away from host communities. Recent instabilities in world politics have highlighted conditions where local resources cannot sustain viable communities. Previously this tended to occur in conjunction with natural disasters. In consequence, unprecedented international call is made on the expertise of emergency responder groups. Traditional emergency services benefits from tried and tested operational practices, but other responder groups may be less experienced or may be deployed (or dispersed on return to base) in a manner that fails to take account of risks of psychological traumatisation. The need to develop and implement credible intervention strategies for all emergency responder groups is therefore more pressing than ever before.

In the aftermath of traumatic incidents, survivors belief systems may have to be reviewed (Janoff-Bullman & Frieze, 1983). Similar radical psychological readjustment may be a requirement of our age given the international changes referred to above. In this chapter, the hitherto unchallenged belief in the value of predominantly clinical perspectives for understanding emergency responders' reactions to critical incidents will be critically scrutinized. Having shown this orthodoxy to be misguided, a new conceptual framework will be proposed that takes account of the special relationship that exists between emergency responders and between emergency services and their host communities. Not only does this alternative conceptualization clarify hitherto neglected functions of various intervention strategies, but it also suggests new approaches to evaluating their impact.

The Psychological Ramifications of Emergency Response

As early as 1954 emergency services workers were cautioned about overextending themselves in disaster situations "lest you become as ill as those who need your help" (APA, 1954, p. 20). This instruction reinforced a confident belief that training of emergency services staff "prepares you to handle your own emotional problems first - and promptly.........and protects you somewhat in times of stress" (p. 20-21). This is consistent with expectations a society will have of its professional emergency services at times of crisis. Wallace's (1956) early review of rescuers' psychological responses to major incidents strongly suggested that neither training or experience render personnel immune to being overwhelmed by some aspects of their work. This was confirmed by other studies of the effect of disasters on health workers (Rayner, 1958; Laube, 1973; Krell, 1974). Subsequent surveys have described psychological risks associated with emergency services work, but it remains unclear to what extent operational procedures can be changed to minimize immediate risks to staff and prevent post incident functional impairments.

Green (1982) has usefully categorized studies of the psychological effects of disasters into three groups according to the type of information they provide and how findings can be used. First of these are clinical descriptive studies that describe the phenomenology of psychological and physical reactions to extreme events. These studies help describe and categorize traumatic stress syndromes and generate data that should guide debate about the nature and significance of observed reactions. The second group of studies endeavor to identify particular features of major incident scenarios that precipitate psychological responses. Included in this group are studies that identify personal characteristics that may make individuals more or less vulnerable to traumatic stress. For instance, knowledge of how incident characteristics such as life threat, identification with victims, or intensity of exposure can impact on staff is as relevant as knowledge about risks pertaining to personal characteristics such as age, sex, years of service, coping styles and social support. Epidemiological surveys constitute the third group of studies. By establishing incidence and prevalence rates of traumatic stress reactions, the course and outcome of this syndrome can be described. This data offers guidance on the extent to that intervention strategies should be provided and the form these may take.

Descriptive Studies of Emergency Responder Groups

Rayner (1958) described nurses implicated in a disaster as inclined to over-intellectualize, rigid in their way of thinking, showing limited capacity to make decisions, and suppressing their emotions in order to cope with the demands of the situation. Some 26 years later, members of a multidisciplinary mental health team providing community support after a disastrous bush fire in Australia initially reported experiencing shock and bewilderment, a need for team support, confusion and uncertainty, depression or sadness and helplessness (Berah, Valent & Jones, 1984). These reactions diminished with time, but depression and sadness plus a need for team support persisted. Later the team reported severe or moderate fatigue. Dyregrov and Solomon (1991) report similar results for 23 mental health professionals responding to community needs after an earthquake in California. Sadness, fatigue, frustration and a sense of unreality predominated during disaster work. Other reactions included anger, anxiety, concentration difficulties and intrusive thoughts that interfered with work. Sadness and concentration difficulties persisted after the disaster, as did 'anxiety for loved ones'. Somatoform reactions such as general illness, muscular discomfort, chest and stomach pains, headaches and respiratory problems have been found to be common after completion of disaster work (Paton, 1989).

In a study of firefighters Fullerton, McCarroll, Ursano, & Wright, (1992) identified four types of cognitive, emotional and psychophysiological responses to rescue work: identification with victims, feelings of helplessness and guilt, fear of the unknown and heightened psychophysiological arousal. Hytten and Hasle (1989) described 58 firefighters reactions to a high fatality hotel fire in Norway. Anxiety, restlessness, overactivity, faintheartedness, high spirit and irritability had been experienced during the incident and up to two weeks thereafter. All the same firefighters claimed they coped 'well' or 'fairly well' with assigned tasks at the time of the tragedy. In contrast, a more recent follow-up report on 519 firefighters called out during the Los Angeles riots in April 1992 (Scott & Jordan, 1993) links reduced post incident job satisfaction to anxiety, tension, anger, irritability, intrusive and repetitive thoughts and a sense of "being on guard for no apparent reason".

Jehu (1989) divided 63 ambulance personnel who had attended to survivors of an aircrash in England into three groups according to operational tasks performed. Two months post incident, those who had worked in the wreckage, transported casualties or had undertaken other duties reported both anxiety and depression at clinically significant levels. On site responders were distinct in endorsing high levels of both anxiety and depression in questionnaire returns. Intrusive psychological reactions not present before the crash included "any reminders brought back feelings about it," "I thought about it when I did not mean to," "pictures about it popped into my mind," and "having trouble falling asleep because of thoughts or pictures about it that came into my mind." Also endorsed were avoidance reactions such as "I have a lot of feelings about it, but I didn't deal with them," "I tried not to talk about it," "I stayed away from reminders of it," and "I tried to remove it from memory."

Police officers reactions to shooting incidents are well documented (Stratton, 1984). To be expected are flashbacks, recurrent thoughts about incidents, sleep problems and fears about legal or disciplinary enquiries instituted after such incidents. In a retrospective study of British policemen involved in "on duty" killings or woundings, Manolais and Hyatt-Williams (1988) reported officers to be either extremely calm and clear headed, or intensely frightened during incidents. After the shooting, reactions varied from relief and elation to "quite serious shock." Several hours thereafter, persistent thoughts about the events started to intrude on consciousness. Subsequently, these largely involuntary thoughts contributed to sleeplessness, sudden waking, coldsweats and nightmares. Typically these reactions disappeared within months of the shooting, but some officers developed severe reactions consistent with a diagnosis of post traumatic stress disorder.

These studies are consistent with Hartshough's (1985) review of data from high casualty situations that concluded:"'emergency workers are affected by certain types of incidents and after intense emergency situations, a majority show evidence of traumatic stress." Psychological reactions to traumatic situations are also experienced by individuals whose role is primarily to support front line workers. These include dispatch workers and control room staff (Doerner, 1987; Holt, 1980; Sewell, Crew, 1984; Weaver, 1987), volunteer workers (Dyregrov & Kristoffersen, 1994; Lundin & Bodegard, 1993) and families of emergency services employees (Robinson & Mitchell, 1993). In a case-study approach involving staff employed in a group clinical practice, McCann and Pearlman (1990) illustrated how severely traumatized patients present a risk of vicariously traumatizing therapists and carers.

But not all psychological reactions are adverse. Emergency responder groups also opinion that major incidents offer opportunities for professional and personal growth. Dyregrov and Solomon (1991) reported that rescue personnel may also discover previously unrecognized strengths in themselves, and a greater sense of appreciation of being alive, and of having a family and a network of friends.

Factors That Precipitate Traumatic Stress Reactions

Duration of exposure and intensity of exposure were the most reliable predictors of post traumatic stress reactions (Green, Wilson & Lindy, 1985). But whereas "duration of exposure" is readily quantified, "intensity of exposure" alludes to the importance of qualitative dimensions and nuances of subjective experience. For instance, identification with victims is consistently associated with greater risk of being distressed (Shubin, 1979; Yager and Hubert, 1979; Fullerton, McCarroll, Ursano & Wright, 1992). Infant deaths, child abuse, mass casualties, disaster and fires in high rise buildings are the most stressful incidents to that ambulance service staff can be called (McGlown, 1981). Incidents involving high mortality rates and body handling are particularly distressing to emergency responders; as reported after the Mount Erebus aircrash in the Antarctic (Taylor and Frazer, 1982) and the Jonestown mass suicide in Guyana (Jones, 1985). A coach crash in a mountainous region of Norway saw volunteer responders reacting more strongly to moving mutilated and severed bodies of children than professionally trained emergency workers (Dyregrov and Kristoffersen, 1994).

The relationship between previous experience of exposure to major incidents and future risk of traumatization requires clarification. Hytten and Hasle (1989) point to risk reduction from previous experience of similar rescue operations. This has to be qualified by considerations of both the nature of the previous experiences and their timing (Robinson & Mitchell, 1993). The absence of experience or training in major incident response is reported to place volunteers at particular risk (Dyregrov & Kristoffersen, 1994). Compounding risks factors arise from role conflict in large scale disasters when responders may themselves also be survivors (Dyregrov & Solomon, 1991; Scott & Jordan, 1993), perceived risk to personal safety during incidents (Durham, McCammon & Allison, 1985; Scott & Jordan, 1993) and individual differences like age, personality and coping strategies (Gibbs, 1989).

Epidemiology of Traumatic Stress Reactions In Responder Groups

As expected, emergency responders typically deal effectively with the situations to which they are called. Received wisdom therefore has it that psychological reactions occur after incidents. At best this is a qualified truth. Several studies (Dyregrov, 1989; Mitchell & Bray, 1989; Ersland & Weisaeth, 1989) list palpitations of the heart, muscle spasms, perspiration, tunnel vision, selective perception, cold rushes and nausea as common on site reactions. Operating under conditions of personal danger due to a risk of being caught in a snow avalanche, 91% of emergency responders reported having felt frightened (Dyregrov, Mitchell & Thyholdt, 1988). Similarly, under threat of gas explosions during an appartment block fire in the United States, 52% of responders acknowledged being afraid (Durham, McCammon & Allison, 1985). Among mental health professionals who cared for earthquake survivors, 74% experienced sadness, 65% fatigue, 48% frustration and 48% had a sense of unreality during their work. Anger was reported by 44%, concentration difficulties by 39%, anxiety by 39% and 35% experienced thoughts or feelings that interfered with maximum operational effectiveness (Dyregrov & Solomon, 1991). During an oil rig disaster in the North Sea, between 64% and 52% of rescue personnel had feelings of discouragement, restlessness, uncertainty, anxiety and irritation (Ersland & Weisaeth, 1989).

The use of humor in the midst of tragedy is a notable behavioral response the adaptiveness of which has been commented on in several studies (Lindstrom & Lundin, 1983; Holen, Sundt & Weisaeth, 1983). Experiencing emotion is clearly not necessarily antithetical to effective emergency response, but the potential of observed reactions to disrupt operational response also warrants acknowledgment.

In the aftermath of critical incidents a range of other, distinct reactions prevail. For four weeks after the Ash Wednesday bushfires, 37% of the mobilized mental health team confirmed having had dreams and thoughts of themselves in a fire situation. A similar number also reported the fire to have reactivated distress felt in association with recollections of earlier life trauma. Forty two percent reported feeling depressed (Berah, Jones & Valent, 1984). Two weeks after an earthquake another mental health team was followed up by Dyregrov and Solomon (1991). The most common reported reactions were sadness (61%), exhaustion (57%), anxiety for loved ones (43%) and anger (30%). Twenty percent reported crying more often, experienced sleep difficulties and suffered impaired general health. After six months, quality of work and family life had not returned to pre-earthquake standards in 26% of team members. Whilst 21% reported no such impact beyond a few weeks, 39% stated full readjustment had taken more than two months. More than one in four (26%) stated the incident had affected their plans for continuing in their chosen profession. Robinson and Mitchell (1993) report 40% of rescue personnel and 51% of welfare and hospital workers stated that critical incidents adversely impact on their family members. Negative reactions included; being urged to get out of the job, partner being distressed, not knowing what to do and the children being badly affected. In some instances, however the change was in a favorable direction; "my partner let me have more time to myself," " family members talked over the incident with me."

Job satisfaction is estimated to have decreased by 10% and morale by 13% among the 519 firefighters surveyed six months after the 1992 Los Angeles Riots. Forty seven percent reported having experienced reactions of anxiety and tension, anger and irritability, being on guard for no apparent reason and having repetitive and intrusive thoughts about the riots that lasted at least one week. Thirteen percent of respondents reported these reactions to have lasted for one to three weeks only; 7% had reactions that lasted between one to three months, and 27% reported their continued persistence six months post incident (Scott & Jordan, 1993). Nine months after involvement in an oil-rig disaster, 24% of rescuers reported "poor mental health condition" attributed to rescue work. In half of these intrusive memories and re-experiencing added to a clinical picture that would have satisfied diagnostic criteria for PTSD (Ersland, Weisaeth & Sund 1989). Two months post incident, clinically significant levels of anxiety and depression was reported in 40% of ambulance personnel who worked on the scene of an aircrash (Jehu, 1989). Amongst those who transported casualties, the rate was 35% whilst for those involved in other duties the rates were 20%. For the three groups Impact of Event Scale (Horowitz, Wilner &

Alvarez 1979) items were endorsed as follows: "any reminders brought back feelings about it" 60%, 36% and 25%, "I thought about it when I did not mean to" 50%, 23% and 5%, "pictures about it popped into my mind" 40%, 18% and 20%, "having trouble falling asleep because of thoughts or pictures about it that came into my mind" 15%, 9% and 10%.

Of 53 professional responders to an apartment building explosion, 21% endorsed symptom constellations that satisfied DSM III criteria for PTSD five months after the incident (Durham, McCammon & Allison, 1985). Most commonly reported reactions were; having repeated recollection of the event (74%), sadness (46%), dreams of the event (15%) and depression (15%). These findings are broadly in line with Raphael, Singh, Bradbury & Lambert's (1984) follow-up study of the Granville rail disaster. In Dyregrov and Kristoffersen's (1994) study of volunteers and professional rescue workers called to a coach crash, the two groups reported reactions of a similar nature but at different rates. At one month, volunteers recorded significantly higher Impact of Events Scale scores (Horovitz, Wilner & Alvarez, 1979) than professionals. Using Horowitz's (1982) criteria for three levels of distress, 66.7% of volunteers fell within the medium and high levels as compared to 43.8% of the professionals. At thirteen months, a significant group difference was maintained only for avoidance subscale scores, but only intrusion subscale scores declined significantly in this time period. A total of 84.2% of the volunteers and 77.3% of the professionals recorded scores in the low distress category at thirteen months. Ersland and Weisaeth (1989) found high levels of uncertainty, anxiety and restlessness during an incident to be predictive of poor mental health in 17% of professional rescue workers and 25% of the volunteers at 9 months. Lundin and Bodegaard's (1993) reported on earthquake rescue workers found professionals endorsing higher distress levels than untrained personnel at one week and one month. At 9 months the group trend was reversed with professionals having achieved a statistically significant reduction in reported distress levels. For volunteers no such reduction was achieved in the timespan of the study.

Not to be ignored are emergency responders' reports of personal development and increased professional confidence through involvement in major incident response. Dyregrov and Kristoffersen's (1994) follow-up survey 13 months post-incident of personnel called out to a fatal coach accident reports 52% of volunteer helpers and 40% of the professionals to have "discovered strong aspects in themselves following disaster work." Among firefighters implicated in the 1992 Los Angeles riots positive effects of emergency response derived from encouragement gained from team members working together under difficult conditions, inter-agency teamwork and perceiving the incident as the greatest fire fighting experience of their career. Also listed was the recognition of having competently met the extraordinary challengesof a complex assignment (Scott & Jordan, 1993). Eighteen of nineteen mental health team members assessed their involvement in early response to a bushfire to have been emotionally valuable to a considerable or moderate degree at four weeks followup (Berah, Jones & Valent, 1984). This proportion is rather higher than the 35% who reported feeling more positive about themselves one year after rescue work during a rail disaster (Raphael, Singh, Bradbury & Lambert, 1984), or the 61% of a group of mental health professionals mobilized after an earthquake (Dyregrov & Solomon 1991).

What Sense Can Be Made Of These Findings?

Lifton's (1964, 1968) explorations of the psychological ramifications of exposure to the consequences of nuclear attack prompted the first systematic attempt to formulate a general theory of traumatic stress in part based on observations of emergency responders. His general theory emphasizes the largely involuntary phenomenon of vivid intrusive images and memories precipitated by exposure to large scale death and destruction. Linked to the same are reactions of extreme fear and a perception of the world as unpredictable and potentially life threatening. Survivor guilt, irritability and rage co-exist with psychic numbing; manifested as a restriction in the range of felt emotion. Human relationships are destabilized by, on the one hand, a desire for support and help and a pervasive scepticism about human relationships on the other. Lifton (1964, 1968) accounts for the genesis and maintenance of these psychological responses to extreme stress in terms of subjective meanings attributed to an event. It is postulated that resolution of traumatic stress reactions occurs in conjunction with individuals ascribing new subjective meanings to these events.

Horowitz (1976) also gives centrality to cognitive phenomena in his conceptualization of psychological responses to traumatic stress. These, it is postulated, are precipitated by information or sensory impressions that are irreconcilable with an individual's schemas of self, others and the world. Such cognitive dissonance engenders a distinct psychological state in that intrusive, vivid and even uncontrollable imagery may abruptly enter consciousness. Co-existing with this propensity to involuntary re-experiencing is a mental state characterized by avoidance and denial. Its features are emotional numbing, attention deficits, constriction of thought processes and amnesia. Sadness over loss may co-exist with fears of identification or merger with victims. Also, an awareness of aggressive impulses, a lowered tolerance threshold for anger and reduced impulse control may generate guilt or shame about apparent change in selfhood. Horovitz (1976) refers to specific existential themes that commonly preoccupy traumatized individuals and links resolution to the individual's adjustment to fears of repetition of the traumatizing event, shame over subjective experiences of helplessness or emptiness and rage at the circumstances or individuals perceived to be responsible for the event.

Drawing on the experiences of health care staff working with trauma survivors, McCann and Pearlman (1990) describe more detailed psychological processes associated with these clinical conceptualizations of traumatic stress. Disruptive psychological reactions are said to be inextricably linked to perceptions of personal safety, dependency and trust in others as well as oneself, how the dynamics of power and control is expressed in relationships, self esteem, intimacy, independence and the idiosyncratic constructs used by individuals to structure experience and make sense of existence.

In the above conceptualizations, the distinctive characteristic of traumatic incidents is alleged to be that they confront emergency responders with sensory evidence which is irreconcilable with previously held beliefs or schemas (whether consciously articulated or not). However transient, intrusive re-experiencing, numbing, arousal and other observed reactions of emergency responders are linked to certain styles of subjective appraisal and belief rather than to objective characteristics of critical events (e.g., duration, extent of damage, number of deaths, degrees of body mutilation). That certain critical or traumatic events consistently impact on the psychological functioning of emergency responders is explained in terms of colleagues sharing similar cognitive schemas rather than some inherent property of these events. Alleviation of traumatic stress reactions is therefore consequent on influences that reduces the discrepancy between an individual's previously adaptive schemata and a new incompatible post incident reality.

Understandably, this conceptualization of critical incident stress reactions as a spiritual crisis is not readily understood or accepted among senior emergency services personnel and represents a major impediment to effecting organizational change. Even clinicians and researchers would acknowledge this rarified conceptualization to be both an oversimplification and an idealization. In the real world denial, cognitive control and avoidance behavior are adaptive first lines of defence for those exposed to distressing events. Also, in our preoccupation with traumatic stress reactions we appear to have lost sight of human distress, sadness, feeling miserable, exhaustion and all their associated physical reactions.

What is required at a service level are studies that inform senior operational staff of preemptive steps to be incorporated in education and training programs (Hytten & Hasle, 1989; Lundin & Bodegard, 1993). Risk reduction can be achieved through informed leadership practices during and after critical incidents (Fullerton, McCarroll, Ursano & Wright, 1992), but the imperative has to be to reduce risk by taking pre-emptive steps that protect responders. To do otherwise in the 1990's is operationally negligent and conflicts with Health and Safety Law in a number of countries (Dunning, 1988 The Times, 1992).

To date, intervention strategies have largely been construed as treatment innovations; their aim being to remove the diverse symptoms of traumatic stress. In part, the rationalization for doing so is that surveys, using methodologies associated with clinical disciplines have revealed levels of psychological distress that if reported in a general population sample would warrant access to clinical services. Given the way these reactions are currently conceptualized the requirement appears to be for intervention strategies that addresses the mismatch between particular belief systems and sensory experience. In other words, the transition to be achieved in the wake of trauma is a personal development from a previously adaptive, but now discredited belief system, to another; the pitfalls of which are not so apparent. Fisher and Fisher (1993) make the point that intervention strategies premised on the above are philosophically bankrupt in so far that it seeks to replace one arbitrary absurdity with another and to this end can resort to no more than make-believe.

In practice, however, advocated intervention strategies are not readily reconciled with this conceptualisation of traumatic stress reactions. Also to be considered is the possibility that distinctive schemata and coping strategies, not shared with the broader public, have evolved in support of personal and professional adjustment of emergency services staff. A degree of social alienation may therefore typify the predicament of emergency responders; a situation likely to be disadvantageous in the aftermath of trauma. Until the implications of this are fully appreciated the manner of delivering critical incident stress management services, their aims and anticipated outcomes cannot be formulated in terms acceptable to the targeted consumer.

Intervention Strategies For Emergency Responder Groups

Early reports describing distress reactions in emergency service personnel used the terminology of clinical science thereby implying a need for special staff care initiatives (Duffy, 1979; Kliman, 1975; Davidson, 1979). Dunning (1989, p. 288-293) offers a useful discussion of issues relating to the establishment of such services, but the extent of acceptance and implementation of critical incident stress management services for responder groups is uncertain. In 1993, 72% of senior officers in United Kingdom emergency services reported at least some critical incident stress provision to have been made within their own local service, but only 28% held the view that sufficient recognition was given this aspect of staff care (Ørner, Paulsen, Thompson, Pickles, Cook, Brown-Warr & Stone, 1993). Reports from other countries have not been published to date.

Critical incident stress management services (CISMS) are categorized by the timing of interventions: pre-incident educational initiatives, interventions incorporated in ongoing disaster response, and post incident follow-up services. The former ought to be integral to basic emergency responder training and should continue in conjunction with in-service training. Central to educational initiatives is the notion of staff being at risk, the normality of traumatic stress reactions, the usefulness of various coping strategies and basic information about CISMS. A core curriculum may therefore impart information about immediate and longer term reactions to critical incidents as they occur at cognitive, physical, emotional and behavioral levels. How such events and reactions impact on immediate family members, colleagues and social networks also deserves recognition. Garrison,(1986) reports using film and video footage taken during major incidents in stress inoculation programs and Solomon (1991) addresses issues of fear and vulnerability in a pre-emptive educational programs for police officers. It is noteworthy that responder groups consistently report degree of relevant preparedness to be associated with less adverse reactions and a positive response-outcome expectancy (Hytten & Hasle, 1989; Dyregrov & Solomon, 1991; Lundin & Bodegaard, 1993). For more senior officers assuming leadership responsibilities during major incidents, Mitchell (1988a, 1988b) advocates preparing stress management protocols. These should be explicit about how and when to arrange rest breaks to limit risk arising from excessive exposure, how to maintain response readiness through appropriate food and fluid intake; and advise on how to engender a protective sense of group cohesion through explicit emphasis on teamwork and mutual support. Also to be explained is the use of on-site psychological support staff, sensible demobilisation strategies, coping strategies that may help to limit adverse psychological reactions in the short term and guidance on post incident psychological care.

An example of how new, improved deployment practices can be informed by such a protocol is given in Alexander's (1991) account of how pre-briefings and explicit emphasis on teamwork were used to good effect with police officers mobilized for body handling duties after the Piper Alpha disaster. Recognizing that early intervention optimizes opportunities for early mitigation (Horowits, 1986) Alexander ensured psychological support staff were available on-site. Daily defusings were held for the whole group. Generally, defusings take place between one and three hours after an incident and should last no more than one hour. They offer an opportunity to discuss events that have made a particular impression on responders is on the assumption this will reduce acute stress and anxiety. The recommended structure for defusings is as follows; a brief introduction describing guidelines for the meeting is followed by a factual exploration of the incident from the perspective of participating responders and the defusing closes with advice being offered that aims to protect staff from potentially disruptive psychological effects of the incident. In particular the value of physical exercise soon after involvement in major incidents is explained (Girdano & Everly, 1986).

Demobilization or deescalation meetings are advocated for larger scale incidents. As responder units step down or disengage from disaster scenarios, staff are invited to attend a ten minutes talk that describes the types of reactions emergency responders experience immediately after involvement in such incidents. Emphasis is placed on the normality of response and practical suggestions about how to cope with these are offered. Along with providing staff with food and opportunity to relax before returning home, demobilization meetings present an opportunity to screen for individuals who may be acutely distressed and who may welcome immediate individual counselling. The introductory talk, plus group activities, need take no more than thirty minutes, and the aim of a demobilization is to ease the transition from major incident response to a more habitual way of life. Protection afforded by peer support is implicit in the tried and tested practice of deploying emergency responders in groups whenever possible. Reflecting a wish to engender such protection to optimal effect during and after critical events, structured peer support programs have gained particular acceptance within United States emergency services (Britt, 1991; Schmuckler, 1991). Drawing largely upon principles of Rogerian counselling (Rogers, 1951) peer support programs aim to provide emotional first aid, facilitate mobilization of coping resources and help colleagues understand or work through their natural responses to traumatic events (Stolz, 1993). Ideally this is provided by peers who have survived similar incidents themselves or who can give account of traumatic stress reactions by referring to their own experience. Fuller (1991) gives a detailed account of the particular considerations that pertain to the establishment of peer support teams within emergency services. Horn and Solomon (1986) offer nine guidelines for good practice: peer supporters should in particular, be conversant with the diversity of traumatic stress responses and take responsibility for initiating contact with colleagues without being intrusive. Non-judgmental acceptance, empathy and support is central to the process of actively listening to colleagues accounts and validating their emotional reactions. Only a limited degree of self disclosure is recommended, except for offering advice about coping strategies that proved useful to the peer supporter. As contact is maintained over time, unhelpful coping strategies should be challenged whilst remaining sensitive to mood and adjustment difficulties. A peer supporter is not considered responsible for how a colleague reacts or adjusts post incident, so intermediate or long term-difficulties should prompt referral to appropriate specialist care. In taking on such a role a peer supporter serves as a model for survival. In an adaptation of these principles Alexander and Wells (1991) incorporated structured peer support during body handling work by pairing less experienced police officers with more experienced ones.

Trained counsellors are not new to emergency services welfare departments. Their remit has now often been extended to providing help in the aftermath of critical incidents (Ørner et al 1993). Usually provided one-to-one, counselling aims to ease the expression of feelings, promote understanding of reactions to critical incidents, the course of these over time and should raise awareness of useful coping strategies. Instillation of hope and a focus on positive achievement is intermingled with a recognition of specific problems the resolution for that is be sought through encouragement of a sense of autonomy and personal control (Alexander, 1990; McFarlane, 1989).

By contrast, psychological debriefing is an intervention strategy developed specifically for emergency responder groups. Its origins can be traced to observations made during military field operations during World War II. Jeffrey Mitchell is rightly deserving of international accolade received for championing this largely prescriptive, task oriented form of group meeting for emergency responders implicated in major incidents. According to Mitchell (1989) 75 critical incident debriefing teams had been established in the United States during the previous six years. Teams are also reported to exist in Canada, Australia, Norway and Germany. Also known as Critical Incident Stress Debriefing it should ideally take place between 24 and 72 hours after events "that have significant emotional power to overwhelm the usual coping mechanisms eg: line of duty deaths, disasters, serious injury or death of children etc.," (Mitchell, 1988a,1988b). Participants should be selected for having broadly similar experiences of a particular incident and meetings may last up to three hours under the stewardship of a team of three trained debriefers. These may be professional care staff or peer supporters who have not themselves been called out to the incident for which the debrief is held. A seven stage debriefing model is implemented to cover; introduction and ground rules, establishing the facts of what happened to participants, description of thoughts about what happened, discussion of the emotions associated with the event, review of signs and symptoms of distress resulting from the event, a teaching phase in which the normality of response is emphasized along with information about useful coping strategies and finally a re-entry phase to address outstanding issues or for the debriefer team to make summary statements and advise on follow-up arrangements (Mitchell & Dyregrov,1993; Mitchell & Everley, 1993). The stated aim of psychological debriefing is to prevent unnecessary complications arising in the aftermath of critical incidents. Variations to this basic model for psychological debriefing has been sanctioned for mass disasters that have involved emergency responders experiencing prolonged exposure (Mitchell & Everley, 1993; Armstrong, Callahan & Marmar, 1991) and for individual therapists at risk of vicarious traumatization (McCann & Pearlman, 1990). In recent years a divergence of opinion about which stage of a debrief is most important has led to other debrief models being advocated and practised (Cohen & Ahearn, 1980; Raphael et al, 1986 Dunning, 1988).

Impact of Critical Incident Stress Management Services

An almost evangelical enthusiasm for developing critical incident stress management services for high risk emergency responder groups (Reese, Horn & Dunning, 1991) has not been matched by a resolve to objectively evaluate their impact. In fact, fifteen years of practice has not generated any studies that adopt methodologies more sophisticated than that required for descriptive surveys.

Lintern (1994) evaluated the impact of an educational program about traumatic stress for emergency services personnel in Lincolnshire, England. The study focused on two groups of firefighters; only one of that had passed through the training module. Information retained over a six month period was monitored along with measures gauging the impact of work related critical incidents. As might have been predicted, firefighters who had structured access to information about traumatic stress achieved significantly higher scores on a written exam type questionnaire than their untutored colleagues. This finding was independent of rank and years of service. As assessed by the Coping Response Questionnaire (Sidle, Moos, Adams & Cady, 1969) the two groups used similar coping strategies, but experienced distress levels measured by the Global Severity Index of the SCL-90-R (Delgado, 1983) and the Impact of Event Scale (Horovits, Wilner & Alvares, 1979) were significantly higher among tutored firefighters throughout the survey period. However, there was no indication of operational readiness being compromized in either service. Consistent with McFarlane (1988), Lintern found those who endorse reactions consistent with a diagnosis of PTSD scored significantly lower on the extraversion scale of the Eysenck Personality Inventory (Eysenck & Eysenck, 1964) and significantly higher on the neuroticism scale when compared to colleagues not so diagnosed.

Psychological support services provided on-site or in the immediate aftermath of major incidents do not appear ever to have been subjected to systematic scrutiny. This is also the case for Peer Support Schemes although Alexander and Wells (1991) report favorable experience with a policy of pairing experienced with less experienced police officers during body handling assignments in connection with the Piper Alpha disaster. Similar mean Hospital Anxiety and Depression Scale Scores (Zigmond & Snaith, 1983) are reported for the two groups soon after the incident and at followup.

Only one report of a systematic evaluation of counselling services for emergency responder groups appears to have been published to date (Duckworth, 1986). After screening all 399 police officers who assisted during the Bradford Football Stadium Fire, thirty four accepted an offer of individual cognitive problem focused counselling specifically tailored to post incident reactions. GHQ-60 (Goldberg, 1978) questionnaire returns at three weeks and six months after completing counselling indicated a satisfactory level of adjustment among the participating officers. Paton (1989) has developed this model of counselling to take fuller account of accumulated knowledge about emergency responders' coping strategies and the effects of individual differences. No systematic evaluation has been reported.

Mitchell (1988a) declaration that much more should be done to evaluate the impact of psychological debriefing has resulted in a number of reports to conferences (Everly & Mitchell, 1992; Scott & Jordan, 1993), one unpublished doctorial dissertation (Rogers, 1992) consumer reports from those who have participated in psychological debriefs (Dyregrov & Solomon, 1991; Dyregrov & Kristoffersen 1994; Robinson & Mitchell, 1993), but not a single controlled long-term outcome study. Surveys bear witness to participants' general satisfaction with the debriefing process. In the absence of systematic comparisons with non debriefed personnel a distinctive impact on long term outcome has not been demonstrated. Recently, Scott and Jordan (1993) presented data which for the first time suggested considerable variation in the perceived value of psychological debriefings organized for firefighters who responded to the 1992 Los Angeles riots. Of the 195 firefighters debriefed after the Los Angeles Riots, 8% rated these as highly effective, 42% as moderately effective, 30% as low in effectiveness and 20% rated effectiveness as very low. Taking all debriefed firefighters together, 48% reported having no residual post incident reactions at three weeks. Among respondents who rated debriefings as moderately or highly effective, approximately one in three (35%) had traumatic stress reactions continuing at six months. Consistent with this trend, 78% of those who rated psychological debriefs as being of low or very low effectiveness confirmed persistent incident related stress reactions over the same time period. In the group reporting low or very low effectiveness only 13% reported no adjustment difficulties at three weeks. The inverse relationship between subjective evaluation of debriefing effectiveness and duration of incident related stress reactions achieves statistical significance.

Possibly, a more optimistic perspective on the effects of psychological debriefing is discerned from Robinson and Mitchell's (1993) follow-up study of 288 emergency, welfare and hospital workers. Of these, 60% returned an evaluation questionnaire eliciting details about the impact of specific critical incidents on themselves and their families; which aspects of these events had precipitated psychological distress and the perceived value of psychological debriefing. Compared to other emergency services staff welfare and hospital personnel consistently reported higher mean ratings of the impact of events at the time of the incidents and when completing the questionnaire. Of the latter, two in every five (41.1%) reported specific events to still have either a considerable or great impact. Interestingly, the group reporting least initial reactions also experiences greatest impact reduction over time with only one in twenty (5.7%) of the least affected initially finding reactions to persist. Satisfaction ratings for the 31 psychological debriefings held were generally high; 51% of emergency personnel and 44% of welfare/hospital staff reported being very happy with the service provided. Particular appreciation was expressed for the opportunity to talk to others about a critical incident, developing understanding of personal reactions to events, being advised about coping strategies and getting a more complete impression of the whole incidents. Criticisms tended to focus on the inexperience of debriefing teams, lack of comfort, the small proportion of all responders who participated in debriefings and the brevity of sessions.

In summary therefore, Mitchell's (1988a) declaration that outcome evaluation of critical incident stress management services should be prioritized has gone largely unheeded. Unconvincing explanations offered to account for the poor quality of outcome research (Robinson and Mitchell, 1993) raises the possibility that the conceptual framework adapted from clinical sciences is too restrictive and may be an impediment to greater understanding of intervention strategies indicated for emergency responder groups.

On The Need For A New Conceptual Framework

A broad consensus exists in clinical and research settings with regards to the "at risk" status of this group, but acceptance within emergency services is still a matter of conjecture. One of the obstacles to affecting organizational change (Ørner et al, 1993) may therefore be that observed psychological reactions in are not readily explained by a conceptual framework that finds favor among senior managerial staff in emergency services. Also, the enthusiastic promotion of psychological debriefing as a cornerstone of critical incident stress management services is not matched by documented proof of its beneficial effects, nor is there a clearly reasoned theoretical rationale for these interventions (Macleod, 1991). Quite simply and sensibly, the premise seems to be that it makes more sense to do something than nothing. No-one can take issue with such a plea, but intellectually such a position is solpsistic.

In view of Baum, Solomon & Ursano's (1993) review of the practical, conceptual and methodological problems inherent in systematically assessing the impact of critical incidents, the notion of generating outcome data at par with that which informs the best of clinical practice is probably overly optimistic. This is not to advocate relinquishing the search for answers to crucial questions about which critical incident management services to deliver, when to deliver these, to whom, and to what end. Rather, it is to argue that the premises which have informed our search for answers to these questions may have been misguided. At issue is the failure to recognize that the phenomenological similarity of post incident reactions among emergency responders, civilian survivors of these events and even patients seen in clinical practice for other reasons has obscured a need to consider these as distinctly different population groups. Among professional emergency responders it may prove more informative to regard immediate and short term reactions as process phenomena contributing to successful psychological and physical adjustment. This is consistent with Mitchell and Dyregrov's (1993) assertion that critical incident stress response and distress is the norm in this group rather than the exception. Also Lintern (1993) report on the impact of an educational program about traumatic stress on firefighters fits with this revised formulation emphasising active psychological processing of extreme experiences.In other survivor groups and clinical populations a conceptualization of functional disorder may be more appropriate. Also of great importance in this regard are the different context within which reactions are experienced and how this affects their course over time.

The confusing ramifications of not making distinctions between distinct groups is most evident in the numerous studies cited above that attribute equal clinical significance to questionnaire endorsements made by emergency responders professionally trained for critical incident response, and those made by unwitting survivors of such events. How misleading this practice is can be illustrated by choosing almost any questionnaire item from instruments commonly used in post incident surveys. For instance, the items of the Beck Depression Inventory (Beck, Rush, Shaw & Emery, 1979) "I am sad all the time and cannot snap out of it. " "I feel guilty most of the time," "I feel irritated all the time;" the SCL-90-R (Delgado, 1983), "I am distressed by repeated unpleasant thoughts that will not leave my mind," "I feel low in energy and slowed down," and "I feel fearful." Interpretation of the clinical significance of questionnaire item endorsements is critically dependent on whether or not a respondent has been implicated in a major event and if so , in what capacity. It is probably a services mistake to assume that a given questionnaire score obtained by an identified patient in receipt of psychological care, and an emergency responder post- incident necessarily carries the same clinical significance. This should also caution against extravagant claims for the therapeutic efficiency of advocated critical incident stress management services. If observed reactions are integral to the psychological process of adjustment following critical events, their elimination through implementation of intervention strategies would be strongly contraindicated. This conceptualization also has significant implications for a reformulation of the aims and objectives of critical incident stress management services and the methods to be used to sensibly assess their impact.

Intervention Strategies As Transitional Rituals

As outlined in the introduction, ceremonies and rituals are integral to the culture of emergency services. They help define the relationship of each emergency service to its host community. Rituals confer special social status on staff within emergency service in recognition of the protective, damage limitation functions they undertake upon completion of specialist training. With accumulated experience they confront and contain dangers that members of the general public are wise to avoid. Within each emergency service rituals simultaneously engender a powerful sense of group identity, and group cohesion, confirm the position and the norm of conformity within subgroups of the command hierarchy and recognizes mutual interdependence in all aspects of operational activity.

Traumatic stress reactions experienced by emergency responders might therefore, first and foremost, be assessed in terms of their repercussions for the organizational imperative of group cohesion and response readiness. This is in contrast to the current practice of relating these reactions to observations made in clinical contexts. From an organizational perspective, adverse psychological reactions marginalize emergency responders operationally and therefore change their roles within core responder groups. Whether this proves to be a transitory or long-term state of affairs it is clearly in the interest of emergency services to facilitate full re-integration of personnel into their peer group. To the extent that critical incident stress management services promote and mark the passage of individuals from one group status to another they are more usefully conceptualized as transitional rituals than treatment interventions.

The merits of this new conceptual framework can be judged by the guidance it gives those providing this type of staff care and the questions it generates for researchers. Whereas a perspective that pathologizes traumatic stress reactions prioritizes the description, classification and elimination of "symptoms", the concept of transitional ritual gives centrality to an understanding of how such reactions compromise operational imperatives at the level of the individual in relation to his or her peer group and this group in relation to the whole emergency service.

This conceptual framework must not be misinterpreted as an attempt to confer respectability on magic and mysticism as associated with religious rituals. A considerable knowledge base underpins the proposed framework. For instance, Lifton (1964, 1968) focuses on the "imprint of death" as a powerful marginalizer of individuals exposed to catastrophies. This is matched by survivors' reports of "feeling alienated or excluded" within communities where previously a sense of integration predominated. Silver and Wilson's (1988) account of native American healing and purification rituals for warriors seeking re-entry into their host tribes draws on exactly the same group focused conceptual framework. In a chapter titled "Tragedy; Outstaring the Gorgon", Taplin (1989) describes how classical Greek Tragedies that incarnate the worst terrors of personal, familial and community catastrophies served as transitional rituals. Sometimes, inspired by contemporary events (e.g., wars), classical tragedies acted out the deepest terrors imaginable and confronted audiences with the almost unbearable. Disasters were lived through vicariously thus easing the process of socially reintegrating survivors. In their shared emphasis on survival and re-integration Greek Tragedies and critical incident stress management services endeavor to achieve the same results.

From a research point of view the notion of transitional ritual generates testable hypotheses about group processes in the wake of major incidents, during the stages of delivering critical incident stress management services, their relationship to operational readiness as well as the course of traumatic stress reactions in emergency responder groups. It should not pass unnoticed that this conceptual framework links directly to the confirmed value of social support after trauma (McCammon, Durham, Allison & Williams, 1988), nuances in the way this support is used (Thoits, 1986) and most specifically the extent to which social support is perceived to be available (Rook, 1990). Rituals make these helpful influences more explicit and readily available. In future therefore, the value of critical incident stress management services might be assessed primarily in terms their impact on group processes, crucial for personal adjustment, rather than traumatic stress symptomology.

Even if emergency responders develop schematas or belief systems that facilitate cognitive processing of most but not all critical events, the truly exceptional and traumatic situations are particularly problematic insofar that they highlight the arbitrariness, both of previous belief systems and any alternatives that may replace the original ones (Fisher and Fisher, 1993). Truth may be the first casualty of war, but notions of absolute certainty do not survive critical incidents. This is of course a matter of degree, but under such conditions of spiritual crisis reassurance is imperative for peace of mind. Although psychotherapeutic approaches may seek to address an individual's cognitive processes through the medium of a person to person relationship, the proposed conceptual framework suggests that reassurance may be more readily forthcoming through intervention strategies that take full account of the power and healing properties of group cohesion and belonging. It may be that these processes, more than any others, help emergency responders effect the tricky transition required to accept, believe in and live by a new but invariably flawed belief system. To seek a rationale for implementing critical incident stress management services in these terms may, in time, lead to more informed notions than "it is better to do something than nothing."

References

Alexander, D.A. (1990). Psychological intervention for victims and helpers after disasters. British Journal of General Practice, 40, 345-348.

Alexander, D.A., & Wells, A. (1991). Reactions of police officers to bodyhandling after a major disaster. A before-and-after comparison. British Journal of Psychiatry, 159, 547-555.

American Psychiatric Association. (1964). First aid for psychological reactions to disasters. Washington, DC: Author.

Anderson, H.S., Christensen, A.K., & Petersen, G.O. (1991). Post traumatic stress reactions among rescue workers after a major rail accident. Anxiety Research, 4, 245-251.

Armstrong, K., O'Callahan, W., & Marmar, C.R. (1991). Debriefing Red Cross disaster personnel: the multiple stressor debriefing model. Journal of Traumatic Stress, 4, 581-593.

Baum, A., Solomon, S.D., & Ursano, R.J. (1993). Emergency-disaster studies: practical, conceptual and methodological issues. In J.P. Wilson & B. Raphael (Eds.), International handbook of traumatic stress syndromes (pp. 125-134). London: Plenum Press.

Beck, A., Ward, C., Mendelson, M., Mock, J., & Erbaugh, J. (1961). An inventory for measuring depression. Archives of general psychiatry, 4, 561-571.

Berah, E.F., Jones, H.J., & Valent, P. (1984). The experience of a mental health team involved in the early phase of a disaster. Australian and New Zealand Journal of Psychiatry, 18, 354-358.

Britt, J.M. (1991). U.S. secret service critical incident peer support team. In J.T. Reese, J.M. Horn, & C. Dunning (Eds.), Critical incidents in policing (pp. 55-62). Washington DC: U.S. Department of Justice.

Cohen, R., & Ahearn, F. (1980). Handbook for mental health care of disaster victims. London: John Hopkins University Press.

Davidson, A.D. (1979). Air disaster: Coping with stress - a program that worked. Police Stress,, 20-22.

Derogatis, L.R. (1983). SCL-90-R: administration, scoring and procedures. Manual II for the revized version. Towson, MD: Reese Psychometric Research.

Doerner, W.G. (1987). Police dispatcher stress. Journal of Police Science and Administration, 15, 257-261.

Duckworth, D.H. (1986). Psychological problems arising from disaster work. Stress Medicine, 2, 315-323.

Duffy, J. (1979). The role of CMHCs in airport disasters. Technical Assistance Centre Report, 2, 7-9.

Dunning, C. (1989). Intervention strategies for emergency workers. In M.Lystead (Ed.), Mental health response to mass emergencies: Theory and practice (pp. 284-307). New York: Brunner Mazel.

Durham, T.W., McCammon, S.L., & Alison. (1985) The psychological impact of disaster on rescue personnel. Annals of Emergency Medicine, 14, 664-668.

Dyregrov, A. (1989). Psychological reactions of helpers during and after catastrophes. Unpublished doctorial dissertation, Bergen University, Norway.

Dyregrov, A. & Kristoffersen, J.I. (in press). Voluntary and professional disaster-workers. Similarities and differences in reactions. Journal of Traumatic Stress.

Dyregrov, A., & Solomon, R.M. (1991). Mental health professionals in disasters:an exploratory study. Disaster Management, 3, 123-128.

Dyregrov, A., Thyholdt, R., & Mitchell, J.T. (1992). Rescue workers' emotional reactions following a disaster. In Engelman, S.R. (Ed.), Confronting life-threatening illness. New York: Irvington Publishers, Inc.

Ersland, S., Weisaeth, L., & Sund, A. (1989). The stress upon rescuers involved in an oil rig disaster. "Alexander Kielland" 1980. Acta Psychiatrica Scandinavica, 80 (Suppl. 355), 38-49

Eysenck, H.J., & Eysenck, S.B.G. (1964). Manual of the Eysenck Personality Inventory. London: University of London Press.

Fisher, S., & Fisher, R.L. (1993). The psychology of adaptation to absurdity. Tactics of make-believe. Hillsdale, New Jersey: Lawrence Erlbaum.

Fuller, R.A. (1991). An overview of the process of peer support team development. In J.T. Reese, J.M. Horn, & C. Dunning (Eds.), Critical incidents in policing (pp. 99-106). Washington DC: U.S. Department of Justice.

Fullerton, C.S., McCarroll, J.E., Ursano, R.J., & Wright, K.M. (1992). Psychological responses of rescue workers: firefighters and trauma. American Journal of Orthopsychiatry, 62, 371-378.

Garrison, W.A. (1991). Modelling inoculation training for traumatic incident exposure. In J.T. Reese, J.M. Horn, & C. Dunning (Eds.), Critical incidents in policing. (pp. 107-118) Washington, DC: U.S. Department of Justice.

Gibbs, M.S. (1989). Factors in the victim that mediate between disaster and psychopathology: a review. Journal of Traumatic Stress, 2, 489-514.

Girdano, D.A., & Everly, G.S. (1986). Controlling stress and tension: A holistic approach. Engelwood Cliffs, N.J: Prentice-Hall.

Goldberg, D.P. (1978). Manual of the General Health Questionnaire. Windsor: NFER.

Green, B.L. (1982). Assessing levels of psychological impairment following disaster. Consideration of actual and methodological dimensions. Journal of Nervous & Mental Disease, 170, 544-552.

Green, B.L., Wilson, J., & Lindy, J.D. (1985). Conceptualising PTSD; a psychosocial framework. In C. Figley (Ed.), Trauma and its wake: The study and treatment of post traumatic stress disorder (pp. 53-69). New York: Brunner - Mazel.

Hartsough, P.N. (1985). Emergency organization role. In: Role Stresses and Support for Emergency Service Workers (pp. 1-20). National Institute of Mental Health.

Holen, A., Sund, A., & Weisaeth, L. (1983). Alexander L. Kielland katastrofen: psykiske reaksjoner hos de overlevende: forelopig sluttrapport. Oslo: University of Oslo Press.
Holt, F.X. (1980, November). The dispatcher & stress. Firehouse (pp.18-21).
Horowitz, M.J. (1976). Stress response syndromes (Second Ed.). Northvale: J. Aronson.
Horowitz, M.J. (1986). Stress - response syndromes: a review of post traumatic and adjustment disorders. Hospital & Community Psychiatry, 37, 241-249.
Horowitz, M., Wilner, N., & Alvarez, W. (1979). Impact of Event Scale: a measure of subjective stress. Psychosomatic Medicine, 41, 209-218.
Hytten, K., & Hasle, A. (1989). Firefighters: a study of stress and coping. Acta Psychiatrica Scandinavica, 80(Suppl. 355), 50-55.
Janoff Bulman, R., & Frieze, I.H. (1983). A theoretical perspective for understanding reactions to victimisation. Journal of Social Issues, 39, 1-17.
Jehu, D. (1989). The impact of the Kegworth Air Disaster on Ambulance personnel. Unpublished manuscript. Lecister University. Department of Clinical Psychology, Leicester, UK.
Jones, D.R. (1985). Secondary disaster victims: the emotional effects of recovering and identifying human remains. American Journal of Psychiatry, 142, 303-307.
Kliman, A.S. (1975). The Corning Flood Project: Psychological first aid following a natural disaster. In H.J. Parad, H.P. Resnik, L.G. Parad (Eds.), Emergency and disaster management: A mental health source book. Bowie, MD: Charles Press.
Laube, J. (1973). Psychological reactions of nurses in disaster. Nursing Research, 343-347.
Lifton, R.J. (1968). Death in life. New York: Random House.
Lifton, R.J. (1964). Psychological effects of the atomic bomb. In Grosser, G.K., Weschsler, H., & Greenblatt, M. (Eds.), The threat of impending disaster. Cambridge, Mass: MIT Press.
Lindstrom, B., & Lundin, T. (1982). Yrkesmessig exponering for katastrof. Nordisk Psykiatrisk Tidskrift, (Suppl. 6), 1-44.
Lintern, J.R. (in press). A study to determine the level of work-related distress that fire-fighters experience and the effectiveness of a post-trauma stress package. British Journal of Clinical Psychology.
Lundin, T., & Bodegaard, M. (1993). The psychological impact of an earthquake on rescue workers: a follow up study of the Swedish group of rescue workers in Armenia, 1988. Journal of Traumatic Stress, 6, 129-139.
Macleod, D. (1991). Psychological debriefing: rationale and application. Practice, 5, 103-111.
Manolias, M., & Hyatt-Williams A. (1988, February). Post traumatic disorder. Triggered reactions. Police Magazine, (pp. 21-28).
McCann, I.L., & Pearlman, L.A. (1990). Vicarious traumatisation: framework for understanding the psychological effects of working with victims. Journal of Traumatic Stress, 3, 131-149.

McFarlane, A.C. (1988). The aetiology of post-traumatic stress disorders following a natural disorder. British Journal of Psychiatry, 152, 116-121.
McFarlane, A.C. (1989). The treatment of post-traumatic stress disorder. British Journal of Medical Psychology, 62, 81-90.
McGlown, K.J. (1981). Attrition in the fire service: a report. Washington, DC: Federal Emergency Management Agency, US Fire Administration.
Mitchell, J.T. (1988,a). The history, status and future of critical incident stress debriefings. Journal of Emergency Services, November, 47-52.
Mitchell, J.T. (1988,b). Development and functions of a critical incident stress debriefing team. Journal of Emergency Services, December, 43-46.
Mitchell, J., & Bray, G. (1989). Emergency services stress. Baltimore: Chevron Publishing Company.
Mitchell, J.T., & Dyregrov, A. (1993). Traumatic stress in disaster workers and emergency personnel. In J.P. Wilson & B. Raphael (Eds.), International handbook of traumatic stress syndromes (pp. 905-914). London: Plenum Press.
Mitchell, J.T., & Everly, T.S. (1993). Critical incident stress debriefing: An operational manual for the prevention of trauma among emergency service and disaster workers. Baltimore, MD. Chevron Publishing.
Ørner, R.J., Paulson, R., Thompson, M., Pickles, M., Cook, C., Brown-Warr, R., & Stone, C. (1993, May). Critical incident stress management services in United Kingdom emergency services. Paper presented at the Second World Congress on Stress, Trauma and Coping in Emergency Service Professions, Baltimore MA.
Paton, D. (1989). Disasters and helpers: psychological dynamics and implications for counselling. Counselling Psychology Quarterly, 2, 303-321.
Raphael, B. (1986). When disaster strikes. New York: Basic Books.
Raphael, B., Singh, B., Bradbury, L. & Lambert, F. (1983-84) Who helps the helpers? The effects of disaster on the rescue-workers. Omega, 14, 8-21.
Raphael, B., & Wilson, J.P. (1993). Theoretical and intervention considerations in working with victims of disaster. In J.P. Wilson & B. Raphael (Eds.), International handbook of traumatic stress syndromes (pp. 105-117). London: Plenum Press.
Rayner, J.F. (1958). How do nurses behave in disaster? Nursing Outlook 6, 572-576
Reese, J.T., Horn, J.M., & Dunning, C. (1991). Critical incidents in policing (Revised version). Washington, DC: U.S. Department of Justice.
Robinson, R.C., & Mitchell, J.T. (1993). Evaluation of psychological debriefings. Journal of Traumatic Stress, 6, 367-382.
Rogers, C.R. (1951). Client-centred therapy. London: Constable.
Rogers, O. (1992). An examination of critical incident stress debriefing for emergency service providers. Unpublished doctorial dissertation, University of Maryland, MA.
Schmuckler, E. (1991). Peer support and traumatic incident teams: A state-wide multiagency program. In J.T. Reese, J.M. Horn, & C. Dunning (Eds.), Critical incidents in policing (pp. 315-318). Washington DC: U.S. Department of Justice.

Scott, M.J., & Stradling, S.G. (1994). Post traumatic stress disorder without the trauma. British Journal of Clinical Psychology, 33, 71-74.

Scott, R.T., & Jordan, M. (1993, May). The Los Angeles Riots April - 1992: A CISD Challenge. Paper presented at the second World Congress on Stress, Trauma and Coping in Emergency Service Professions, Baltimore, MA.

Sewell, J.D., & Crew, L. (1984.) The forgotten victim: stress and the police dispatcher. FBI Law Enforcement Bulletin, 53, 7-11.

Shubin, S. (1979, January). Rx for stress - your stress. Nursing, pp. 53-55.

Sidle, A., Moos, R., Adams, J., & Cady, P. (1969). Development of a coping scale: A preliminary study. Archives of General Psychiatry, 20, 226-232.

Solomon, R.M. (1991). The dynamics of fear in critical incidents: Implications for training and treatment. In J.T. Reese, J.M. Horn, & C. Dunning (Eds.), Critical incidents in policing (pp. 347-358). Washington D.C.: U.S. Department of Justice.

Solomon, R.M., & Horne, J.M. (1986). Peer support: A key element of coping with trauma. Police Stress, 9, 25-27.

Stolz, P. (1993, December). Peer support and other post-trauma intervention strategies. Paper presented at the meeting of the Lincolnshire Emergency Services Initiative, Lincoln, United Kingdom.

Stratton, J.G., Parker, D.A., & Snibbe, J.R. (1984). Post traumatic stress: study of police officers involved in shootings. Psychological Reports, 55, 127-131.

Taplin, O. (1989). Greek fire. London: Jonathan Cape.

Taylor, A.J.W. & Frazer, A.G. (1982). The stress of post-disaster bodyhandling and victim identification work. The Journal of Human Stress, 8, 4-12.

Taylor, W.C. (1987). Stress and the EMS dispatcher. Emergency Medical Services, 16, pp. 18, 21, 23, 25-26.

The Times. King's Cross fireman awarded £147,000 for trauma injuries. November 5, 1992.

Wallace, A.F.C. (1956). Human behaviour in extreme situations, a survey of the literature and suggestions for further research: (Report No. 390.) Washington, DC: Committee on Disaster Studies, National Academy of Sciences - National Research Council.

Yager, J., & Hubert, D. (1979). Stress and coping in psychiatric residence. Psychiatric Opinion, 16, 21-24.

Zigmond, A.S. & Snaith, R.P. (1983). The Hospital Anxiety and Depression Scale. Acta Psychiatrica Scandinavica, 67, 361-370.

CONCLUSIONS: ADDRESSING COMMUNITIES UNDER EXTREME STRESS

Stevan E. Hobfoll, Kent State University, Kent, Ohio, USA
Marten W. deVries, University of Limburg, Maastricht, the Netherlands
Rebecca P. Cameron, Kent State University, Kent, Ohio, USA

Perhaps because we can watch any war, disaster, or tragedy worldwide from our home television sets, we have become increasingly aware of the urgency of addressing the mental health needs of those affected by such events. Moreover, the interest in and advances made on the individual level in traumatology have made it possible to provide a more advanced level of care to victims of extreme community stress. However, it has been the thesis of this volume that approaching extreme community stressors from an individualized perspective alone will lead to underservice of the population, possible interference with cultural imperatives, and potential psychological harm to the service providers themselves.

    To begin to adequately address these issues, we must move from the individual to the group as the unit of analysis. As we make this shift, community-level aspects of extremely stressful events become more salient. Very different services are required and can be offered if two percent, or fifty percent, of the population is deeply affected by an event (McFarlane, this volume). The presence or absence of collateral physical and property damages also affects the signature of the event. Resource theories (Hobfoll, Briggs, & Wells, this volume) can be applied to aid assessment of community-level existent, damaged, and lost resources, and can guide the efforts of interventionists and researchers. An understanding of how social support operates and is sustained on the group, organizational, and community level (Sarason, Sarason, & Pierce, this volume) is critical. Thus, it becomes clear that we need to learn much more about how support systems are influenced and changed during and following periods of extreme stress. Understanding the culture of those affected will underlie any further insights into how resources will be utilized and how professionals can direct community efforts without becoming negative agents themselves (de Jong, this volume; deVries, this volume). Yet, few Western programs in psychology or psychiatry train professionals in the anthropological perspectives that facilitate cultural understanding.

Moving from an individual to a collectivist perspective also requires changes in perspective at another level (Riger, 1993; Triandis, McCusker, & Hui, 1990). Specifically, the very factors that we look toward, even when we examine groups or communities, are individual variables. Along these lines, research by Hobfoll, Dunahoo, Ben-Porath, and Monnier (1994) has found that the "preferred" modes of coping--action coping and problem solving--are often accompanied by antisocial behavior that may affect others negatively. For example, when individuals seek to evacuate from a disaster area (problem solving), they may ignore others in need, clog roads against emergency instructions, and even trample others to seek their own safety. Yet, current coping models would evaluate this as positive coping because coping measures tap coping behavior narrowly, and from an individualistic perspective, never asking about the consequences for others of particular coping behaviors. This stems from a Western bias that favors agentic behavior and values individualistic goal-seeking without regard for the well-being of the larger group.

Indeed, those who are more communal are often denigrated in Western mental health. For example, when women stay with their alcoholic partners as pressed to by religion, society, and their upbringing, they are called co-dependent. Support-seeking is even classified as a passive behavior on some coping scales (Endler & Parker, 1990). The experiences of people from non-Western cultures and of women and some ethnic minorities within Western countries may fit less well with this agentic model (Riger, 1993).

In many cultures, individual survival and psychological well-being are much more deeply entwined with the collective. The following case may illustrate this point (I. Hobfoll, 1986):

> A large group of Adolescent Ethiopian Jews arrived in Israel without their families. They were sent ahead of their parents and extended families because elders had decided that only the young and the strong could make the perilous journey across the Sudan. Because children, the sick, and the elderly could not make the journey, adults stayed behind to care for them. This very decision strategy underscores the need of the collective to survive and the fact that individual families did not seem to even consider a plan of action different than that decided by the group.
>
> Adolescents had a long trek across the Sudan. At times they were attacked by marauders who robbed, raped, and murdered. They arrived in Israel tattered and exhausted and at this point they were split and sent to different group homes in medium size groups (approximately 20 to 50). Rather quickly it was apparent how high was their mental health risk. Rates of suicide climbed, psychosomatic illnesses were frequent, and psychological breakdown was common.
>
> Despite language difficulties, most centers attempted to treat the adolescents from a case by case perspective, typically hospitalizing

those in need or attempting individual crisis intervention. Instead, one center attempted a communal strategy, allowing culturally-based care to take precedent over individualized medical decision making. Instead of hospitalization, group watch was placed on suicide risks. Instead of psychotherapy treatment, the few Rabbis and elders from the Ethiopian community already in Israel were called on to consult about cases. Rather than dismissing psychosomatic illnesses, those afflicted were surrounded by friends who helped them mourn and console them for their illness through visits to the sick bed, until the sickness was "treated" and the ill person arose to reenter the group.

It would have been easy to treat them all as children. Instead, older and more mature young adults, sometimes only in their late teens, were given added responsibility and allowed to serve as "elders" of the group. They did so quite successfully.

Although still deeply affected by their enormous trauma, no suicides occurred at this center. Few hospitalizations were required and illnesses were reduced. Overall, morale and spirits rose quickly and the business of education, necessary health care (many adolescents had serious illnesses), and absorption into their new country were allowed to proceed more smoothly.

A number of community psychologists have evoked broad concepts that may help us obtain greater insights into community processes. S. Sarason (1974) developed the construct of the psychological sense of community. He defined this as a sense that people feel supported and esteemed by a group with which they are affiliated. Iscoe (1974) took more of an action orientation in his conceptualization of the competent community. The competent community acts on behalf of its members and forms a supportive net for residents. Even in community psychology, however, the individual perspective adopted by most psychologists has prevented significant development of ways to foster, manage, or even study these concepts. The cascade method developed by deVries (this volume) may help pave the way for a clearer elucidation of how this can be done. In this model, natural cultural healing methods are studied and integrated with relief efforts. Mini-tests of model interventions are then conducted before attempts are made to generalize these models to large-scale interventions. DeVries and his colleagues' own work in war-torn areas should prove adaptable for many types of community stress.

Finally, we should remind ourselves that the individual should never be lost in the study of extreme community stress. The affected child, adult, and family will continue to be in need of both our care and our increased efforts to understand their immediate, midterm, and long-term distress. However, losing the individual does not seem to be the risk. Western models of training are so ingrained in professionals, even those trained in non-Western countries, that individual distress quickly and almost uniformly becomes the focus of attention. We need to learn much more about processes affecting the well-being of groups; for example, how the dissemination of information affects people's cognitions (Meichenbaum, this volume), group reactions to catastrophe (Weisæth, this volume), and group trends in development of post trauma disorder (Solomon, this volume). We are beginning to become aware that much of the clinical folklore of traumatology must give way to empirically-based research findings (Solomon, this volume; Wortman, Carnelley, Lehman, Davis, & Exline, this volume). However, in order to advance our empirical knowledge of traumatic community events, we must learn to work flexibly under very difficult research and intervention conditions (Bromet, this volume; Norris, Freedy, DeLongis, Sibilia, & Schönpflug, this volume). Certainly we can borrow at times from individually-based theories, but events of the magnitude addressed here reverberate and shape the communities and even the cultures of those afflicted (Lomranz, this volume; Figley, Giel, Borgo, Briggs, Haritos-Fatouros, this volume). We must be aware of where individualistic theories are not only not utilitarian, but where they may interfere with understanding and intervention.

Despite the conceptual and methodological shifts that are required to make real progress in this area, clinicians and social scientists should not leave this work to others, as we are the professional groups most likely to champion mental health as critical. We can do this best by joining with communities in need and offering our expertise in a sharing fashion. We must be aware that although our agendas are important and well-meaning, there are other important agendas operating that are intertwined with our own. Pynoos, Goenjian, and Steinberg (this volume) make this point very well in their discussion of mental health professionals' need to support school administrators and to work together with them on our mutual agenda of providing care and education for children during periods of war and disaster and their aftermath. We must act not only as direct agents of intervention, but also as catalyzers of community support by working to facilitate the salutogenic processes that already exist or that may be instilled in the community (Milgram, Sarason, Schönpflug, Jackson, & Schwarzer, this volume). Through this entire process, research and intervention must proceed hand in hand, as there is great danger of losing credibility if we practice interventions that are found to be faulty (Ørner, this volume). As a group, we hope that this volume will work to catalyze advances in research and intervention and will contribute to the growing knowledge base that will inevitably continue to be in demand due to the tragic consequences of extreme community stress.

References

Bromet, E. J. (this volume). Methodological issues in designing research on community-wide disasters with special reference to Chernobyl. In S. E. Hobfoll & M. W. deVries (Eds.), Extreme stress and communities: Impact and intervention. Dordrecht, the Netherlands: Kluwer.

de Jong, J. T. V. M. (this volume). Prevention of the consequences of man-made or natural disaster at the (inter)national, the community, the family, and the individual level. In S. E. Hobfoll & M. W. deVries (Eds.), Extreme stress and communities: Impact and intervention. Dordrecht, the Netherlands: Kluwer.

deVries, M. W. (this volume). Culture, community and catastrophe: Issues in understanding communities under difficult conditions. In S. E. Hobfoll & M. W. deVries (Eds.), Extreme stress and communities: Impact and intervention. Dordrecht, the Netherlands: Kluwer.

Endler, N. S., & Parker, J. D. A. (1990). Multidimensional assessment of coping: A critical evaluation. Journal of Personality and Social Psychology, 58, 844-854.

Figley, C., Giel, R., Borgo, S., Briggs, S., & Haritos-Fatouros, M. (this volume). Prevention and treatment of community stress: How to be a mental health expert at the time of disaster. In S. E. Hobfoll & M. W. deVries (Eds.), Extreme stress and communities: Impact and intervention. Dordrecht, the Netherlands: Kluwer.

Hobfoll, I. H. (1986). Ethiopian Jewish adolescent refugees' adjustment to Israel. Presented at the meeting of the Stress and Test Anxiety Research Society (STAR), Dusseldorf, Germany.

Hobfoll, S. E., Briggs, S., & Wells J. (this volume). Community stress and resources: Actions and reactions. In S. E. Hobfoll & M. W. deVries (Eds.), Extreme stress and communities: Impact and intervention. Dordrecht, the Netherlands: Kluwer.

Hobfoll, S. E., Dunahoo, C. L., Ben-Porath, Y., & Monnier, J. (1994). Gender and coping: The dual-axis model of coping. American Journal of Community Psychology, 22, 49-82.

Iscoe, I. (1974). Community psychology and the competent community. American Psychologist, 29, 607-613.

Lomranz, J. (this volume). Endurance and living: Long-term effects of the Holocaust. In S. E. Hobfoll & M. W. deVries (Eds.), Extreme stress and communities: Impact and intervention. Dordrecht, the Netherlands: Kluwer.

McFarlane, A. C. (this volume). Stress and disaster. In S. E. Hobfoll & M. W. deVries (Eds.), Extreme stress and communities: Impact and intervention. Dordrecht, the Netherlands: Kluwer.

Meichenbaum, D. (this volume). Disasters, stress and cognition. In S. E. Hobfoll & M. W. deVries (Eds.), Extreme stress and communities: Impact and intervention. Dordrecht, the Netherlands: Kluwer.

Milgram, N., Sarason, B. R., Schönpflug, U., Jackson, A., & Schwarzer, C. (this volume). Catalyzing community support. In S. E. Hobfoll & M. W. deVries (Eds.), Extreme stress and communities: Impact and intervention. Dordrecht, the Netherlands: Kluwer.

Norris, F. H., Freedy, J. R., DeLongis, A., Sibilia, L., Schonpflug, W. (this volume). Research methods and directions: Establishing the community context. In S. E. Hobfoll & M. W. deVries (Eds.), Extreme stress and communities: Impact and intervention. Dordrecht, the Netherlands: Kluwer.

Ørner, R. J. (this volume). Intervention strategies for emergency response groups: A new conceptual framework. In S. E. Hobfoll & M. W. deVries (Eds.), Extreme stress and communities: Impact and intervention. Dordrecht, the Netherlands: Kluwer.

Pynoos, R. S., Goenjian, A., & Steinberg, A. M. (this volume). Strategies of disaster intervention for children and adolescents. In S. E. Hobfoll & M. W. deVries (Eds.), Extreme stress and communities: Impact and intervention. Dordrecht, the Netherlands: Kluwer.

Riger, S. (1993). What's wrong with empowerment? American Journal of Community Psychology, 21, 279-292.

Sarason, I. G., Sarason, B. R., & Pierce, G. R. (this volume). Stress and social support. In S. E. Hobfoll & M. W. deVries (Eds.), Extreme stress and communities: Impact and intervention. Dordrecht, the Netherlands: Kluwer.

Sarason, S. B. (1974). The psychological sense of community: Prospects for a community psychology. San Francisco: Jossey-Bass.

Solomon, Z. (this volume). The pathogenic effect of war stress: The Israeli experience. In S. E. Hobfoll & M. W. deVries (Eds.), Extreme stress and communities: Impact and intervention. Dordrecht, the Netherlands: Kluwer.

Triandis, H. C., McCusker, C., & Hui, C. H. (1990). Multimethod probes of individualism and collectivism. Journal of Personality and Social Psychology, 59, 1006-1020.

Weisæth, L. (this volume). Preventive psychosocial intervention after disaster. In S. E. Hobfoll & M. W. deVries (Eds.), Extreme stress and communities: Impact and intervention. Dordrecht, the Netherlands: Kluwer.

Wortman, C. B., Carnelley, K. B., Lehman, D. R., Davis, C. G., & Exline, J. J. (this volume). Coping with the loss of a family member: Implications for community-level research and intervention. In S. E. Hobfoll & M. W. deVries (Eds.), Extreme stress and communities: Impact and intervention. Dordrecht, the Netherlands: Kluwer.

Index[1]

action control, 163
action-outcome expectancies, 162
acute:
    reactions, 230, 231
    trauma, 430, 436
adaptation, 14-24, 290, 294, 295
    processes, 165, 167, 169, 173
adult development, 347, 348
adults, 307-310, 314-318, 320, 323
    and children, 307, 310, 314, 317, 318
agency beliefs, 163, 176
aggression, 427, 428
aging, 325, 326, 330, 332-334, 342, 345-350
alcoholism, 277, 280
ambulance personnel, 501, 504, 519
animistic, 379
anxiety, 163, 164, 167, 174, 176
    reduction, 191, 192
appraisal, 107, 108, 113, 114, 127
attention, 179, 180, 183, 185, 187, 192
attribution, 160
attributional response style, 160
autonomic hyperarousal, 425

behavior disorders, 66-78, 81
bereaved, 83, 84, 86-96, 98, 100-102
bereavement, 85, 86, 93, 100-103
bias, 268, 272, 275
    interviewer, 268
    nonresponse, 268
    perception 160
    selective mortality 268
biography, 334, 336
brief therapy, 456, 465, 469
Buffalo Creek:
    dam collapse, 312, 321
    Disaster, 307, 312, 321
buffer mechanisms, 169

career, 332, 333
cascade, 385, 386, 388, 389
catalyzing, 473, 474, 481, 482, 487
ceremonies, 499, 515
Chernobyl, 267-272, 275-281
child sample, 316, 318
children, 268-281, 445-451, 453, 454, 456-463, 465-471
co-morbid conditions, 461
cohort, 340, 349
collective perspective, 407
combat stress reaction, 229, 231-2, 245-6
communal coping, 109, 110
community, 105-127, 129, 207-210, 213-227, 247, 250-252, 254, 255, 259, 262, 264, 283-299, 436, 473, 474, 476-487
    altruistic communities, 120, 121
    context, 284, 285, 287-290, 299
    host communities, 499, 500
    specific community setting, 288
    stress, 105-113, 115-119, 121-123, 126, 137-139, 141, 142, 144, 146, 149-154, 267, 269, 279, 489, 490, 497
    stressors, 353, 361, 363
    subcommunity, 291, 292
    support, 473, 474, 480, 483, 487
    values, 480
community research:
    conducting, 284
    studies of multiple communities, 289, 292
    single community studies, 289
compassion fatigue, 496, 497
Conservation of Resources (COR) Theory, 138, 286, 290, 291
    COR, 137-140, 142, 144-147, 149, 152

constructive narrative perspective, 34, 38, 44, 48
context(s), 11-18, 20-22, 24, 490
continuity of risk, 313
control group, 272
    comparison group, 274, 278
controllability, 421
coping, 83-86, 90, 95-98, 100-103, 105, 107-112, 115-120, 122, 124-128, 179, 185-188, 191, 192, 194-196, 325, 326, 328-335, 337-342, 345-349, 401, 404, 406, 408-410, 413, 417, 476, 478, 488, 490, 492, 496
    multidimensional, 337
    public, 109-111
    resources, 161, 169, 172
    style, 161
critical incident stress management services, 508, 511, 513-516, 520
cross-national:
    studies, 355
    validity, 272
cultural:
    pluralism, 22
    responses, 378
culture, 11-17, 20-22, 24, 325, 326, 329, 336-339, 341-343, 490, 497
cycling of resources, 16-18, 290

death, 84-88, 91, 93, 97, 98, 100, 101
debriefing 447, 450, 457-460, 510-513, 517, 519, 520
    individual, 459-460
deconditioning, 431-433
denial, 84, 85, 97
depression, 160, 163, 165, 167-169, 172, 174-176, 453, 461, 462
development, 421, 428, 430
developmental, 445, 451, 453-458, 460-467, 470, 471
Digo, 380-383

disaster(s), 33-37, 39, 42, 45, 46, 49, 54, 60, 105, 106, 110-112, 115, 116, 119-122, 125-128, 207, 208, 210, 214, 216-218, 221-224, 247-256, 258-265, 267-269, 272, 275, 277, 279-281, 283, 286, 289-294, 296-299, 401-414, 416-418, 445-451, 453-463, 465-467, 469-471, 474-486, 488, 489-497
    medicine, 407, 417
    research, 267, 269, 279
    training, 409, 411
dissociation, 422, 423, 427, 432, 440-443
distrust, 271, 278
    of authorities, 271

East German migrants, 164, 167, 169, 172, 176
ecological:
    context, 287, 289
    environment, 13
    metaphor, 11, 13, 15-18, 21, 25
emergency responder groups, 499-502, 508, 510-513, 516
emotional well-being, 165
employment, 164-169, 172, 175
    status 167, 169, 175
environment, 64, 67-74, 76, 79
    predisposing, 69-71, 73, 74, 76
    protective, 69, 76
epidemiologic research, 267
epidemiology, 267, 273-275, 279, 280, 503
ethnic conflicts, 356
evacuation, 270-272, 274, 277
evacuee:
    children, 274
    families, 273
evacuees during the Gulf War, 231
expectancies, 159, 161-163, 175
expectancy-value theories, 162

experience sampling, 386, 387
explanatory style, 159-161, 175
exposure, 449, 451, 456, 460-462, 465-467, 469, 470

facilitation, 377
family, 207, 209, 211, 214, 215, 217, 219-224, 327, 328, 332-335, 340, 343
firefighters, 501, 504, 505, 511, 512, 514, 518, 519
focus groups, 385-388, 392

gain cycles, 143, 146
generativity, 336
gerontology, 330
gourd dance, 384, 387, 391
grief, 83, 84, 86-90, 94, 100-103, 449, 450, 453, 456, 458, 460, 462, 464, 466, 469
grieving, 85, 86, 93, 94
group (psycho)therapy, 435, 440, 442, 466
Gulf War, 339, 346-348

health, 159-162, 164-169, 172, 175-177, 353, 358-362, 366, 370-373
  complaints, 167-169
helplessness, 91, 98, 102, 160, 163, 174
hidden populations, 386, 391, 393
Holocaust, 325-339, 341-343, 345-348, 350
hope, 163, 176

ideographic, 330
ideology, 336-339
illness, 160, 161, 164, 165, 168, 175

impact, 249-256, 259, 263, 264
  of setting on disaster effects, 311
  on mental health, 307
inconsistencies, 340-342
individual, 105-115, 117-119, 123, 124, 126, 127, 207-210, 221, 223-225, 247, 250, 251, 253, 258
induction, 377, 379
information processing perspective, 37, 38
Information Support Center, 413
informed consent, 272
  procedure, 272
integration, 422, 431, 433, 434, 442
interdependence, 11, 16, 18, 19, 23, 290-292
  principle, 18, 19
intergroup conflict, 353, 356, 360
(inter)national, 207, 209, 211, 213, 214, 224
interpersonal, 325, 331, 337, 338, 340, 341
intervention(s), 140, 146-149, 151-153, 155-157, 207-210, 213, 214, 216, 217, 220-224, 226, 473, 474, 476, 478, 482, 486, 487, 499-501, 507-510, 513-517, 520, 521
intrusive memories, 34, 44, 46
inventory and rescue ,255
Israel, 333, 336, 338, 339, 342, 343, 345, 346, 348

Kiev, 270-2780

language, 335, 339, 343
learning difficulties, 426
life:
  perspective, 165
  review, 334, 345
  transition, 164, 165, 169

long-term effects, 325-327, 329-331, 336, 339, 341, 342
long term sequelae, 233
longitudinal:
    findings, 316
    perspective, 248
loss, 490-492
    and life events, 376
    cycles, 143-147, 151

maintenance, 377-379, 384, 387, 388
man-made, 207, 208, 217, 221, 224
Masai, 380
meaning, 334, 336, 338, 342, 345, 346
means-ends-beliefs, 163
measurement, 248, 253, 262
media, 481-486, 495, 496
memory disturbances, 427
mental health effects, 268-270, 272, 275, 278, 279
    distress, 272, 276, 277, 279
    impairment, 267, 272, 281
    phobias, 276
    radiophobia, 276
    somatic complaints, 276
    somatic symptoms, 271, 276
mental health expert, 490
mental health, parental, 277
metaphors, 34, 37, 38, 40-43, 45, 47
methodologic issues, 317, 318
methodology, 248, 253, 326, 327, 329-331, 343, 344
migration, 164, 165, 168, 172, 173
mitigation, 401
model for studying the psychological impact, 308
modified cohort design, 267, 269
motivation, 161, 163, 176
mourning, 272, 492
multimethod, 385
multi-modal, 207, 208, 224

national identity, 338, 341
natural, 207, 208, 214, 217, 218, 220, 224
    disasters, 307-309, 320
    experiments, 269
nomothetic, 330, 331, 344
numbing, 421, 424-426, 428, 437
nurses, 501, 519, 520

optimism, 159-163, 172, 174-176
    defensive, 160
    dispositional, 160-162, 172, 175, 176
    functional, 159, 160
    learned, 160, 176
    unrealistic, 163
optimistic:
    action beliefs, 164
    bias, 164
    resource beliefs, 164
    self-beliefs, 159, 164, 168

participant observation, 385, 387, 388
partner, 165-169
    support, 166, 167
partnership, 166-169, 172
pattern:
    of concern, 120
    of neglect, 120
    of relationships, 292
performance, 163, 175
personal:
    efficacy, 169
    resources, 159, 174
personality, 325, 326, 330-332, 334, 337, 340-343, 345-348
pharmacotherapy, 466
physical symptoms, 165, 167-169, 172
police officers, 502, 508-510, 512, 517, 521
population at risk, 272

positive illusions, 163
post-disaster, 289, 293
post-traumatic stress, 493
post traumatic stress disorder, 88, 439-441 (*See also PTSD*)
posttraumatic stress reactions, 453-455, 461, 462, 466, 467, 470, 471 (*See also PTSR*)
pre-disaster, 293
predictability, 421, 422, 430
preparedness, 401, 402, 404, 406, 411
pressure cooker effect, 149
prevention, 195, 207, 208, 210, 211, 213-227, 401-404, 411, 414, 415, 417, 419, 489, 490, 495-497
preventive, 207-210, 213, 214, 216-222, 224, 226
    psychosocial intervention, 401
primary, 207, 210, 221-227
Pripyat, 270-273, 275-277
protective resource factors, 165
psychiatry, 401-404, 416-418
psychological first aid, 461, 471
psychosomatic, 426, 428
PTSD, 88, 248, 249, 251, 252, 257-262, 403, 404, 407, 409-411, 414, 415, 421-434, 436-439, 441, 442 (*See also post traumatic stress disorder*)
    delayed, 236, 237, 243
    transgenerational impact, 241
PTSR, 327, 328, 332, 333, 337, 340, 341 (*See also posttraumatic stress reactions*)
public awareness, 109-111
pulsed interventions, 456-457

Quality of Relationships Inventory, 182

racially stratified society, 361
racism, 353, 355-363, 365-373

radiation, 269, 270, 274, 276-278
reactions of civilians during the Gulf War, 230
reactivation:
    of CSR, 238
    of stress response, 238, 240
readjustment, 164-166, 168, 169, 172
recall bias, 268
recover, 87, 88, 90, 96, 98
recovery, 85, 87-89, 91, 94, 101, 103
refugees, 167, 169, 173, 207, 208, 210, 213, 217-220, 225-227
religion, 334-336, 341
religious rituals, 40
relocation, 164, 166
remedy and recovery, 256
rescue work, 457
research, 325-331, 333, 334, 337, 340, 341, 343, 344, 346-348, 350
    directions 319
resilience, 36, 84, 97
resolution, 87-89, 91, 92, 102
resolve, 87, 98
resolving, 83, 84, 88
resource(s), 66, 79, 105, 108, 110-113, 120, 122, 124, 126, 137-144, 146-152, 154, 155, 159, 161, 164-166, 169, 172-174, 285, 286, 290, 291, 293, 295, 297, 473, 475, 477-479, 482, 484, 485, 490, 492, 493, 497
    characteristics, 286, 290, 296
    conditions, 286, 291, 295, 296
    energies, 286
    investment, 141, 146, 150
    mobilization, 108, 110, 115
    objects, 286
restitutive experiences, 435
restructuring, 434
Reverberation Theory of Stress and Racism, 353, 360, 361, 368-370

risk:
    factors, 307, 310, 316, 319
    groups, 169, 475
rituals, 379, 380, 382
rule of relative needs, 120

sample of convenience, 273, 274
schema-based perspective, 38
school personnel, 447, 456, 457
screening, 404, 408, 413-415, 446, 449, 450, 459, 471
scrotal hernia, 383, 384
secondary, 210, 211, 216, 218, 222, 224
    trauma, 260
    traumatization, 229, 240-242, 246
self, 328-331, 333-335, 337, 340-342, 346, 347, 349
self-efficacy, 159, 160, 163-169, 172, 174-176, 435
    generalized, 163, 164, 167, 172
    perceived, 159, 160, 163, 166, 169, 176
self-esteem, 163, 164
self help, 377, 380, 383, 384, 388, 389, 493, 494
self-regulation, 161, 174
self-serving attributions, 160
sequelae, 325, 332, 345, 347
situation-outcome expectancies, 162
sleep problems, 426
snowball sampling, 386-388, 391, 392
social integration, 165-169
social network(s), 159, 165, 166, 172, 180, 184, 186, 192, 195, 197, 386, 391, 490
    disruption, 165
social relations, 340
social resources, 169
social security, 376-378, 380-382, 388

social support, 108, 111, 119-128, 159, 165, 166, 172, 174-177, 179-197, 432, 434, 436, 492-494, 497
    buffering hypothesis, 185, 194
    functions, 180
    global, 179, 182, 184, 187
    interactional-cognitive view, 183
    perceived, 181, 182, 184, 186-188, 195, 196
    provisions, 180, 181, 197
    received, 181, 184, 197
    relationship-specific, 179, 182, 185, 187
    role in obstetrics, 190
    sense of acceptance, 184, 196
somatic response, 423
sorrow, 88
stabilize, 436
stress, 63-69, 71, 73-81, 105-113, 115, 117-119, 121-129, 179, 180, 184, 185, 188, 189, 191, 192, 194-197, 207, 208, 210, 214-216, 218, 222-227, 247-251, 253, 257-260, 263-265, 267-270, 274-281, 283-286, 288-292, 294-299
    coping with, 63, 64, 66, 79
    consequences of, 63, 66, 67, 69, 74, 75, 77
    costs of, 66
    daily, 392
    psychological, 269, 276
    state of, 63-68, 74
stressful life transitions, 159, 175
stressful transition, 164
stressor(s), 75, 76, 81, 473, 474
    criterion, 249, 259, 262
subordinate groups, 353, 357, 358, 361-363, 367, 369, 370
succession, 16, 19-21, 290
    succession principle, 20, 21
support, 402, 404, 406, 408, 411-415, 418
supportive networks, 430

symbolic, 378, 379, 388
symptomatology, 423, 424, 431, 434, 438

taxonomic incorporation, 377, 380
taxonomy, 405
technological events, 308
temperament, 63, 64, 67-81
    difficult, 67, 68, 76-78
Temperament Risk Factor (TRF), 67-73, 75-76
tertiary, 211, 223, 224
theory, 327, 330, 334, 340, 341, 344, 346-348
threat, 247-255, 260
Three Mile Island, 267-270, 272, 279
thyroid disease, 269, 276
time, 329-333, 336, 337, 339-343, 347, 348
traditional:
    healer, 380, 382, 383
    medical system, 380
transitional rituals, 515
trauma, 83, 87-90, 92, 93, 95, 100-102, 325-343, 346-349, 421-428, 430-436, 438-442
    mass, 325, 329, 338, 339, 341-343
    response, 248, 253, 258, 259
    transmission, 333
traumatic, 83, 84, 88, 89, 92-94, 98, 99, 102, 490, 496-497
    events, 107, 111, 128
    loss, 83, 84, 92, 98, 99
    reminders, 450, 451, 454-458, 460, 461, 463-466
    stress, 328, 335, 341, 343, 346-349, 402-404, 408-415, 417, 418
    stress reactions, 501, 502, 506-508, 510, 512, 515, 516
traumatized, 90, 93

treatment, 421, 423, 430-434, 436-442, 489, 490, 493, 495, 496
    phase oriented, 430
    psychopharmacological, 436
two-stage household sampling procedure, 273
types of outcomes, 309

Ukraine, 272, 273, 276, 278
unemployment, 165, 166, 168, 169, 174-177
urban-rural differences, 274

verbalizing, 432
victimization, 91, 93
victims, 87, 93, 98, 100, 102, 103, 492, 493, 495
Vietnam, 380, 384
volunteers, 477-480, 482, 484
vulnerabilities, 165
vulnerability, 91, 93, 98, 165, 169, 174, 176, 332, 335, 336, 338, 341, 342, 410, 414, 438
vulnerable, 93, 98

within-disaster, 293
wives of CSRs, 242
work, 327, 332-334, 343, 348
working group, 283-285, 287, 289, 295

Zionism, 336

[1]The index contains words and phrases chosen by the authors of each chapter.